BY VICKI LANSKY & CONSUMER GUIDE® EDITORS

# COMPLETE PREGNANCY & BABY BOOK

PUBLICATIONS INTERNATIONAL, LTD.
SKOKIE, ILLINOIS

Manufactured in Yugoslavia by CGP Delo

ISBN: 0-453-00554-3

Front cover photo: Wayne Sproul/International Stock Photography

Back cover photo (left): Gerber Products

Back cover photo (right): Steven Feinberg

Photos pages 6-7, 10-11, 56-57, 72-73, 104-105, 136-137, 156-157, 186-187, 278-279, 304-305, 334-335, 396-397, 414-415: Gerber Products

Photo pages 376-377: David Rees

Photos page 15: From Moore, K. L.: *Before We Are Born. Basic Embryology and Birth Defects.* 3rd ed., 1982. Courtesy W. B. Saunders Company, Philadelphia, Pennsylvania.

Illustration page 16: From Moore, K. L.: *Before We Are Born. Basic Embryology and Birth Defects.* 3rd. ed., 1982. Courtesy W. B. Saunders Company, Philadelphia, Pennsylvania.

Illustrations: Mike Muir; Dori Gordon; Teri J. McDermott, M.A., Medical Illustrator

# Editor

VICKI LANSKY's first book, *Feed Me! I'm Yours,* was published in 1975. With nearly two million copies in print, it is now the most popular baby and toddler cookbook in the country. Her second book, *The Taming of the C.A.N.D.Y. Monster,* was published in 1978 and quickly became a #1 *New York Times* best-seller. In 1979, Ms. Lansky launched the acclaimed *Practical Parenting* newsletter, which inspired a syndicated radio show and a book, *Practical Parenting Tips.* In addition, she has written a series of Practical Parenting books on specific topics, including *Toilet Training, Welcoming the 2nd Baby,* and *Traveling with Your Baby.* A familiar face on such television shows as *Today, Donahue,* and *P.M. Magazine,* Ms. Lansky is currently a member of the Board of Directors of MELD, a parenting support group. She is a graduate of Connecticut College, and the mother of two children.

# Contributors

LIBBY BOTWICK studied counseling at the University of Maine and has attended numerous workshops on family therapy. She is currently a family counselor, a freelance writer, and the managing editor of *Pediatrics for Parents.*

GILLA DAVIS, M.D., is an Associate in the Department of Psychiatry at the Northwestern University Medical School and is Director of Consultation Liaison Psychiatry at Evanston Hospital.

AGNES E. DILLON is a freelance writer who has published in *Redbook, Parade,* and numerous other magazines. She was educated at the University of Kansas City Dental School, and is a member of the American Medical Writers' Association.

JEFFREY W. ELLIS took his M.D. degree at the University of Illinois. He is Assistant Professor, Department of Obstetrics and Gynecology, at Northwestern University Medical School. Dr. Ellis is also Medical Director, Planned Parenthood of Chicago, and an Associate Attending Physician, Obstetrics and Gynecology, at Northwestern Memorial Hospital. He was a medical consultant to CONSUMER GUIDE®'s *The New Illustrated Family Medical & Health Guide.*

ANN KEPPLER is an R.N. and holds a Masters in Nursing degree from the University of Washington. She has taught pediatric nursing at the Catholic University of America in Washington, D.C., and at the University of Washington in Seattle. Ms. Keppler is co-author of *Pregnancy, Childbirth and the Newborn,* and is presently Education Director for the Childbirth Education Association of Seattle. Ms. Keppler contributed to the nutrition, diet, and colic sections in Chapters 2, 8, and 9 of this book.

JAMIE CONROY MERRELL took her degree in journalism from Michigan State University. She writes regularly on parenting, financial planning, and other topics for the *Chicago Tribune,* writes a weekly column for Chicago-based Lerner-Life Newspapers, and contributes to *Chicago Parent.*

MARGERY LEWY RIEFF received her Ph.D. in Educational Psychology from Northwestern University. In addition to teaching courses at Barat College and National College of Education near Chicago, she is a Board Member for the Arlyn Day School, a private alternative school for learning disabled and behaviorally disordered adolescents.

KATHRYN RING holds a B.A. in Journalism from the University of Minnesota and has served as writer and editor for best-selling parenting and nutrition authors.

RICHARD J. SAGALL, M.D., is editor of *Pediatrics for Parents* and writes a monthly column for *Parents* magazine. After graduating from Antioch College, Dr. Sagall did graduate work in genetics at Ohio State University, and later graduated from the Medical College of Ohio at Toledo. He is in private practice in Maine.

PENNY SIMKIN, R.P.T., has been a childbirth educator and lecturer for eighteen years, and is president and editor of Pennypress, Inc., publishers of books and pamphlets on childbearing. She is the editor and author or co-author of numerous articles, pamphlets, and books, including *Pregnancy, Childbirth and the Newborn* and *Episiotomy and the Second Stage of Labor.* Ms. Simkin serves on the Board of Consultants of the International Childbirth Education Association and the Seattle Midwifery School. Portions of Chapters 3 and 5 of this book were written by Ms. Simkin.

EMILY SOLOFF is a writer, mother of three children (one of whom is hearing-impaired), and a founding member of LISTEN, a parent-support group for families with deaf children.

LINDA BLACHLY WHITE, M.D., is a contributing editor of *Pediatrics for Parents* and a part-time faculty member at Denver's Metropolitan State College, where she teaches human physiology. She has a B.S. and an M.S. in Biology from Stanford University, and an M.D. degree from the University of California at San Diego.

RULENA WHITE, R.N., is an ASPO Certified Childbirth Educator with fifteen years of childbirth and fitness education experience. She holds a Bachelor of Science in Nursing degree, and is Clinical Director of The Woman's Hospital of Texas Fitness Center in Houston. Ms. White designs fitness programs, lectures, writes, and offers Teacher Training Programs on pregnancy and new-mother fitness.

JODY W. ZYLKE took her M.D. degree from Harvard Medical School. She was a Resident in Pediatrics at UCLA Hospital in Los Angeles, and is currently a pediatrician with the Child Life Center near Chicago.

The editors especially wish to thank Dr. Jeffrey Ellis, Dr. Linda White, and Dr. Jody Zylke for their medical expertise.

# Contents

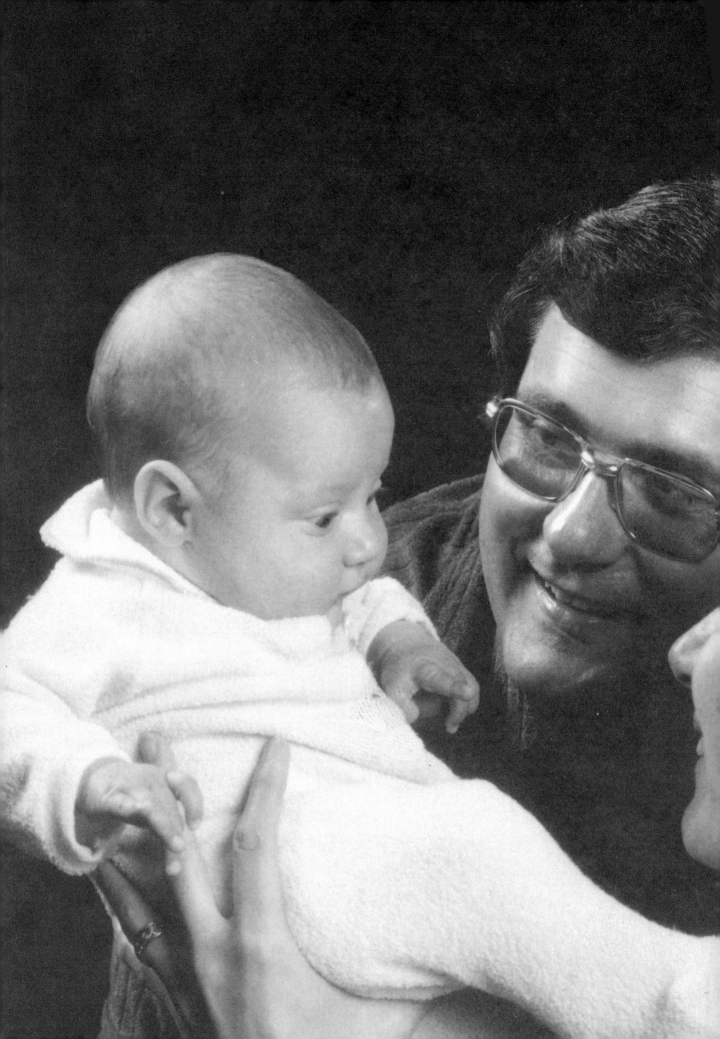

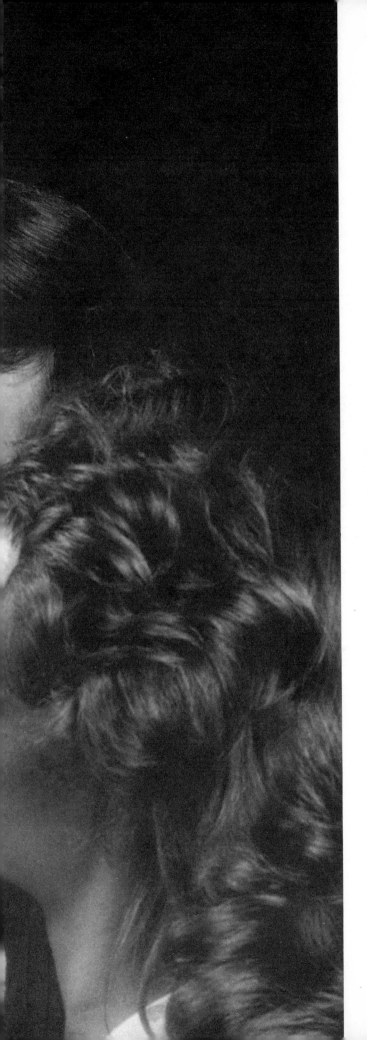

# Chapter 1:
# The Adventure
# of Parenthood

## The Family

The earliest human families were formed in response to deep biological drives and emotions that are not too dissimilar from the drives and emotions that we feel today. In a hostile, intimidating prehistoric world, men, women, and children found physical and psychological support in the family unit. Early families not only ensured the survival and growth of the human species, but established a social structure as well. Over the centuries the specific social structures that have grown to preserve and protect the family unit may look different, but the central concept remains quite similar.

The modern family provides us with many of the benefits enjoyed by our ancestors. Though now existing in a multiplicity of forms, the family remains a central element of society. We all seem to return to

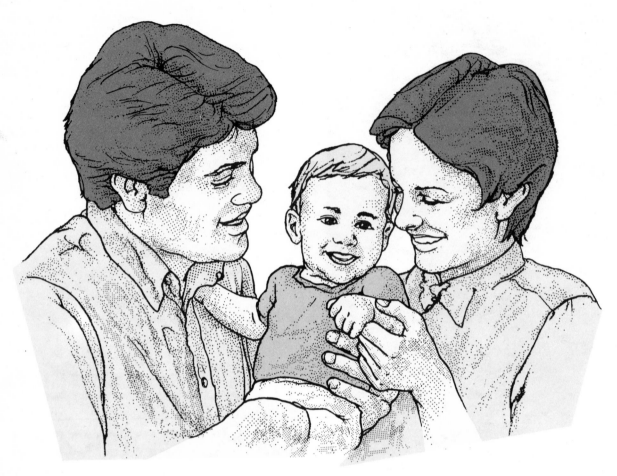

*The family is a vital element of modern society.*

the family unit again and again: for rejuvenation, for pleasure, for safety. The family continues to serve as the vehicle with which we feel most comfortable as we bring children into the world. Whoever has claimed that the family structure is disappearing is very wrong. The family—restructuring itself to fit modern-day life—is alive and well!

## Becoming a Parent

Children are the special elements of family life. Out of apparent nothingness, a human being is created—a miracle that is rediscovered by each of us at childbirth. Your child is inextricably bound to you, yet wholly different.

When we create children, we create hope and pride, and achieve a subtle sort of immortality. When we accept the responsibility of parenthood, we participate in the oldest of human traditions.

Nothing can take the place of parents who are concerned, loving, and involved. To be a parent is to engage in a privileged and special occupation—one that is heavy with responsibility but full of joy. You will work long and hard at parenting, and make many sacrifices—and with no guarantee that your child will become the person you had envisioned. Still, it's a fascinating and challenging journey that puts us in touch with the whole continuum of life and the human species—both past and future. You will begin to see your own parents in a new light.

Each person's parenthood will share much in common with others who have traveled the same road, but will still be different because each child, each mother, each father is a different and unique person.

You will be your baby's focal point—his or her whole world. You'll have many moments of well-deserved happiness, and times when you must live with mistakes you'll have made. And we've all made them.

Babies, unfortunately, don't arrive with an instruction booklet attached. There is a lot we need to learn in addition to on-the-job training. There are times when you will need help with particular questions or problems.

## Help When You Need It

To provide that help is why we have created this book. It has been designed to be the most complete single-source book of pregnant mother, infant, and toddler care yet published. Generously illustrated, it is a compilation of expert opinion, clearheaded objectivity, and practical information.

It has been a privilege for me to participate in this project. You will see that we have no axes to grind, no pet theories to push. Our goal is simply to inform—to help you make decisions that will be the best for you, your new family, and your new baby.

Obviously, not all babies—or parents for that matter—are identical. We realize that broad generalizations just don't hold water in most instances. Babies develop at varying paces. Their environments differ, and the philosophies of you and your spouse may be radically different from one another and from those of other parents. Because we understand this, the book has been written to cover a wide range of topics with discussion of the full spectrum of alternatives.

Inside, you'll find complete, straightforward information covering the span from the inception of your pregnancy to your baby's third birthday. Careful attention is given to the vital third trimester of pregnancy; selecting the right doctor; proper prenatal care (including mother's diet); and good general health care. Special sections recommend programs of exercise and fitness for pregnant and new mothers. Also discussed are the progression of pregnancy and the miracle of birth, and options in birthing techniques and environments.

Once your baby has arrived you will have information available to you on newborn care; the changing roles of fathers; how to adjust to your new baby; common infant and toddler ailments and emergency treatment; baby's diet and exercise; and the learning process.

You'll find authoritative consumer guides that will assist you in the selection of your baby's clothes, furniture, toys, and equipment. We discuss variations in product quality and features to look for, and how to select products that will be the best and safest for your baby.

We've made a special effort to look at your baby in the context of your family, *however* your family may be structured. Modern society and styles of living are changing with great rapidity, and we've reflected those changes with informed discussions of working parents, single-parent families, young and older parents, and other variations of the "traditional" family unit. Whatever your lifestyle, you'll find that the book offers a wealth of relevant, practical information.

It is not a book that, we think, is to be read from cover to cover at one sitting. Keep it out and within reach. Delve into it in bits and pieces as the need arises and when time permits.

It's our hope that the *Complete Pregnancy & Baby Book* will grow *with* you and your baby, and that your copy will become well-thumbed. The book can be your companion on a great and remarkable adventure—parenthood.

Vicki Lansky, editor

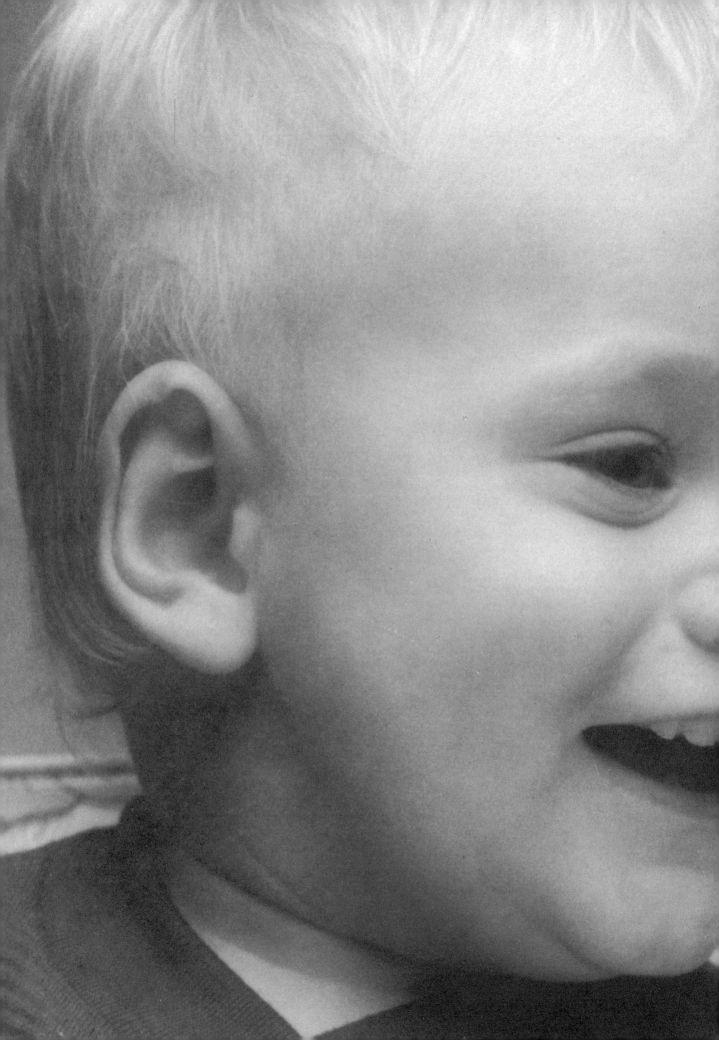

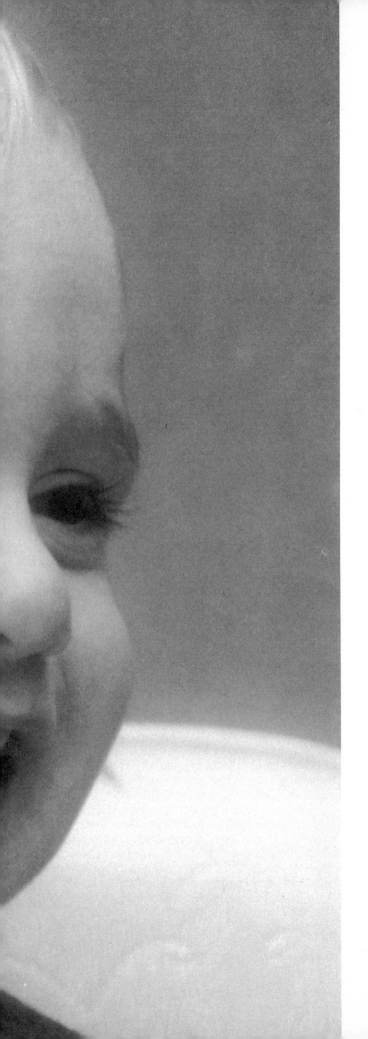

# Chapter 2: Prenatal Care

### Determination of Pregnancy

You've made the decision to have a baby. Your menstrual period is late. Should you be elated, or is cautious optimism in order? You may suspect you are pregnant by the way you feel, or your doctor may suspect it by findings on a physical exam. But symptoms and signs are just suggestive—the possibility that you are pregnant should be confirmed by a urine or blood test. If the result of one of these tests is positive, you can start rejoicing.

In the first few weeks after conceiving, you may notice changes in your body and in the way you feel. A late menstrual period is often the first hint you are pregnant. However, many other conditions, from stress to infections, can delay the onset of menses, so a late period is not a reliable sign until at least two weeks after the expected date.

On the other hand, you can have spotting while pregnant, so the presence of some bleeding doesn't eliminate the possibility.

You may notice more fatigue than usual in the first weeks. You may experience nausea or vomiting, especially in the morning, a week or two after your missed period. Your breasts may have some tingling or tenderness and may even enlarge. The *areolae* (the areas around the nipples) may darken. If you have been having trouble getting pregnant and are recording your basal body temperature, you may find that the temperature continues to be elevated. Just as with a late period, all of these signs and symptoms, if they occur at all, can be attributed to other causes. By themselves, they do not prove, but just suggest, that you are pregnant.

If you go to see your doctor when your period is two weeks late, he may find physical changes that suggest you are pregnant. Your vagina and cervix may be a blue to purplish color because of increased blood flow. This is known as Chadwick's sign. The uterus may feel softer, larger, and rounder. Your doctor may be able to feel intermittent contractions, called Braxton Hicks contractions, even though you may not recognize them.

Many women know they are pregnant before they see their obstetrician, however, because they run a pregnancy test themselves at home. Nonprescription home pregnancy tests are available in any pharmacy and cost about ten dollars. These tests are designed to detect the presence in the urine of human chorionic gonadotropin (HCG), a hormone produced by the embryo shortly after fertilization.

Home pregnancy tests on the market today vary in sensitivity. Some can detect HCG one day after the missed period. Others require one to two weeks. Some tests must be done on a urine specimen obtained in the morning, when the concentration of HCG is the highest; others can be performed on any urine specimen. Some react within ten minutes, but others require one to two hours. No matter which test you use, if the directions are followed carefully, the results are ninety to ninety-five percent accurate.

The tests are easy to perform. You add a few drops of urine to a test tube containing a protein, called an antibody, that reacts specifically with HCG. If you are pregnant and HCG is present in the urine, it will bind to the antibody, forming a complex. If you are not pregnant and no HCG is present, the antibody will remain free in the solution. Different chemical reactions are used in the different test kits to indicate whether a complex or free antibody is present. Positive tests usually are indicated either by formation of a circle at the bottom of the tube or by a color change in the solution.

Even though these tests are extremely sensitive, there are a few other things that, when present in the urine, will cause a positive test result even though the woman is not pregnant. Luteinizing hormone (LH) is one of the hormones that regulate the menstrual cycle. It can cross-react with HCG and give a positive test result. Ordinarily, it is not present in the urine in detectable amounts. However, menopausal women have a high level of LH and can have a falsely positive test result. Women with protein in their urine can have a similar reaction. Protein may be present because of infection or kidney disease or because certain medications, such as tranquilizers, thyroid medications, and seizure drugs, have been taken. More common than a false-positive test result is a false-negative one—that is, the test result is negative even though the woman is pregnant. This usually occurs when the test is done too early after the missed period, when the level of HCG is too low to be detected. Low levels of HCG may also be caused by an ectopic pregnancy (a pregnancy that develops outside the uterus). If the first test result is negative and your period doesn't start, repeat the test in five to ten days. If it is still negative, consult your doctor.

If you go to your doctor two weeks after your missed period, he or she will probably perform a pregnancy test on your urine that is similar to the home pregnancy tests. The "rabbit test" is no longer used because of the greater speed, convenience, and accuracy of modern tests.

If your doctor needs to know if you are pregnant at a time before the urine test can be used or if he or she suspects a false-negative test result, a blood test that is more sensitive and specific may be used. It measures a part of the HCG molecule known as the beta-subunit. Since LH doesn't have a beta-subunit, this test can distinguish between LH and HCG. Because it can measure very small amounts of HCG, it can be used to diagnose pregnancy before a missed period (by seven to nine days after fertilization) or to diagnose a tubal pregnancy (one that develops in one of the fallopian tubes). The test takes longer (twenty-four to forty-eight hours) to complete, and it is more expensive because it requires special equipment and personnel. Therefore, it is not used routinely to diagnose pregnancy.

When you finally know for sure that you are pregnant, the next question will undoubtedly be "When will my baby be born?" Delivery usually occurs 280 days after the first day of the last menstrual period. An easier way to calculate the delivery date, or due date, is to count back three months from the first day of your last period and add seven days. Most women don't give birth on the exact date, but eighty-five percent do within two weeks of it; delivery is earlier for ten percent and later for five percent. As your pregnancy progresses, your due date can be double-checked by the timing of certain events. For example, the baby's heart is usually heard at ten to twelve weeks. The level at which the top of the uterus can be palpated (felt) by the doctor can also be used; at twenty-four weeks, for example, it is usually at the umbilicus (navel). If your obstetrician performs an ultrasound study, a measurement of the baby's head can be taken and compared with standard tables to estimate gestational age.

Discovering that you are pregnant is an exciting moment. The next nine months will be filled with excitement both for you and your family as the changes of pregnancy take place.

## Choosing an Obstetrician

Your pregnancy involves many other people besides yourself and your baby. Your family, of course, is affected. You may have a Lamaze teacher and an exercise instructor. And you will certainly have a doctor. Your obstetrician is a partner in your pregnancy. He or she will have the responsibility for your and your baby's health, so you want to be sure the doctor is qualified and competent. In addition, he or she will intimately participate in a very special event in your life—you want someone with whom you can cooperate and feel comfortable.

Finding the right obstetrician may take some work. You may need to talk to people and may visit a number of doctors before you are satisfied. You can get recommendations from many different sources. Friends and relatives may suggest their obstetricians. Another doctor, such as your internist, may provide a name. Maternity nurses or obstetrical residents (doctors in training) at your local hospital often know which obstetricians in the community are good. You can ask the department of obstetrics and gynecology at the nearest

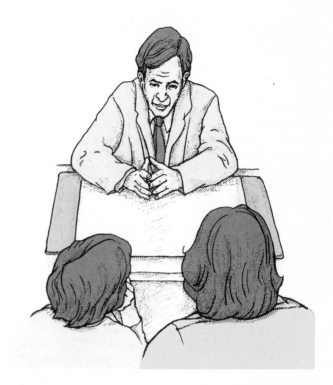

*Meet and talk with a number of obstetricians before choosing one.*

university hospital for the names of graduates or faculty members who work in your area. If these avenues fail, try contacting a childbirth education group, such as the International Childbirth Education Association, a local Lamaze instructor, or your La Leche League chapter.

When you have the name of an obstetrician who sounds promising, your next step is to find out more detailed information about her. To be sure she is a competent doctor, check out her training. An obstetrician should have completed an obstetrics residency at a registered hospital and should be certified by the American Board of Obstetrics and Gynecology.

Next, find out which hospital she is affiliated with. The hospital should be accredited by the Joint Commission on Accreditation of Hospitals (JCAH). Find out whether the hospital is a teaching institution. If it is, be sure you understand how residents will participate in your delivery. The hospital should be convenient for you, and it should have the facilities you want or need for your delivery. Some hospitals have only the traditional separate labor and delivery rooms. Others have elaborate birthing centers. If you are at risk for having problems during pregnancy or delivery, the hospital should have an infant intensive care nursery.

Find out about the people the doctor works with. If she works with a group of doctors, they probably take turns being on call at night. If you go into labor on a night when your doctor is not on call, will she come in or will one of her partners perform the delivery? If one of her partners may deliver your baby, you will have to be sure that you are comfortable with the other members of the group and that they have the same attitudes toward childbirth as your doctor. Otherwise, the delivery you've so carefully planned may be changed at the last minute. Some obstetricians employ nurse practitioners or midwives to do checkups or even perform uncomplicated deliveries. If this is the case, be sure you understand and are comfortable with the arrangement.

Finally, don't be afraid to ask about finances. Be sure your insurance will cover the doctor's charges and find out how and when payment is expected. Find out what happens to the charges if there are any complications.

When you have collected your information, you are ready for your first meeting with the doctor. It is a good idea for your husband to accompany you so that he can ask questions and form an opinion about the doctor as well. If you haven't been seeing an internist or gynecologist regularly, it is a good idea to choose an obstetrician before you attempt to conceive; arrange a prepregnancy appointment to be sure there are no medical conditions that make pregnancy inadvisable at the time. If you have been receiving regular medical care, your first appointment should occur as soon as you think you are pregnant, usually two weeks after the missed period. During the first visit, the doctor will take a complete medical history, including discussion of past and present illnesses and past pregnancies. A complete physical exam, not only a pelvic exam, should be done. You should then have an opportunity to discuss with the doctor issues about your pregnancy and delivery. Be prepared for this part of your visit. Make a list of questions you want to ask. The obstetrician should be willing to answer any questions and to discuss the type of care you will receive. She should be flexible about issues that are important to you, but if she feels that something you want will compromise your care, she should be willing to explain to you why.

You will want to talk about both pregnancy and delivery. Important issues during pregnancy include nutrition, exercise, illness, and monitoring the baby's development. Discuss with the doctor what you should eat. How many more calories will you need? How does she feel about your drinking coffee or other caffeinated beverages? What about alcohol consumption? She will probably recommend vitamins and calcium supplements. Discuss with her how much exercise you should get. Would she recommend an aerobics class? Find out what you should do if you become ill. What medicines can you take and what should you avoid? The obstetrician can monitor a pregnancy with blood tests, urine tests, ultrasound studies, and amniocentesis. What does she think is appropriate for you?

There are many decisions regarding delivery that should be made beforehand. You need to decide where you want to give birth—in a regular delivery room or in a birthing center. If you want your husband or other children there, be sure your doctor agrees. If you have strong opinions about the medical treatment during labor and delivery, be sure to discuss them with your doctor. For example, some women do not want an intravenous line, anesthesia, or an episiotomy (a surgical incision to enlarge the external opening of the birth canal and make delivery easier). Fetal monitoring is another topic you may wish to inquire about. You may want to find out your doctor's opinions about inducing labor and about cesareans. Ask her how many cesareans she performs. If her rate is high, try to find out why. Does she have a high-risk population or is she just quick to operate?

By the time you are finished discussing all of these topics, you should have a good idea how well you like the obstetrician. Do you feel at ease with her? While you may not agree on every subject, you should feel confident that you can develop a working relationship and that you can discuss a problem and reach a compromise that will be satisfactory to both of you.

Finding an obstetrician may be easy, or it may require a search. Because the doctor plays such an important role in your life at this time, it is worth the effort to find someone you like as well as trust. Only in this way can you be sure that your pregnancy and delivery will be as safe and joyful as possible.

## Physical Changes During Pregnancy

The physical changes that occur during pregnancy, both in the baby and in the mother, are dramatic and wondrous. Two cells join, and an entirely new person is created. A complex array of body systems is formed in just a few short months.

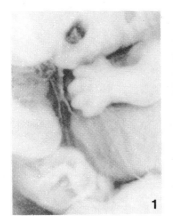
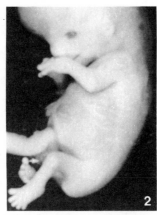
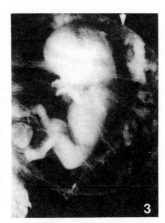
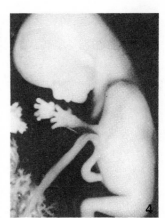

1: *A normal human embryo at about thirty-eight days. Already the ears, nose, and fingers are distinguishable.* 2: *At about forty-eight days, toes are clearly evident.* 3: *Notice the thin amniotic sac that surrounds this nine-week-old fetus, as well as the umbilical cord that attaches to the placenta (left).* 4: *Normal fetus at approximately eleven weeks. Notice the relatively large head.*

The changes in the mother's body to accommodate this new life are no less amazing. A combination of hormonal actions and physical pressures cause major alterations in her physique. While medical science may not know exactly why pregnancy advances as it does, a lot about what unfolds during those nine months has been discovered. Although it is sometimes complex, it is well worth the effort to try to understand these changes.

## Changes in the Baby

Conception occurs two weeks after the woman's last menstrual period. The egg and the sperm fuse to produce one cell. In the first three months, or *trimester,* the embryo takes shape and all the organs are formed. In the last six months, the fetus grows and matures.

In the first weeks after conception, the single cell rapidly divides into many cells. A hollow ball of cells is formed and becomes attached to the womb. Some of the cells will become the placenta; the rest will become the embryo. The latter group of cells develops into a four-layered disc. Each layer will be converted into different areas of the body. The outer layer, or ectoderm, for example, will develop into skin, hair, nails, and the nervous system. The inner layer, or endoderm, will develop into the intestines and lungs. The middle layers will develop into the heart, bones, and muscles.

By three weeks after fertilization, or about one week after the first period is missed, the embryo already is one-tenth of an inch long and has an oval shape. In the next few weeks, it becomes more curved in shape, and a head and tail become discernible. The beginnings of the spinal cord and brain take shape. A tubular heart begins to form. Tiny eyes can be seen. Arms and legs begin to bud.

By the fourth week after fertilization, traces of all the organs of the body are present. Bulges that will become the ears and nose appear. The gut is formed from blind pouches within the embryo; these push forward, creating an opening in the head that will become the mouth. A crude face begins to take shape. At this point, the embryo is only one-quarter of an inch long.

The embryo is called a *fetus* at the seventh to eighth week. It has grown to a length of one inch. The head is disproportionately large because of the size of the developing brain, while the abdomen seems large because of the growing liver. Fingers and toes appear. The rudiments of all the major hormone-producing glands—the pituitary, thyroid, and adrenal glands—are present. Amazingly, the tiny heart begins to beat.

By the end of the third month, the fetus is two to three inches long and weighs less than an ounce. Nails form on the fingers and toes. The bones begin to calcify. The male or female sex organs begin to develop. The tooth buds form in the mouth. The fetus begins to make breathing movements and starts to swallow amniotic fluid. The muscles of the intestines contract and relax, as if digesting food. Skeletal muscles begin to work as well, so the fetus can move in response to local pressure.

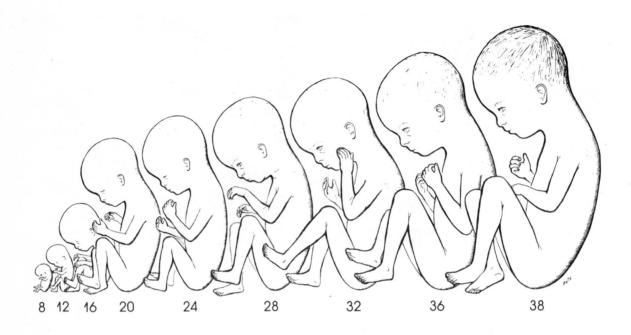

8  12  16  20    24      28      32      36      38

*In just a few short weeks, a microscopically tiny embryo grows and develops into a complex and fully formed infant.*

Although all the organs are present by the end of the first trimester, the fetus is not yet able to live outside the mother's body. The second trimester is devoted primarily to maturation of the organs. By the fourth month, the fetus moves spontaneously but is too small for the mother to feel. The fetus is four to five inches long and weighs three ounces.

By the fifth month, however, the baby is six inches long, weighs one-half pound, and is strong enough to make his presence felt. The mother's perception of the baby's movement is known as *quickening.* In the fifth to sixth month, the body becomes covered with fine hair, or *lanugo,* and coarser hair appears on the head.

The baby is fully developed by the beginning of the third trimester. The last three months, therefore, are devoted to growth. The fetus is about ten inches long and weighs one to two pounds by the seventh month. The skin is red, wrinkled, and thin. It becomes covered with *vernix,* a thick, white, sticky material composed of skin cells, lanugo, and oily skin secretions. If the baby were born at this time, he would have a fifty percent chance of survival, provided he received appropriate medical care. Babies born this early can respond to taste, light, and sound.

If the baby is born during the eighth month of gestation, his chance of survival increases to ninety percent. By this time, he is ten to twelve inches long and weighs three to four pounds.

The final preparations for independent existence occur during the ninth month. Surfactant, a substance that lines the lungs and allows them to expand easily, develops. Fat is stored, and its deposition under the skin smooths out the wrinkles. Much of the lanugo disappears.

By the final month of pregnancy, the fetus is usually fourteen to sixteen inches long and weighs seven to eight pounds. He is large and strong enough for the next step—birth and independent life. That one cell has come a long way, from embryo to fetus to newborn baby.

## Changes in the Mother

The change from a microscopic cell to a seven-pound baby requires substantial alterations in the body of the mother carrying the baby as well. However, while the baby changes most rapidly in the first few weeks, the mother undergoes her most dramatic changes in the later stages of pregnancy. In the first six weeks, the mother's physical changes are due primarily to alterations in hormone levels. These changes are subtle, and she may not even realize she is pregnant. She may have few symptoms or may easily attribute them to other causes. After this time, the mother's physical changes are partly dependent on the growth of the baby and become more noticeable as the baby gets larger and larger. Although the most obvious changes occur in the uterus and abdomen, almost all of the organs in her body are altered.

When a woman becomes pregnant, her uterus is the part of her body that is affected first and that undergoes the most significant changes. It increases to five to six times its original size, twenty times its original weight, and one thousand times its initial capacity. The amount of muscle, connective and elastic tissue, blood vessels, and nerves increases. The shape changes from elongated to oval by the second month, to round by midgestation, then back through oval to elongated at term. The uterus softens beginning at the sixth week. It changes position as it increases in size, ascending into the abdomen by the fourth month and eventually reaching to the liver. It also becomes more contractile, with irregular, painless Braxton Hicks contractions beginning in the first trimester. These contractions may be felt in the last weeks of pregnancy, when they are known as false labor.

Other parts of the reproductive system change along with the uterus. The cervix and vagina have increased blood supply, which causes a darkening in color. This is apparent by the sixth week. The amount of elastic tissue increases to prepare the way for the stretching that will be required during delivery. Secretions increase, and a mucous plug develops in the cervix. The fallopian tubes, ovaries, and ligaments supporting the uterus all enlarge and elongate. The ovaries, of course, cease to ovulate.

During the fourth month, the uterus will grow into the abdomen, causing the abdominal wall to expand to accommodate it. The connective and elastic tissues are stretched and straightened, creating thinned areas called *striae* (stretch marks). Unfortunately, while the color of the striae may fade, scars remain after delivery. In fifty percent of women, striae will develop in the third trimester. Late in pregnancy, the internal pressure from the large uterus may even cause the muscles of the abdominal wall to separate.

A woman's breasts must undergo many changes during pregnancy to be able to produce milk. In the first two months, the breasts may feel sore or full. They will increase in size, and veins may become visible on the surface. Striae can de-

velop. The nipples also increase in size and usually darken in color. By mid-pregnancy, colostrum (a thick, yellowish fluid) can be expressed, but milk is not produced until after delivery.

Since the baby is being fed by the mother's blood supply and the mother's enlarging reproductive organs require more blood flow, the amount of blood must also increase. During pregnancy, blood volume expands by twenty-five to forty percent, but the number of red blood cells (the oxygen-carrying component of blood) increases to a lesser extent. Therefore, pregnant women are relatively anemic—that is, their blood's oxygen-carrying ability is somewhat decreased.

To pump an increased amount of blood around the body, the heart must work slightly harder. The heart pumps more blood per beat and beats slightly faster. Heart murmurs attributable to the increased flow through the heart may develop.

The blood vessels are also affected by pregnancy. The enlarging uterus presses on veins in the pelvis, increasing the pressure in the veins from the legs. This increased pressure causes the leg veins to enlarge, producing varicosities (areas of enlargement). It may also cause fluid to leak out of the veins and into the tissues, causing swelling of the feet and ankles. Late in pregnancy, the uterus can also compress a major vein, the vena cava, in some women when they lie on their backs; if this occurs, blood is prevented from returning to the heart, and a feeling of faintness results.

The enlarging uterus not only pushes forward on the abdominal wall and down on the pelvic veins, but it also pushes up on the bottom of the rib cage and on the diaphragm (the muscle that stretches across the bottom of the chest cavity and assists in breathing). The rib cage widens, and most women breathe slightly faster. Some feel short of breath.

Urination and digestion are also affected during pregnancy. The urinary tract is changed both by pressure from the uterus and by hormonal influences. The uterus presses against the bladder, which may cause a pregnant woman to urinate more frequently. Hormones cause the ureters (the tubes conducting urine from the kidneys to the bladder) to distend (widen) and the flow of the urine in them to slow. The sluggish urine flow predisposes a pregnant woman to infection. Hormones, along with the increased blood volume, also cause the kidneys to filter more blood. How-

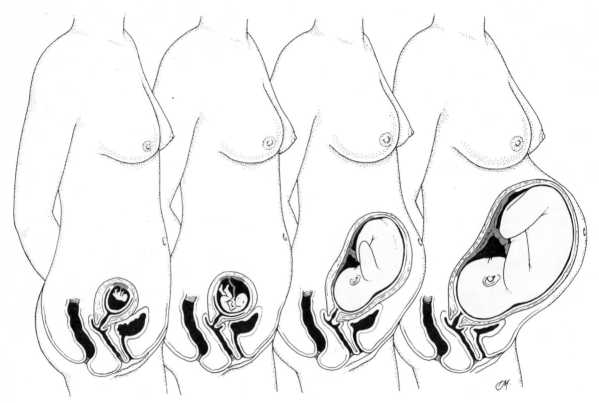

*As the fetus grows within the uterus, the mother's body changes both internally and externally.*

ever, the kidneys may not reabsorb sugar and protein efficiently because of this increased work load, and these substances may spill into the urine. Since the presence of sugar in the urine can also be caused by diabetes and the presence of protein can be caused by infection, most doctors screen the urine frequently during pregnancy and may do other tests if any abnormality is found.

The changes in digestion associated with pregnancy are well known and frequently kidded about. A pregnant woman's craving for pickles and ice cream has been the premise of many a joke. Women may have unusual cravings, and may also notice changes in the senses of smell and taste, which may cause them to alter eating habits. During pregnancy, women often produce more saliva, and the saliva will be more acidic, which promotes tooth decay. The gums are more sensitive and may swell and bleed easily. In the first trimester, a woman may have morning sickness, characterized by vomiting and a poor appetite. She may also be constipated. One of the pregnancy hormones causes the muscles of the digestive tract to relax, and they therefore pass digesting food more slowly through the intestines. In

addition, the uterus can press on the colon, inhibiting passage of feces. Similar mechanisms produce heartburn. The muscles at the junction of the esophagus and the stomach relax and the uterus presses on the stomach from below, causing the stomach contents to flow back into the esophagus. In late pregnancy, the stomach may even be pushed all the way up into the chest, producing a hiatal hernia.

A number of changes are necessary in the structures supporting the uterus to stabilize it as it grows. The ligaments in the pelvis and abdomen stretch to accommodate the uterus. In late pregnancy, the upper part of the spine bends backward to compensate for the enlarging abdomen. Hormones loosen the joints of the pelvis in preparation for childbirth.

Hormonal influences are also responsible for changes in the skin. Pigmentation of the nipples, vulva (the external genital organs), the center of the lower part of the abdomen, and the umbilicus increases. Darkening across the face may appear; this is known as *chloasma*, or the mask of pregnancy. Hormones can also cause reddening of the palms and the appearance of small red spots on the skin; these are nests of blood vessels, which are known as *spider nevi* or *telangiectasias*. Sweat and oil glands also become more productive.

One of the most important changes during pregnancy is the increase in metabolism, which is necessary to provide nourishment to the fetus. A woman must eat more to supply adequate protein, carbohydrates, and fat to the fetus and to her own enlarging body. Most women gain about twenty-five pounds, three pounds in the first trimester and ten to twelve pounds in each of the second and third trimesters. The placenta, fetus, and amniotic fluid and the increased volume of blood and breast and uterine tissue account for twenty pounds of that weight gain. The rest of the weight is fat and extra fluid. A pregnant woman must also take in more vitamins and minerals for the growing fetus. Calcium, which is needed for developing bones, and iron, which is used to make new blood cells, generally need to be ingested in greater amounts from the fourth month of pregnancy on.

The physical changes during pregnancy are miraculous. Amazingly, though, the physical alterations in the mother reverse after birth, and her body returns to its normal state. For the baby, however, the process of change started nine months before has just begun.

## Discomfort During Pregnancy

The sudden and dramatic changes that occur during pregnancy may make a woman feel that her body is alien to her. Her body looks different and feels different. Often, those feelings are uncomfortable. Carrying twenty-five extra pounds around inside one's abdominal cavity puts a strain on the legs and hips, not to mention the pressure on other organs.

She may experience pain in the lower part of the abdomen, especially on the right-hand side, beginning at about twenty weeks. This is caused by the stretching of the ligaments that support the uterus. There may also be pain in the upper front part of the thigh, which is caused by the uterus pressing on a nerve that passes over the rim of the pelvic bone. These pains can be relieved by lying down.

Pain can also occur in the upper part of the abdomen. It is often due to heartburn, which can be relieved by sitting upright after meals, eating smaller quantities, and taking antacids (with doctor's permission). However, serious complications of pregnancy, such as gallstones, may also cause upper abdominal pain, so it is best to check with your doctor.

She may experience other sorts of discomfort besides pain during her pregnancy. Hormonal changes in the first trimester may cause morning sickness, with nausea, vomiting, and loss of appetite. It may help to eat something bland, such as a cracker, first thing in the morning. Eating small, frequent meals may also ease the sensation.

Constipation can be an uncomfortable side effect of pregnancy. It can lead to hemorrhoids, which may result from straining while eliminating. Hemorrhoids may also appear because of increased pressure from the uterus on the pelvic veins. Alterations in diet to increase the amounts of fruit and fiber may help, but often laxatives and stool softeners are needed. Sitz baths, lubricating creams, and suppositories may be used for hemorrhoids, but a pregnant woman should check with her doctor before using any medication.

The uterus also exerts pressure on the veins to the legs, especially in the third trimester. This causes varicose veins and leg swelling. Wearing shoes may become difficult. Elevating the legs and wearing elastic stockings helps.

Late in pregnancy, a woman may have pain in her pelvis or feel as if her pelvis is separating. Hormonally induced loosening of the ligaments is responsible for this. The best remedy is to avoid activities that strain these ligaments.

She may also have backaches. These are due to the change in posture required by the enlarging abdomen. A good exercise program (with doctor's approval) to strengthen the abdominal and back muscles may help prevent backaches; rest and a heating pad will help relieve them when they occur.

The changes of pregnancy can be uncomfortable. By being aware of the potential for pain and taking the appropriate steps to avoid it or relieve it when it occurs, it is possible to get through the nine months in relative comfort.

## Mother's Diet

The attention you give to good nutrition during your pregnancy does make a difference for your

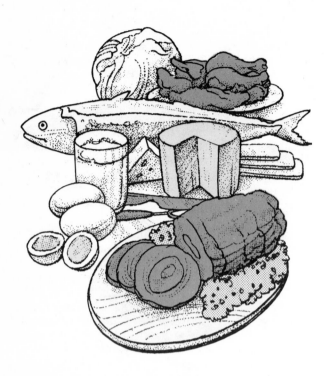

*A healthy, balanced diet during pregnancy is vital for the well-being of mother and baby.*

baby's health and yours. Your diet before you were pregnant and now during your pregnancy provides the essential building blocks for your developing baby's healthy growth. Just as you would choose the very best yarn to knit a sweater or special ingredients to make a birthday cake, you will want to consume the most nutritious foods you can during pregnancy to build your baby's heart, lungs, brain, and skeleton. Eating well during pregnancy is a gift to your baby for life and a way of nurturing yourself as well. Eating well makes you feel good, and it contributes to a healthy pregnancy.

Ideally, nutrition for pregnancy begins before conception, as you maintain your stores of iron, calcium, and other nutrients. But it is never too late to pay attention to what you eat. You will feel better and your baby will benefit from your good diet.

Today, we know how important good nutrition and adequate weight gain during pregnancy are for producing a full-term, vigorous infant and for contributing to a healthy pregnancy. In years past, however, nutrition advice to pregnant mothers differed greatly from what you will be told today. Weight gain was severely limited, salt was eliminated from the diet, and diuretics, laxatives, and even diet pills were routinely prescribed.

You can feel comfortable gaining more weight than your mother might have been allowed, and you can be assured that your abstinence from alcohol and certain drugs is of utmost benefit to your developing baby.

## Weight Gain During Pregnancy

From the early 1950's until the early 1970's, pregnant women were advised to gain ten to fifteen pounds during pregnancy. Limited weight gain was thought to help keep the baby's weight low to reduce problems with delivery of a large baby and to avoid the matter of a mother having to lose weight after the birth of her child.

Concern about adequate weight gain during pregnancy was highlighted by the Task Force on Mental Retardation commissioned by President Kennedy in 1962. The task force found that prematurity and low birth weight were major factors in infant mortality (death) and morbidity (disease). Their findings led to the development of the federal Maternal and Infant Care Program, which stressed good nutrition during pregnancy.

Since that time, many researchers have focused on the relationship of weight gain and pre-pregnancy weight to pregnancy outcome. We now know that poor weight gain, especially in the third trimester, is associated with low birth weight and neurological deficits in the baby. Low birth weight is associated with a higher incidence of infant mortality and morbidity, mental retardation, learning disabilities, and inadequate growth than is adequate birth weight.

Still other studies have correlated height and pre-pregnancy weight with the baby's birth weight. Mothers who are ten percent or more below the standard weight for their height are at a significantly greater risk for producing low-birthweight and premature infants.

Research has also shown that large women tend to produce large babies. The birth size of an infant is related to the size of his mother and is not influenced greatly by the size of his father.

How does all this information affect recommendations for weight gain during pregnancy? Advice about weight gain for pregnant women today reflects an individualized approach based on the mother's height and her pre-pregnancy weight, and whether the mother is a teenager or is pregnant with more than one baby.

## Components of Weight Gain (in pounds)

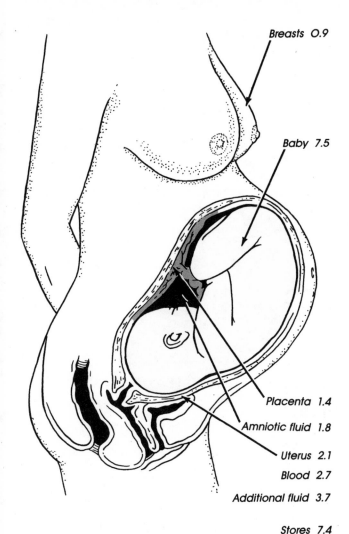

Breasts 0.9

Baby 7.5

Placenta 1.4

Amniotic fluid 1.8

Uterus 2.1

Blood 2.7

Additional fluid 3.7

Stores 7.4

*Total weight gain: approximately 27.5 pounds*

You will be advised to gain between twenty and thirty pounds during pregnancy. If you are underweight, you will probably be encouraged to gain closer to thirty pounds. If you are of normal weight, you will ideally gain between twenty-four and thirty pounds. If you are overweight (weigh more than thirty-five percent above the ideal body weight), you may be urged to gain between fifteen and twenty-four pounds. If you are pregnant with more than one baby, you will be advised to gain an even greater amount of weight. If you are a teenager, you will need special guidance to get enough calories and nutrients to satisfy your growth needs as well as the needs of your baby.

Where does the weight gain go? Some goes to the growth of your baby and some goes to the body changes necessary to support your pregnancy.

## Pattern of Weight Gain During Pregnancy

Weight gain during pregnancy occurs in a predictable pattern. You will gain only a little weight the first trimester and will have a more rapid gain during the second and third trimesters. Your weight gain will be plotted by your doctor at your prenatal visit on a chart similar to the one that follows.

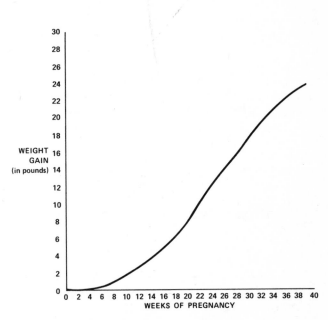

The chart helps your doctor detect some potential pregnancy problems. If weight gain is too slow, nutrition counseling may help. If weight gain suddenly rises, especially in the latter part of pregnancy, it may be the result of edema (swelling), which could be an indication of pre-eclampsia, or it may be the result of extra calorie consumption or decreased activity.

Morning sickness in early pregnancy may affect weight gain temporarily. Continued vomiting throughout pregnancy is more serious and requires treatment. Activity level may also affect weight gain during pregnancy.

Today, an increasing number of women worry about the effects of anorexia or bulimia on their pregnancy. Women who are or have been anorexic or bulimic have a more difficult time accepting the weight gain and body changes that are a normal part of pregnancy. Counseling can be very helpful. Most large metropolitan areas have bulimia and anorexia support groups. Since eating well is so critical during pregnancy, getting help is crucial.

Keep in mind that there is a wide variation in weight gain and pattern of weight gain among pregnant women. The weight gain suggestions reflect *average* weight gain ranges and are a guide for you and your doctor. Your weight gain may not follow these guidelines, but if you are making an effort to eat a quality diet with adequate calories, you can feel comfortable knowing you are doing what you can to ensure your health and your baby's.

## Good Nutrition During Your Pregnancy

What should you eat in order to be healthy during pregnancy and how much should you eat? You will want to pay special attention to certain nutrients and add about three hundred extra calories to your diet. The recommended daily caloric intake during pregnancy is 2,100 to 2,400 calories. Your weight gain is a good guide to how well you are meeting your caloric intake.

# DAILY FOOD GUIDE

Use the following guide to help you decide if your daily diet is sufficient for pregnancy. Pay specific attention to serving size and to variety in your diet. The sixth column ("Servings Needed") will help you decide if you need to alter your diet. Several times during pregnancy, analyze your diet over a period of days.

| FOOD CATEGORY | PRIMARY NUTRIENTS OR NUTRITIVE ROLE | NUMBER OF DAILY SERVINGS | EXAMPLES OF SINGLE SERVINGS |
|---|---|---|---|
| **Dairy** | Calcium, phosphorus, vitamin D, protein | 4 | 8 oz. milk, 1⅓ cups cottage cheese, 1½ oz. cheese, 1½ cups ice cream |
| **High-quality protein** | Complete protein, iron, folate, vitamin A, B-complex vitamins | 3 to 4 | 2–3 oz. meat, 2 medium eggs, 8–12 small oysters or clams, 1 cup baked beans or dried peas, ¼ cup peanut butter, ½ cup nuts, 1 cup tofu |
| **Grains and breads** | B-complex vitamins, incomplete proteins, iron (also provide energy and fiber) | 4 or more (as needed for calories) | 1 slice bread (whole-grain or enriched), ½ cup cooked cereal, 1 tbsp. wheat germ, ½ cup brown rice or macaroni, 1 tortilla or bagel, 1 pancake (5-inch) |
| **Green and yellow vegetables** | Vitamin A, folate, vitamin C, vitamin E, riboflavin, iron, magnesium | 1 to 2 | 1 stalk broccoli, 1 small sweet potato, ¾ cup carrots, ½ cup spinach, 3½ oz. romaine, ½ cup squash |

## Protein

Protein intake should be increased during pregnancy to provide for the growth of your baby, breasts, uterus, and placenta; for the increased blood volume; and for the production of amniotic fluid. Recommended daily amounts of protein increase dramatically, from forty-six grams before pregnancy to seventy-six to one hundred grams during pregnancy.

## Iron

Iron is an important nutrient during pregnancy for three primary reasons. First, iron is necessary for the formation of maternal and fetal hemoglobin, the oxygen-carrying component of blood. Since your blood volume increases considerably during pregnancy and your baby is manufacturing his blood cells too, your need for iron increases. Second, during the last trimester, your baby draws from you some of the iron reserves that will help to keep him from becoming anemic during the first four to six months after birth. Third, your increased blood volume and iron stores help your body adjust (to some degree) to the blood loss that occurs during childbirth.

You may wonder why your prenatal vitamin contains thirty to sixty milligrams of iron when the recommended amount during pregnancy is just

| NUMBER OF SERVINGS YOU HAD TODAY | SERVINGS NEEDED TO MEET REQUIREMENTS | FOOD CATEGORY |
|---|---|---|
| | | Dairy |
| | | High-quality protein |
| | | Grains and breads |
| | | Green and yellow vegetables |

continued

## DAILY FOOD GUIDE continued

| FOOD CATEGORY | PRIMARY NUTRIENTS OR NUTRITIVE ROLE | NUMBER OF DAILY SERVINGS | EXAMPLES OF SINGLE SERVINGS |
|---|---|---|---|
| **Citrus fruits; fruits and vegetables rich in vitamin C** | Vitamin C, folate | 1 to 2 | 1 orange, 1/2 cup grapefruit, 1/2 cup orange juice, 3/4 cup strawberries, 1 cup tomato juice, 1 large tomato, 1/2 green pepper, 3/4 cup cabbage |
| **Potatoes and other fruits and vegetables** | Vitamins (also provide energy and fiber) | 1 or more as needed for calories | 1 potato, 1/2 cup cauliflower, 1/2 cup beets, 1/2 cup corn, 1/2 cup eggplant, 1/2 cup celery |
| **Fats** | Vitamin A, vitamin E (also provide energy) | 1 to 2 | 1 tbsp. oil, fortified margarine, butter, mayonnaise, or salad dressing |
| **Fluids** | Necessary because of increased metabolic rate (also increases comfort) | 2 to 3 quarts (drink to satisfy thirst) | 1 glass (8 oz.) of water, juice, or other beverage (avoid alcohol and caffeine) |
| **Iodine-containing foods** | Iodine | Salt to taste at table or in cooking | Iodized salt (avoid excessive amounts), seafood |
| **Foods consisting primarily of nonnutritious calories** | (Provide energy) | In moderation, and only after daily nutrient requirements have been satisfied | Candy bar, jam, sugar, honey, syrup |

over eighteen milligrams a day. Because iron is not totally absorbed from supplements, you must ingest about sixty milligrams of iron to ensure that you actually absorb the required amount.

Iron supplements are best absorbed if they are taken with foods rich in vitamin C, such as orange juice, grapefruit, and strawberries. Absorption is impaired if you take them with an antacid. Iron supplements sometimes cause an upset stomach, constipation, or nausea. If that is the case for you, remember that you can get much of the iron you need from the iron-rich foods you eat. Good food

sources of iron include organ meats, red meat, egg yolk, and legumes.

### Calcium

Your calcium needs increase during pregnancy from eight hundred to twelve hundred milligrams a day. Calcium is essential for the development and growth of your baby's skeleton, heart, muscles, and tooth buds. Inadequate calcium intake results in your own stores of calcium being depleted.

| NUMBER OF SERVINGS YOU HAD TODAY | SERVINGS NEEDED TO MEET REQUIREMENTS | FOOD CATEGORY |
|---|---|---|
| | | Citrus fruits; fruits and vegetables rich in vitamin C |
| | | Potatoes and other fruits and vegetables |
| | | Fats |
| | | Fluids |
| | | Iodine-containing foods |
| | | Foods consisting primarily of nonnutritious calories |

Milk and milk products (such as yogurt and cheese) are the best sources of dietary calcium. Tofu and canned whole fish (with bones) are good secondary sources of calcium. If you are milk-intolerant, a calcium supplement prescribed by your doctor may be necessary.

## Vitamins

The recommended daily allowances of nearly all vitamins increase in pregnancy by twenty-five to fifty percent. The recommended allowance for folic acid doubles. A high-quality, varied diet will supply most of the vitamins you need for a healthy pregnancy, with the probable exception of folic acid. Folic acid supplements of two hundred to four hundred micrograms are recommended to provide for the large increase in the folic acid requirement during pregnancy.

Folic acid is important for the synthesis of all cells and for the production of DNA and RNA. Folic acid deficiency can cause megaloblastic anemia in the mother, characterized by the development of abnormal red blood cells.

Since adequate folic acid intake is so important for your baby and you, choose a diet high in foods containing this essential vitamin. Liver, lean beef, legumes, egg yolks, and leafy dark-green vegetables are good food sources of folic acid.

## General Guidelines

Using the freshest foods you can; choosing a varied, high-quality diet; and preparing the foods carefully ensures your getting the most nutritional value from your food. Vitamins, especially the water-soluble vitamins (folic acid, niacin, vitamin C, and the B vitamins), are easily destroyed by overcooking. Uncooked vegetables and fruits have the highest vitamin content. Next best is using very little or no water to cook and cooking for a very short time.

The chart on pages 26–31 can help you to understand the increased need for nutrients during your pregnancy.

## A Daily Food Guide

Food may be divided into various groups. Using the "basic four," as in the past, may not provide for all the essential nutrients you need. Instead, using the following approach of dividing foods into seven food categories and three nonfood categories may better ensure your getting the nutrients you and your baby need.

# NUTRIENTS FOR PREGNANCY

| NUTRIENT | RECOMMENDED DAILY AMOUNT FOR PREGNANCY | WHY IT IS IMPORTANT | GOOD FOOD SOURCES |
|---|---|---|---|
| *Calories* | 2,100–2,400 calories | Necessary for energy because the basal metabolic rate is increased<br><br>Necessary for growth of maternal and fetal tissues | Proteins, carbohydrates, fats |
| *Protein* | 74–76 grams | Necessary for growth of baby and placenta<br><br>Necessary for production of amniotic fluid and increased maternal blood volume<br><br>Necessary for growth of uterus and breasts | Meat, poultry, fish, cheese, eggs, grains, nuts, milk, legumes |
| *Vitamins: Vitamin A* | 5,000 international units | Contributes to maintenance of healthy skin and mucous membranes<br><br>Necessary for development of tooth buds and bone growth<br><br>Stored by the developing fetus | Butter, fortified margarine, cream, dark-green and deep-yellow vegetables, liver, fish-liver oils, yellow noncitrus fruits |

Daily meal planning is sometimes a task that takes place in the grocery store as you choose the foods that are the best buys and the most appealing. You can be assured that you are choosing the best food by shopping mostly on the perimeter of the store, where you find the fruits, vegetables, meats, and dairy products. The inner aisles contain the breads and grains you need, but try to avoid the heavily processed and highly salted foods you see.

Use the "Daily Food Guide" chart on pages 22–25 to record your daily diet and assess where changes need to be made. Keep track of your intake for several days, and then use the chart to analyze your diet. Are you missing certain food groups? Are you not getting enough of certain kinds of foods? (At first glance, the recommended numbers of servings may seem like too much food. However, on checking the size of the sample portions, you will find that the amount of food recommended is not at all excessive.)

Sometimes your capacity or appetite is diminished, especially during late pregnancy or if you are experiencing heartburn or nausea. Eating several small meals during the day instead of three large meals may help to alleviate these symptoms.

Let your weight gain be a guide for how much food to eat. Any concerns you have about the amount of food you need should be shared with your doctor.

| DEFICIENCY OF NUTRIENT DURING PREGNANCY | EXCESS OF NUTRIENT DURING PREGNANCY | NUTRIENT |
|---|---|---|
| May contribute to poor pregnancy outcome<br><br>May contribute to low birth weight | May contribute to obesity | *Calories* |
| Affects pregnancy outcome since it affects growth of the baby and changes in the mother | Highly controversial, but retarded fetal growth and increased risk of prematurity have been reported | *Protein* |
| Has been related to abnormalities of the eyes and impaired vision in offspring<br><br>Impaired resistance to infection in offspring | Has been associated with some congenital anomalies | *Vitamins:*<br>**Vitamin A** |

continued

## NUTRIENTS FOR PREGNANCY continued

| NUTRIENT | RECOMMENDED DAILY AMOUNT FOR PREGNANCY | WHY IT IS IMPORTANT | GOOD FOOD SOURCES |
|---|---|---|---|
| Vitamin $B_1$ (thiamin) | 1.5 milligrams | Necessary for energy metabolism | Pork, liver, enriched and whole grains, legumes, nuts |
| Vitamin $B_2$ (riboflavin) | 1.5 milligrams | Necessary for protein and energy metabolism | Milk, liver, lean meats, eggs, enriched grains, cheese, leafy dark-green vegetables |
| Vitamin $B_6$ (pyridoxine) | 2.6 milligrams | Necessary for protein metabolism and fetal growth | Pork, liver, bananas, fish, whole-grain cereals, legumes |
| Vitamin $B_{12}$ (cobalamin) | 4.0 micrograms | Necessary for protein metabolism and formation of red blood cells | Milk, eggs, liver, meat, fish, cheese, legumes |
| Vitamin C | 80 milligrams | Necessary for maintenance and growth of tissues<br><br>Increases iron absorption | Citrus fruits, strawberries, tomatoes, melons, leafy green vegetables, broccoli, potatoes |
| Vitamin D | 400–600 international units | Aids absorption of calcium and phosphorus<br><br>Helps with mineralization of fetal bones and tooth buds | Fortified milk, margarine, fish (especially herring, mackerel, salmon, sardines), fish-liver oils |
| Vitamin E | 10 milligrams | Necessary for tissue growth and integrity of red blood cells and other cell membranes | Vegetable oils, egg yolks, liver, leafy green vegetables, milk, butter, peanuts, wheat germ and whole-grain products |
| Folate | 800 micrograms | Necessary for synthesis of RNA and DNA and cell division<br><br>Necessary for production of hemoglobin<br><br>Helps prevent megaloblastic anemia | Liver, leafy dark-green vegetables, legumes, whole grains, egg yolks, lean beef, melon, orange juice |

| DEFICIENCY OF NUTRIENT DURING PREGNANCY | EXCESS OF NUTRIENT DURING PREGNANCY | NUTRIENT |
|---|---|---|
| Associated with congenital beriberi if deficiency is severe | Unknown | **Vitamin B$_1$ (thiamin)** |
| May be associated with higher incidence of vomiting in pregnancy | Unknown | **Vitamin B$_2$ (riboflavin)** |
| Associated with inflammations in mouth<br><br>May be associated with increased incidence of depression | Unknown | **Vitamin B$_6$ (pyridoxine)** |
| Pernicious anemia in mother | Unknown | **Vitamin B$_{12}$ (cobalamin)** |
| Severe deficiency associated with maternal scurvy | May contribute to neonatal scurvy if infant has been conditioned to receive large amounts of vitamin C | **Vitamin C** |
| Associated with rickets in offspring and loss of calcium from maternal bones | Has been associated with some congenital abnormalities | **Vitamin D** |
| No clear result of deficiency | Unknown | **Vitamin E** |
| Associated with maternal megaloblastic anemia | Unknown | **Folate** |

continued

## NUTRIENTS FOR PREGNANCY continued

| NUTRIENT | RECOMMENDED DAILY AMOUNT FOR PREGNANCY | WHY IT IS IMPORTANT | GOOD FOOD SOURCES |
|---|---|---|---|
| Niacin | 15 milligrams | Necessary for protein and energy metabolism | Lean meats (especially pork), poultry, fish, organ meats, peanuts, beans, peas, enriched grains, eggs, milk |
| Minerals: Calcium | 1,200 milligrams | Necessary for formation of fetal skeleton and tooth buds | Milk, cheese, tofu, canned fish (with bones) |
| Iodine | 175 micrograms | Necessary for increased thyroid hormone production | Iodized salt, saltwater seafoods (especially clams, oysters, sardines) |
| Iron | 18+ milligrams | Necessary for production of increased maternal blood volume and fetal and maternal hemoglobin

Necessary for fetal liver iron storage | Liver, other meats and poultry, egg yolk, whole or enriched grains, prunes and prune juice, leafy dark-green vegetables, nuts, legumes, dried fruit, blackstrap molasses, fish and seafood (especially oysters, clams, shrimp, sardines) |
| Magnesium | 450 milligrams | Necessary for protein and energy metabolism

Necessary for tissue growth, cell metabolism, and muscle action | Nuts, soybeans, cocoa, seafood, whole grains, dried beans and peas, leafy dark-green vegetables |
| Phosphorus | 1,200 milligrams | Necessary for formation of fetal skeleton and tooth buds | Milk, cheese, lean meat, legumes, whole-grain products |
| Zinc | 20 milligrams | Necessary for insulin production

Necessary to help maintain the acid-base balance in body tissues | Oysters, other seafoods, liver, other meats, eggs, whole-grain products |

| DEFICIENCY OF NUTRIENT DURING PREGNANCY | EXCESS OF NUTRIENT DURING PREGNANCY | NUTRIENT |
|---|---|---|
| Severe deficiency associated with pellagra (characterized by dermatitis and diarrhea) in the mother | Large excess associated with flushing and pruritus (a skin condition) in mother | **Niacin** |
| May be associated with diminished bone density in mother and offspring<br><br>Implicated in toxemia | None known | *Minerals:*<br>**Calcium** |
| Associated with goiter in the mother and decreased thyroid function in the infant | May be associated with congenital goiter and hypothyroidism in infants | **Iodine** |
| Increased incidence of anemia in offspring in the first year<br><br>May be associated with greater incidence of prematurity | None known | **Iron** |
| Potential interference with tissue growth | None known | **Magnesium** |
| Potential interference with development of fetal skeleton and tooth buds | Unknown | **Phosphorus** |
| Associated with fetal anomalies of the central nervous system | May be associated with prematurity | **Zinc** |

Some doctors will prescribe prenatal vitamins, while others may prescribe only folic acid supplements or iron supplements. Remember that these supplements are not a substitute for good food. They supply only some of the nutrients needed for health. The rest you must get from the nutritious food you eat.

## Discomforts of Pregnancy

### Nausea and Vomiting

Nausea and vomiting are common discomforts of early pregnancy. They may result from some of the hormonal changes of pregnancy. They may be set off by an empty stomach (which explains why they often occur in the morning), certain odors, fatigue, or certain foods. Fatty foods, spicy foods, and caffeine are often the culprits.

Nausea and vomiting usually disappear without treatment by about the fourth month of pregnancy. To be more comfortable until this passes, you might try the following:

- Put some crackers by your bed at night to eat before getting out of bed in the morning.

- Eat high-protein foods throughout the day. This prevents a drop in your blood sugar level, which is thought to be linked to nausea.

- Take your vitamins or supplements with your largest meal to help avoid an upset stomach.

- Carry a high-carbohydrate snack (such as fresh fruit, bread, or crackers) with you during the day and eat it when you begin to feel nauseated.

Severe nausea and vomiting are less common and will be treated by your doctor.

### Heartburn

During pregnancy, the cardiac sphincter (the opening between the esophagus and stomach) is relaxed due to the effects of progesterone. Heartburn occurs when some of the contents in your stomach rise up into the esophagus, causing a burning sensation. You might want to try the following to ease heartburn:

- Eat several small meals instead of three large ones during the day.

- Avoid eating or drinking right before bedtime.

- Drink liquids in small amounts frequently during the day.

- Elevate the head of your bed on two- to three-inch blocks.

### Constipation

This is a common complaint during pregnancy, resulting from the relaxation of the smooth muscle in your digestive tract. It may be aggravated by iron supplements, lack of adequate fluid intake, and inactivity. The following may relieve constipation:

- Increasing the fiber in your diet

- Consuming two to three quarts of liquid a day

- Having some form of daily exercise, such as walking

- Drinking prune juice

## Special Nutritional Concerns

### Vegetarian Diets

Vegetarians may need some help with diet planning during pregnancy. General guidelines include the following:

- Weight gain is a good indicator of adequate calorie intake.

- If you do not eat dairy products, vitamin $B_{12}$, calcium, and vitamin D supplements may be necessary.

- Pay special attention to getting enough protein by making meals with complementary proteins.

- Let your doctor know you are a vegetarian.

### Teenage Pregnancy

An adolescent needs special guidance during pregnancy because her diet must supply the nutrients and calories necessary to meet her own growth needs as well as her baby's. Teenagers would benefit from individualized nutritional counseling aimed at meeting their nutritional requirements and matched to their lifestyles.

## Multiple Pregnancy

If you are expecting two or more babies, you should consume more calories and nutrients. Seek the advice of your doctor or a registered dietitian.

## Caffeine

Caffeine is a substance naturally found in coffee, tea, cola drinks, and chocolate. It may also be found in some medications. Careful label reading will alert you to its presence.

Caffeine readily finds its way to the fetus, and the concentration of caffeine in fetal blood will be about the same as the level in maternal blood. Studies have not shown an association between caffeine consumption and fetal abnormalities, but it is known that caffeine is a powerful stimulant. Caffeine also increases production of stress hormones, causing constriction of uterine blood vessels, which lessens the blood flow to the uterus and temporarily decreases the amount of oxygen reaching the fetus.

Large amounts of caffeine cannot be good for your baby or you. Since this substance has not been proved safe for the developing baby, little or no caffeine consumption during pregnancy is wise.

## Artificial Sweeteners

Little is known about the long-term safety of nonsugar sweeteners, such as saccharin and aspartame. (NutraSweet is the trade name for aspartame.) Saccharin has been associated with bladder cancer, and no one is sure about the long-term effects on the baby of early intra-uterine exposure to saccharin. NutraSweet has not been proved unsafe, but there are no long-term studies that show it is safe for the developing fetus. Probably the best advice is to consume these products in moderation or to avoid them altogether.

## Herbal Teas

Some herbs and herbal teas contain drugs (see the section that follows for more information on drug use during pregnancy). Ginseng tea contains a small amount of estrogen. Chamomile tea contains ragweed, which can cause severe allergic reactions in some people. Teas made from juniper berries may cause stomach irritation. Just because herbal teas are considered to be "natural" does not mean they are safe for pregnant women. You might check with your doctor or pharmacist about the safety of particular herbs before you take them.

## Smoking, Drinking, and Drugs

### Cigarettes

Cigarette smoking poses a serious threat to the well-being of your baby. Mothers who smoke have smaller babies than mothers who do not smoke. Smoking is also associated with a greater incidence of miscarriage, prematurity, stillbirth, and death of the baby soon after birth. According to congressional testimony of members of the American Academy of Pediatrics and the American College of Obstetricians and Gynecologists, nearly fourteen thousand perinatal deaths per year are attributable to smoking by pregnant women. Further, smoking by mothers has been shown to be associated with impaired intellectual and physical development in their children.

Still, if you have always smoked, it may be difficult to stop during pregnancy. If you cannot stop entirely, just cutting down is helpful since the harmful effects of smoking are dose related.

The following tips may help you cut down or quit smoking:

- Cut down on the number of cigarettes you smoke each day. Try to continue to reduce the number of cigarettes a little more each week.

- Cut each cigarette in half and smoke only the half with the filter.

- Choose a brand that is lowest in tar and nicotine.

- Take fewer puffs on each cigarette you smoke.

- Use a water filter, which can be purchased at the drugstore.

- Consider entering a program designed to help you quit. The American Lung Association can help you find one.

If you cut down on your smoking or quit altogether during your pregnancy, try not to resume the habit after having your baby—children of smokers have been shown to have a greater susceptibility to respiratory diseases.

## Marijuana

Marijuana use has been associated with pulmonary cancer. It has been shown to have negative effects on memory and can cause menstrual irregularities.

Studies in animals have shown that the active ingredient in marijuana crosses the placenta and accumulates in the fetus. Effects on the offspring include intra-uterine growth retardation, low birth weight, and changes in secondary sex characteristics. In humans, precipitate labor (which ends with rapid expulsion of the fetus), prolonged labor, low birth weight, prematurity, and a greater risk of fetal distress have been associated with marijuana use.

## Cocaine

Cocaine has profound effects on the mother and her fetus. It causes an increase in maternal heart rate; constriction of the blood vessels of the placenta, allowing less blood to reach the fetus; increased secretion of stress hormones, which cause constriction of uterine blood vessels; and increased uterine contractility.

It has been difficult for researchers to isolate the effects of cocaine since so many users take other drugs as well. However, cocaine use is also thought to be related to a high incidence of spontaneous abortion and to placental abruption. Infants whose mothers used cocaine have a difficult time adjusting to environmental stimuli after birth and may be addicted to the drug.

## Alcohol

Heavy drinking during pregnancy (more than five or six drinks daily) puts the baby at risk for fetal alcohol syndrome. Affected babies are born with physical malformations, including microcephaly (abnormally small head), certain heart defects, and often subsequent mental retardation.

Even moderate (one or two drinks per day) and social (three to four drinks per day) drinking have been associated with problems. Some research points to a higher miscarriage rate among women who drink moderately. Other studies associate this level of drinking with a more frequent occurrence of birth defects and lower birth weights.

No safe level of alcohol consumption has been established yet. As a result, it is probably best to take a cautious approach to alcohol consumption by abstaining or by drinking very little and very infrequently. Probably the best way to handle social situations is to choose a nonalcoholic substitute, such as tomato juice, sparkling water, or fruit juice.

## Other Medications and Drugs

Pregnancy is a time for prudent use of drugs. Since no drug has been proved safe for the unborn child, and some drugs have been proved unsafe, you will want to be cautious about the medications you take. Drugs and medications include any over-the-counter remedies you may buy as well as prescriptions authorized by your doctor. Your doctor can help you to decide when medications are indicated for you during pregnancy.

# Fitness for Expectant Mothers

### Finding the Right Prenatal Program

Being pregnant doesn't mean being fat. It doesn't have to mean being tired all the time, nor does it mean looking dumpy and saggy as a new mother. The way you feel (terrific or fatigued) and the way you look (sleek or bulgy) depend to a great extent on actions you take during pregnancy regarding diet and exercise. By eating a wide variety of wholesome foods and by exercising aerobically on a regular basis, you can maintain or improve your fitness and health during this time of extra demands on your body.

Decide how you want to look and feel after delivery. Then accept the challenge of making necessary changes in eating and exercise. That's the first step. Look at your schedule and make changes to include sensible eating and an exercise program. The two go hand in hand. Just because you're pregnant doesn't mean you're fragile. Give your exercise time top priority. Plan your day around your exercise program, not the other way around.

This section describes a safe and effective fitness program for pregnant women at any level of fitness. The emphasis is on aerobic exercise, with some discussion of the other important components of a complete fitness program—stretching and strengthening exercises.

## Starting an Exercise Program for the First Time

Becoming fit during pregnancy requires safe, regular, sustained, moderate exercise—not embarking on a new sport or doing strenuous workouts. Even if you have never exercised regularly before, you can safely begin a workout program during pregnancy. The safest and most productive activities during pregnancy (especially for the woman exercising for the first time) are swimming and brisk walking. They are best because they can usually be continued until almost the day of delivery, and carry little risk of injury that would prevent further exercising. All you need before beginning is a sound program, appropriate clothing, and a health clearance from your personal physician.

## Continuing Your Current Program

Most obstetricians, midwives, and specialists in sports medicine agree that if you are already regularly engaged in a sport or an exercise program when you become pregnant, you can continue it during pregnancy. Depending on the activity, you may need to modify, slow down, or change activities due to fatigue in early pregnancy or due to added weight and the normal softening of joint ligaments as your pregnancy advances. Your body is your best guide and usually responds with pain or fatigue if an activity becomes inappropriate. Pay attention to these signals. Be especially aware of your lower back, hip joints, and pelvis—they are your most vulnerable parts.

## General Guidelines

- *Exercise regularly.* You can't make up for lost time, and you shouldn't push too hard to catch up. Plan ahead and take this special time for yourself without fail. Make exercise a habit! (Half-life of exercise theory: By allowing more than two and a half days to elapse between exercise sessions for the same muscle group, you lose the benefits of the first exercise session!)

- *Stop if you feel pain.* Modify your exercise program if necessary or substitute other forms of exercise. Check with your physician before resuming your program, but do it right away—don't waste precious time.

- *Finish eating at least one to one and a half hours before working out.* Otherwise, you may experience burping, belching, or abdominal discomfort as a consequence of exercising on a full stomach.

- *Drink water before, during, and after your workout.* Replace the liquids lost through exertion. Without sufficient fluid, your body becomes slow to react and easily fatigued. Drink four to eight ounces frequently, rather than one long drink.

- *Don't diet during pregnancy.* This is very dangerous for your baby. Do, however, eat a nutritious pregnancy diet.

## Cautions

**Every pregnant woman should consult her physician before beginning an exercise program.** It is particularly important that you not begin exercising on your own if:

- You have any type of heart or respiratory condition

- You have diabetes that developed before or during pregnancy

- You have high blood pressure, whether the onset was before pregnancy or occurred as a symptom of toxemia

- You have a history of premature labor

- Your placenta is implanted completely over or near your cervix (placenta previa)

- You have physical impairments or musculoskeletal disease that would prevent exercise even in the nonpregnant state.

Should any of the above conditions apply, consult your physician and follow his or her guidelines. In some instances, a stretching program or a modification of the program suggested here may be appropriate. (Maintaining flexibility should increase comfort.) But again, seek medical guidance first.

## Appropriate Clothing

- Wear loose-fitting, comfortable clothes. Stay cool. Comfort is more important than glamour.

- Wear a good support bra while exercising. In pregnancy (and postpartum, if nursing), your breasts are larger, and the supporting structures may be somewhat relaxed due to hormonal influences. For exercising, an adequate bra (1) provides firm support; (2) limits bouncing; (3) is made of firm, mostly nonelastic, nonchafing, sturdy, nonallergenic materials; and (4) fits well, especially around the edges of the breasts beneath the arms. "Sports bras" that meet all these requirements are available in all large sports and department stores. If your breasts are very large and heavy, wear two bras for extra support and comfort during your workout. Wearing a nursing/maternity bra beneath a sports bra (or vice versa, if that's more comfortable) works very nicely to minimize bouncing and increase comfort.

- Wear good shoes. This is very important! Walking and aerobic dancing (even without hopping, jumping, kicking, and skipping) involve contact with relatively hard surfaces. Proper shoes provide protection, support, cushioning, traction, and flexibility. Ordinary tennis shoes are not adequate. What you need is a good pair of walking shoes or aerobic shoes with adequate arch supports, heel cushioning, and lateral support. These are available from stores specializing in athletic or sports equipment. Describe the type of exercise you will be doing, so the clerk can help you select the most appropriate shoes.

## Guide for Safe and Effective Exercise

For anyone engaged in an exercise program, it is important to know if you are under- or overworking your heart. If you underwork your heart muscle, you won't build stamina or endurance. If you are overworking your heart, you could become short of breath, dizzy, nauseated, or faint.

During pregnancy, it is especially important not to overwork. There are many internal body changes taking place that require oxygen and energy, in addition to the fact that you are growing a whole new person! That is why you should learn how to measure your body's responses to exercise.

One sign of overworking aerobically is shortness of breath. If you are working at just the right pace, you should be able to carry on a normal conversation while exercising (the "talk test"). But to be more accurate, you can learn to use your own pulse to tell you exactly how your body is responding to exercise.

## Taking Your Pulse

Your pulse varies according to your activity level; it is lowest when you are least active. It also varies in response to illness and emotions. Your pulse can tell you about your physical fitness level, too. The more fit you are, the lower your resting pulse rate. Most women have a resting pulse rate of seventy-two to eighty beats per minute (bpm), but this may decrease as their level of fitness improves. During pregnancy, the resting pulse normally varies within the same day and from day to day. As pregnancy advances, the pulse rate usually increases just slightly.

There are many pulse locations you can use, including the ones at your temples, your wrists, and inside your upper arms. Do not use the carotid artery (the pulse at the side of your throat). Pressing this artery often alters the pulse beat, giving an inaccurate reading. Also, if you should accidentally press too hard or "massage" your neck trying to locate the pulse (especially during a workout), you may alter or decrease the blood flow to the brain, making yourself feel faint or dizzy. Never take your pulse with your thumb. There is a pulse in your thumb, and it is easy to confuse that pulse with the one in the artery you are trying to measure.

For practice, try to find the pulse in your wrist right now. To locate it, look on the thumb side, just below the small, round bone on the side. Press firmly with your index and middle fingers. You should feel it beating. If not, get up and move briskly around the room for a couple of minutes and try it again. Practice several times during nonexercise times to become proficient at locating and counting your pulse.

## Pulse Monitoring During Your Workout

Three or four times during your workout, monitor your pulse. If you are attending an aerobic dance or exercise class with an instructor, monitor your own pulse whether or not the instructor has the entire class doing it. You should check your pulse after each aerobic dance or exercise segment, approximately every four minutes. After a while, you will be able to "read your body" and will know when your pulse is at the right level. You will then be able to check your pulse less frequently. But at first, be consistent in checking your pulse often.

Try to keep moving while you check your pulse. It will take practice to become proficient at doing this, but it is very important. Each time you stand still to take your pulse, it drops or changes. At the same time, the blood has a tendency to pool in the lower part of your body, affecting the blood pressure, and you may become dizzy or light-headed. So, keep moving to get an accurate pulse. (Of course, if biking is your aerobic activity, you will have to stop to take your pulse. "No-hands" biking is *not* a good idea! Try jogging in place to keep your pulse rate up.)

The most precise way to count your pulse is to use a digital watch turned face up on the inside of your left wrist. Place the index and middle fingers of your right hand on your left wrist, finding your pulse beat. Keep moving as you begin counting (to yourself) how many times you feel the beat. The first beat you feel is called zero, followed by one, two, three, and so on. For six seconds, count each beat. Then simply place a zero after the number of your count. For example, if you counted to twelve, your pulse is 120 bpm.

## Finding Your Target Heart Rate Zone

Which pulse range is right for you? In order to improve the heart muscle and receive the other benefits of exercise, you must keep your pulse within your individual "target" heart rate zone. This target zone (in pregnancy and until approximately twelve weeks after delivery) is achieved when the heart is beating at between sixty and seventy percent of your safe maximum attainable heart rate (SHR).

A formula is used to determine each person's target zone: 220 (which is considered the highest pulse) minus your age equals your SHR. Multiply that by sixty and seventy percent to get the limits of your target zone. The chart that follows contains target zones for pregnant women of all ages. Use it to determine your own target zone. If you cannot carry on a conversation in your target zone, you should reduce your activity, lowering your pulse to the level at which you are able to converse comfortably.

Use your target zone to help you regulate your activity during exercise. If your pulse is below your target zone, you need to work harder. If it is above your target zone, you are working too hard for your fitness level; you need to slow your activity to bring your pulse down to your target zone.

## Target Heart Rate Zones for Pregnant Women and New Mothers*

| Age | Target Heart Rate Zone (in beats per minute) |
|---|---|
| 15 | 123–140 |
| 20 | 120–140 |
| 21 | 119–139 |
| 22 | 118–138 |
| 23 | 117–137 |
| 24 | 117–137 |
| 25 | 116–136 |
| 26 | 115–135 |
| 27 | 115–135 |
| 28 | 114–134 |
| 29 | 113–133 |
| 30 | 113–133 |
| 31 | 112–132 |
| 32 | 111–131 |
| 33 | 110–130 |
| 34 | 110–130 |
| 35 | 109–129 |
| 36 | 108–128 |
| 37 | 108–128 |
| 38 | 107–127 |
| 39 | 106–126 |
| 40 | 106–126 |
| 41 | 105–125 |
| 42 | 104–124 |

*Target heart rate is calculated at sixty percent to seventy percent of the safe maximum attainable heart rate. In pregnancy, maximum heart rate should never exceed 140 beats per minute.

Stamina and endurance are achieved sooner by working at the lower end of your target zone, not the higher. Therefore, don't try to rush yourself to fitness by overworking, because it doesn't work and could cause harm.

Remember that your target zone is just for you. If you haven't exercised regularly before, you may have to do very little to zoom your pulse up. The more fit you become, the harder you will have to work to get your pulse in the target zone. Do not compare yourself with others; there is no norm to achieve. Each pregnant woman should work at her own individual level.

Memorize the low and high numbers of your target zone. If you are above the high number, you need to slow yourself down—by walking, pedaling your bicycle more slowly, or reducing the vigor of your arm and leg movements. Unless you believe you are going to collapse or faint, do not stop moving or sit down. Keep yourself moving until your pulse drops to your target zone and you are ready to resume exercising.

If at any time during exercise you begin feeling faint, dizzy, light-headed, nauseated, clammy and cold even though you are sweating, or extremely fatigued, stop exercising, but walk around for a while and then have a seat. If you are in a structured class, talk with the instructor before leaving—let her know that you are feeling unwell. She may want to keep an eye on you for a bit, or she may want to help you seek medical assistance. Also, see your physician before resuming exercise. These are warning signs. Listen to your body. There may be a very simple cause or one that is complicated and serious. *Your physician, not your fitness instructor or you, should determine the cause.*

## Aerobic Exercise

What is aerobic exercise? Is it calisthenics? Isometrics? Slimnastics? Working with weights? Sports like racquetball, golf, softball, tennis? No! It is lap swimming, jogging, walking, biking, rowing, dancing, cross-country skiing, and so on. Aerobic exercises differ from other exercises in that they center upon your heart, lungs, and circulatory system (collectively called your cardiopulmonary system), while other forms of exercise concentrate primarily on your muscular system. An activity or exercise is aerobic if it (1) makes your heart work harder than usual over an extended period of time and (2) creates an increased demand for oxygen, (3) making you breathe more deeply and rapidly to meet your body's increased metabolic demand.

### The Benefits of Aerobic Exercise

What can aerobic exercise do for you? Everyone benefits from such exercise because it is indi-

vidualized to each person, whatever the level of fitness, whether pregnant or not. Aerobic exercise during pregnancy has not been widely studied, but a knowledge of maternal and fetal physiology, as well as the few studies that have been done, indicates that aerobic exercise during pregnancy is safe and effective in improving maternal fitness. Among the benefits reported are the following:

- You have more energy. You feel less tired and fatigued.

- Your heart muscle becomes stronger, meaning that it beats fewer times each minute and rests longer between beats.

- The walls of your blood vessels are toned and strengthened, becoming more flexible. This enhances circulation throughout your entire body.

- Your lung capacity increases, opening up unused air sacs. This brings in more oxygen for your blood to distribute to all parts of your body, including the uterus, the placenta, and your baby.

- Your stamina and endurance increase, enabling you to do more without tiring as quickly. Stamina and endurance are especially important during labor and birth. Although fitness does not guarantee a quick, easy, or painless labor, aerobically fit women seem to experience less fatigue during and after labor.

- Recovery after birth is generally quicker for physically fit women than for physically unfit women.

If you are building your fitness level, you must exercise a minimum of three times a week. Four to six times is even better.

## The Aerobic Exercise Session

Each workout or exercise session should consist of three parts: a warm-up period, the aerobic workout, and a cool-down period.

## The Warm-Up

Don't neglect this. No aerobic workout should be started on a "cold" body. Warm-up moves (1) signal your body that more vigorous activity is coming and (2) prevent injury by releasing muscle tension and making the body more flexible. Spend a minimum of five minutes (ten minutes is much better) stretching and limbering up. Stretch just to the point of mild tension (not pain), and then hold the stretch for a slow count of ten. Release and repeat, three times in all. *No bouncing!* It will only make your muscles tighter. Concentrate stretches mainly on the lower body (legs, ankles, hips, knees), but don't completely neglect the upper body (arms, shoulders, neck). If you are lap swimming, walking, biking, or engaging in some other independent activity, spend another five minutes moving slowly, and then gradually move faster and faster toward your target zone. In other words, don't stretch and then try to "burst" into your pulse range.

## The Stretches

*Hold each for ten seconds.*

### Calf Stretch

1.  Face a wall for support. Stand a little distance from the wall and rest your forearms on the wall. Place your forehead on the backs of your hands, and keep your back flat.

2.  Bend one knee and bring it toward the wall. The back leg should be straight and your foot flat, heel pressed into floor. Create an easy feeling of stretch in your calf muscle.

3.  Hold an easy stretch for ten seconds, then increase the stretch feeling just slightly for another ten seconds.

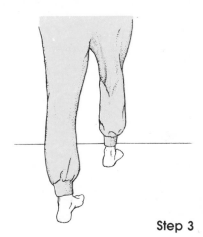

**Step 3**

### Soleus (Deep Calf) and Achilles Tendon Stretch

1.  Start in same position as for the calf stretch.

2.  Lower hips downward as you slightly bend your knees. Be sure to keep your back flat. Your back foot should be slightly toed-in or pointing straight ahead during the stretch. Keep heel pressed down.

*Note: This is good for developing ankle flexibility. The Achilles tendon area needs only a slight feeling of stretch.*

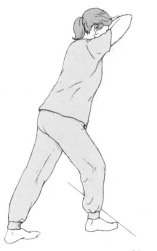

**Step 2**

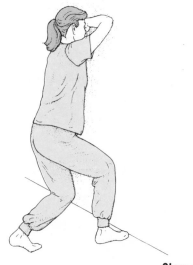

**Step 2**

### Back, Calf, and Hamstring Stretch

1. Sit with one leg bent and the other leg stretched out forward. Straight leg should have back of knee flat on floor.

2. Find an easy stretch. Lean forward from the hips to increase the stretch.

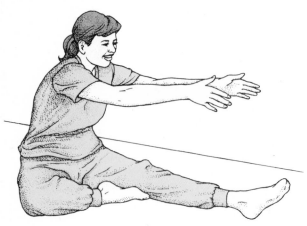

**Step 2**

## The Aerobic Workout

Spend a minimum of twelve minutes with your pulse in your target zone. Be aware that you may need to spend a little longer than twelve minutes

### Walking Program for Expectant Mothers

| Warm-Up Stretch | Walk | Cool-Down Stretch |
|---|---|---|
| 5-10 minutes | 5 minutes slowly<br>15 minutes briskly*<br>5 minutes slowly | 5-10 minutes |

*Remember: Walk with your pulse in your target heart rate zone. Never exercise to exhaustion. End your workout at the point at which you feel you could go on for another ten minutes.

in your activity to meet the twelve-minute requirement. For instance, you may have to bike twenty minutes to actually keep your pulse within your target zone for twelve continuous minutes, or walk briskly for fifteen to twenty minutes to satisfy the twelve-minute minimum. (The accompanying chart shows a recommended walking program.) Recently, the American College of Obstetrics and Gynecology recommended no more than fifteen to twenty minutes of aerobics in your target zone during pregnancy. This amount of time is sufficient, when repeated three times a week, to develop or maintain aerobic fitness. Until you increase your body awareness and know the internal feelings that mean you are in the correct pulse zone, depend on your watch, frequent pulse checks, and the talk test.

## The Cool-Down

Once you stimulate your circulation and complete your twelve-minute workout, slow down your activity gradually, over a five-minute period. Before you actually sit down (or begin strengthening exercises), your pulse should be below your target zone of 110 bpm or lower. Then stretch again for five minutes (ten minutes is even better), and you're done! You will feel warm, full of energy, and virtuous!

## Strengthening Exercises

Strengthening exercises, or calisthenics, can be fun as well as beneficial when done to music. They tone, strengthen, and increase your muscle mass to help you perform better in physical activity and look glowing in pregnancy and sleek after delivery. The exercises that follow will strengthen all muscle groups.

### Cautions

During pregnancy, do not perform an exercise that calls for you to lie on your back for more than one minute. If repetitions are not complete in one minute, by the clock, go to the next exercise and then come back to the previous exercise to complete repetitions.

When a pregnant woman is lying on her back, the uterus (with the weight of the baby) presses on the vena cava, a large blood vessel directly behind the uterus. This pressure decreases blood flow to the lower part of the body and inhibits returning blood flow to the upper body and heart. Blood flow (and therefore oxygen supply) to the pelvic region, where baby growth is in progress, is decreased. Blood pressure drops, while the pulse increases. In early pregnancy, these changes may be slight and barely noticed by the mother. After the fourth month, however, these changes are more pronounced. Even if the mother does not experience symptoms or if the symptoms are not strongly felt, the physical changes still occur, compromising the well-being and physical and mental health of the growing baby.

Symptoms range from a feeling of vague discomfort to shortness of breath, dizziness, anxiety, and even fainting. All symptoms can be relieved (and avoided) by turning on the side, especially the left side, which allows the uterus to roll completely off the vena cava.·

Lying on your back should be avoided during exercise except for one minute, by the clock, to perform abdominal exercises. If you choose not to lie on your back at all, exercise the abdominal muscles by using the Pelvic Rock on All Fours and Sit-Backs exercises. These are not as efficient for strengthening the abdominal muscles but will still allow you to exercise them while avoiding the supine position.

Situations other than exercise may also cause the vena cava to be compressed. Try to sleep on your side at night, and avoid flopping back in chairs and propping yourself up at an angle when sitting on the floor.

Remember, before beginning *any* exercise program, it is important to check with your doctor.

## Strengthening Exercises for Pregnancy and After Delivery

All exercises should be performed at least three times a week, on alternate days, on a firm surface. Perform in order. Be sure to breathe normally during all exercises; don't hold your breath. During abdominal exercises, it may be easier to exhale on exertion, that is, inhale when you are down and exhale briskly as you perform the lift. Remember, don't lie on your back for longer than one minute by the clock. The following exercises work all major muscle groups. Don't skip any!

### Hamstring Lift

*Start with five, increase to twenty.*

1.  Rest on hands and knees, with back flat and abdominal muscles squeezed tightly (do not let abdominal muscles "hang loose").

2.  Extend left leg straight behind with foot flexed (do not point).

3.  Keeping back flat, lift leg up until it is level with back. Weight should be shifted to left arm.

4.  Lower leg. Repeat several times.

5.  Change sides and repeat, shifting weight to right arm.

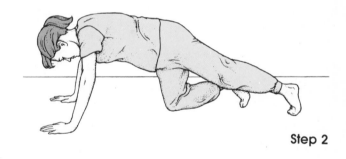

**Step 2**

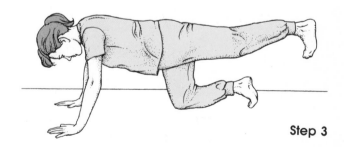

**Step 3**

## Inner Thigh Lift

*Start with five, increase to twenty.*

1. Lie on side with bottom leg straight, inside of leg toward ceiling. Bend top leg with foot resting, flat, in front of bottom leg at the thigh. (Alternatively, top leg may be bent with foot resting *behind* bottom leg.)

2. With foot flexed, lift bottom leg slowly two to three inches (as far as is comfortable).

3. Lower bottom leg slowly to the floor—do not drop it!

4. Repeat several lifts. Be sure to stay on your side, not rolling back on your buttock.

5. Change sides and repeat.

## Outer Thigh Lift

*Start with five, increase to twenty.*

1. Lie on side, head resting on hand, body straight (no flexion of hips). Bottom leg may be bent at a forty-five-degree angle for balance.

2. Slowly lift top leg straight up and slightly back. Hold for a slow count of five, then lower slowly.

3. Repeat several times. Change sides.

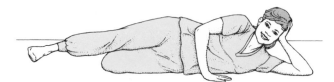

Step 1

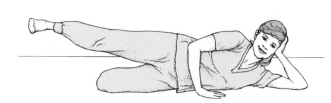

Step 2

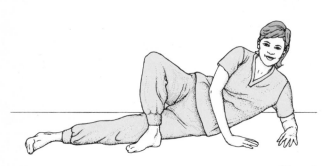

Step 1

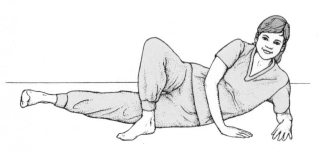

Step 2

## Chest Muscle Exercise

*Start with five to ten, increase to twenty.*

1. Raise elbows to shoulder height, place palms together.

2. Press palms together for a slow count of five.

3. Locking fingers, pull against fingers for a slow count of five. *Do not hold your breath.* (This stage of the exercise actually strengthens muscles in the upper back.)

## Pelvic Rock on All Fours

*Start with five, increase to twenty.*

1. Rest on hands and knees, with back straight and knees comfortably apart.

2. Picture yourself as having a tail. Tuck your "tail" between your legs, rocking your pelvis under and arching your lower back. Hold for a slow count of four.

3. Return to starting position, without allowing your back to sag. Tuck and release slowly; do not jerk. Hold the tucked position for a full count of ten. Squeeze your pelvic floor at the same time for an added benefit.

*Note: Do not allow the lower back to cave in.*

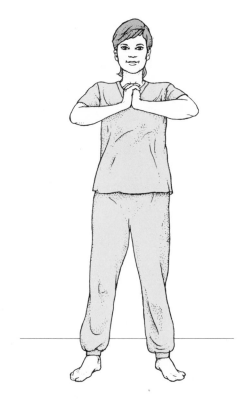

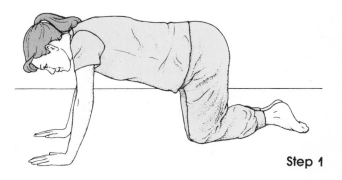

Step 1

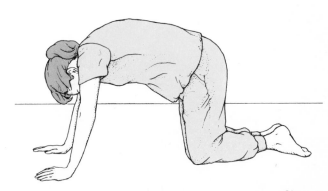

Step 2

### Diagonal Knee and Arm Reach

*Five to ten times.*

1.  Lie flat on back, with knees bent and feet flat.

2.  Flatten lower back to floor, then raise head (straight up toward ceiling, not with chin down on chest), shoulders, right arm, and left knee *all together* slowly.

3.  Lie back slowly. Arms may reach and be crossed on chest or behind head (do not pull on neck!).

4.  Repeat, raising left arm and right knee.

### Plié

*Start with five, increasing gradually to twenty.*

1.  Stand, with feet about two feet apart and toes turned comfortably out.

2.  Slowly bend the knees, keeping back flat. Buttocks should never be lowered past the knees. Knees should be over toes—don't let them roll in.

3.  Rise slowly, concentrating on the leg muscles as you push upward. Heels should remain flat during the entire movement.

*Note: To advance the exercise, stay down for fifteen to thirty seconds, then rise slowly.*

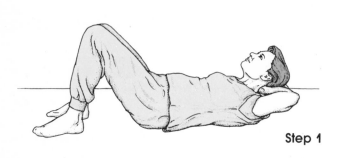

Step 1

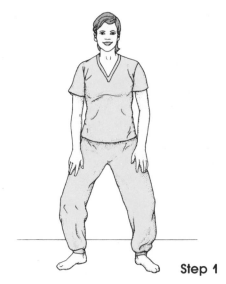

Step 1

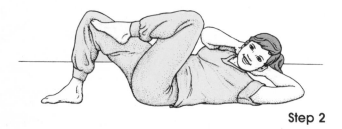

Step 2

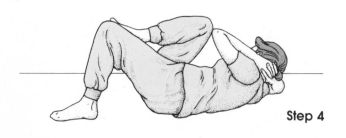

Step 4

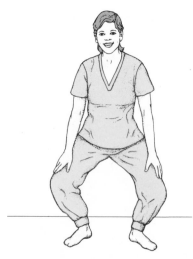

Step 2

## Sit-Back

*Start with five, increase to twenty.*

1.   Sit with soles of feet together and comfortably away from body, arms held parallel to the floor in front of you.

2.   Tuck chin to chest and curl back slowly until you are half to three-quarters of the way down, keeping edges of feet on the floor and back rounded. (Do not attempt this with a straight back!)

3.   Return to sitting position. Exhale as you curl back. (If this is easy to perform, do the exercise with arms crossed over the chest.) Do *not* try to curl back to the floor and up again.

## Curl-Up

*Five to twenty times.*

1.   Lie on back, with knees bent and feet close to buttocks. Press back down. Inhale slowly and deeply.

2.   Exhale slowly; at the same time, lift head and shoulders. Perform slowly and with control (no jerky movements). Head stays in line with spine; do not throw head forward! Relax jaw and neck muscles. The "lift" comes from the shoulders and should be *straight up,* with face toward ceiling.

3.   Slowly return to starting position; inhale as you do so.

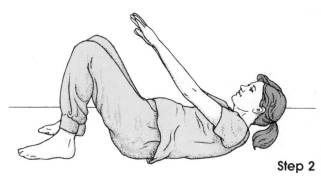

Step 2

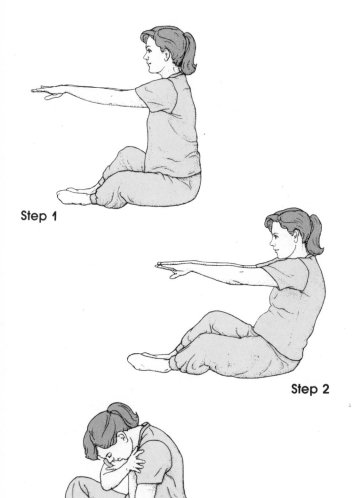

Step 1

Step 2

Step 3

### Pelvic Floor Squeeze (Kegel Exercise)

*Twenty sets per day.*

1.   Sit or stand comfortably (you can do this exercise in most positions). The farther the legs are apart, the more challenging.

2.   Thinking about the vagina and perineum, tighten the pelvic floor as if to lift the internal organs or to stop urination in midstream. Hold as tightly as possible for a slow count of five (be sure to breathe).

3.   Relax completely.

*Note: Because these muscles fatigue easily, repeat in sets of three or four squeezes throughout the day anytime, anywhere. Concentrate on the sensations of tension and lifting, relaxing and lowering within the pelvis.*

## Trunk Roll

*Five to ten times.*

1.  Lie on back, with hips flexed, knees bent, shins parallel to the ceiling, and arms on floor straight out from your sides. Feet may be off floor, as shown, or, alternatively, on the floor.

2.  Keeping shoulders down and knees together, roll legs over to the left, touching left leg on floor.

3.  Roll legs back to the starting point, and then to the right. Make sure knees are not bent too close to the chest.

## Push-Away

*Start with five, increase to twenty.*

1.  Stand, with hands on wall slightly farther apart than shoulder width. Move feet back from wall about two to three feet. Hold arms and body straight, and tuck hips under body.

2.  Lean toward wall, allowing arms to bend. Touch one cheek to the wall.

3.  Push body (still straight) away by straightening arms. *Do not arch your back.* Hands should stay in contact with wall at all times.

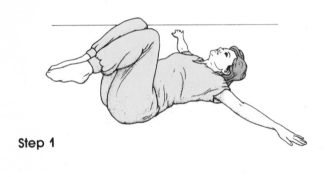

**Step 1**

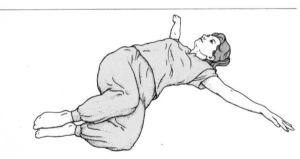

**Step 2**

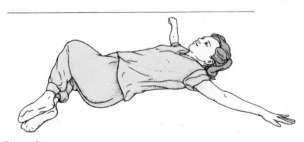

**Step 3**

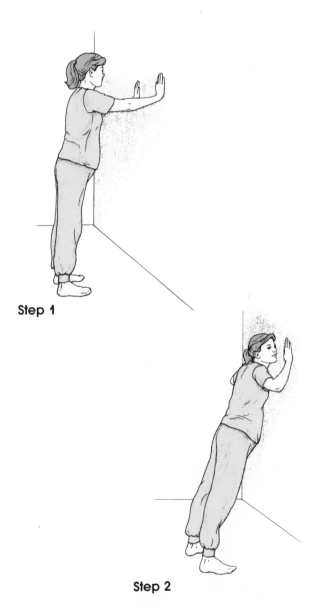

**Step 1**

**Step 2**

## Exercises to Avoid

If you are pregnant, avoid the following exercises and heed precautions until after delivery.

- **Double-leg raises** (any exercises in which both legs are raised or lowered together): This exercise puts too much strain on the lower back and on the ever-thinning abdominal muscles. In fact, double-leg raises are not recommended for anyone, pregnant or not.

- **Full sit-ups:** They can strain the lower back. Also, in pregnancy, a full sit-up may pull on the round ligaments in front of the uterus, causing a sharp, off-to-the-side abdominal or groin pain. Halfway up and halfway back is enough to strengthen abdominals any time.

- **Any exercise that causes swayback** (requires that you arch your back).

- **Jumping, hopping, skipping, and bouncing:** These may cause strain or pain in hip and pelvic joints, especially in late pregnancy. If you are in an instructor-led class for non-pregnant persons, perform these movements with *one foot firmly on the ground.* Don't try to be the perfect example or "Superwoman and pregnant, too"; be sensible and listen to the messages your body sends you.

- **Exercise/dance movements that require good balance and quick moves:** Your center of gravity shifts as the baby grows, and all joints (including knees and ankles) are looser and less stable.

- **Any exercise that requires you to be on your back for a prolonged period of time** (over one minute).

## Choosing an Exercise Class

Above and beyond the physical benefits, there are many emotional and social benefits to be gained from joining an exercise program especially for pregnant women and new mothers. Pregnancy fitness classes build a marvelous sense of camaraderie and support. They help you keep your sense of humor about your rapidly changing body and bolster your commitment to exercise because of the structure and community spirit.

In evaluating a pregnancy fitness program, use the following checklist questions:

- Do the women consult their physicians before enrolling in the exercise class? Do they have to present their physician's consent *in writing* before participating in the first class?

- Are they told that if they have any bleeding, cramping, or other symptoms, they should stop the exercise or activity and consult their physician immediately?

- Do the exercise classes start with a warm-up period consisting of mild to moderate stretching and light exercise?

- Do the exercise classes end with a cool-down period consisting of less strenuous exercises and stretching or relaxation exercises?

- Do the exercises include bouncing? (There is a chance of overstretching the uterine ligaments when there is too much bouncing. Also, it is an incorrect technique for increasing flexibility.)

- Do the exercises stress correct posture and body alignment?

- Do the exercises avoid severe stretching? (Ligaments in pregnancy loosen, and joints are less stable.)

- Are participants encouraged to breathe deeply and not hold their breath during the floor exercises?

- Do the exercises include calf stretches to help prevent and help treat leg cramps?

- Are pelvic floor (Kegel) exercises incorporated into the class exercises?

- Are abdominal strengthening exercises included? (They should not be strenuous.) Are the women told to protect their lower backs during these exercises by doing a pelvic tilt and by using slow, controlled moves? Is there prolonged exercising while lying on the back? (Such a position should be maintained for one minute at the maximum, by the clock; then the position should be changed.)

- Do the classes include aerobic or cardiovascular exercises (twenty minutes at the *maximum*) along with muscle strengthening and stretching? (If not, the class is incomplete.)

- Is the exercise program pulse-monitored? If not, why not?

- Are the women taught correct body mechanics and energy-saving techniques (for example, for lifting, walking, standing, sitting, cleaning, and getting out of bed)?

- Are any exercises done with the women on their hands and knees? (This is an excellent position to relieve back pressure and to increase circulation to both mother and fetus. Abdominal and hip exercises can be done in this position. The abdomen should be kept tight—don't let the baby hang down.)

- Are exercises included to strengthen the pectoral muscles? (This is important to lend support to the breasts, and to aid in lifting the baby later.)

- Does the class include exercises to stretch inner thigh muscles and to limber up the hip joints (which will allow a woman to be more comfortable in the lithotomy position—on the back with the feet up and knees spread wide apart—if it is used during delivery)?

- Are shoulder stretches or relaxation exercises taught? (Most new mothers complain of pain in this area due to constant lifting.)

- What are the teacher's educational qualifications? Did the instructor complete a training program to qualify her to teach exercises? Where? How long was it?

- How long has she been teaching pregnancy fitness classes?

- Who designed the exercise program? Who is responsible for safety?

- What is the cost of the exercise program? How many classes are included in a series?

## Psychological Changes in Parents-to-be

Pregnancy will be an experience full of growth, change, enrichment, and challenge. It is a time when you as a couple will confront your fears and expectations about becoming parents and will begin to determine your own parenting style.

## Mind-Body Interactions in the Mother-to-be

Although there are certain general similarities in all pregnancies, each pregnancy is special. Shifts in your body image, changes in your hormones, and your attitude toward cultural pressures and expectations will all combine to make your pregnancy unique.

Each of the physical landmarks of pregnancy is accompanied by specific psychological issues that will affect your perception of that particular part of your pregnancy. For example, if your pregnancy was planned and wished for, you and your partner will respond with joy and anticipation to the news that you have conceived. If the pregnancy was unexpected, you will initially have mixed feelings about it.

Interactions between your body and your mind will occur throughout your pregnancy. For example, a high level of stress in your life or negative feelings about being pregnant may contribute to some of the nausea that occurs in the first trimester (three months). Conversely, the nausea and vomiting may make you feel less than enthusiastic about your pregnancy. The important thing to remember is that because of this interaction between mind and body during pregnancy, trying to maintain a positive outlook may actually alleviate some physical ills.

## Dreams During Pregnancy

During pregnancy you may find that you are much more vulnerable to certain fears and concerns. For example, pregnant women are often more anxious about the possibility of bodily harm. Things ordinarily taken for granted, such as riding in a car or engaging in sports, may provoke some anxiety. These anxieties may surface in your dreams. Dreams may be realistic representations of your fears, or they may take the form of surrealistic nightmares. Dreaming about your worries is normal and may help you to deal with them during the day. Be reassured that dreams do not represent life as it is—or as it will be once the baby is born.

There is a progression of changing themes in dreams that may occur throughout your pregnancy. Dreams about pregnancy and babies often begin in the first trimester. Uncertainties about your new role as a mother may surface in dreams about not being able to care properly for your baby. Such dreams are normal.

Pregnant women often dream of being trapped, and in many ways this is a direct representation of fears and concerns about the future. Especially if you have worked outside the home, you may be frightened about what having a baby will do to your ability to continue your outside interests.

Many mothers-to-be dream about having a child of one sex or the other. These dreams may reflect your preference for a child of a particular sex, as well as your concerns about your own sexual identity.

Another common theme in dreams is looking for a child or having lost a child. These dreams usually occur toward the end of the pregnancy, when you begin to anticipate the delivery of your child. In reality, a loss *is* about to occur: the loss of the fetus who will become your baby.

Assault is another theme that may occur in your dreams about pregnancy, reflecting your worries that if you were to be assaulted or injured, the consequences might be harmful to your baby, as well as to yourself. Also, as the pregnancy continues and your body enlarges, you may worry that you will not be able to react quickly in a dangerous situation.

Perhaps the most relevant anxiety about assault that a pregnant woman has to deal with is the loss of control over her body. Clearly, you are not in control of your body's changes during pregnancy. Especially for the first-time mother, these assault dreams may reflect your fears about what labor and delivery will be like. Then, too, the assault dreams may reflect your feelings about the "stranger" that is within your body.

Remember, having these frightening dreams is normal and should not worry you. In fact, because of the love you feel for the baby inside you, your concerns about his or her fragility, as reflected in your dreams, are not at all unusual.

## Psychological Changes in the First Trimester

Numerous psychological changes occur once you are aware that you are pregnant. Although

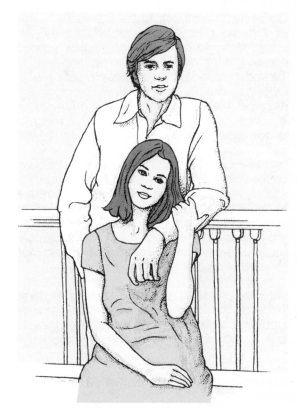

*Forthcoming parenthood brings psychological changes in both mother and father.*

you may not look any different to other people for weeks to come, you start to feel a number of changes beginning. A rapidly changing emotional state is one of them. Your usual emotional highs and lows will be magnified at this time, and if this is your first pregnancy, these feelings may confuse you. Things that normally would not bother you provoke you to tears or cause you to become depressed or angry, even at those you care about.

These sudden emotional swings are more pronounced in some women than in others. This depends on your personality structure, the kind of stress that you are experiencing, and the emotional support that you are receiving, as well as hormonal changes in your body.

Since the risk of miscarriage approaches twenty percent in the first trimester, you may worry about whether the pregnancy will continue. If you have had a previous miscarriage, this will be a time of heightened stress and anxiety.

Talking to a friend or a counselor might be very helpful at this time, especially if the feelings of anxiety and tension appear to be significantly interfering with your day-to-day activities. Also, it is important to try to get as much rest as you can during the first trimester because rest will help you feel better. If there is a lot of stress in your life, you may want to modify it, if possible, or attempt to learn some relaxation techniques to help you cope with it. Meditation, yoga, and relaxing fantasies can help.

Your feelings about your own sexuality and your desire for sexual activity may change during this time. Many women report a diminished desire for sex in the first trimester because of fatigue, nausea, and sore breasts. Sexual desire usually returns to pre-existing levels or may even increase in the second trimester, only to diminish again in the third trimester as one's size increases.

A virtually universal fear is concern about injuring the fetus during intercourse. In most instances, intercourse is safe throughout the pregnancy, but make sure that you discuss it with your doctor.

## Psychological Changes in the Second Trimester

During the second trimester (months four through six), a sense of general well-being develops. The fear of miscarriage has usually disappeared, and the physical discomforts of the first trimester have diminished.

The most overwhelming event during the second trimester occurs at the time of fetal movement. In first-time mothers this generally occurs at about twenty weeks. It can occur a little bit earlier if this is a second or subsequent child. Psychologically, you may begin to feel an increased dependency toward your partner. You have more needs than usual, and you may worry about whether your partner will be available, interested, and able to support you during this time of change.

During the second trimester, both vaginal lubrication and blood flow to the pelvic region are increased. These changes, plus the diminishing of the nausea and breast sensitivity of the first trimester, may increase your desire to have sex with your partner. You may wonder if he still considers you attractive. Some women and men, particularly in this weight-conscious society, associate weight gain with unattractiveness. Talking to each other about this should help alleviate many of your fears and misconceptions, so that you and your partner

can enjoy a healthy sex life during your second trimester.

## Psychological Changes in the Third Trimester

The third trimester is the time of anticipation. Soon the nine months will come to an end, and your baby will be born. First-time mothers usually have increased anxiety and concern about labor and the delivery. Prepared childbirth classes, usually begun in the seventh or eighth month of pregnancy, are very helpful in educating parents-to-be about what they can expect.

Usually by the time the third trimester has arrived, any ambivalent feelings about the pregnancy have been resolved. During this time, you may feel very special. If you have had difficulty with infertility, the pregnancy may take on more than the usual significance.

During the third trimester, the baby begins to take on an identity of his or her own. This is when a nursery is often set up, and the parents-to-be begin to decide about names for their child.

Some people treat a pregnant woman in a deferential way. They may offer her a chair in a crowded room or a seat on a crowded bus. However, this deferential treatment has some negative aspects as well. If you are still working outside the home, you may be concerned about how others see you and may worry about whether you are competent to continue functioning in your professional capacity. Most women, unless there are medical complications, can work until their delivery date. Other women find that they want some transition time away from their employment before their child is born.

Whether or not you work until your due date is strictly a decision to be made by you, your partner, and your physician. There are no right or wrong answers to this question. What is important is that you make a choice based upon your own needs. Many first-time mothers report that their co-workers become increasingly anxious as the delivery date approaches, and you may find yourself needing to reassure co-workers that you are feeling fine. Talking with a colleague who has been through a pregnancy and continued working can be particularly helpful. She may be able to share with you what was helpful in dealing with her work situation.

How you feel about the physical limitations of the third trimester will be a reflection of your concerns and feelings about impending motherhood. First-time mothers have a great deal of anxiety about whether they will know when labor will start. In women who have had previous children, Braxton Hicks contractions may be so strong that they also may not know when real labor has started.

During this time, you may need extra attention from your partner, your family, and your friends. You may need reassurance regarding your physical appearance, especially if your sex drive has diminished again, as well as reassurance regarding your ability to be a good parent.

## Psychological Changes in the Father-to-be

As a father-to-be, you may also undergo a psychological process during a pregnancy. Although there is no physiologic basis for this, it is nevertheless very real and to some degree predictable. A father-to-be, particularly in the third trimester, may feel a need for a creative outlet. You may want to paint or decorate the nursery, make a cradle, or begin a garden as a way of becoming involved in the forthcoming birth.

Men, as well as women, bring to a pregnancy their own emotional "baggage," as well as the echoes of their childhood fantasies about the mechanics and significance of pregnancy, birth, and parenthood. How the father-to-be perceived his own parents can directly affect his feelings about becoming a parent himself. For some men, being able to father a child may also create a sense of heightened self-esteem regarding their masculinity. Conversely, if there were previous losses or a history of infertility, the father-to-be may see the creation of life as a fragile phenomenon.

Impending fatherhood also seems to bring with it all the memories and emotions of a man's childhood relationship with his father. In some ways, becoming a father means giving up the idea of being a son. It also means reconciling the experience that one had as a child with being a father. It seems that these feelings are stronger during the pregnancy than during the months following the birth of the child.

During most men's childhoods, there was little emphasis on learning fathering functions, except perhaps for the provider role. Television and cartoons from the 1950's and early 1960's portrayed fathers as helpless and inadequate in handling a young child. Women were seen as having the primary duty of raising their children.

For fathers-to-be, there is no internal reality—no physical changes to feel. You must rely on your partner's reports about her feelings in experiencing the pregnancy. Perhaps not until fetal movement is obvious will you perceive the fetus as a growing child, and often this does not occur until the seventh month of gestation. Participating in prenatal visits may be a way to allow greater awareness of the reality of the pregnancy. If an ultrasound study is indicated, viewing the ultrasound scans can be an invaluable experience because on the screen you will have visual confirmation of the existence of your baby.

Pregnancy can elicit feelings even in a man who has had previous children. It provides an opportunity to think about the kind of father he has already been to the children that he has, as well as the increasing responsibility he will be facing. If the father-to-be is proud of his prior fathering experience, and if the new child is wanted, he may feel extremely happy about the new pregnancy.

It is still rare for men to admit openly that they have concerns, fears, and perhaps ambivalent feelings about their partners' pregnancies, yet these feelings are nearly universal. Studies indicate that more than one out of ten men will have psychogenic (having an emotional or psychological origin) physical symptoms in relation to a pregnancy. These symptoms tend to appear by the beginning of the second trimester of the pregnancy. There may also be increased feelings of anxiety and depression.

The relationship between you and your partner may also undergo profound changes from your perspective. Previously, you may have had a sense of predictability in your partner's reactions, but her reactions may change significantly during the pregnancy. You may also have significant feelings about the changes in her bodily proportions, as well as her shifting sexuality. While you are wrestling with feelings about the added responsibilities of fatherhood, you may have to simultaneously "mother" your wife. This is particularly true in our culture, where the extended family is often not readily available to provide support.

The father-to-be's tasks during the first trimester include both acceptance of the pregnancy and provision of some emotional support for his wife. Many men are ecstatic about being prospective fathers, but some may be frightened by this as well. The mother-to-be plays a role in shaping her partner's attitude and initial reaction, but mutual support, open lines of communication, and reassurance are the responsibilities of both partners.

By the end of the first trimester, the obligations of becoming a father may begin to weigh on you. You may reevaluate your job, salary, and savings. It is important for you and your partner to begin talking with each other about your fantasies, anxieties, and expectations at this time.

During the second trimester, you will be able to feel the baby moving. Concerns about sexual activity may begin during this time, and obtaining reassurance from the doctor can be very important. On the other hand, a man may not be sexually attracted to a woman whose body seems to be so different from that of the woman he married. It is critical that you and your partner talk about your sex life if you are having problems adjusting to the pregnancy.

During the third trimester, many couples experience a renewal of their relationship in a romantic bond that may have been missing during the previous few months. However, the woman's increasing size may present an obstacle to comfortable sexual activity. A physician or childbirth educator may be able to offer some suggestions for coping with this temporary problem.

If you participate in a prepared childbirth class, you may have some heightened concerns about your ability to coach during labor. Again, talking with men who have previously had this experience can be valuable. Often, childbirth education classes provide this opportunity.

Just as it was assumed in the 1950's that no father could adequately participate in the labor and delivery experience, it is now assumed that most fathers should. If you, however, feel that you will not be able to participate in the labor and delivery, this should be discussed and resolved prior to the event. Further, you should not feel that your decision is in any way wrong.

## Expectations and Realities

For many expectant first-time parents, the impending birth of their baby makes them acutely aware that they will never be simply a couple again, but that they are about to become a family. Other parents-to-be try to convince themselves that life will be unchanged after their child is born. This is not realistic. The birth of a child will bring with it multiple changes, both in the couple's relationship and in the reality of their activities and what they can plan, at least on a temporary basis. It is critical that a couple discuss these issues before their child is born. A couple who have convinced themselves that nothing will change will be in for a massive disappointment and many frustrations. The idea that they are in control of so profound an experience will be a disappointing fantasy once their baby is brought home from the hospital. On the other hand, the couple who have realistic expectations about the pregnancy and life with their newborn will enjoy the changes in their relationship as they become a family. See Chapter 12 for a helpful list of support groups for parents and parents-to-be.

## Infertility

About one of every five couples who want to conceive a child are unable to do so. During the last ten years or so, medical science has made tremendous progress in diagnosing and treating causes of infertility and thus has given new hope to childless couples. Improved testing procedures, new drugs that stimulate ovulation, and surgical techniques that can correct female and male structural problems and sometimes successfully reverse sterilization procedures have enabled many couples to become parents.

Infertility is defined as a couple's failure to conceive a child after one year of regular sexual intercourse without birth control. In about forty percent of all cases of infertility, the problem lies with the man; in about sixty percent, it lies with the woman or with both partners.

Infertility is not sterility. The term infertility implies that the condition can be treated and reversed; the term sterility is applied to a permanent, irreversible inability to have children.

### Causes of Male Infertility

One of the major causes of male infertility is a low sperm count. The sperm count is determined by measuring the number of active sperm present in a milliliter (less than one-half teaspoon) of semen (the fluid ejected from the penis during intercourse). An average sperm count is ninety million sperm per milliliter; a count of forty to sixty million is thought to be necessary for conception. If a man's sperm count is less than twenty million, it is highly unlikely that he will be able to father a child (although since only one sperm is needed to fertilize an egg, it is still possible).

A low sperm count can be caused by low levels of testosterone, the male sex hormone; by exposure to chemicals, pesticides, or radiation; by very frequent sexual intercourse, which depletes the sperm supply too quickly; and by heat (which slows sperm production) generated by wearing tight underwear or pants, sitting for long periods in hot cars or trucks, or working near ovens and kilns. Also, a man's fertility declines after the age of forty, although men can remain fertile into old age.

Infertility can also result if sperm cannot propel themselves through the female reproductive tract to reach the egg, or if sperm are irregularly shaped (only sperm with oval heads can fertilize an egg).

In addition to problems with the sperm themselves, male infertility can be caused by any obstruction in the tubes that convey the sperm from the testes to the penis. Infertility may also be caused by varicose veins in the scrotum (the pouch containing the testes), perhaps because the increased blood flow in these swollen veins brings extra heat to the area, or by a local infection or injury. Such infertility problems may often be reversed when the underlying condition is corrected.

Surgical removal of part of the prostate gland, as well as the use of certain drugs for high blood pressure, can lead to retrograde ejaculation (a disorder in which the semen is passed backward into the bladder, to exit with the urine, rather than out through the penis during ejaculation).

## Causes of Female Infertility

A woman may be infertile because of a variety of conditions. Age is one factor: recent research has shown that a woman's fertility decreases significantly between the ages of thirty-one and thirty-five and continues to decline thereafter until menopause, when it ceases. An imbalance of the female hormones estrogen and progesterone or of other hormones secreted from the pituitary or

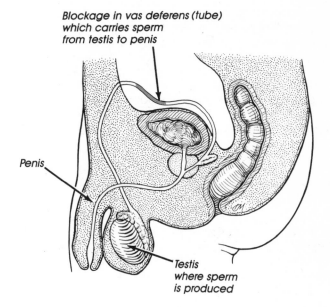

*Blockage in vas deferens (tube) which carries sperm from testis to penis*

*Penis*

*Testis where sperm is produced*

*Male infertility can be caused by a blockage anywhere in the tubes that convey sperm from the testes to the penis.*

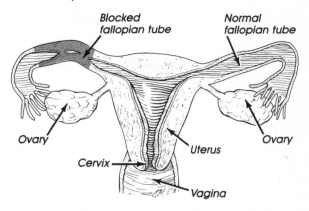

*Blocked fallopian tube*

*Normal fallopian tube*

*Ovary*

*Uterus*

*Ovary*

*Cervix*

*Vagina*

*Female infertility can be caused by an obstruction in the fallopian tube through which the egg passes from the ovary to the uterus and in which the sperm and egg are united at conception.*

thyroid glands can interfere with the reproductive cycle. It may also be that she is not ovulating (releasing an egg each month); this is true in about twenty-five percent of all infertility cases.

Structural problems are often the cause of infertility. The fallopian tubes (through which the egg travels on its way from the ovary to the uterus) may be obstructed, often as a result of pelvic inflammatory disease, which inflames the tubes and causes the formation of scar tissue. *Endometriosis* (displacement of tissue from the lining of the uterus to outside the uterus) may also cause the formation of scar tissue that blocks the fallopian tubes. A weakness in the cervix (the neck of the uterus), sometimes resulting from a previous abortion or other surgery, may render it unfit to hold the weight of a pregnancy. A "hostile" cervix (one that creates an environment that in some way prevents sperm from surviving) may also be the cause of infertility.

## Symptoms

The major "symptom" of infertility is the failure to conceive a child after regular sexual intercourse without birth control for a year. Whether there are other indications depends on the cause of the infertility.

## Diagnosis

A couple who are experiencing difficulty in conceiving will most likely be referred to an obstetrician/gynecologist or a urologist who specializes in infertility. Diagnosis of the reason for the infertility problem will usually begin with physical examinations and complete medical and sexual (and, in the woman's case, menstrual) histories of both partners.

A fresh sample of the man's semen will be examined under a microscope to determine the quantity and quality of the sperm. This will provide a sperm count and will also determine whether the sperm are adequately mobile and have oval heads, both of which characteristics are necessary for conception to occur.

To determine whether ovulation is taking place, the woman's basal body temperature (the body temperature upon awakening, before eating or drinking) will be taken every morning for several months. If the temperature rises by six-tenths of a degree to one degree for a few days in the middle of the menstrual cycle, ovulation is probably taking place. An endometrial biopsy (in which a sample of the lining of the uterus is obtained) can also indicate whether ovulation is occurring.

Obstruction of the fallopian tubes can be diagnosed by injecting a dye into the reproductive tract and then performing an x-ray study. Another test consists of injecting carbon dioxide gas into the fallopian tubes and waiting for the patient to feel discomfort in the upper body, which indicates that the gas is passing through the fallopian tubes and that there are no obstructions.

A weakness in the cervix can be diagnosed through a physical examination and an x-ray study. A hostile cervix can be identified by a microscopic examination of the mucus in the cervix shortly after sexual intercourse to determine the rate of sperm survival. Endometriosis is diagnosed by inserting into the woman's abdomen a small, lighted instrument (a *laparoscope*), through which the doctor can actually see the uterus, fallopian tubes, ovaries, and any displaced endometrial tissue that may be causing the infertility.

Hormonal imbalances in both men and women may be diagnosed with blood tests.

## Treatment

Treatment for a low sperm count caused by a testosterone deficiency usually consists of hormonal therapy to increase testosterone levels. If the low sperm count is due to exposure to chemicals, radiation, or excess heat, the causative situation needs to be corrected or avoided. If the sperm count is low for some unknown reason, there may be little that can be done.

If male infertility is caused by varicose veins, surgery may be necessary. If an obstruction exists somewhere in the tubes leading to and through the penis, microsurgery to open the blockage may correct the problem.

In women, failure to ovulate is often treated with a fertility drug called *clomiphene*, which stimulates the production of hormones that regulate ovulation. About sixty percent of women treated with this drug become pregnant, and the chances of multiple births are very low. A stronger drug, which is a combination of certain pituitary gland hormones, may also be prescribed, but it carries a greater risk of multiple births.

A hostile cervix may be treated with the female hormone estrogen, which stimulates the increased production of the mucus necessary to transport the sperm. Sometimes sperm can be placed directly into the uterus, bypassing the cervix completely.

Endometriosis may be treated by the surgical removal of displaced tissue and the scar tissue that has formed around it. Hormonal imbalances may be corrected with hormone therapy.

Obstruction of the fallopian tubes may necessitate microsurgery to open the blockage or a new procedure in which an egg is removed and replaced beyond the point of the obstruction, where it may be fertilized normally.

Test-tube, or *in vitro*, fertilization is a relatively new technique in which an egg is removed from the woman's ovary and is then placed in a test tube or special sterile dish containing the husband's sperm. Once the egg has been fertilized, it is then placed into the woman's uterus, where it will continue to grow. This technique is used primarily in women whose blocked fallopian tubes cannot be opened by surgery.

Although recent advances in treating infertility have led to greater and greater success, about fifteen percent of all female infertility problems and about ten percent of all male infertility problems remain undiagnosed and therefore untreatable.

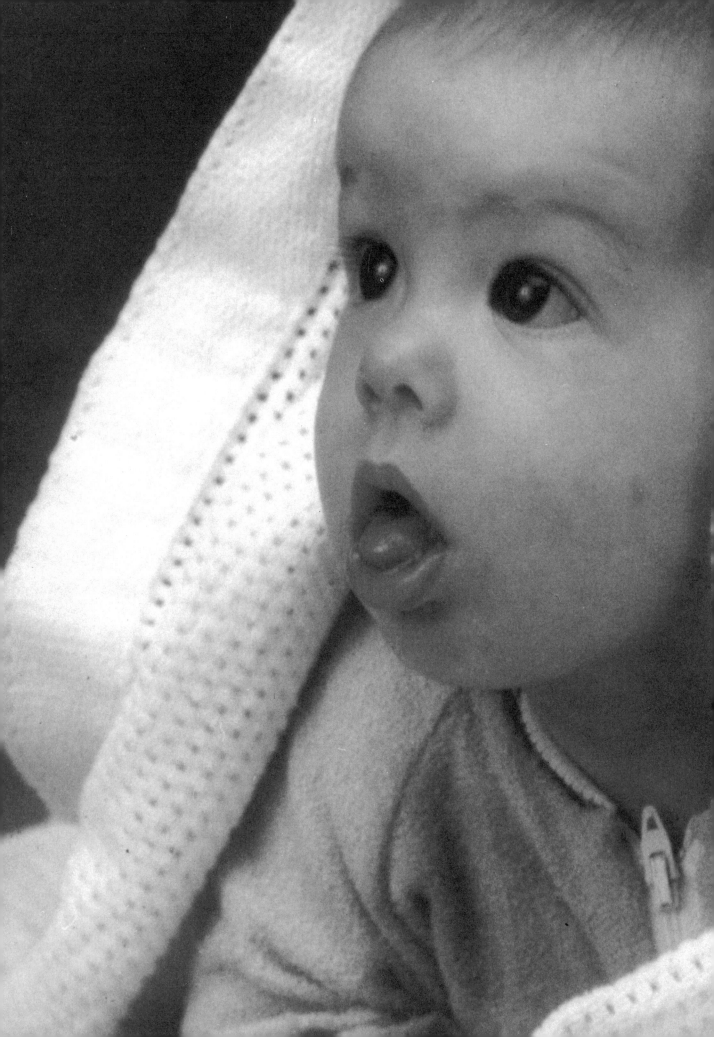

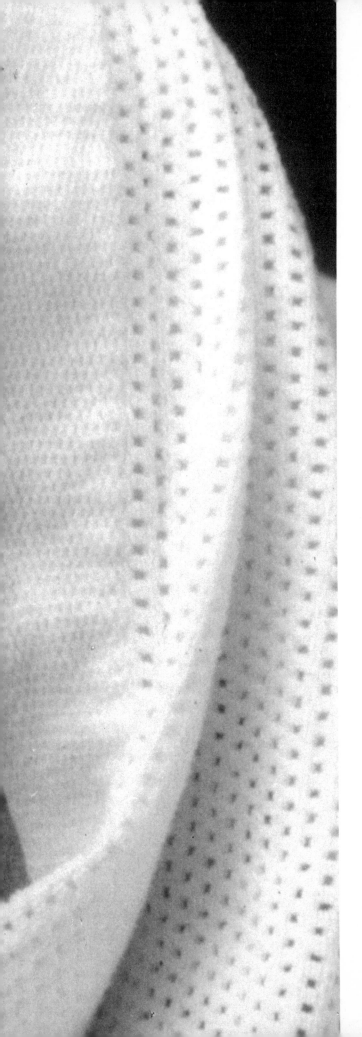

# Chapter 3:
# Birthing
# Alternatives

### Recent History

Our attitudes toward pregnancy and childbirth form over a lifetime, shaped by the values and beliefs of our families and our culture. The way a baby is born reflects not only personal and family beliefs, but also the prevailing cultural attitudes.

Since the turn of the century, the ways of birth have undergone continuous change, as has society itself. When you talk to your mother and grandmother about childbearing beliefs and practices when they were having children, they probably will not tell you it was wonderful "in the good old days." Most people believe that childbirth today is much better managed than it was one or two generations ago.

In looking back, we see that until the mid-1930's, childbirth was truly dangerous. High percentages of women and their infants died during or soon after childbirth. Determined to correct this persistent problem, organized medicine took many steps to lower mortality rates. A new medical specialty, obstetrics, was founded, and an aggressive effort was made to eliminate risky practices (for example, lack of cleanliness and infection control, and overuse of drugs to speed up labor and obliterate pain) and to improve the training of physicians. Prenatal care also gained recognition for its benefits in preventing death. Childbirth moved from home to hospital, with the promise of more efficient and controlled conditions for birth.

With these efforts, along with general improvements in public health (for example, improved working conditions, public sanitation, family nutrition, and better control of some chronic illnesses), came a reduction in the danger of death in childbirth.

The 1940's brought such advances as antibiotics and blood banks, as well as improvements in surgical techniques and anesthesia, which further increased the safety of childbirth.

But by the 1950's, routine maternity care, originally designed to improve safety, had become almost too rigid. For example, the fear of infection, a major killer of mothers and babies, led to such practices as taking away all a woman's personal belongings when she entered the hospital; shaving all her pubic hair; administering large, uncomfortable enemas; prohibiting fathers and other loved ones from entering the maternity area; keeping babies in nurseries, away from their mothers; and handling babies as little as possible. Bottle-feeding was believed more sanitary and superior in almost every way to breast-feeding.

In addition, heavy use of pain medications often took away mothers' ability to control their behavior and to understand and remember labor. They often remained drugged and sleepy for hours or days after birth.

In response to these hospital routines, women protested that such practices were not necessary or beneficial; and they began seeking other, more satisfying ways to give birth. Fortunately, concerned and enlightened professionals joined them in their quest.

Thus began the natural childbirth movement and the movement toward family-centered maternity care. The 1960's was a time when national and international organizations were founded to make these changes. Women and men wrote and read books describing more humane, satisfying ways to give birth. Mothers attended childbirth classes, involved their loved ones in their support and care, breast-fed their babies, and spent more time while in the hospital caring for their babies.

These improvements in care and in safety have continued until the present. As the individuality of each woman was recognized, so was the uniqueness of each labor. It became clear that not all women need or want the same kind of care.

The 1970's saw the re-emergence of the midwife as a popular and trusted care-giver for healthy women wanting more participation in their own care, more emphasis on prevention of problems, and more recognition of their emotional needs. This was also the time when alternative settings for birth—at home or in a birthing center—surged in popularity.

Hospitals also joined the ranks, offering more flexible, family-centered care and more comfortable, home-like rooms for birth. The role of the physician changed from being in complete control of the birth to being more sensitive and responsive to each woman's needs and wishes.

All this is to say that today there are many different approaches to maternity care. There is no single correct way. In this chapter we will describe and discuss many of these choices to help you decide what kind of care you think will be best for yourself during your pregnancy and birth.

## Informed Consent

There is one concept that you should understand because it is an important principle underlying health care in the United States and Canada today. The legal concept of *informed consent* designates the patient as the decision-maker in medical care.

What is informed consent? It means simply that a patient understands and agrees to any treatment or procedure that is done for medical purposes. Her care-giver is legally responsible for giving her full information about any procedure before she consents to it. This is because there are often risks as well as benefits associated with medical treatments, and the patient (who has the greatest stake in the decision) has the right and responsibility to decide whether the risks are worth taking.

The principles underlying informed consent are really the features of any good relationship between patient and physician. Discussion, understanding, and agreement are the hallmarks of optimal care. Many of us, however, feel we do not know enough to have an intelligent discussion with our care-givers, and are a little insecure trying to do it. There is no need to feel that way, however, and the following general guidelines for discussion may give you more confidence in discussing your care.

- If your care-giver (doctor or midwife) suggests a test, a treatment, or a procedure, the first thing you should know is why.

- Is it because you have or may have a problem? If so, what is the problem and why does it need to be detected or treated? How likely is it that you have the problem—one chance in ten? in a hundred? in a thousand?

Is it a routine procedure or test that your care-giver always uses? Why?

- Then you want to know about the procedure itself. What is it, how is it done, and what does it cost?

- What are the benefits and advantages of the test or procedure and how will the results influence your care-giver's management? In other words, what will happen next if a test result is positive or a procedure or treatment is done?

- What are the risks and disadvantages of the test, procedure, or treatment? How reliable or successful is it? Is it painful? What problems can it cause and how often?

- What are the alternatives to the suggested test, procedure, or treatment (including doing nothing)? The risks and benefits and the advantages and disadvantages of the alternatives should be discussed also.

When you have discussed these issues, then you can make an informed decision.

All this may seem very complex and time-consuming. It occasionally is, especially if it is a major procedure or if you have a serious condition. Usually, however, this kind of discussion is fairly straightforward and not too time-consuming, especially when care-givers are in the habit of informing their patients or clients as they go along, discussing what they are doing and why.

Of course, there are situations when it is not possible to become fully informed. If a mother is in an emergency situation, or if she is unable to comprehend the facts, due to either medication or illness, then a family member is consulted for consent, or the care-giver simply does the procedure because of the need for speed.

The concept of informed consent is based on the principle that you have not only the right but the responsibility to make decisions regarding your care. This is not to say that you have to make these decisions all by yourself. Besides asking your care-giver what he or she thinks ought to be done, consult friends, family, consumer groups, childbirth educators, or other care-givers for help. This book and others will provide much background information to help you ask the right questions and gain the information that you need to make informed decisions.

## Choosing a Doctor or Midwife

When you become pregnant or suspect that you are, your first decision will be what care-giver to go to. (The word *care-giver* refers to a person—physician or midwife—who cares for pregnant and laboring women.) This decision is more important than most people realize. Care-givers may differ vastly in their philosophies and beliefs about pregnancy and birth and in their level of skill. This section provides a description of the specialists who provide maternity care and the types of care they offer. You will also find a list of questions to ask as a way to help you decide if a care-giver will be right for you.

### Physicians

Medical doctors (those with a Doctor of Medicine, or M.D., degree) provide most of the maternity care in North America. All medical doctors have completed college and medical school; most have further residency training. Those who care for pregnant women specialize in either perinatology, obstetrics and gynecology, or family medicine.

Obstetrician-gynecologists provide most of the maternity care in the United States, while in Canada it is the general practitioners and family physicians. In order to become a specialist in obstetrics, a physician has to pass a board certification examination administered by the American College of Obstetricians and Gynecologists or the Royal College of Obstetricians and Gynaecologists in Canada. (See Chapter 2 for information on choosing an obstetrician.)

The most highly specialized obstetrician is the perinatologist. Beyond medical school and obstetrics residency, the perinatologist takes further training in the care of high-risk pregnant women: those who have underlying illnesses, such as diabetes, heart disease, and high blood pressure, and those who have complications during their pregnancies or who had complications with previous pregnancies. Perinatologists tend to practice in large cities. Most of their patients are referred to them with complications requiring not only their special expertise but also the facilities of a large hospital with all the latest technology.

Family physicians care for pregnant women as well as other family members, from infancy through old age. They tend to refer difficult maternity cases to obstetricians or perinatologists. While the family physician is the practitioner who provides most of the maternity care in Canada, the number of family physicians in the United States who provide maternity care is relatively small and seems to be decreasing. People who choose family physicians for their maternity care appreciate the fact that the physician can take care of them throughout pregnancy and birth and then continue to care for the baby and family members.

Osteopathic physicians (those with a Doctor of Osteopathy, or D.O., degree) also provide maternity care and care for the entire family. Osteopaths differ little from medical doctors in training and practice, and have about the same legal scope of practice.

## Midwives

The other large category of care-giver is the midwife. In many countries of the world, midwives are the primary care-givers for pregnant and laboring women. In North America, their place is not as well established. All states have provisions for the legal practice of midwifery. In Canada, most provinces have active midwifery promotion groups who have made significant efforts in establishing midwifery as a legal form of maternity care.

The emphasis of the midwife's training is that birth is a normal physiologic event. They learn methods for supporting and promoting women's physical and emotional health to optimize the reproductive process. The care they give consists of thorough physical assessment and prevention of complications through education in self-care, emotional support, and nurturing of the woman throughout her pregnancy and labor. Midwives do not care for women with complications of pregnancy, underlying illnesses, or other high-risk conditions. Should any of these problems arise, a midwife will refer the woman to an obstetrician.

Within the broad category of midwife, there are several subcategories. In the United States, certified nurse-midwives are the most numerous. They are registered nurses who have taken an additional one or two years of training in midwifery. Many receive master's degrees when they complete their nurse-midwifery training. They usually practice in close cooperation with physicians in hospitals, birthing centers, and the home setting. Nurse-midwives are certified after passing an examination administered by the American College of Nurse-Midwives.

In some states, other types of midwives are recognized and are licensed to provide maternity care. Licensed midwives practice in at least seven states. They receive training that is more comparable with that in midwifery training programs in Europe. They are called direct-entry midwives, and do not necessarily possess a background in nursing. They usually have received some college education followed by a two- to three-year program in midwifery training. At present, most licensed midwives practice outside the hospital, providing care for home births and birthing-center births. Their orientation and pattern of care are similar to those of nurse-midwives.

In addition, lay midwives, sometimes called empirical midwives, practice in a number of states. Most of them have received informal training—apprenticeship to an experienced midwife, participation in short courses or study groups, or extensive independent study. Their qualifications, experience, and standards of care vary; some practice within the law, and others practice without legal sanction. Lay midwives emphasize the spiritual aspects of birth, as well as the physiologic and psychosocial.

## Questions to Ask

With all the choices available, how are you going to decide what kind of care and what person will be best for you? Following are some questions you can ask to help determine whether the care-giver you are considering provides the kind of care you need or want. Begin by "shopping" over the phone and talking with the office nurse. You might ask about the background and training of the care-giver, how long he or she has been in practice, in which hospitals he or she has privileges, and the cost of care. If the person you are considering provides home birth or birthing-center care, ask about backup arrangements—which hospital and physician are used if transfer or consultation becomes necessary. If the care-giver is involved in a group practice, find out how likely it is that your own care-giver will see you during your prenatal appointments and be present for your birth. In some group practices, you meet all members of the group; in others, you see only one, even though the others may attend your birth. Some groups are so large that the chances of a woman's having her own care-giver during the birth are really quite small. If you do not like that, and there are no other overriding reasons for choosing such a group, you might decide to look for a smaller group or an individual practitioner.

Other questions for the office nurse concern the prenatal appointments themselves. How much time is scheduled for each prenatal appointment? Who sees you if your birth attendant is called away during office hours? Sometimes a colleague sees you; sometimes the office nurse sees you. In both those instances, the substitute care-giver may not be willing or able to answer questions about policies, philosophies, and usual practices. Sometimes, in a busy practice, a woman comes in several times without seeing her own care-giver. This can be very frustrating, especially if her partner has arranged time off from work in order to meet the care-giver, or if she has questions that only the care-giver can answer.

Ask whether the care-giver encourages natural or prepared childbirth, if that is a desire of yours. Also ask if your partner is welcome to attend prenatal appointments with you.

If your phone conversation with the office nurse gives you a positive impression, make an appointment with the care-giver. (You do pay for these appointments.) Plan to use this appointment as an interview rather than a first prenatal visit, which includes an extensive physical exam and many costly laboratory tests. Make it clear when setting up the appointment that you are in the process of choosing a care-giver, and would like the opportunity to meet and ask a few questions of this person. The charge for such an appointment is usually less than an initial prenatal appointment.

During such an initial interview, ask the care-giver questions about topics important to you. You might want to know how he or she feels about a birth plan prepared by you. (Birth plans will be discussed later in this chapter.) You might ask what interventions and diagnostic screening are normally used during labor. For example: Do all women receive intravenous fluids and electronic fetal monitoring? Are women free to walk, move, and take showers throughout labor? What about the use of medication and anesthesia? How often does the care-giver perform cesarean sections? Are episiotomies usually done? Does the care-giver recommend childbirth preparation classes, and if so, which ones? Other questions might center on the father's or partner's participation throughout labor and birth, even cesarean birth. Are other support people also welcome? When does the care-giver normally arrive during labor and how much time does he or she spend by the bedside during labor? If not the care-giver, who provides professional support and care during labor?

Other questions might be about level of skill and training, ability to detect problems (prenatal and neonatal), and policies on induction of labor. You might ask how often and for what reasons labor is induced, and what precautions are taken to avoid prematurity with induced labor.

If you are planning a home birth, ask when your care-giver normally arrives during labor. You will want to know what equipment your care-giver carries for normal care and for emergencies and what his or her policies are on transfer to the hospital if problems arise. Can the care-giver continue to provide your care in the hospital or remain as a support person and advocate while an obstetrician takes over the management? Or does he or she not accompany you in the hospital?

You also will want to know any limitations on the scope of practice of your care-giver. For example, only some family physicians and no midwives perform cesarean sections. Few physicians attend out-of-hospital births. Midwives do not provide care in complicated labors, nor do they use forceps. Some midwives cannot perform episiotomies or repair either episiotomies or lacerations. Who would do these things if they are outside the scope of your care-giver's practice? Some midwives cannot give pain medication during labor.

Finally, ask questions about the routine care of the newborn immediately after birth. Does the newborn usually stay with the parents, or is the baby taken to the nursery very soon after birth? For how long? For what reasons? Can some newborn procedures be delayed, especially those that interfere with the contact that allows "bonding" to take place between parents and baby? These include the use of eye ointments (which can blur the baby's vision), the use of nursery heaters to maintain body temperature, and the immediate admission of the baby into the nursery for routine procedures, such as weighing and measuring. Some of these can be delayed, which would give the parents time to admire and cuddle their new baby, if the baby's condition permits. What about circumcision? Ask if your care-giver recommends it and, if so, why? Does he or she do circumcisions? (See Chapter 5.)

## Choosing Health Care for Your Baby

Ideally, you should choose health care for your baby (a pediatrician or other care-giver) before your due date, so that you have someone to turn to right after birth, if necessary. During late pregnancy, ask for recommendations from friends, other physicians or midwives, and childbirth educators, or call local reputable hospitals and find out which doctors and pediatric nurse practitioners have privileges there. After some screening for location (medical care close to home, if possible, is a real advantage), you can make one or several prenatal appointments to discuss your questions and concerns. In many communities, an interview to select a doctor for the baby is free. Find out before making very many appointments.

There are several types of health-care providers available for babies and children; each has its own advantages.

Pediatricians specialize in the care of children only; they have more training in childhood illness than any of the other providers. Their staffs and their waiting rooms are geared for children. They have completed medical school and three years of residency training in pediatrics.

Family physicians can care for the entire family, including the children. Those who have completed family medicine residencies have had several months' training in pediatrics, but probably would refer any serious illnesses to a physician with more pediatric training.

Pediatric nurse practitioners are registered nurses who have taken additional training in clini-cal pediatrics. Most work in clinics or groups, with physicians available for consultation and referral. They specialize in well-child care and the treatment of common illnesses. They tend to be very capable in the areas of children's development and emotional needs and parenting concerns, and do a lot of teaching in these areas. They refer serious problems to pediatricians.

Private care tends to be more personalized, more convenient, and more expensive.

Children's health clinics cost less to those with low incomes and usually offer good care, although there may be more waiting and less continuity of care with the same practitioner. Children's health clinics are largely staffed by physicians taking their specialty training in family medicine or pediatrics.

Well-child clinics, such as those sponsored by the public health department, provide free or low-cost checkups and immunizations, but usually no care for the sick child.

After looking into the types of care, decide which you want to investigate and make appointments to get to know the people involved. Ideally, try to do this at least a few weeks before your baby is due.

In a prenatal appointment (they usually last ten to fifteen minutes), you will not be able to discuss all your questions (see "Choosing a Baby Doctor" in Chapter 8). Decide on a few areas that interest you the most and discuss those. Pay as much attention to how your questions are answered as to what is said. Do you feel secure picturing this person as your child's health-care provider? Are his or her style and philosophy compatible with yours?

## Where to Have Your Baby

Another basic decision is choosing where you will give birth. Most women choose the hospital. Some give birth in freestanding birthing centers or at home. Your decision on where to have your baby is made in much the same way you choose your care-giver. You find out what is available and ask questions that are important to you.

### The Hospital

If you prefer a hospital birth, the next question is, which hospital? Most care-givers have privileges

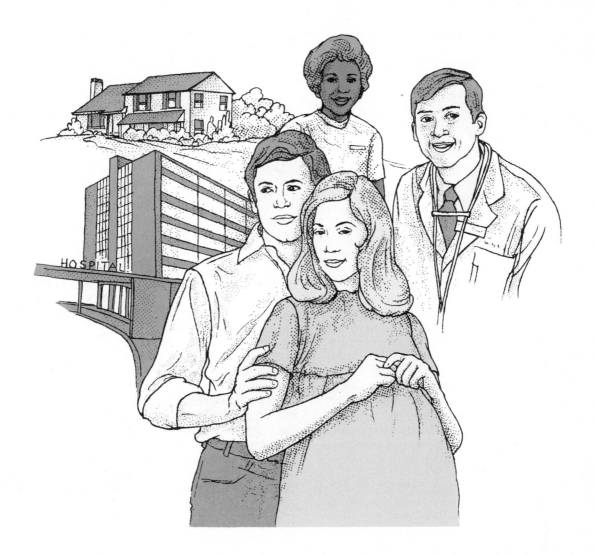

*Among the important decisions to be made by expectant parents are the choice of a care-giver, and where to have the baby.*

in one hospital, but some use more than one. Tour each of the hospitals your care-giver uses. It also may be useful to tour other hospitals—for comparison purposes, if nothing else. You might discover that you prefer a hospital where your care-giver does not have privileges; if so, and if you do not feel a strong tie to your care-giver, you might decide to change care-givers in order to use the facilities that appeal to you. If your community has more than one hospital, you might be surprised at how different they are from one another in their facilities, policies, and philosophies of care. Most hospitals offer tours of their maternity ward. You should call the hospital itself to sign up for a tour.

What do you look for when touring a hospital? First of all, simply observe the atmosphere. Many

hospitals have attractive private labor rooms and bathroom facilities. What provisions are there for the mother's comfort? Some have very comfortable labor beds, while others have very narrow, hard labor beds. Some provide nice touches like rocking chairs, couches where the partner can rest, showers and tubs to use for pain relief, and beanbag chairs for getting into comfortable positions. Others make no provisions at all for the comfort of either mother or father.

Does the hospital have birthing rooms (attractively decorated rooms where the mother can labor, give birth, and spend time with her newborn afterward)? In some hospitals, the birthing room is the only room the mother will be in throughout her entire hospital stay. In others, she labors and gives birth in the birthing room, and then goes to a post-partum room for one, two, or three days before going home. In still other facilities, she labors in one room, is moved when she is about to deliver, may go to another room to recover, and then goes to still another room for the rest of her hospital stay. Currently, many hospitals are beginning to convert their maternity facilities so that a woman can labor, deliver, and recover in the same room (a so-called LDR room).

Check the nursery. What does it look like? Are the mothers encouraged to keep their babies with them in their rooms, or do the babies spend most of their time in the nursery? Do the nurses seem friendly and warm? What about the person leading the tour? Is she friendly and does she answer your questions, or is she simply herding you through brusquely? (Some hospitals are so busy that they don't take potential clients on a tour of the actual facilities. In place of a tour there will sometimes be a slide show and discussion of policies and procedures with a member of the staff.)

Ask some specific questions about admitting procedures. Ask to see the general consent forms that require your signature when you arrive at the hospital. Be sure to read these in advance and clarify any questions you may have. It is certainly not easy to read consent forms carefully if you are already in labor.

Questions about hospital procedures need to be carefully worded. For example, if you ask, "What usually happens to the baby after he or she is born?" you will learn more than if you ask, "What is the hospital's procedure for routine newborn care?" There are few hospital policies on these kinds of things, but there certainly are customs, and those are what you want to know about. You might ask for a step-by-step description of what usually happens after a woman in labor arrives. Do most women have a nurse assigned to them, or do the nurses take care of more than one laboring woman at a time? Are they understaffed sometimes, and what do they do if this happens? Do women usually receive pain medications, or do many women use little or no pain medication? If a woman desires an unmedicated childbirth, is she actively encouraged and supported in this by the nurse? Do most women receive intravenous fluids, continuous electronic fetal monitoring, rupture of the membranes, oxytocin, and episiotomies? Does the hospital have a high rate of cesarean births? Ask how cesareans are usually done (for example, what type of anesthetic is usually used, and is the father encouraged to be

present?). Can a woman have a vaginal birth after a previous cesarean? How long is the usual hospital stay? Is there a short-stay or early-discharge program that allows mothers and babies to go home within a few hours after the birth? Does the hospital provide any kind of follow-up?

Clarify the costs of labor and delivery rooms, nursery charges, postpartum care, and so forth. You also, of course, will want to check your insurance policy, if you have one, to see how much you will have to pay.

## Out-of-Hospital Birth

If you are considering giving birth outside the hospital, find out what services are available in your community. Are there competent people offering home-birth care? Is there a licensed birthing center in your area?

Out-of-hospital birth is a choice only for women who are in good health and who have had normal pregnancies. Interventions are often not necessary for healthy women having normal labors, but if the need arises, the woman is transferred to the hospital. Those planning out-of-hospital births, therefore, expect to labor without pain medication and without medical intervention. It must be remembered that care-givers in out-of-hospital settings have fewer facilities (and possibly less skill) should emergency situations arise. Minutes count. How long will it take to receive adequate care?

Many women, of course, are not comfortable giving birth away from the emergency medical facilities available in hospitals. This disadvantage of out-of-hospital births should be carefully considered by all women contemplating birth outside the hospital.

## Risks With Out-of-Hospital Birth

Just what are the risks in giving birth outside the hospital? There are two classifications of risk: true obstetric emergencies, and other conditions that might require a less critical transfer to the hospital for assistance with the birth.

Even though true emergency conditions are uncommon, they are factors that must be considered by anyone who is contemplating an out-of-hospital birth. (See Chapter 6 for more information on complications of pregnancy and labor.)

It should also be remembered that even in a normal pregnancy and labor, unexpected situations could arise *after* delivery. For example, respiratory distress or cardiovascular problems of the newborn infant are true emergencies that can best be dealt with in a hospital setting.

## Nonemergencies Requiring Transfer to the Hospital

Women are also transferred to the hospital for conditions that are nonemergent in nature. Sometimes, if a complication (such as anemia, high blood pressure, diabetes, twin pregnancy, or breech presentation) is discovered during pregnancy, the woman is no longer a candidate for out-of-hospital birth. If labor is prolonged or if it looks as though the mother will need pain medication, forceps assistance, or other intervention, she is transferred to the hospital. Under these circumstances, the transfer is not an emergency, and there is usually time to try various solutions and, if necessary, decide whether and when to go to the hospital. While it is never pleasant to have to give up plans for an out-of-hospital birth, and transfer is uncomfortable and worrisome for the parents, it is not usually associated with danger for either mother or baby. Of women who choose out-of-hospital birth, approximately fifteen to twenty-five percent of first-time mothers and five to fifteen percent of second-time mothers are transferred to the hospital during labor or after delivery. The possibility of transfer should be considered when parents are deciding on the merits of an out-of-hospital birth.

When inquiring about out-of-hospital birth services, find out what drugs and technology they use in their birth practices, such as pain medications, intravenous fluids, oxytocin, and fetal monitoring. Ask what emergency equipment they have with them for all births. You will want to know about the backup hospital and the backup or consultant physicians. You should know about transfer arrangements. For example, is an ambulance available? Or are the automobiles of the staff and clients the usual transportation in case of transfer? How far away is the backup hospital?

## Advantages of Out-of-Hospital Birth

The advantages of out-of-hospital birth are that parents may have more control over their birthing experience. There are few routines that must be followed. Parents have the freedom to move around, visit with friends, go outside the home, and do household activities and other things during labor as much as they like. In addition, few interventions are used. Contact with the baby after the birth is unlimited and in accordance with the parents' wishes.

Women who choose birthing centers often find a sense of community and fellowship. Classes and social gatherings are often held at the birthing center, contributing to a sense of security and friendliness. Women who choose home births tend to find great appeal in the complete familiarity of their own surroundings.

The costs associated with home birth are by far the lowest of the three environments; birthing centers usually cost less than hospitals. Those parents for whom finances are an important issue need to look into the actual costs involved in all three options.

Many uninsured people with low incomes find home birth to be the only affordable option. But if a planned home birth winds up as a transfer to the hospital, it may turn out to be more expensive than a planned hospital birth.

Some health insurance policies do not cover home-birth or birthing-center care, even though it is much less expensive. If you have insurance, make sure to investigate ahead of time the possibility of being reimbursed for those expenses.

## Disadvantages of Out-of-Hospital Birth

The major disadvantages of out-of-hospital birth are primarily related to the lack of available appropriate medical care should emergencies occur. Such situations can arise quickly (for example, hemorrhage, seizures, mucus aspiration, or any severe fetal or maternal complication that might place either baby or mother in jeopardy). The value of proximity to the full range of modern medical care should not be underestimated.

See Chapter 6 for more information on complications of pregnancy and labor.

## Childbirth Classes

By choosing your care-giver and the place where you will give birth, you will have made the two choices that will most greatly affect your birth experience. Besides those, however, there are oth-

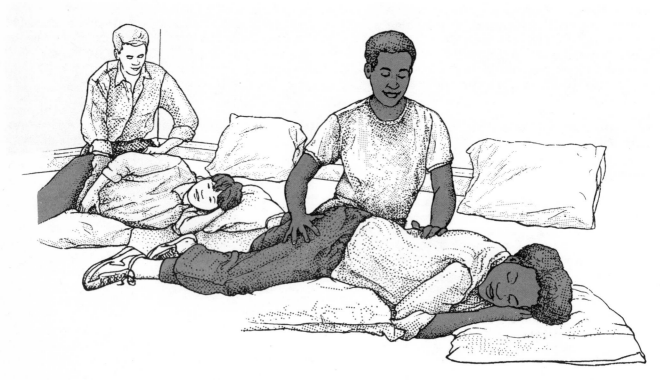

*Childbirth classes provide expectant parents with valuable information and moral support.*

ers that also make a big difference. For example, your choice of childbirth classes will influence your feelings of confidence and readiness as you approach the birth and early parenthood.

The idea of formal classes to prepare women and their partners for childbirth came to North America in the early 1950's when the work of Grantly Dick-Read, an English obstetrician, became publicized. Dick-Read was the real pioneer of natural childbirth techniques in the Western world. As a young man in the 1920's and 1930's, he presented a new approach to childbirth management. He used education, relaxation, slow abdominal breathing, and caring labor support to combat the three-way cycle of fear, tension, and pain that fed on itself and escalated during labor to the point where a woman had to be heavily medicated. His belief that childbirth pain is unnatural and unnecessary guided him in the development of the Read method.

In France in the 1940's and 1950's, Dr. Fernand Lamaze developed another, quite different system of childbirth preparation, which was widely practiced in France and later in North America. Lamaze called his method psychoprophylaxis—literally, "mental prevention." He emphasized complex distraction methods and the dominant role of a professional "coach" to reduce a laboring woman's awareness of pain.

Both the Read and the Lamaze methods thrived, although there has always been some competition and rivalry among proponents of the two different methods. They thrived because they appeared at a time in our history when many women were heavily drugged and unconscious through labor and delivery. These methods of "natural" childbirth appealed to women who wished to be more in control during labor.

Childbirth education has evolved over the years, with major modifications contributed by prominent childbirth educators and obstetricians. Among them is Robert Bradley, the American obstetrician who brought the father into the birth situation as a labor coach. Fathers had traditionally been prohibited from attending births, but Dr. Bradley felt not only that the father's presence was his right, but also that his role as labor coach was an appropriate one for him to play, helping his wife through the labor process.

Sheila Kitzinger, a well-known British anthropologist and childbirth educator, brought a woman's perspective to childbirth preparation, emphasizing body awareness, innovative relaxation techniques, and breathing patterns that harmonize with the intensity of a woman's contractions. Rather than distracting the woman from her labor pain, Ms. Kitzinger said that labor pain is nothing to fear; it is "pain with a purpose." By accepting her pain and working with it, a woman can cope successfully and reap great psychological rewards from her active participation.

The popularity of natural childbirth led to the founding of several national and international organizations devoted to promoting family-centered maternity care, parent participation in childbirth, and childbirth education classes. The International Childbirth Education Association (ICEA), the American Society for Psychoprophylaxis in Obstetrics (ASPO), and the American Academy of Husband-Coached Childbirth (AAHCC) were founded in the early 1960's to give parents a greater voice in maternity care. A closely related issue, the promotion of breastfeeding, became the cause of La Leche League International (LLLI), also founded in the early 1960's. These organizations and others contributed to effective change in maternity care in favor of more consumer involvement and choice.

In the 1970's, Dr. Frédéric Leboyer drew our attention to the newborn baby and what he or she goes through during the birth process. He promoted "birth without violence," or gentle birth. He said that the baby should be helped to a gentle and calm transition from life in the uterus to life outside the mother's body. He advocated a warm, quiet room with dim lights for the birth and a warm bath for the baby shortly after birth.

Also during the 1970's, the term "bonding" was coined after it was discovered that when newborn babies stayed with their mothers for extended periods of time, the behavior of the mothers seemed to be more loving and maternal than that of mothers whose babies spent most of the time in the nursery. The work of Leboyer and others focused the attention of parents and care-givers on the early care of the newborn and early interaction between parents and newborns.

In the 1980's, investigators with training in psychotherapy focused on the healing potential (and, conversely, the potential for emotional trauma) of the profound experience of childbirth, and incorporated counseling and stress reduction measures into childbirth preparation. Some have urged more spontaneity in childbirth and less emphasis on intellectual preparation and prescribed responses to labor contractions. Childbirth education continues to evolve as we learn more, as people's tastes change, and as maternity care changes.

Finding the right childbirth class for you may require some comparison shopping. Some classes teach only one method (Lamaze or Bradley, for example). Others provide a broader, more individualized kind of preparation, drawing from these methods and the other innovations to provide a framework of relaxation techniques, patterned breathing, massage, visualization, music, sound, and other pain-reduction methods, along with guidelines for adapting them to suit the individual. The goal of these classes is to enable women and their partners to discover their own style for labor.

Many communities have independent, consumer-based childbirth education groups that provide classes. Most hospitals and some groups of physicians or midwives also sponsor childbirth classes for their patients or clients.

## Where to Start

You can begin the search for classes by asking your care-giver, your friends with babies, or the hospital's maternity department for suggestions. Then call and ask the providers of childbirth education to describe their classes. Find out who the teachers are. Is it possible to interview the teacher before registering in a class? You can learn a lot in a brief phone conversation. Is the teacher an independent certified childbirth educator who subcontracts her services? Or is she an employee of a hospital or group? Does she belong to one or more of the local and national organizations of childbirth educators?

Ask about the teacher's qualifications. Some sponsors require a medical background, such as nursing or physical therapy. Others require a college degree, sometimes in a related field, such as psychology, social work, education, or biology. Some have no specific educational requirements. Many sponsors require that their teachers have a child. In addition to background requirements, most teachers have received training in childbirth education. Training may be minimal (for example, the teacher may be required only to observe a series of classes) or it may be rigorous. Certification by one of the national or international childbirth education organizations may be required. Some community childbirth education organizations provide their own training and require their own certification. The certification process may include classroom sessions or workshops, written work, examinations, observations of childbirth classes, attendance at births, and teaching under supervision.

Find out the number of classes in a series. They range from about four weekly classes to as many as twelve. Classes may last one and a half to two and a half hours. What topics are covered? (Possible topics include self-care in pregnancy, preparation for normal and complicated childbirth, cesarean birth, newborn care, breast-feeding and bottle-feeding, and the beginnings of parenthood.) You should know how much time is spent on learning and practicing techniques for coping with labor, such as relaxation, breathing patterns, massage techniques, and methods of visualization and focus.

How large are the classes? Classes may range in size from private sessions for one or two couples to very large classes for forty to fifty couples. A small, intimate class may be important to you, or you may prefer a more diverse, larger group. If the group is large, does the teacher have one or more assistants to provide more personal contact with the students? Is there room for everyone on the floor? Is personal contact by phone or private consultation available if you wish it?

Will there be a reunion of the group after the babies have been born? If so, it indicates that the teacher is aware of the importance of group support. It also shows that the teacher has an interest in following up on her students.

## Specialized Classes

In many communities, specialized classes are offered—for example, early pregnancy classes; home-birth classes; refresher classes (a shortened series for those who had childbirth classes during a previous pregnancy); cesarean preparation classes; classes for single mothers, lesbians, parents with a language barrier, parents with impaired hearing or vision, and teen parents; classes for women planning to give up their babies for adoption; classes on vaginal birth after a previous cesarean; sibling preparation classes for other children in the family; grandparent classes; adoptive parent classes; and breast-feeding classes. Postpartum classes for parents with their infants are also offered in many communities.

## Professional and Other Labor Support

Professional staff provide one kind of support during labor; their expertise and perspective give a woman confidence that she may not otherwise feel. But professionals are also busy with other responsibilities, such as recording information in the chart, listening to fetal heart tones, taking blood pressure, doing vaginal exams, placing electronic fetal monitors and intravenous tubes, preparing for delivery, and even caring for other women at the same time. Nurses may not be able to supply very much emotional support because of the other demands on them. Today many women are also supported through labor by one or more loved ones, in addition to a nurse or midwife. These support people, if prepared, can do things the nurse does not do—for example, give the woman exclusive, continuous, loving encouragement; help with creature comforts, like rubbing her back, mopping her brow, and bringing her water or juice; and help with relaxation and with techniques for coping with labor.

## The Birth Plan

One problem that keeps coming up in patient-physician relations is communication. Physicians are busy people, and one of the most common complaints about them is that they are always rushed and do not have time to answer or discuss questions. Sometimes the physician is not even present; the office nurse is the one who sees the woman if the physician is tied up at the hospital. Poor communication and misunderstandings lead to depersonalized and sometimes unsatisfying care.

There are solutions to this problem. One is to seek a care-giver who is not so busy (physicians who are just starting a practice often have more time) or who schedules appointments long enough to get to know each woman. Midwives are such care-givers, but they are few in number. Some established physicians also plan more time for individual appointments.

Another solution, which has many other advantages, is the birth plan. What is a birth plan and why is it worthwhile?

A birth plan is simply a written description of your priorities and preferred options during labor and birth and afterward. The plan may be placed in your chart, where it can be read and consulted by those involved in your care. The por-

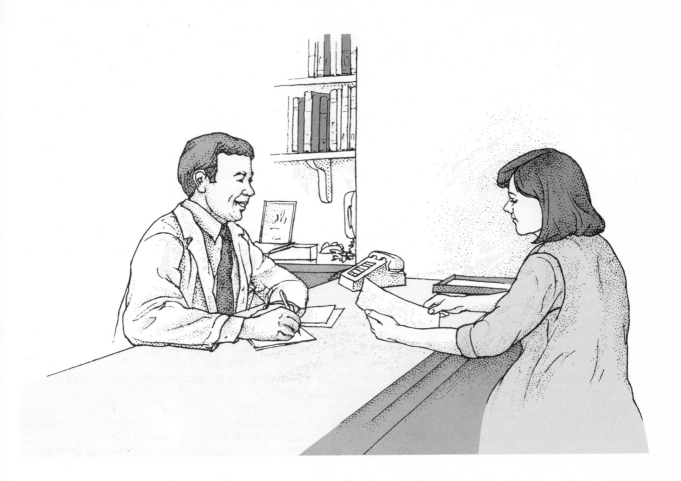

*A thoughtful birth plan will help you communicate your wishes to your physician and other care-givers.*

tion that pertains to the care of your baby (the baby care plan) can be placed in the baby's chart, which is separate from your own.

A birth plan has many advantages. Simply preparing a birth plan helps you focus your learning on the various options (for example, natural versus medicated childbirth, circumcision versus no circumcision, breast- versus bottle-feeding). It encourages you and your partner to discuss your worries and expectations, and to come to agreement on what is important. During labor, of course, the benefit of the birth plan is that you do not have to take the time and trouble to tell each staff member your wishes on every option as it comes up.

Birth plans also help your care-giver. If you prepare a rough draft and go over it with your caregiver, he or she will know you better and will know how to help you in labor. He or she can also help you modify options that may seem unwise or inappropriate. Potential misunderstandings can be de-

tected in advance, so that neither of you is caught by surprise when the stress of labor makes discussion difficult. Your care-giver may be willing to initial your plan, indicating to hospital staff that he or she agrees with it. It is not a legal agreement or a contract. It is simply a statement of your wishes.

For the nursing staff and other people who will be caring for you during labor, the birth plan makes you less of a stranger to them. It is a shortcut to communication and lets them know what is important to you and how they can help.

Your birth plan should be flexible, taking into account not only a normal, or "textbook," labor, but also the possibility of a difficult labor, complications, or other unexpected events.

## Components of the Birth Plan

Your birth plan might begin with a brief paragraph describing yourself and anything that you feel would help the staff to understand you better and to understand your birth plan. For example, if you had a long period of infertility before your pregnancy, if you have had miscarriages in the past, or if you previously experienced a tragedy associated with childbirth, it will help for the staff to know that. If you have a fear of hospitals or medications, or if you have had unpleasant experiences in hospitals in the past, tell them. If a natural birth is extremely important to you, let them know so they can offer you maximum support in that effort. If avoidance of pain is a high priority, let them know. If you have religious preferences, if yours is a "blended" family with other children, if you have impaired hearing or vision, if this has been a particularly difficult pregnancy—knowing these things will help the staff to meet your needs. You might simply want to state that you will appreciate their help, advice, and expertise.

The next section of the birth plan is a straightforward list of your preferences for a normal labor and birth. Include only items that you care about. You do not have to hold an opinion on everything. See Chapter 5 for helpful information about common procedures and when they might be indicated and when optional. At the moment, you may feel you do not have enough background to decide your preferences on these procedures. Childbirth classes and discussions with your caregiver will give you the needed information.

If your labor is prolonged or more painful than expected, if the baby isn't tolerating labor, or if you develop complications that make intervention necessary, your ideal birth plan may have to change. Let it reflect a recognition that these things can happen and that you are flexible enough to be able to accept changes in the plan if they are necessary for your sake or your baby's.

Sometimes a cesarean birth becomes necessary for any of a number of reasons (see Chapter 6 for a discussion of cesarean section). It helps if you acknowledge the possibility of a cesarean birth in your birth plan, and indicate your preferences if it does indeed happen to you. For example, you might state that you prefer to remain awake, to have your husband present, or to touch and nurse your baby as soon as possible after the surgery.

## The Newborn Care Plan

Your birth plan should also include a newborn care plan. Many mothers wish to hold their baby skin-to-skin immediately after birth. Skin-to-skin contact provides warmth for the baby and satisfaction for the mother. Some parents want their baby to have a relaxing float in a Leboyer bath soon after birth. The baby might be placed in a heated unit in the nursery if the mother prefers or if the baby is chilled.

What about feeding your baby? Do you prefer to breast-feed or bottle-feed? Do you want to provide all the feedings for your baby (which would mean that the baby should receive no water or glucose water from a bottle)? Do you want to feed on demand (that is, whenever and for as long as the baby seems to want to nurse)? Many nurseries restrict demand feedings unless the mother states that demand feeding is her preference.

How much contact do you want with your baby? Some hospitals provide a private postpartum room, and even allow the father to rent a cot and stay all night. Other options are to have the baby with you during the day only or for feedings only. The less time you spend with your baby, the less well you will know her personality and how to care for her.

It should be remembered, however, that the amount of time you will spend with your baby is dependent on several factors. The most important of these are the health of the mother and the health of the baby. For example, it may be medically necessary for a premature infant to be placed in the hospital nursery, where her condition can be carefully and continually monitored.

What about circumcision of your baby boy? This surgical procedure involves removing the foreskin of the penis. Since the procedure is optional, it deserves your consideration. This and other routines and alternatives, such as eye care and blood tests, are discussed in Chapter 5.

When will you and your baby leave the hospital? You can stay a few hours to a few days after the birth. An early discharge, or short stay, means that you leave within six to twenty-four hours after the birth. One obvious advantage is the financial savings involved. Hospitalization costs are calculated by the day or fraction of a day; obviously, the longer you spend in the hospital, the more it costs. Find out how the billing is done so that you won't inadvertently stay longer than you can afford. Other considerations besides costs, however, are your need for rest, your need for medical care, and your desire for teaching and medical supervision for the first couple of days. Find out if your hospital sends a nurse to visit all women who have had a short stay, or if they at least make a phone call to check on them. Is instruction available for those wishing a short stay, so that you know what observations to make to be sure everything is going well for both of you? Another factor in your decision is whether you will have help at home. Sometimes the father can take time off from work, or a relative or friend can come in and help extensively; sometimes parents hire helpers to come in daily for a week or two after the birth. In the absence of any help, you might prefer to spend a couple of days in the hospital before going home to all that responsibility.

If your baby is premature or ill and needs extensive medical care, she will either stay in the nursery or be transferred to a different hospital with more sophisticated facilities for newborns. Time with the baby and breast-feeding may be postponed until she recovers or becomes strong enough to suckle. State in your birth plan if you want to feed the baby yourself and if you want to spend as much time as possible with your baby.

### Unexpected Loss of a Baby

One of the greatest difficulties we face is the possibility that the baby may not live. Every prospective parent worries at times about losing a child. Although it is uncommon, some babies die. This very sad ending to the pregnancy leaves the parents stunned, grieving, depressed, and angry. After losing a child, parents are in no state to make important decisions. If you have thought through how you would want a newborn death handled, then, should a death occur, such decisions will have already been made by you at a time when you were calm.

Many counselors recommend that couples have private time together with their baby who died. Seeing and holding the child gives the parents a chance to say good-bye to the baby. In addition, pictures, footprints of the baby, and perhaps a lock of hair are mementos that mean a great deal later.

Having a memorial service or a funeral for the baby allows friends and relatives to also acknowledge the baby's life and death. Formal ceremonies can often give people a vehicle through which to express their grief and their support for the bereaved parents.

The question of an autopsy often comes up. If the cause of death is unclear, sometimes an autopsy is beneficial, both in answering questions and in possibly preventing the same thing from happening in the future. It would be worthwhile to think through in advance whether you would consent to an autopsy in such a case.

### The Value of a Birth Plan

In summary, a birth plan represents your thinking on the various possibilities regarding normal labor, postpartum, and newborn care. It also includes your preferences even if the process does not follow a normal course. Because you prepare it when you are calm and rational, it tends to reflect what you really desire. Once completed, it becomes a valuable guide for you and for your care-givers during a stressful period when you might not be thinking clearly.

## Choosing Freely

This chapter has provided some background on maternity care in North America and a description of some very important choices for prospective parents to make. These choices require thought and discussion and careful planning. They can make a great difference in your ultimate sense of satisfaction and fulfillment in giving birth. There is so much more to giving birth than simply having mother and baby come out of it alive. The emotional and physical quality of the experience will have an impact on you and your family for a very long time to come.

There is not one universally correct way for all women to give birth. The choices are numerous, and there are no conclusive studies to date that indicate that one place of birth or one type of care-giver has a better safety record than another as long as women are well cared for throughout pregnancy and have access to hospital facilities and obstetric care when needed. That still leaves a lot of room for parents to freely choose the type of care that seems best for them. It is well worth the time and trouble to choose carefully.

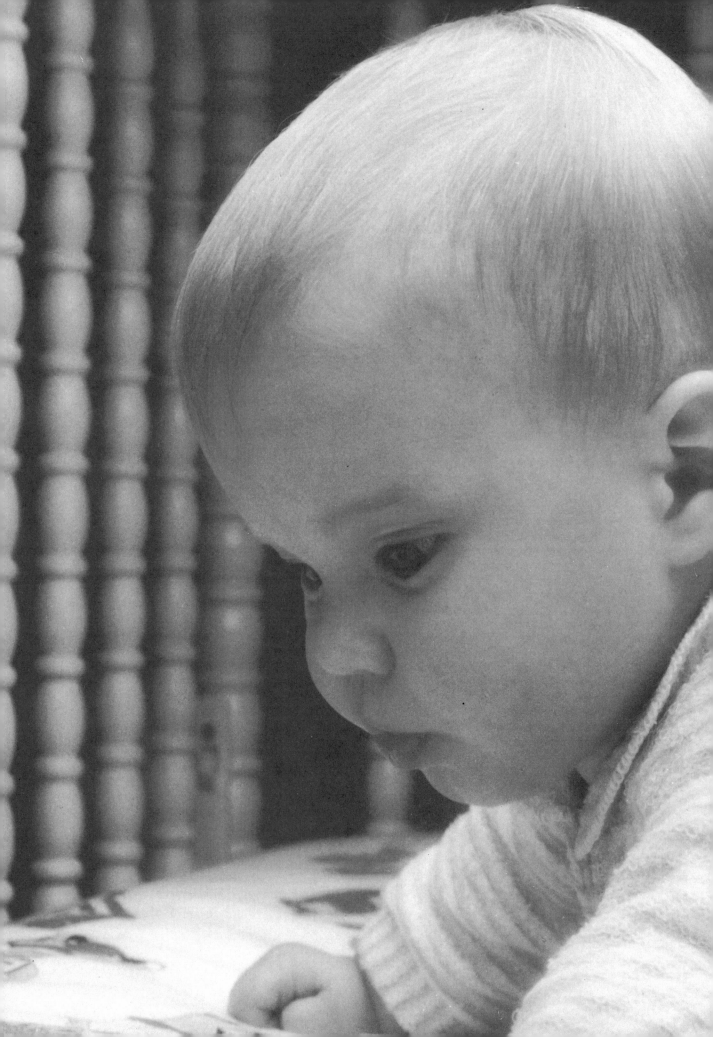

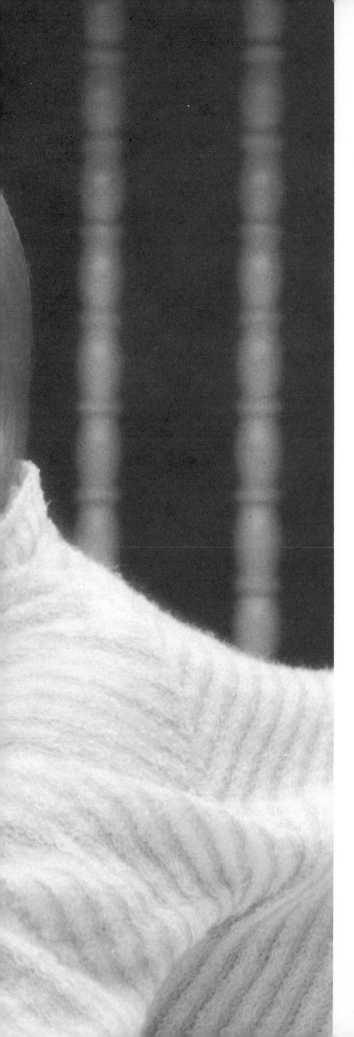

# Chapter 4: Preparing for Baby

## Naming Your Baby

Choosing an appropriate name for your baby may not be as easy as you expected. Husbands and wives are not always in agreement about the choice of a first name, or even a middle name. You will certainly have plenty of names—and suggestions of names—from which to choose. Sometimes, compromise is the best solution.

Naming customs vary from culture to culture, yet name giving is as universal as language. In America we are very democratic about naming babies: mothers and fathers listen to family, friends, strangers, and their own impulses before bestowing a name on their newborn.

Many of our names come from the Bible, which means they are often of Greek or Hebrew origin. Our most common biblical names—John, James,

Mary, Ruth, Mark, Rebecca, Joseph, Susan, David, Daniel, Jason, Matthew, Judith, and their variations—account for more than fifty percent of our forenames. Another large group is derived from the Teutonic (or Germanic) languages. These include such names as William, Brenda, Roger, Frederick, Caroline, and Emily.

Our last names, or surnames, have long been used as first or middle names. English, Teutonic, and Norse surnames, including Ashley, Marion, Clayton, Kimberly, Adair, Shirley, and Mildred, are commonly given as first names. And the lines between masculine and feminine names are also blurring. Names like Pat, Chris, Leslie, Robin, Sidney, Lee, and Hilary could all raise the question of whether a letter should begin "Dear Ms." or "Mr."

Along with the Bible, our families frequently provide the source for baby names. These traditions can pass on such interesting first or middle names as Taylor, Tyler, and Huntington. And the maiden name of the mother is often given to a child as a middle name to keep the mother's family name alive.

While you are free to name your child according to tradition, family custom, or creative impulse, consider first your responsibility in bestowing an appropriate name, and then think about the following:

- Is the name easily spelled and pronounced?

- What nicknames or pet names can be derived from it?

- Do the initials form a word? Is that word objectionable or apt to be embarrassing?

- Is the name so unusual that it will draw undesired attention?

- Be sure the name fits the gender of the child.

- Give full names rather than diminutives; Robert Joseph is preferable to Bobby Joe.

- Use care in naming your baby for well-known personalities; celebrities fade or fall out of favor, and your child will be left with a dated or unpopular name.

- Consider how your choice of a first name flows into the last name, particularly if your last name is hyphenated.

- Avoid choosing a first name that becomes "cute" in conjunction with your last name (Barbie Doll, Sandy Rhodes, Holly Wood).

- Finally, both parents should agree on the name—as much in advance of the delivery as possible.

Many baby-name books are available, should you feel a need for outside help in your decision. Read them, make notes, and discuss your reactions with your partner. Your child will appreciate your thoughtfulness.

## Budgeting for Baby

You already have some idea that raising a child is going to be expensive—in fact, a reasonably reliable rule of thumb for figuring the direct costs of raising a child from birth to the age of eighteen years is that the amount will be roughly three to four times a family's annual income. But how much will child-rearing cost during the first year of your baby's life? What kinds of things do you need to take into consideration when preparing a budget?

The figures we offer here are based on national averages, and they're based on the assumption that items are purchased new. Costs can be trimmed by buying used equipment and furniture, or perhaps borrowing items from friends and family.

The medical costs of having a baby in the United States average more than three thousand dollars. This is based on figuring in the costs of a three-day hospital stay, doctors' fees, anesthesia, sonograms, vitamins, prenatal laboratory work, and birthing classes. Pediatric care in the first year, assuming your baby is well and needs only routine checkups and vaccinations, will cost, on average, between two hundred and three hundred dollars. But most babies experience colds and other common ailments during the first year that will probably bring you to the doctor more often.

Check your insurance. Some policies don't cover obstetrics, and even when they do, there's usually a deductible of about two hundred dollars. Family health insurance, if you have to pay for it, will cost between two thousand and three thousand dollars annually; most policies do not cover checkups and vaccinations. If you have access to a health maintenance organization (HMO), you will have to pay nearly two hundred dollars a month, an amount that covers virtually unlimited medical care.

In the first year, you may spend between four hundred and five hundred dollars on basic dressing furniture and at least another two hundred dollars on bathing and bedding equipment. Toiletries will average about twenty dollars a month. Other major and miscellaneous items, such as cradle, carriage, toys, and nursery lamps, will amount to roughly five hundred dollars.

If you choose to buy cloth diapers and wash them at home, you will spend about four hundred dollars during your baby's first year. Diaper services will cost at least five hundred dollars a year, and disposable diapers between five hundred and six hundred dollars.

Bottle-feeding is considerably more expensive than breast-feeding—about six to eight hundred dollars as opposed to about two hundred dollars a year—and commercial baby food, when it is added to your baby's diet, will cost between one and two dollars a day. Other expenses related to your baby's diet include a breast pump, nursing bras and pads, bottles, and nipples.

If both you and your spouse will be working, child-care costs can be considerable. Expect to pay at least two hundred dollars a week to someone who will come to your home to care for your baby full-time, or close to two hundred dollars weekly (plus board) if you want that person to live in. Frankly, these options are beyond the means of most new parents. More feasible is a day care center, which (for full-time care) can cost up to one hundred dollars a week. A family day care situation (day care in a private home) usually costs between fifty and sixty dollars a week. See Chapter 7 for additional information about day care.

While you probably can't cut the costs of food and medical care, you can indeed cut the costs of your baby's equipment and clothing. Postpone buying such items as stretch suits, sweater sets, and blankets because your baby may receive these things as gifts. And should you end up with an overload of sweater sets after a baby shower, many baby stores will allow you to exchange them for other things you need.

Talk to friends and relatives—they will probably know someone who has next-to-new things that her children have outgrown. Also, don't be afraid of thrift shops.

Know that a lot of the equipment and furniture we mention in the following pages is not absolutely necessary, and that what's necessary and what's not is in many cases a matter of personal preference. Just remember that no single item will make or break your child's first three years, so don't feel guilty if there are some things you simply can't afford.

As we will point out numerous times, don't assume that the so-called top-of-the-line items are necessarily of the best quality; the best is not always the most expensive. Indeed, if you read the following pages carefully, you should feel more confident in your ability to select equipment regardless of its price, brand name, or previous usage. It's entirely possible that the next-to-new crib your sister retired a few years ago meets federal safety standards. And, while you will probably find the lowest-priced products to be less than satisfactory, you will also find a lot of moderately priced equipment to be safe and durable.

## Baby's Room

Your baby's room will most likely contain a crib and a chest of drawers. You may choose to buy a rocking chair for nursing and feeding the baby, and you may also have a changing table, but neither of these is essential.

### Cribs and Bedding

For the sake of the consumer, a lot of attention has been paid to crib safety, so that any crib manufactured after February 1974 has to conform to strict safety codes. If you are considering an older crib, perhaps one that has been in your family, you will want to compare its features with the current safety standards, which were necessitated by a large number of serious crib accidents.

Crib slats must be no more than $2^{3}/_{8}$ inches apart to prevent babies from getting their heads or limbs caught in between them, which could result in strangulation or injury. Never use a crib if it has missing slats or spindles!

Make sure the metal hardware on the crib you buy or borrow has no rough or sharp edges, in case your baby falls against it. Also, check out the

## Crib

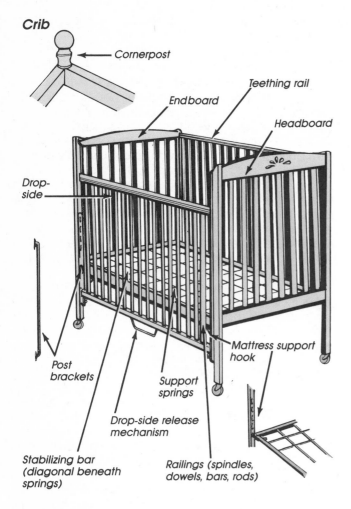

Cornerpost

Teething rail

Endboard

Headboard

Drop-side

Post brackets

Mattress support hook

Support springs

Drop-side release mechanism

Stabilizing bar (diagonal beneath springs)

Railings (spindles, dowels, bars, rods)

locks and latches on the drop-side of the crib to be sure your baby won't be able to accidentally release them from inside the crib and fall out. Many cribs have double release mechanisms—you must use a foot release as well as release the side of the crib—which are even safer. And once released, make sure the sides of the crib move up and down easily.

You want to be sure your baby will not be able to climb out of the crib. There should be no bars or other surfaces on railings or end panels that the baby could climb on.

Another crib danger of the past was mattresses that didn't fit snugly in cribs. Babies would get their heads caught between the mattress and the crib frame and suffocate or strangle. Now all crib mattresses are a standard size: they must be $27\frac{1}{4}$ by $51\frac{5}{8}$ inches and not more than 6 inches thick.

When you go out to buy a crib, don't be fooled into thinking that if you spend enough money,

you'll be assured top quality. That simply isn't the case. While currently manufactured cribs generally meet minimum safety standards, some cribs are shoddy and some manufacturers have poor quality control. There's no substitute for your careful inspection of the floor model and a repeat inspection upon delivery.

Look for a crib that has at least one stabilizing bar beneath the springs; two are even better. Make sure the finish of the crib is smooth and evenly painted. If it's an older crib, be sure it's not finished with a paint containing lead. If you suspect that the paint contains lead, ask your local health department where you might have paint chips analyzed for lead content. Do not use a crib finished with lead-based paint—babies gnaw on crib railings; lead poisoning can cause brain damage and even death.

The crib's railings should be sturdy; you shouldn't be able to flex them. Round railings are better than decorative spindles or those with protruding edges or corners. The teething rails should run the length of the railing tops and should not be cracked or have any jagged edges. Specialty stores sell new teething rails for older cribs. Corner posts should not extend more than $\frac{5}{8}$ of an inch above the end panel, since these knobs can catch clothing and cause strangulation. If you already have a crib with longer corner posts, either unscrew them or saw them off and sand them smooth. The endboards should be straight and functional and should have no decorative open spaces that the baby could climb on or get caught in. Avoid decals; they may have a lot of initial appeal, but they don't hold up well.

*Crib mattresses* must meet federal flame-retardancy standards. They are available in three types: innerspring, hair block, and all foam. Other variables include the thickness of the outer fabric, the number of vents, and the type of edging used around the borders.

Innerspring mattresses vary in the number of coils they have, the type of cushioning on top of the springs, the presence or absence of a metal grid across the springs or additional metal supports, and the type of covering and venting. Although they are widely advertised, they don't hold up to the wear and tear of a bouncing toddler. Protruding metal parts is a common complaint.

Hair block mattresses are constructed of molded animal hair. Because of allergic potential, they are not recommended.

Your best bet is a high-density foam mattress, which will not be bouncy and also won't have any inner parts that can break. Make sure the sides are well vented to allow air to flow in and out under pressure, since a poorly vented mattress will trap air inside and could pop, tearing the vinyl cover. A torn vinyl cover could prove dangerous to your inquisitive baby. A firm foam mattress will fit a crib more tightly than an innerspring mattress. Foam mattresses are often thinner than innerspring mattresses, allowing for extra space between the mattress and the top railing, thereby making the crib more difficult to climb out of.

*Crib bumper pads* provide extra protection for your baby at three or four months. They guard against her becoming accidentally wedged between the mattress and the crib side or between the bars. The pads should cover all four sides of the crib and tie onto the crib bars securely in at least six places. You'll want to remove the pads as soon as your baby begins to use them to pull herself up to stand—at this point, they can collapse and cause her head to be thrown into the bars. Also, they could be used as a prop in an attempt to climb out of the crib.

Bumper pads tend to be of poor quality, and there are frequent reports of elastic snap ties tearing from pads, snaps pulling off, and vinyl seams ripping and exposing foam interiors, which can then be ingested. Tie cords may be long enough to tangle around your baby's neck. Try to buy a firm bumper pad that's covered with washable fabric. Clip tie cords after you've fastened them to the crib bars, leaving only an inch or so of excess cord.

The following list is a rough guideline for bedding: three fitted crib sheets, two crib-sized mattress pads, one vinyl or plastic crib mattress protector, two crib-sized, flannel-covered rubber pads, two small washable quilts, and one set of bumper pads.

*Pillows* are often sold as baby gifts, but they should never be used. They can suffocate a baby or cause postural stress to her neck.

*Portable cribs* are smaller and narrower than regular cribs. Many of the regulations that cover full-size cribs are similar for portable cribs, but don't apply to mesh-sided or tubular-frame portables. While some families appreciate being able to collapse their portables and take them along, there are frequent problems with portables that should be mentioned: shoddy construction often causes legs to crack or collapse; bottoms that aren't well supported fall through; teething bars splinter; and very often these cribs just aren't as portable as they appear.

If you're going to buy a portable crib, look for a wooden one that has no protruding wing nuts that can loosen easily. Make sure the floor supports are sturdy, and check to see that the mattress pad is well finished and firm. The bars should be straight on all sides. Avoid one with latching gates, which can be climbed on or present a pinching hazard to a baby's fingers. Avoid models that have mesh sides or, worse yet, mesh-supported floorboards, since the mesh can tear and cause your baby to fall. Once your baby is sitting up, remove the leg supports from the crib and allow it to sit directly on the floor, or retire it from use, since portable cribs are meant for newborns and very small babies.

---

### Guidelines for Crib Safety

- Set the mattress at the lowest possible level to give maximum side-bar protection.

- Always keep the drop-sides of the crib up to safeguard against accidents caused by faulty hardware or forgetfulness.

- Use bumper pads for the first five months.

- Use the crib for sleeping only. Never allow jumping or playing in or around the crib.

- Place the crib away from walls and furniture to eliminate the danger of entrapment in case the baby falls from the crib. Also make sure the crib is not near curtain or blind cords, which could entangle or strangle a child, and make sure these cords are out of the baby's reach.

- Keep loose clothing and large, soft toys out of the crib; they could cause suffocation. As the baby gets older, remove toys that could be used by him as stepping-stones for climbing out.

- Once your baby appears able to climb out, buy hospital netting to cover the top of the crib or consider another sleeping arrangement, like putting the mattress right down on
continued

continued

the floor or on a small frame designed for a baby mattress.

- Do not use plastic bags as mattress covers, especially dry-cleaning bags or others that could cause suffocation.

- Remove mobiles once a baby can sit up, since a baby could be hanged on the side straps of one. Mobiles are designed for visual stimulation, not handling.

## Changing Tables

Changing tables provide a safe place to diaper and dress your baby. However, if you don't want to spend the money, an alternative will do.

To be functional, a changing table should be at a height comfortable for handling a baby without having to lean over. It should have a waterproof pad and enough space for open storage of shirts, plastic pants, and diapers, or you'll waste time gathering needed items for each change. There should be a safety belt that is wide and easy to use (but not so easy that the baby can release it). Never use the table without using the safety belt—it takes only a few seconds for the baby to fall when your back is turned. However, don't trust a "belted" baby to be safe if left unattended.

Commercially available changing tables usually have a long, slender, padded area for changing and an area of open shelves underneath for storage. Most of these changing tables fold for storage.

When buying a changing table, look for one that has high sides around the changing area to prevent your baby from rolling out. The covering on the foam pad should be of thick, smooth vinyl, which will make it easier to clean. Make sure the table is sturdy and doesn't wobble or tip over easily. Many parents find it extremely frustrating to assemble these tables and get the legs balanced, so we suggest you purchase yours preassembled. Shelves should be spacious and open and very easy to use; many popular models have small, narrow, half-open boxes for shelves, which can be very hard to use. Look for a model that features stable side shelves for holding washcloths and

other items. Attachable side pails for soiled items are also very useful.

A changing table is useful only for about the first two years, so if you're on a tight budget you may want an alternative. You can use a wide table or even the padded top of a dresser instead. You can buy a special top that secures to a dresser to convert it to a changing table. But if you're going to use the top of a dresser, don't put your baby's things *in* the dresser—it's dangerous to go rummaging through drawers to find things while holding the baby steady on the table with one hand. You will want some sort of an open-shelf system nearby instead. Some parents construct a wall-to-wall shelf in a closet at the appropriate height and top it with a vinyl-covered pad; you might also use a portable crib raised to its highest position.

When using a changing table, keep diapers handy and ready for use, but keep all pins closed and out of the baby's reach. Have a container of water handy. A roll of toilet paper attached to the wall and out of the baby's reach and a wastebasket nearby will make the arrangement even more workable.

## Drawers and Shelves

What you use for drawers and shelves is up to you. There are lots of nice baby chests on the market. Don't feel you have to buy one; it's largely a matter of taste and budget. If you've already opted to buy a changing table, there may be enough space in the shelves below it, and you won't need additional storage. If not, consider purchasing a used baby chest, or perhaps a used dresser that you can refinish for your baby's room.

If you're buying a new chest, shop as you would for any other piece of furniture. Look at the workmanship inside and out. Are you planning to have a large family? If so, you may want to invest in a high-quality chest to use for each infant. If you're not planning a big family, will you want to use the chest as the child gets older? If so, you may want to buy something that will eventually look good in an older child's room.

If you are using a chest of drawers, it's a good idea to install safety latches so a small child can't pull the drawers out and have them fall on her. Also, once your baby is walking, you'll want to be sure you don't leave things, like pins, on top of the dresser that your child could reach or pull down on herself.

## Bassinets

If you're looking for a bassinet, here are some general guidelines to keep in mind:

- Make sure it's stable and not shaky.

- There should be no sharp edges.

- Check for any hinges or clips that your baby could catch her fingers on.

Since many bassinets are wicker or rattan, you'll want to be sure there are no sharp or rough areas that could be itchy or scratchy for a baby; adding a bumper pad to the inside may help. If the bassinet folds up, make sure the legs have an effective locking mechanism, so they don't accidentally fold when the bassinet is being used. Also, periodically check to be sure all screws and bolts are tight.

Remember that a bassinet's usefulness is limited because your baby will quickly outgrow it. If you must watch your budget, you probably will not wish to buy a bassinet.

## Rocking Chairs

Some mothers could not do without a rocking chair; others couldn't care less about them. Again, it's a matter of personal choice, taste, and budget. You can buy one new or used. If it's going to be in the baby's room, you'll probably want a style that fits in well with the decor and other pieces of furniture.

The major thing to consider if you're buying a rocking chair is comfort. Will it be a comfortable place for you to nurse? How will it feel to sit in the chair and hold your baby? You'll probably want one with an armrest.

A drawback to having the rocking chair in your child's room is that once he can crawl, there's a possibility he might get caught in the frame or push the chair and get hit in the head by it. There's also the possibility that he will put his tiny fingers under the rocker while the chair is moving. For this reason, you might want to remove the rocking chair from his room once he is crawling and walk-

ing, or be certain you are keeping a careful watch on his activities. Or you can make special stops that prevent the chair from rocking all the way forward or backward.

## Cradles

Cradles have a romantic aura about them, perhaps because they're historically associated with mothers and babies. They provide a gentle rocking motion, which can lull a baby to sleep.

If you're buying a cradle, or if you inherit one, look for the following safety features: The slats should be no more than 2 3/8 inches apart, like crib slats. Cradles are commonly suspended by hooks, which can sometimes stick out and can injure your baby as you put her in or take her out of the cradle. Make sure the hooks don't protrude. A locking mechanism is a definite plus; it will prevent an unattended cradle from rocking and possibly causing a sleeping baby to become wedged against the side of the frame due to the shifting weight.

## Furniture and Furniture Safety

### High Chairs and Feeding Tables

There are a number of consumer safety standards for high chairs. Nonetheless, there are still a large number of injuries, but these are more often the result of careless use than of poor design.

Many babies stand up in and fall out of high chairs, but this could be prevented by using the restraining straps. Adults often think the feeding tray is sufficient for restraining the baby, but it's not. The tray and the baby can fall together; when this happens, injuries can occur if the baby hits the sharp edges of the overturned tray. Other high-chair accidents include finger and hand injuries from the collapse of a chair that folds with the baby in it, cuts to fingers from the pincers on some tray latches, and foot injuries that result from tripping over the chair's extended legs.

Old high chairs can be unsafe for a number of reasons. One is that if the chair was made before 1976, it probably doesn't conform to the current high-chair safety standards. Many of these older chairs are top-heavy and tip over easily. Some lack adequate straps to hold a baby in securely. Some of the hinged trays on them can come

*High chair*

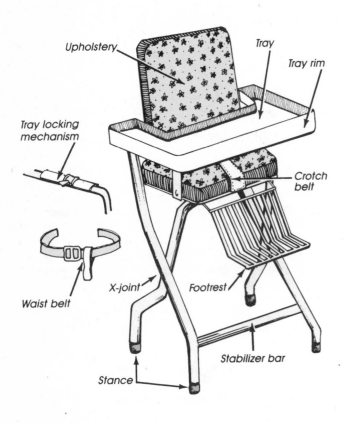

Upholstery

Tray

Tray rim

Tray locking mechanism

Crotch belt

Waist belt

X-joint

Footrest

Stance

Stabilizer bar

• Assembly and usage instructions are easy to understand and follow.

• The following warning is provided: "WARNING: The child should be secured in the high chair at all times by the restraining system. The tray is not designed to hold the child in the chair. It is recommended that the chair be used only by children capable of sitting upright unassisted."

Safety standards aren't enough. You're going to have to examine the chair to see if it seems durable, easy to use, easy to clean, and comfortable.

Look at the frame. The legs should be widely separated. You should jiggle the tray and tip the chair over from the rear and front to check for stability and collapsibility. (You'll find that folding models, which are easier to store, will not be as sturdy.) The front or the rear legs, or both, should have a stabilizing crossbar. The chrome finish should have an even, glossy look and feel.

Pinch the vinyl in the seat padding between your thumb and index finger. If you can pull the vinyl up off the padding, chances are it's too thin and will eventually tear with use. The foam padding should be firm. Make sure heat-sealed edges on the upholstery aren't scratchy. Avoid chairs that have decorative welting, which will trap food particles and make cleaning difficult (it won't take you long to realize that food gets caught everywhere it can).

Look for trays that have spill-resistant rims rather than trays without rims or trays with chromed railings and decorative plastic beads. A large wraparound tray that gives support to the child's elbows is best. Remove the tray and put it back on several times to see if it's easy to use. Test its fastening strength by first locking the tray and then trying to remove it from a number of positions while it's locked. If the tray latches with wide coils, they should be covered, so small fingers can't possibly get caught in them. Avoid chairs with trays that require you to bend over in order to place the tray correctly on its railing. Check the underside of the tray for sharp edges, pinching latches, or vinyl parts that may tear where they are bolted to the tray. Look for small pieces that could break off the tray if it should fall. And choose a tray that is dishwasher-safe, immersible, and resistant to scratches. A vinyl tray creates a quieter surface for a beginning drummer than does a metal one.

The chair should have both waist and crotch belts—preferably a pair in which the waist belt

crashing down on a small head or hand when hit by an active baby.

If a high chair does meet the safety standards (which are voluntary), it will have a label saying it complies with the F-404 Safety Standards for High Chairs as certified by the American Society for Testing and Materials. Chairs meeting safety standards will incorporate these safety features:

• There is a locking device to prevent a folding chair from accidentally collapsing when it is in the sitting position.

• The joints of the frame have no scissoring action that could cause injury when the chair is being collapsed.

• It has sturdy restraining straps.

• The chair is stable and will not topple if a child climbs up by the footrest.

• It can support up to one hundred pounds on the seat and fifty pounds on the footrest.

threads through the crotch belt. These prevent dangerous falls and entrapment of a baby between the seat base and the tray, which can be fatal. Try the belting system. It should fit over the baby's abdomen, not her legs; it should be easy to thread; and the belt latch should hold securely when you push it up or down or pull it outward, as a baby will.

You can also purchase a fabric "safe chair" in a well-stocked baby shop. It can be used in high chairs in restaurants, where there are often no straps, or it can be used to convert an ordinary chair into a high chair.

The high chair's footrest should be adjustable so that it can be used comfortably by a six-month-old as well as a two-year-old. Wire footrests are more durable than flexible vinyl ones, which tend to tear when weight is put on them. Check the finishing on the wire edges and avoid those with sharp undersides. The footrest should be removable or should flip out of the way under the chair to accommodate an older child; however, it should not be so easy to remove that it can't be trusted to hold the weight and movement of a climbing tot.

A few other things to consider: If there are caps protecting sharp edges or points, make sure they're difficult to remove. Evaluate the chair without the tray, too, since you'll probably want to use it at the dinner table before your toddler graduates to a regular chair.

Although wooden chairs are superior in stability and durability, they are plagued with problems. They tend to be difficult to clean, and there are frequently problems with latches breaking. The seat measurements on wooden chairs tend to make them uncomfortable for one- and two-year-olds, and they often have nonadjustable footrests that are far too low on the chair to service babies. They seldom have adequate crotch belts, and tend to rely on snap-on leather straps to connect the tray and seat. Wooden chairs with padded seats tend to have staples that fasten vinyl skirts to the seat. Unless you're willing to add extra padding for comfort and a harness or other restraining device, we don't recommend wooden high chairs.

You may want to use a feeding table instead of a high chair. They are closer to the ground, so there's less distance to fall; and since the child is propped in the middle of the square table, there is less chance of his falling in the first place. One

disadvantage is that you can't pull it up to the table when you want the baby to join the rest of the family for dinner. In addition, feeding tables are much larger than high chairs, and they can be awkward to have in small kitchens, even when they can be stored under the kitchen table when not in use. Bending over to feed a baby at a feeding table can be hard on the back, and getting a baby in and out of one is more difficult than with a high chair.

## Playpens

Playpens, now euphemistically referred to as "play yards," were once an essential part of standard baby equipment, but research shows they can actually inhibit a baby's mental development because they don't provide for continuous and varied stimulation. Playpens block the inborn drive to touch, to move, and to see. In fact, the "good" babies who sit quietly in the playpen for hours are the very ones who need more human contact and stimulation than the babies who object to confinement in the playpen.

That's not to say a playpen has no use. It's a good place to put your baby when momentary restraint is needed for a phone call, meal preparation, or perhaps housework. But it should be used sparingly. The ideal arrangement is a carefully child-proofed house where a younger baby can be allowed to exercise on a blanket on the floor and an older baby to roam under watchful eyes. It's important for babies to be able to practice pulling up and crawling in an unrestrained environment. You can talk to your baby as you work around the house and give him physical freedom. This will provide an excellent learning environment for him.

Many families find that the playpen soon becomes a bulky, possibly unsafe toy depository that takes up space in the living room or nursery. Indeed, there are over three thousand playpen injuries every year that are serious enough to require emergency room treatment. Safety standards for playpens are voluntary, so manufacturers aren't required to meet them; those that do tag their products to notify buyers.

There are two basic types of playpens: those constructed of wood and those made with metal tubing and nylon mesh. Wooden playpens are usually heavier than mesh-sided playpens; they fold down when their two hinged sides sandwich inward as the two floor panels lift up from the cen-

### A dangerous mesh playpen

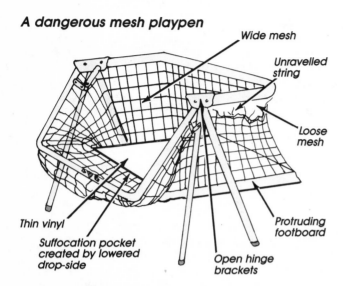

Wide mesh

Unravelled string

Loose mesh

Thin vinyl

Suffocation pocket created by lowered drop-side

Protruding footboard

Open hinge brackets

### A safe mesh playpen

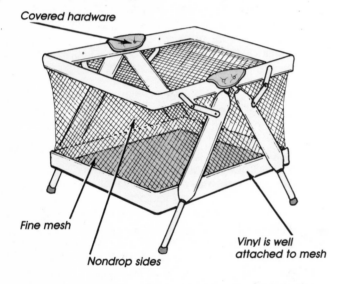

Covered hardware

Fine mesh

Nondrop sides

Vinyl is well attached to mesh

ter. Mesh-sided playpens call for a variety of folding maneuvers, in some cases even requiring that the playpen be turned completely upside down.

Mesh-sided playpens come in a variety of sizes and shapes, from rectangular crib-size models to larger square and multipaneled designs. The supportive tubing of the playpen is usually constructed of chrome, chrome-plated metal, or aluminum. Some models have straight legs with caps to protect the floor, while others have a bent-tube design; some of the latter may have uncovered metal U-joints that cause floor abrasion and rust stains.

Most soft-sided playpens use vinyl with heat-welted seams for a border at the base of the mesh

(providing draft protection) and at the top of the playpen to cover the hinge assembly and the bars. More expensive models have thick foam padding between the vinyl and the bars to prevent injuries to babies should they fall.

If you decide to buy a playpen, keep the following points in mind:

*Railings*
- Railings should be able to support fifty pounds without breaking or bending.

- There should be a locking device to prevent the playpen from collapsing accidentally.

- Side railings should be at least twenty inches tall to prevent a baby from climbing out.

- The playpen should come with a locking device to prevent it from accidentally folding up or the sides being lowered by the baby.

- Unlocking the sides should require a dual action.

- There should be no scissoring, cutting, or pinching potential at the hinges.

*Vinyl*
- Older models and second-hand vinyl-covered playpens often have vinyl on the top rail that, if torn, the baby could bite off and choke on.

- Make sure the vinyl upholstery is thick, is not torn, and has no holes. There are hundreds of incidents every year of babies biting off sections of vinyl and ingesting or aspirating them. Pinch the vinyl between your fingers. Thick vinyl is difficult to crease and will feel heavy when separated from the padding; thin vinyl will crease easily and is less durable.

- Make sure vinyl seams are heat-welted or stitched. Look for seams that are smooth to the touch. Heat-welted seams should appear even to ensure there's no problem with splitting. Machine-stitched seams should leave no dangling threads, gaps, or holes where the stitching has missed the vinyl.

*Floors*
- Floors should be strong enough to withstand eighty pounds of static weight.

- Floors should be able to withstand fifty pounds of bouncing weight without giving way.

- Be sure there are no metal staples or hardware in the floor that could be pulled loose and swallowed.

- See that there are no sharp bolt heads that your baby could fall on if the padding were to slip out of place.

*Edges*
- There should be no sharp edges, protrusions, or points that could hurt a baby.

## On wooden playpens:
- Slats should be spaced no more than 2³/₈ inches apart (like crib slats).

- Wooden surfaces should be finished well and be splinter-free.

- Wooden playpens provide babies with a better view, back support, and bars that can help them pull up into a standing position.

- As with cribs, there is the potential that babies can hit their head on the bars.

- Wooden playpens are heavy and awkward to move, but much safer than mesh ones.

- There should be teething rails on all four sides, and they should adhere securely so little fingers cannot get under them.

## On mesh playpens:
- Be sure the mesh is tightly woven so clothing can't catch in it, which could result in strangulation.

- When the mesh is woven tightly enough to be safe, the baby's view is limited, and the world outside the pen will be a blur.

- There is a potentially fatal suffocation pocket between the mesh and the mattress when the drop-side is down. Also, with the drop-side down, children have cut or pinched their fingers in the locking mechanism.

## Equipment and Equipment Safety

### Strollers and Carriages

Having a stroller will make long walks a lot easier. If you're going to be packing the stroller in the

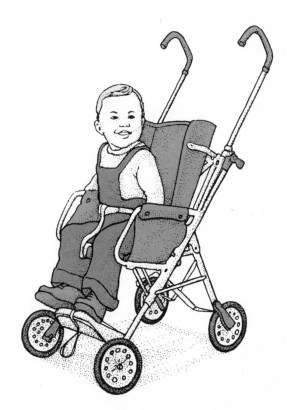

*A well-made stroller is an invaluable piece of baby equipment.*

car, you'll want to invest in a high-quality, lightweight model. These strollers are known as umbrella strollers because of the handles, which look like umbrella handles. They have lightweight aluminum frames and weigh as little as five pounds.

If you live in the city, and you'll primarily be using the stroller for walks over cracked sidewalks and curbs, you may want a standard-size stroller for its sturdiness. The larger models will also hold more packages than umbrella strollers, and they often have trays that hold toys or snacks, sunshades, multiple-position reclining seat backs, and plastic windbreakers to cover the sides.

You can get both the collapsibility of the lightweight umbrella-handle strollers and the postural support and durability of the larger, heavier models by buying one of the new medium-weight models.

Strollers are not without hazards. In one recent five-year span, there were more than forty thousand stroller-related emergency room visits in the United States. The major cause of injury is from babies falling out of strollers and hitting their heads.

Babies' fingers can become entrapped or crushed in the scissoring action of the joints as the stroller is being folded. Babies have also been injured by falling into protruding sharp edges of bolts and other metal parts. Also, many strollers, particularly the umbrella styles, are unstable and can fall over backward when a baby stands or attempts to stand up in the seat.

The Juvenile Products Manufacturers Association has established a voluntary safety standard for strollers and carriages. Since these standards are voluntary, not all stroller manufacturers have adopted them. And don't be lulled into thinking that the standards are what they could be. There are no provisions for the quality of the restraining belt or latch. While the standards require brakes, there are no safety measures to prevent another child from accidentally releasing them. Also, there is no protection offered from the scissoring action of joints or from sharp holes in the metal tubing that could capture a child's finger, nor is there any specification for how securely caps or other pro-

tective devices must be attached to the stroller's tubing and hardware.

Strollers and carriages that do meet safety standards:

- Shouldn't have any exposed coil springs that could pinch or otherwise injure a child.

- Should have a locking device that prevents accidental collapse.

- Should come with safety belts that are attached securely to the frame or the upholstery.

- Should be stable and unlikely to tip over when on an inclined surface with a child inside.

- Should have a permanently attached warning that reads: "Caution: Secure child in the restraint. Never leave child unattended."

When shopping for a stroller, look for the following features:

- *Steering ease*—Try pushing the stroller around to see how well it turns corners and how easily it maneuvers if you use only one hand. The stroller should handle well without veering to either side. A stroller with a single crossbar is easier to handle than one with umbrella-type handles.

- *Stability*—The stroller should be stable and unlikely to tip over when in use. If the stroller has a reclining seat, it should not be able to tip backward when the baby lies down.

- *Collapsibility*—Don't hesitate to try opening and collapsing the stroller before you buy it. You should be able to fold the stroller and open it up again in one or two steps while you hold your baby. If a stroller is going to be difficult and time-consuming to operate, you need to know that before you buy it. Make sure there's a locking device so the stroller can't collapse accidentally.

- *Seating*—Compare the thickness of vinyl upholstery on several different models by pinching it. The vinyl should be thick, and all seams should be well finished. The crotch belt, in particular, should be reinforced where it joins the seat. The seat should be shallow enough to provide back support for a six- to eighteen-month-old baby.

### Stroller

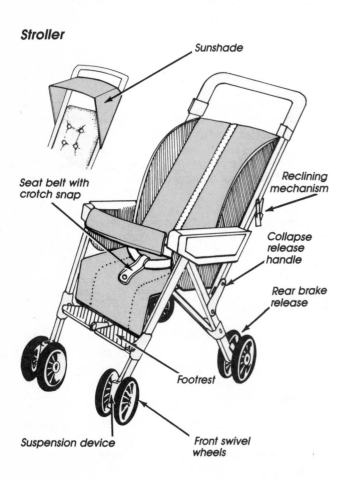

Sunshade

Reclining mechanism

Collapse release handle

Rear brake release

Seat belt with crotch snap

Footrest

Suspension device

Front swivel wheels

- *Reclining feature*—Very young babies tend to hunch forward in a sling-type stroller seat. Tots, too, have a hard time napping in an upright position. It's useful to be able to move the stroller seat into a reclining position. If the stroller does recline, it should have sides to prevent the child from rolling out, even in the lowest position.

- *Seat belt*—The seat belt should actually make contact with even the smallest baby's waist. The belt material should be strong, and the latches either heat-welted or sewn with multiple seams. The latch should be simple for you to operate and yet require enough pressure to open so a curious tot couldn't release it accidentally.

- *Front padding or tray*—Some strollers have plastic trays. Those that feature small balls fastened by plastic or thin wire aren't satisfactory since the balls could splinter or be ingested if they were pulled loose. If a bumper pillow replaces the tray, check underneath to see that it's securely fastened to the front bar. Pads often pull off, tearing out the screw bed so they can't be refastened.

- *Sunshade*—Some strollers come equipped with a sunroof, though often the roof is placed so high that it's useful only during the noon hour. If you plan to use the stroller in the sun, you may want to invest in a flexible-arm umbrella shade, which is offered as an option by some manufacturers.

- *Wheels and suspension*—Wheels with plastic spokes do not hold up well. Opt for steel or aluminum hubs. Suspension systems are seldom available on medium-weight strollers, but heavyweight models may offer springs or other types of shock absorbers, which will give your baby a less jarring ride.

- *Brakes*—Brakes should offer a positive grip on the tires so they can't be dislodged. The child should not be able to release the brakes while seated in the stroller.

Baby carriages conjure up images of prams and nannies and walks in the park. A carriage allows you to take long, leisurely walks, even when the baby is very small. Its high sides and hood help protect the baby from side drafts and bright sunlight, and the soothing bounce from the carriage springs often helps babies sleep.

### Carriage

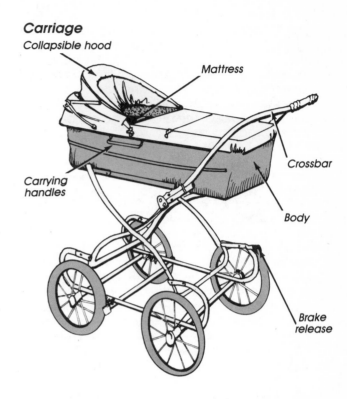

Collapsible hood

Mattress

Crossbar

Body

Carrying handles

Brake release

However, before you run out to buy a carriage, consider a few things: Carriages are quite expensive, and you'll use a carriage for only the first few months. They weigh quite a bit, making them awkward to use and awkward to store. If you're bringing one along on a trip, you'll have to collapse it to get it into the trunk of your car. Unless you live where there are winding country roads, traffic and curbs present maneuverability challenges for carriages.

If you decide to purchase a carriage, look for the following features:

- *Fabric*—Choose a thick, moisture-resistant fabric, such as one coated in vinyl that can be easily wiped clean.

- *Steering*—Try rolling the carriage around to see how easily it maneuvers. When you press on the bar, you should be able to raise the front wheels high enough to get up and over curbs.

- *Mattress*—If the mattress pad is covered in vinyl, test the thickness of the vinyl by pinching it between your fingers; it should be difficult to crease. Check the finishing on the pad to see that the seams are tightly sewn, with no danger of unraveling. The pad should fit flush against all sides of the interior of the carriage.

- *Brakes*—The brakes should hold firmly, preferably on both back wheels, and should not disengage even when you attempt to push the carriage forward. The brake handle should be easy to reach without having to let go of the carriage handle.

- *Interior safety*—There should be no sharp edges from frame hardware inside the carriage bed that could hurt a baby's head if she's jostled during maneuvering.

- *Folding ease*—The most economical unit is a two-piece carriage that doubles as a carry bed. Try collapsing and setting up the carriage to see how easy it is to handle. Examine the safety locks to be sure that they will prevent the carriage from folding accidentally and will hold the carry bed securely. There should be no sharp edges that could hurt your baby's fingers or your own.

- *Frame safety*—Avoid carriages that have a sharp scissoring action of metal against metal X-joints. These joints can cause crushed fingers when collapsed.

Whether you choose to buy a carriage or a stroller, you can protect your investment from rust by coating chrome areas lightly with petroleum jelly.

## Car Seats

Car seats save lives and prevent serious injury to infants and small children. While states regulate their use, the federal government regulates the construction of car seats. Child seats must meet federal standards that are based on dynamic, rather than static, testing.

Car seats come in three basic designs: *infant seats, shields,* and *harnesses.* Infant seats position the baby in a half-upright position, facing rearward. The baby is secured in the carrier by a harness, and the carrier is strapped to the seat with a lap belt. These seats are usually placed in the front passenger seat. When the child is old enough to sit unsupported, he should be placed in a seat that sits him straight up, facing frontward. The carrier should be placed in the back seat. Either a shield or harness seat can be used. The shield type has a protector, which is lowered in front of the child. It is padded on the inside surface to guard the child in a crash. Because it requires only the safety belt to lock it in place, it is easy to use. Older children can get in and out themselves, which is an advantage for the busy mother. For younger children, though, the shield type can be uncomfortable, because there is little arm room and it is difficult to see above it.

The harness type holds the child in the seat with two shoulder straps, two lap straps, and one crotch strap, all of which converge on a buckle. The seat itself is held in place by the lap belt and may have a tethering strap as well. It is comfortable for the child, but adjusting the straps can sometimes be a nuisance. There are other seats that combine the harness and shield, so that the adjustment difficulties of the harness and the discomfort of the shield are minimized.

When buying a car seat, there are a number of factors to consider. Besides looking for the best seat at the lowest price, you will need a seat that will be comfortable for your child, that can be secured in your car, and that is easy to use. First,

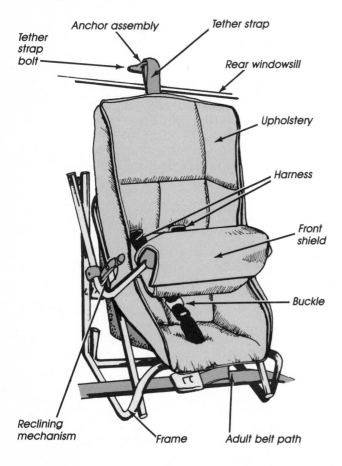

*Tether strap bolt*

*Anchor assembly*

*Tether strap*

*Rear windowsill*

*Upholstery*

*Harness*

*Front shield*

*Buckle*

*Reclining mechanism*

*Frame*

*Adult belt path*

**Car seat**

check the construction of the seat. Be sure it meets federal standards (car seats that do are labeled as such). The most durable seats are those with molded seat shells and tubular steel underframing. To save money, consider buying a convertible seat, with dual positions for infants and children, rather than buying two separate seats. Next, check the seat to be sure your child is comfortable in it. She should have enough arm room, and the seat should be high enough so that she can see out the car windows easily. This not only helps keep her entertained, but helps to prevent car sickness. Be sure the seat fits in your car and that your lap belts are long enough to secure it. Some seats require a tether. While this type of seat is superior in safety, it does require the installation of a bolt in the car to anchor it. Be sure you can, and want to, install this. Check the number of straps, and be sure they are easily adjustable. Check the latch of the seat for ease of operation.

Whichever kind of seat you choose, be sure to use it each and every time your child is in the car—and use it properly. The seat must be anchored appropriately to the car, including using the tether strap if applicable, and the child must be secured correctly in the restraint. Improperly used, a seat becomes a missile, causing more injury than if the child were unrestrained.

There are other advantages to car seats besides safety. Children in car seats are better behaved than unrestrained children. While this is a benefit in itself, well-behaved children are also less of a distraction to the driver and thereby contribute to overall auto safety. In addition, children accustomed to riding in car seats are more likely to use seat belts when they get older. Teaching your children good habits now thus may contribute to their future safety.

You should exercise similar care when shopping for and when using other safety restraint items, such as baby bicycle seats (the kind that attach behind your own) and bicycle helmets. Never scrimp on quality in order to save a few dollars. Solid construction and secure fasteners are vital.

## Backpacks, Slings, and Wrap Carriers

Devices that allow the baby to be carried directly on the parent have been around since ancient times, when people found ways to strap their babies to their bodies so they could free their hands and arms for other tasks. The rhythmic movement of the parent can be relaxing to a col-

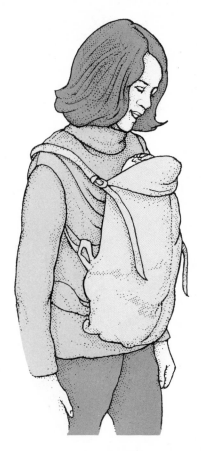

*A soft carrier will free your hands and soothe your newborn or young baby.*

icky or distressed baby, and at the same time can evoke a feeling of tenderness in the parent.

Wearing a frontpack or backpack requires gradual muscular adjustment on the part of the parent. The packs don't lessen the sense of weight; they simply place all the weight on the shoulders instead of the arms. Over time, this strengthens a parent's leg, neck, and shoulder muscles.

Packs function best on hikes and long walks, and are terrific in places where strollers and carriages would be bulky and awkward. But they can be clumsy in confined situations, such as in stores or at home.

Once a child can sit up, a backpack is more comfortable for the parent than an infant carrier and also allows the child to have a view of more than just his parent's shirt. Backpacks are made to accommodate children weighing up to twenty-five pounds.

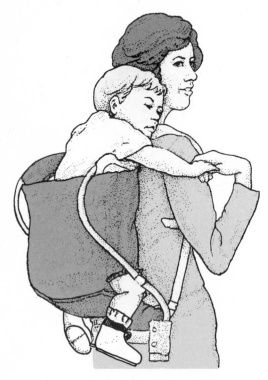

*An older baby can see the world from a tubular-frame backpack.*

Getting the baby in the pack and putting it on will take practice and, initially, someone else's help. Most parents balance the pack on a knee and place one arm into the appropriate strap before swinging the baby and pack around to put the other strap on. Others back into the pack, which they have placed in a chair with the baby already in it. All packs come with directions to help you adjust the pack to fit and to guide you in learning to shift the baby and the pack onto your back. Brisk walking with a baby in a frame carrier is far more comfortable than passive activities that require standing still with the pack on.

There are two basic types of packs: those made solely of fabric and those with tubular metal frames.

*Soft carriers* are especially useful for the newborn and the young baby, who will usually be soothed by the involvement with your body's rhythmic movement. Some are designed to have the baby facing outward, away from your body, but most carriers snuggle your baby close to your chest, which is preferable for a very young baby. While you can use a fabric carrier with an older, heavier baby, it will feel like a heavier burden on your shoulders.

*Tubular-frame backpacks* are made especially for babies over six months of age, who can sit up and like viewing the world over your shoulders. The frame helps to redistribute some of your baby's weight off your shoulders and onto your back or hips.

When shopping for a soft carrier, look for the following:

- The fabric should be heavyweight and completely washable. Corduroy, cotton, polyester, and denim are excellent.

- Seams should be well finished, especially at stress points, such as where the straps are fastened to the pack.

- The carrier should be easy to put on, and it should fit. Some models will have shoulder straps that are spaced too far apart or are too long. Try it out in the store.

- The strap fastening should be heavy-duty, preferably made of metal. It should be easy to adjust and should be able to hold the baby's weight securely.

- The crotch width of the seat should not force the baby's legs into an uncomfortably splayed position, and the leg holes should be very soft and should not be higher than the seat, which could cut off circulation to the baby's legs.

- The carrier should adjust to accommodate a growing baby, either by letting out seams or by adjusting straps. Read the directions and experiment before you buy it.

- The shoulder pads should be thick and firm for maximum comfort.

- There should be a head support built in to prevent the baby's head from flopping.

- Some carriers have discreet zippers for nursing so you don't have to take the baby out. Other carriers have instructions for how to use the carrier while breast-feeding.

A tubular-frame pack should offer:

- Very thick shoulder pads to keep the straps from gouging your shoulders.

- A good fit—try the pack on to see how its length and width fit your body size. It should feel comfortable with the baby in it; you shouldn't feel the top rail digging into your backbone or the frame interfering with your arm movements.

- Correct strap positions—the straps should hit you directly on top of the muscles halfway between your neck and the end of your shoulders. If the straps are too widely set, it will cause undue postural stress. If they are too narrow, they may cause chafing and constriction around your neck.

- Seat design and leg holes that are comfortable for your baby—the crotch of the seat should be narrow enough not to force the baby's legs too far apart. The leg holes of the seat should be flush with the seat, not higher than the seat, so circulation to the baby's legs won't be cut off. The rims of the leg holes should be soft, not scratchy.

- There should be a sturdy, easy-to-operate seat belt to prevent your baby from standing up in the carrier.

- There should be padding on the front rail to protect your baby's gums and teeth when she mouths the front bar of the carrier frame as you walk.

- The fabric should be sturdy, stretch-resistant, and easy to clean. Make sure the seams, especially those around the top rail of the pack, are reinforced around high-stress points. This will ensure your baby's safety.

- A storage section at the base of the pack is a helpful feature.

- A pack with a padded pelvic belt helps to redistribute the weight from your shoulders onto your less vulnerable pelvic area. This is a worthwhile feature if you're going to be hiking or camping.

- Support stands are often pushed as a desirable feature. Some manufacturers claim the stand enables you to use the pack as an infant carrier. It doesn't. While the stands do help when putting the baby in the pack and mounting it on your back, they shouldn't be used as infant carriers because they're unstable and can topple over easily. If you do buy a pack with a stand, examine the hinge mechanism to be sure it can't capture or crush fingers in its scissoring action.

## Infant Seats

Infant seats are made from rigid molded plastic shells on plastic stands or are cloth, hammock-like seats sewn onto round frames. They hold the baby in a semi-upright position that is convenient for feeding and interaction, and they're easy to carry because of the rigid support they provide. Some infant seats are even designed to fit into the carts at the supermarket. They are good for infants up to five or six months of age.

As far as safety goes, there are about one thousand emergency room visits every year due to injuries, mostly to the head, when these seats slip off high surfaces, such as counters and tables. Occasionally, the seat supports give way, or the baby's movement causes the seat to fall. Many of these injuries could have been prevented if the baby had been properly fastened into the seat.

It's never a good idea to put an infant seat on a high surface; if you do, make sure the surface isn't slick, like the top of a washing machine. If you're going to turn your back, even for a second, put the infant seat down on the floor. Avoid buying infant seats that come with rockers or slender wire frames in the rear—they are potentially unstable. Also, never carry an infant seat by carry handles, which can fail or cause the seat to accidentally swing into a wall or a door. Infant seats, unless specified, cannot double as car restraints.

Look for an infant seat that has a nonskid bottom, so it won't slip off any surface. For greater stability, the base should be wider than the seat, and there should be some sort of supporting device in the back to prevent it from collapsing. There should be an adequate crotch and body belt with latches that won't slip. A seat that has several adjustable positions will be most useful. And look for one that's easy to clean, made of vinyl or other water-resistant material, so you can easily remove spills and crumbs.

## Jumpers and Swings

A jumper is a fabric or plastic seat that is suspended from a metal clamp on a door jamb via a combination of chains, springs, or rubber and fabric strips. The baby bounces from it, pushing off from the floor. Some babies don't like them; others do, and they will enjoy them until they can walk.

The problem with jumpers is that the clamp can release or the straps can fray and break, causing the baby to plunge to the floor or strike the door frame. Some of the seats put too much pressure on the baby's inner thigh, causing red marks or circulation problems. They're hard to set up, too, and prolonged use has produced vertigo, similar to seasickness, in babies. There's also a danger of whiplash. We don't recommend them.

Swings are a useful luxury item, especially for a colicky or fussy baby; they can be very soothing. There is usually a small seat, sometimes a mesh-sided bed, suspended from a four-legged metal stand. There is either a wind-up handle or a large plastic knob that tightens an interior spring mechanism that makes it swing. Some are battery-operated. The rhythmic motion soothes the baby—and the parents. One of the biggest drawbacks to swings is that they don't get used for very long, and they take up lots of room, which can be difficult in an apartment.

Swings should be used with proper belting and supervision. There is a danger that an unbelted baby can fall forward into the padded front bar and suffocate. They shouldn't be used with babies more than six months old, who may try to climb out or grab the sides, potentially causing the entire swing to fall. There have been a few reports of springs shattering, resulting in assembly parts in the top bar flying out, and of support legs collapsing. Parents have also reported bumping the baby's head in the process of getting her out of the seat.

Look for a swing that has the longest possible running time for each winding. It can be frustrating to get your baby lulled to sleep and have the swing stop, especially since many of the winding devices will startle the baby—so also look for one with a quiet wind-up mechanism. There should be padding on the front bar of the seat, and leg holes no higher than seat level, with smooth edging. Make sure the frame is wide and stable, preferably with locking side bars. Don't bother with an awning; you'll seldom use a swing outside, so the awning serves no purpose.

## Walkers

Walkers don't help babies walk any sooner. In fact, the leg actions required for a baby to use a walker have nothing to do with walking. Keeping a baby in a walker may actually impede the natural transition a baby will make from crawling to walking. Besides that, walkers can be downright dangerous. Each year, there are thousands of walker-related emergency room visits, many a result of walkers tipping over or falling down stairs. In the past, many injuries resulted from fingers getting caught in X-frames that collapsed. New regulations in 1972 required that all parts that could crush, lacerate, or sever fingers be covered, and that walkers be protected against accidental collapse.

The major problem with walkers is that the baby's mobility is increased and parents can't keep up with him. The baby can very quickly tip the walker over in the process of moving it over rugs, cords, or other obstacles. If you turn your back to answer the door, your baby could be heading for the stairs.

Walkers do give eight- to ten-month-olds an early taste of mobility, but the high risk of injury and the short period of time that they're even appropriate makes walkers a poor investment.

## Gates

For the most part, gates aren't safe, especially the kind with rubber gaskets that can fall down the stairs along with the baby, causing more injuries than if the baby fell alone. Gates with mesh can be climbed if the mesh isn't fine enough. Accordion-style gates present a tremendous pinching hazard to little fingers, and they're also quite climbable.

If you must gate off an area, the U.S. Consumer Product Safety Commission recommends gates that are made of climb-resistant mesh in a small diamond pattern and that have a straight top edge. These gates should be attached firmly to the wall with screws, not rubber gaskets. If you do use an accordion gate, use one that doesn't have to be stretched much; select the longest gate that will fit the doorway in the closed position (so the openings can't be climbed in), and install it with screws. A homemade gate of plywood with no crossbars will also work, as will a locking screen or wood door. All gates should be installed with minimal space between gate and floor so the baby can't get trapped trying to crawl under it.

If you're going to use a pressure gate, which we don't recommend, make sure the pressure bar side of the gate is away from the child, who could use it to climb on.

The best alternative to gates is to teach your baby to manage stairs as soon as she can crawl and have her practice with supervision. Install railings on the stairway at a height accessible to children who are eighteen months to five years old.

## Medicines, Toiletries, and Health Aids

Your initial supply list will look something like the one below. We've noted the reasons for some items, and we've also listed other items parents frequently assume they will need, along with our reasons for *not* having them on hand.

- Syrup of ipecac (replace every three years)

- Children's acetaminophen

- Children's aspirin (Never give a baby with a suspected viral infection aspirin. It has been implicated as a possible cause of Reye's syndrome.)

- Rubbing alcohol

- Petroleum jelly

- Baby lotion and baby oil (optional)

- Cornstarch or baby powder (To use, dust it onto your hands and then spread it on the diaper area. Never pour or squirt it on. If inhaled, the particles can be very irritating to the lungs. Also, keep the container out of baby's reach.)

- Ointment for diaper rash (After *thoroughly cleaning* the diaper area, ointment should be applied heavily to protect irritated areas against urine. Application without cleansing merely seals irritants against your baby's skin.)

- Cotton balls (NEVER use cotton swabs to clean nose or ears. Swabs may introduce infection and even puncture eardrums.)

- Diaper pail (and disinfectant if you're using cloth diapers)

- Plastic garbage bags to line diaper pail (if you're using disposable diapers)

- Diaper liners (helpful in early weeks if you're laundering diapers at home)

- Toilet paper for changing table (easier on plumbing than towelettes or tissues)

- Nasal aspirator

- Rectal thermometer

- Vaporizer, cool-mist type (optional)

- Baby scissors with rounded points

- Bar or liquid soap (Liquid soaps are easy to use with one hand. All soaps should be used sparingly to preserve the baby's own skin oils; a mild, nondrying soap is best.)

- Washcloths (six is a good number to start with)

- Hand towels (two or three)

- Baby shampoo

- Brush and comb

- A Bathinette or portable baby bath

A word or two about bathing. Newborn infants do not appreciate baths because of the abrupt temperature change. It's important to keep newborns warm and secure during bathing; sponge baths given under a blanket or a towel are best for the first month.

You don't really need to go out and buy a special tub for your baby. You can use the kitchen sink. However, specially designed baby bathtubs have slanted support areas for the baby that are covered with nonslip foam pads; these may be more comfortable. Their disadvantage is that they're difficult to move once they're filled, but if you can place the tub on the counter next to the sink, it won't be a problem.

When buying a baby bathtub, look for one with smooth, rounded edges. Don't buy one with all-sponge cushioning, since the sponge part can be torn off and eaten. Make sure the support area has a nonslip surface, and check to see that the tub is sturdy and will hold its shape when full. It will be a plus to find a tub that has recessed water channels on the sides so you can bathe the baby without immersing him. For more information about bathing your baby, see Chapter 7.

## Feeding Implements

Your basic shopping list will look something like this:

- Bottles or nursers (which you'll need for juice and water even if you're breast-feeding): one or two 8-ounce bottles and one 4-ounce bottle if you're breast-feeding; four to six 8-ounce bottles and two 4-ounce bottles if you'll be using formula

- Nipples to go with bottles and nursers, as well as some extras and one orthodontic nipple

- One long-handled feeding spoon (select one with a tiny bowl) and one short- or curve-handled spoon. The long-handled spoon will be easier for you to use while feeding your baby. Later, when the baby begins to feed herself, a stubbier spoon will prove easier for her tiny hands to grasp and control

- One bottle and nipple brush (One that has a large brush for bottles on one end and a smaller brush for nipples on the other end is handy.)

- Bibs—six of soft plastic, and three of firm, molded plastic with trough bottom for when baby gets a little older. Make sure any bib has well-finished edges and adjustable neck straps, not strings.

- Baby food grinder or strainer (optional)

- Vegetable steamer (This is useful if you're going to make your own baby food. You can buy these in a housewares department or in a health food store.)

- Blender (an excellent investment if you'll be making baby food; three speeds will suffice)

- Bottle warmer (optional, but may be useful in the first months or if the baby's room is far from the kitchen)

- Sterilizer kit

- Presterilized disposable nurser kit

- Baby dishes, electric or hot-water

- Measuring spoons and cups

- Pacifier (can help meet the baby's strong sucking needs and soothe him while he waits for the bottle)

- Training cup

Today, you can get clear and opaque plastic bottles as well as glass ones. Few parents still use the glass ones, but they do have their advantages. They're easier to clean, but, needless to say, they're breakable. The plastic ones tend to retain food odors. The opaque ones stain easily, and you can't see the amount of liquid in them. We recommend the clear plastic bottles. Don't bother with novelty bottles that come in fun shapes; they're very difficult to clean.

If your doctor recommends that you sterilize your baby's bottles, there are two ways it can be done. The sterile-field method involves sterilizing empty bottles and equipment and takes as little as twenty minutes. The terminal method involves sterilizing bottles already filled with formula, and takes sixty to ninety minutes. Either type of sterilization requires two hours cooling time. There are stove-top and electric sterilizers. Stove-top sterilizers are quicker. The danger with either type of sterilizer is that if the water totally evaporates, the plastic parts can ignite. Some electric models have safety cutoff mechanisms to prevent overheating; we think these are worth paying for.

You can skip the entire process by buying premixed prebottled formula, but you really end up paying for the added convenience. If you go this route, shop around and buy in quantity.

Nursers are bottle-like frames that hold plastic bags filled with liquid. They use wide-necked nipples that attach to the top of the frame and hold the bags in place. Their advantage is that they eliminate the need for scrubbing, but the bags can be damaged if liquids poured into them are too hot. Also, they've been known to leak, and it's hard to measure the amount of liquid in them.

Not all nipples are the same. The bottom line is to use the nipple your baby prefers. Nipples come in different lengths, and smaller babies will prefer shorter nipples—they may gag on nipples that are too long. Babies of breast-feeding mothers tend to accept nipples designed for premature babies more easily. If the hole in the nipple is too large, the baby may choke or thrust her tongue forward attempting to cut off the excess supply of liquid. If the hole is too small, she may be frustrated. You can enlarge a too-small hole by boiling the nipple for five minutes and then cooling it for three minutes with a toothpick lodged in the hole; if you make it too big, boil it again.

Orthodontic nipples have been touted as more natural, more like a mother's breast. They have bulbous tips with protruding rims that must be positioned at the top of the baby's mouth. They tend to deteriorate more quickly than other nipples because they're harder to clean.

All nipples will deteriorate over time as a result of exposure to saliva and milk products. Throw out nipples that show signs of stretching, peeling, or stickiness. Careful cleaning, thorough rinsing, and proper storage of them in a cool, dry place will prolong their life.

Breast-feeding, as pointed out at the beginning of the chapter, is more economical than bottle-feeding. It also provides the baby with more intimate contact, and research has shown it releases hormones in the mother that stimulate maternal, tender feelings. Human milk is especially suited to human babies, is easy to digest, and actually helps protect the baby from getting sick.

Breast-feeding supplies are minimal:

- Breast creams—aren't necessary. If your breasts get sore, the best healer is fresh air and pure hydrous lanolin.

- Rubber nipple shields—don't work well and interfere with the natural toughening process that eventually makes nursing more comfortable.

- Nursing bras—come in a variety of styles that either fasten in the front center or have fold-down flaps. Flaps are easier. Some women prefer to use an ordinary stretch bra that they simply lift up. Whatever your choice, wait until your ninth month of pregnancy or until after the baby has been born to find your size, since you won't be at your maximum size until then. If the bra is too tight, it will interfere with the downflow of milk and be uncomfortable. Look for a bra that is machine washable. If your breasts are very heavy, select one with large, wide straps and extra support, like underwires. Try on several types and buy up to six of the one that's most comfortable, since milk leakage during the first few months will necessitate frequent washing (a damp bra can stimulate bacterial growth).

- Breast pads—for milk leakage. You can use men's cotton handkerchiefs tucked into your bra or mini-pads cut in half. Commercial breast pads are more expensive, but those that are made of washable layered fabric aren't a bad investment. Disposable breast pads usually have plastic liners, which can irritate sore nipples by keeping moisture in.

- Breast pump—You may need to pump milk if you're going to be separated from your baby for prolonged periods. It's best to pump while the baby is nursing on the opposite breast. There are four kinds of breast pumps. Hand-operated pumps work with a rubber bulb for suction and can be purchased in drugstores. The problem with these is that they usually don't work well. To get them to work at all, you must use an intermittent, gentle, tugging action rather than continuous suction. Breast pumps that use piston or syringe cylinders also work with an intermittent tugging action, but are designed to be more effective than hand-operated pumps. Get one that has adapters for different breast sizes and bottles for storage. You may prefer a battery-operated pump; these are somewhat more expensive than hand-operated or piston pumps, but are quicker and easier to use. Electric pumps are very expensive and are usually used by hospitals. They can be rented by the month; if you have a premature baby in the hospital you want to be breast-feeding, this may be the way to go until he is home.

All babies have sucking urges that go beyond feeding, and this sucking urge is at its highest between three and seven months. By the age of two, most babies have lost the urge, except when they're under stress. Pacifiers may prevent thumb sucking and other undesirable sucking habits. However, there is the danger that the pacifier will come apart and pieces will become stuck in the throat. There have also been strangulations from ribbons or cords when pacifiers were hung around the baby's neck. New regulations require that there be two ventilation holes in the pacifier for air passage. The protrusions on the backs of shields must be a specific size to prevent ingestion, and the pacifier must be tested for durability to ensure that it won't come apart. There is also a warning on pacifiers that tells you not to tie the pacifier around your baby's neck because of the strangulation danger.

Once your baby gets a little older, you'll want to get her a training cup to make the transition from the bottle. The cup should have a snap-on lid with a narrow spout and wide handles. Look for cups that are dishwasher safe and preferably transparent. Avoid cups that look like toys; they will encourage play, not drinking.

You'll also want baby dishes. You can choose either electric or hot-water dishes. The electric ones should have temperature regulators to prevent overheating, and they should have a cold section. If you're using an electric dish, always unplug the cord from the wall socket before unplugging the dish. If you use a hot-water dish, make sure the spout cap locks firmly so that the baby can't pull it out and ingest it. Either kind should be completely immersible and preferably dishwasher safe, for easy cleaning. Dishes with steep sides and suction bases to prevent sliding will be easier for self-feeding. Feeding spoons used for a child who is beginning to feed herself should have semi-flat bowls and weighted handles that can be easily gripped by chubby little hands. Avoid spoons with rubber bowls; they taste bad.

## Additional Equipment for Ages One Through Three

### Toilet-Training Equipment

Successful toilet training will be a combination of good timing (the child must be ready) and the parents' understanding of the complexity of the process (being able to break it down into a series of simple tasks). For most children, the ideal time is around two years of age—a time when they can follow verbal instructions, have good muscle control, and take pride in doing things by themselves. The how-to's of toilet training are covered in Chapter 11.

What you'll need is really not much. Training pants aren't necessary, because they shrink a lot when washed, making them hard to take off. They're also bulky, like diapers—a child may forget that wetting her pants is no longer acceptable. Buy regular children's underwear to mark the transition and instill some pride in your child about growing up.

You can buy either a potty that sits on the floor or a seat that adapts to the adult flush toilet. There are arguments for and against each. Generally, children who have older siblings are more motivated to use the adult toilet because they want to be grown up like their brothers and sisters; they often do very well with the adapter seat. Children who don't have older siblings often experience a fear of heights on the adapter seat, and some have a real fear of all that flushing. The adapter seat is more portable and obviously doesn't involve emptying, but if it fits poorly, it can slip or break, causing the child to fall off or in. Also, children often tend to urinate off to the side, wetting the adult seat or the floor. No difference in ease of training has ever been found between adapter seats and potties, so the choice is yours.

Go on a preliminary shopping trip for the potty or seat. When you've whittled it down to two choices, bring your child with you to assist in the final selection. Have your child sit on the seats to see which is most comfortable. This will give him an investment in what's about to take place.

If you're looking at adapter seats, take them from the package to be sure the edges are smooth and round and not sharp. There should be a flexible front shield for boys, preferably of a rubber-like material that won't hurt if your son bumps against it. The catches holding the seat on should be rubberized or of some other nonscratch material to prevent damaging the adult seat. If you're buying an adapter seat, you'll also need to buy a footstool so your child can climb up to the seat.

Potties are portable and easy for children to use. Look for one with a seat top that can later be used as an adapter seat. Potties with plastic seats are superior to those with wooden ones; they're easier to clean and fit children better. Find one with a wide base for increased stability. Also, rubber tips under the potty will prevent it from sliding as your child backs onto it. Make sure all edges are smoothly finished, and check to see that the splash guard is flexible. Potties with top loading chambers are best because they're easier to empty without spills; in fact, children can eventually learn to empty these themselves.

### Table and Chair

Get rid of the high chair as soon as you can, since all high chairs present a risk of falls. Besides, once your child is two, she will consider the high chair a prison. Having a chair and table of her own will allow a child to spread out her things for work, play, or eating, making it a very important piece of equipment.

Buy the largest table you can afford or have room for, definitely no smaller than twenty by thirty inches. Many suppliers make sturdy tables and matching chairs for children. Some even have adjustable legs. But you don't have to buy something that's sold as a child's table. One mother covered a Parsons table with oilcloth and then bought a few sturdy child-size chairs to go with it. The chart that follows specifies heights for tables and chairs at different ages, but if you can afford only one set, and you can't find one with adjustable legs, go with a table that's at least twenty-two to twenty-four inches high and a seat that's about thirteen inches high. There should always be eight to ten inches of room between the chair seat and the table.

| Age (in years) | Table Height (in inches) | Chair Seat Height (in inches) |
|---|---|---|
| 1½ to 2 | 17 | 9 |
| 2 to 3 | 18 | 10 |
| 3 to 4 | 20 | 12 |
| 4 to 5 | 26 | 17 |

*Shelves for Toys, Books, and Other Belongings*
Buy sturdy shelves with no sharp edges. The shelves should be affixed low on the wall, so a child can't pull things down on his head. It's a good idea to store soft things, like stuffed animals, on the highest shelves.

*Toy Chests*
Though toy chests are immensely practical (and useful for teaching a small child to put her belongings away), they are not without hazards. The two most prominent dangers are *sharp edges* that could injure your baby if she should fall against the toy chest, and a *tight-fitting lid* that could fall and trap your baby inside, suffocating her. Though the possibility of the latter may seem remote, it is a very real danger.

When choosing a toy chest, look for the following features:

• Sturdy construction

• Smooth surfaces, with no sharp corners or edges

• A gap of at least a half-inch between the closed lid and the chest

• A hydraulic closure that will prevent the lid from slamming onto your baby's head

Be sure that the inside of the box has no latch or other locking mechanism that could trap your child inside. Ideally, the chest's lid should be light enough for a baby to push it upward with little effort.

If you're unable to find a commercially manufactured toy chest that suits your specifications,

consider making one yourself, or having one custom made. Finally, don't pass your own old toy chest (or anyone else's) on to your baby unless you are certain it is safe.

## The Diaper Dilemma

When you figure you're going to go through approximately six thousand diapers in the first two and one-half years of your baby's life, it makes sense to spend some time focusing on what you're going to use for diapers. There are three alternatives: disposables, cloth diapers that you launder yourself, and diaper services that supply and launder cloth diapers for you, and offer pickup and delivery service.

Since you'll be going through about sixty-five diapers a week during the first year, it makes good sense to use a diaper service, which would save you either laundering time or the extra expense of that many disposables. During the second year, when laundering cloth diapers doesn't require the extra rinses that may be necessary for some hypersensitive newborns, laundering your own diapers might be more practical. Then, in the third year, until toilet training is complete, disposables will be handy and lessen your impatience about the training process, taking the pressure off your child. When it's all over, the old diapers make wonderful cleaning rags!

Regardless of what you use for a diaper, you'll inevitably run into diaper rash. It's caused by a combination of moisture, warmth, and contact between the skin and irritants in urine and stool. Plastic or rubber aggravates it; cool, dry air makes it better. Most experts assert that disposable diapers, which don't "breathe" like cloth ones, lead to more frequent and more severe diaper rash. So, if you're using disposables and your baby gets diaper rash, you might want to switch to cloth for a while.

Another diaper danger is the substances that your baby may eat or inhale in the process of diapering. Usually what happens is that the "diaperer" hands the baby something to hold for entertainment, or the baby grabs it himself. The baby then ingests or inhales the baby powder, the ointment or cream, or the baby wipes. Symptoms can include coughing, wheezing, choking, shortness of breath, and vomiting. It's important to keep these products away from the baby while diapering. For additional information about diapers and diapering, see Chapter 7.

## Disposables

Environmentalists have raised a lot of questions about disposables because they are not biodegradable and can't be recycled. They also cause a public health hazard, since viruses present in excrement can be spread to those who collect the trash. And after disposable diapers are dumped at a landfill site, viruses can be carried into water supplies.

Some disposables (particularly generic brands) keep the skin warmer and moister than cloth diapers (no brand has been found that really keeps a baby dry), and may cause more frequent and more severe diaper rash. Disposable diapers in general can be expensive—up to thirty-two cents per diaper.

On a more positive note, disposables do save a lot of work, and they are more convenient. They eliminate the need for plastic pants, and they're much easier to use when traveling. Because there are no pins, less experienced family members are often more willing to change them.

If you choose to use disposables, here are some guidelines:

- Sample different brands. Start with a variety in the newborn size until you find one that fits well and has the softness and quality you like. Name brands will usually be more consistent in quality.

- Don't use brands that clump, shred, or bunch up when wet, since your baby could ingest loose paper pieces.

- Brands that don't allow any plastic to touch the baby's skin are better for preventing rash.

- Once you've found a brand you like, shop around for a good discount, and then buy by the case.

- Inspect each diaper for impurities, discolorations, and foreign materials in the paper padding.

- Create air holes. Since air circulation is the biggest problem with disposables, pinch out a piece of the plastic liner in the seat area. This will allow air to circulate, and it will also make it easier for you to tell when the baby needs to be changed.

- Use the weight and size charts on the box to determine fit. Diapers with elastic legs aren't necessary, but they do help prevent leakage. As you fasten the diaper, make sure the leg holes are not too constricting.

- Some disposables supposedly have parts that can be easily flushed. These don't work well. Nonetheless, you should try to flush as much from the diaper as possible. Then tightly roll up the diaper so the soiled area is not open to the air, and seal the diaper with diaper tape before throwing it out.

- Garbage cans should be lined with plastic bags, which should be tied and sealed tightly for disposal. Garbage cans that have locking lids are good; they keep curious tots out.

- Diapers with refastenable tape are convenient, but not necessary if you keep a small roll of strapping or masking tape and safety-tipped scissors handy.

## Home-Laundered Cloth Diapers

Buying diapers and washing them yourself is the cheapest way to resolve the diaper dilemma. You can cut costs even more by:

- Using ordinary detergent (instead of special detergent for diapers);

- Avoiding fabric softeners, which can trigger skin reactions in your baby;

- Using bleach sparingly. Never pour it directly onto diapers; concentrated bleach decreases the life of the diaper fabric.

To help prevent diaper rash, be sure to *thoroughly* dry diapers before folding them and putting them away.

Diapers come in three different types of fabric: bird's-eye, gauze, and flannel. Bird's-eye is the softest and most absorbent. It's a tightly woven, textured cotton, usually in a diamond pattern. It's either sealed on the edges or pinked. Gauze is a fine, loose, open-weave fabric, usually with pinked, unfinished edges. Flannel is thick and has a soft nap to it. Babies find it the most comfortable.

There are two styles, flat and prefolded. The flat diapers are a single, large piece of fabric. They are more absorbent, they dry more quickly, and, because you fold them to fit, they can be more easily adjusted as your baby grows. But, they're also more difficult to use since they require some know-how to fold, and they take up more storage space. The prefolded style has folds that are stitched in place. There are usually several layers in the center and fewer at the sides, for comfort. They're much easier to use.

If you're using cloth diapers:

• Start with about three dozen regular-size diapers. You'll have to fold them double for newborns, but you'll be able to use them throughout babyhood.

• Select heavier-weight fabrics. Diapers come in packages of a dozen, so compare package weights.

• Waterproof pants are essential for keeping bedding and clothing dry. You'll need three pairs in the newborn size to start with. The kind that snap are easier to put on and provide for more air circulation than the pull-up type.

• Diaper liners are disposable inserts that are handy for night diapering, eliminating the need for double diapering.

## Diaper Services

Diaper services are not nearly as expensive as disposables, but are more costly than home laundering. They're a good compromise between buying more than two years' worth of disposables and the cost and labor of home laundering.

Diaper rash is less of a problem with diaper services because of the high temperatures and strong detergents they use. If your baby is having chronic diaper rash problems, it might be a good idea to switch to a service for a while. Also, using a service during the first year, when laundering can be very labor-intensive, makes a lot of sense.

Most services allow you to choose diapers for your baby that will be exclusively yours while you use the service. They usually pick up and drop off diapers once or twice a week, and provide you with a diaper pail, a mesh bag, and deodorant cakes. You can call to reserve the number of diapers you'll need before your baby comes home from the hospital.

## Diaper Fasteners

Diaper pins carry with them the danger of a puncture injury to your baby. When diapering, always be sure to keep your finger between the pin and the baby's skin to avoid an accidental stabbing. Most accidental injuries occur when the pins get dull and the diaperer is using extra pressure to get the pins through the diapers. Occasionally sticking the pins in soap or petroleum jelly will help, but dull pins and pins that show signs of rusting should be discarded and replaced.

The best pins are those with safety locks that snap down over metal latch sections. Buy several pairs. Avoid diaper pins that have plastic tops in decorative shapes. These are unsafe because the plastic becomes brittle and chips off, exposing the sharp edge of the pin.

## Clothes and Clothing Safety

New parents usually receive a lot of clothes as gifts. Unfortunately, some of the more popular gift items aren't very useful to or popular with babies. If you receive things you don't need, try to take them back to the place of purchase and exchange them for things you do need.

When purchasing baby clothes, it's a good idea to stick to one color scheme. Bright colors are unisex, more easily seen, and less easily soiled than pastels. They're a really good idea for outerwear—it's a lot easier to see a child wearing a bright red jacket in a busy supermarket than one wearing light pink.

Be practical. Babies aren't neat, so you're going to want everything to be machine washable, no matter how cute it is. And speaking of cute, fancy clothes aren't practical at all since they often interfere with movement and aren't comfortable. Clothes made of cotton and other natural fabrics are more comfortable, especially in hot weather. Clothes that have buckle fasteners are better than those with buttons; buckles can be adjusted as the child grows, but buttons have to be moved.

When shopping, keep in mind that more expensive clothes are not necessarily better. You'll have to examine each item, especially since baby sizes are not standardized. Don't be afraid to remove items from plastic packaging. Check to see if the seams are well finished and the stitching is strong. Knit fabrics should be strong, not flimsy.

Good sources of clothes are thrift shops and other parents who won't be having any more children. Both will often have infant wear that's next to new. You'll want to thoroughly wash previously used items once or twice and perhaps use a little bleach.

The problem with hand-me-down or used sleepwear is determining whether it was treated with a fire retardant, and what the retardant was. One retardant, Tris, was banned by the U.S. Consumer Product Safety Commission in 1977 because it causes cancer in animals; anything made before 1977 may contain it. Also avoid sleepwear containing acetate, triacetate, polyester, or polyester-cotton combinations in which Tris or Fyrol may have been used.

If you purchase new sleepwear, ask the salesperson whether the garment was chemically treated. Some fabrics, such as modacrylic, vinyon, matrix, and wool are inherently fire retardant. Your best option in sleepwear is going to be cotton, which unfortunately shrinks, or the inherently fire-retardant synthetics (which don't "breathe" and often have strong chemical odors). Stay with trusted brand names.

## Infant Clothing (Birth to Six Months)

What you'll need initially will be determined by the time of year your child is born. Obviously, you won't be needing blanket sleepers for a baby born in July. Your initial shopping list will probably include undershirts, possibly a footed sleeper for your baby to wear home from the hospital, sleeping gowns, a hat, warm blankets, a bunting, and socks.

*Shirts*—Buy undershirts in the three-month or six-month size for newborns. It's better to buy them too big. A shirt and a diaper will usually be enough to keep your baby warm around the house; in the summer, you can even dispense with the shirt. Buy pure cotton shirts for maximum absorbency and washability. Shirts with a side tie are excellent because they eliminate snaps that are uncomfortable for a baby to lie on, and they expand as she grows. Babies don't like pullovers at all. Shirts that have tabs on the side for pinning them to the diaper and long-tail shirts that pull through the legs and fasten over the diaper may look like a good idea, but the tabs and tails may act like wicks, drawing up moisture from the diaper, and therefore shouldn't be used.

*Sleepwear*—Footed stretch sleepers are more popular with parents than with babies. Parents feel secure knowing that their baby is warm, but for the baby, the stretch sleeper may be constricting and may mask the incoming stimulation that is so important for body awareness. Heavy blanket sleepers, which make blankets unnecessary, are good for winter, but if you plan to use them, make sure the baby's room is not excessively warm. For a winter baby, you might want one in a three-month size. Less expensive brands tend to shrink, especially around the zipper and snap tabs. After washing either type of sleeper, turn it inside out and look for hanging threads that could wrap around a toe or finger and cut off circulation. Avoid buying sleepers that have vinyl inlays, which are sticky and uncomfortable, and sleepers made of brushed nylon, which loses its soft, furry finish and wears out at the toes. Look for sturdy, well-made items with finished seams.

For a tiny infant, a gown with a string-tied bottom in a pure cotton knit makes the most sense as sleepwear. Gowns keep a baby's feet and legs covered and make changing easier. Also, as your baby grows, the gown can still be used without the strings; once your baby can crawl, you won't want her in a bag-type gown. Avoid any gown or shirt with elasticized armbands, which can constrict and scratch.

In the summer, your baby will be comfortable sleeping in just a diaper and a shirt or kimono.

*Buntings*—A bunting is essentially a quilted or knitted zip-up bag with a hood. Buntings are handy when you want to go out and don't have time to dress your baby. On the other hand, buntings are impractical in situations where your baby must be strapped in for safety, as in a car seat or stroller; the bag will prevent the proper use of restaining belts and straps. If you choose to make one from a pattern, know that most patterns tend to be too wide in the chest and too long in the arms, and adjust accordingly.

*Blankets*—Receiving blankets are useful with newborns. They can be used to wrap up a new baby and make him feel secure. They can also be used as a light cover for sleeping or as a shoulder cover for burping. All-cotton ones are softer, more absorbent, and easy to fold. Heavy blankets and quilts are useful in the winter. Stay with natural fibers; synthetics don't wash well—they shrink and mat. After laundering, always watch for strings, which pose a strangulation danger.

*Sweaters, hats, and booties*—Sweater sets are favorite shower gifts, but unfortunately they're not really useful. If you're going to use a sweater, make sure it's tightly knit; wide-woven knits may entangle fingers and toes. Sweaters that have back zippers or large buttons with bound buttonholes are easiest to put on. Make sure any sweater you use is machine washable.

Make sure hats and hoods are small enough so that they can be placed well away from your baby's face, so he can't turn his head and suffocate in them.

Booties are cute, but they just don't stay on. Parents tend to think babies need to have something on their feet because their feet are cold, but babies' feet are naturally cool to the touch. Some babies don't like having things on their feet, but if you do need to put something on them, try fuzzy baby socks that have stretch cuffs; they stay on better.

## Crawler Clothing (Six to Twelve Months)

At this age, it is very important to have functional clothes so your baby's explorations and movements aren't inhibited. Your shopping list should include overalls with snap crotches, tops, undershirts (dependent on the climate), a jacket, a sweater, and footed sleepwear or nightgowns.

*Daywear*—For daytime, bright T-shirts with shoulder snaps and straight-cut overalls with adjustable straps are best. Pants that have elasticized waists are too constricting on a baby's abdomen. When you buy overalls, make sure there's reinforcement where the straps join the bib and in the crotch snap area. You can sew on knee pads with foam or cotton stuffing to protect your baby's knees on outdoor crawling expeditions.

*Sweaters and jackets*—The easiest sweaters to put on will be those that slip over the head and have side buttons at the neck. Make sure any sweater you buy is machine washable. Jackets that zip or snap in the front will be best. If you need to buy a snowsuit, buy one that is in two pieces, so you can use just the jacket in warmer weather.

*Sleepwear*—For this age group, footed pajamas that have snaps between the shirt and the pants work well. Heavier blanket sleepers can eliminate the need for blankets in the winter, but they're hot and should be used only if you keep your house fairly cool. Watch for shrinkage in any of these.

The most practical sleepwear choice for boys and girls is a cotton flannel nightgown. Such a nightgown tends to fit longer and makes diaper changing easier.

## Toddler Clothing (One to Three Years)

Once your child begins to walk, you'll want to add shoes and boots to his wardrobe. You'll also be buying a raincoat. As your child gets toward the toilet-training age, you'll need to buy underpants.

*Daywear*—Once your child is walking, T-shirts and snap-crotch elastic-waist pants are a good choice for everyday wear. Often, the T-shirts sold for children of this age are too short and tend to pull up, and pants with a snap crotch are sometimes hard to find in sizes big enough to fit comfortably over diapers. For girls, a jumper with shoulder buttons and large pockets is a nice dress-up alternative. Most of the expensive coordinated outfits sold for children of this age are a waste of money; they may actually tear more easily, and can shrink and fade like anything else.

In hot weather, it's okay to dress your toddler in just underpants or shorts, or you can get sleeveless tank tops to go with knit pull-on shorts. To protect your toddler from heat and glare, buy a small-brimmed washable hat.

*Coats and winter wear*—A machine-washable coat with a drawstring hood will be most practical. Those with large buttons or loops and toggle buttons are excellent because eventually your child will be able to manage these herself. Make sure coats are not so bulky that your child can't move in them. Actually, a few thin layers are more comfortable and just as warm without the bulk. Your toddler will be happier.

For very small toddlers, buy thumbless (whole-hand) mittens; they're warmer than gloves. Older toddlers will prefer mittens with thumbs for increased dexterity. Mittens that have a connecting string that gets threaded through the sleeves of a coat are a good idea. Suspender clips to attach mittens to coats have pinching potential (the mittens usually get lost anyway). In any case, buy two pairs of mittens in the same style since it's not unlikely that at least one mitten will get lost.

Never use long scarves with preschoolers since they pose a strangulation risk should they get caught on something as the child moves by.

*Rainwear*—Old-fashioned yellow raincoats with hoods and ponchos with hoods are good at this age. The old-style clasp latches are much more manageable for tots than zippers. Don't buy vinyl coats; they tear quickly, especially under the arms and at the snaps. When you fit the coat, get it large enough that your child can wear it over a winter coat if necessary.

Galoshes are a favorite with tots, probably because they are one of the few kinds of shoes they can put on by themselves. Buy the kind that are worn without shoes, preferably with an inner lining and a waterproof fabric neck that ties with a drawstring. These will be very practical for the mud and puddle stomping that is a natural part of being a tot.

Never buy a child-size umbrella; the sharp points can be dangerous, and the opening mechanism can pinch a small child.

*Underwear*—Don't purchase training pants; they shrink. Let your child graduate into regular cotton underpants when training time comes. It's essential to buy pure cotton; synthetics aggravate rashes and infections. Unless you live in a cold climate or house, undershirts aren't necessary.

## Socks and Shoes

You don't need to have shoes for your baby before he can walk. In fact, small babies are better off barefoot since they get a lot of sensory input through their feet. Also, feet have natural nonskid surfaces, and toes can grasp as your baby pulls himself up. Before your baby walks, you may want to buy shoes only for protection, and cheap sneakers or leather moccasins will do the job.

When your baby is just starting to walk, lighter leather shoes are probably better—she's less likely to trip. Later on it makes little difference whether you choose leather shoes or sneakers. If, however, your child has a problem with foot perspiration, you should keep in mind that leather breathes. Sneakers and athletic shoes are generally made of synthetics, which will keep your child's feet moist.

If you're going to fit your baby's shoes yourself, allow half an inch between the big toe and the end of the shoe. Test this while your child is standing. The shoe should fit firmly against the back of the foot with no gaps. Make sure the sides of the shoe are low enough not to rub against the ankle bone. Avoid artificial arches and raised heels. Look for shoes with nonskid bottoms. Keep in mind that buckles or Velcro closures are much easier for a child than laces.

Once your baby is walking, you'll need to buy new shoes every four to six months, which gets fairly expensive no matter what you spend. Though expensive shoes are not necessarily better, children's shoe stores stock the hard-to-find sizes, and you will have to go to one (and pay more) if you can't fit your child in a self-service store. If your child is easy to fit, you can get away with sturdy sneakers, which provide traction for climbing and running, unless your doctor says otherwise.

An oxford-style shoe provides more toe room than other styles. Mary Janes and other dress styles are good for special occasions but not all the time because they constrict the toes and are often stiff.

You need to pay attention to socks, too, since a sock that is too tight is just as bad as a shoe that is too small. To absorb moisture, socks should be mostly cotton, but fleecy acrylic socks don't shrink as much. If you buy all socks in the same color and weave, you'll have less difficulty matching them up when they come out of the wash. Stretch tights are a waste of money because children soon outgrow them; also, tights get runs, and their elastic waistbands stretch out when washed. They're not a substitute for pants as far as warmth is concerned, either.

## Toys and Toy Safety

The first time you look through the toy department you may be struck by how much more expensive toys are today than you remembered. Toys don't *have* to be expensive, though. And with toys, expense has nothing to do with quality. We've all heard the story about the parents who bought their child an expensive toy, and all the child wanted to do was play with the box. Once you're familiar with toy safety issues, you can find good toys at local yard sales or thrift shops. Some parents even set up informal toy "libraries," or exchange systems. If you're going to purchase new toys, there are many safe, good toys available at all prices, and it doesn't make sense to invest a lot of money in a toy that will be appropriate for only a short period of time.

A good toy for one child won't necessarily be a good toy for another child. When you get a toy for your child, you need to consider her personality, likes, and dislikes.

Generally speaking, a good toy should challenge a child at his level of development. If it's too sophisticated, it will frustrate the child; if it's too simple, it will bore the child. For that reason, it's important to observe the age ranges on packages.

A good toy requires the child to actively play with it; if the toy does the playing, it won't interest the child for very long.

## Toy Safety

Every year about 130,000 children are injured by toys that cut, puncture, burn, shock, or choke them. Many times the cause is a lack of supervision, misuse of the toy, or use of a toy that is not age-appropriate.

While there are mandatory federal standards and voluntary industry standards for toy safety, these are no guarantee, since safety testing is only done at random or after children have experienced injuries from a particular toy. So you, the consumer, need to do your own testing before you acquire a toy.

Before buying a toy, check for the following:

- *Strong construction*—Try to pull off eyes, buttons, parts, pieces, and ornaments to be sure a small child will not be able to pull them off and choke on them.

- *Breakability*—Make sure the toy won't shatter if it's dropped or thrown onto a hard surface from a child's height.

- *Paints*—New toys must be painted with nontoxic paints, but antiques or hand-me-downs may not be coated with a safe paint.

- *Cloth and stuffing*—should be flame-resistant.

- *Sharp or pointed edges*—Run your fingers over metal or plastic pieces to see if they will cut or scratch. Sharp ridges on molded plastics can be filed down. On wood toys, be sure there are no edges that are splintering. Be sure there

are no points or propelling objects that could cause eye or puncture injuries.

- *Sitting toys*—Place these large toys on the floor and try to push them over. They should be broad-based for stability.

- *Nonelectric*—Avoid electric toys for toddlers since they may attempt to eat batteries or get hurt while attempting to plug in or unplug the toy. Toys that have heating elements are unsafe for children under eight years old.

- *Hardware*—Make sure hardware is not rough and does not have a scissoring action that could pinch.

- *Noise toys*—Activate toys that make noise and be sure they won't damage hearing if held close to the ears. Avoid any toy that emits a continuous, loud pure tone; such a noise can damage the ears. Teach your child to keep noise-making toys away from her ears. Even proper use of toy guns (which many parents avoid on general principle) can cause ear damage—they should be avoided.

- *Parts*—Make sure there are no parts small enough for a child to ingest. If there are moving parts, be sure they are securely enclosed.

- *Strangulation dangers*—Ropes or strings on toys should be no more than twelve inches long, and loops should not be big enough to fit around a child's neck.

- *Outdoor play equipment*—Should be purchased for your child's age and size. There should be no rough edges or exposed hardware. Make sure these toys are assembled properly, according to the manufacturer's instructions. Swings should be more than six feet from houses, trees, and other obstructions and should be set on soft surfaces, not concrete. Sandboxes should be filled with fresh, clean sand, and should be covered when not in use. Sandboxes are not recommended for children in the "let's-taste-everything" stage of development. For reasons of sanitation, keep pets away from the sandbox.

## Age-Appropriate Toys

*Infant toys (birth to one year)*—The major safety concern during this period is choking and suffocation.

Stuffed toys should be nonflammable, nontoxic, and washable. Stuffed animals that are all one piece are best; if there are limbs, they should be securely attached. Features should be painted or embroidered, and should not be embellished with glass eyes or whiskers that can be pulled off and swallowed. Small, lightweight toys will be easier for infants to hold and cuddle.

Mobiles help develop a baby's ability to focus attention on objects, but they are meant to be looked at only—not handled. Once your child is old enough to reach up and grab the mobile (usually at about four to five months), it should be removed.

Rattles and teethers must be unbreakable and washable, have no loose parts, and have rounded stems. No part of a rattle should be small enough to fit in a baby's mouth. To test this, draw an oval that is 1 3/8 inches by 2 inches on a piece of paper and cut it out. If the rattle or any part of it can pass through the hole to a depth of 1 3/16 inches or more, the rattle could choke your child. Rattles can be purchased in a variety of shapes, sizes, and colors. The size and weight should be compatible with your child's ability to grasp it in one hand.

Crib and playpen exercisers enhance pulling and grasping. They usually stretch across the crib or playpen, and should be removed before babies are big enough to use them to pull themselves up.

Special balls that make noise and have moving pieces inside provide motor, visual, and aural stimulation and help develop eye movement, crawling, and gross motor skills. Be sure that moving pieces cannot be removed from the ball and swallowed.

Mirrors delight infants. But make sure they are unbreakable, have no sharp edges, are light enough for your baby to pick up, and are large enough not to be swallowed.

*Twelve to eighteen months*—At this point, babies can stand and sit, but may not yet walk by themselves. They have no sense of danger and enjoy moving objects, especially push/pull toys that make sounds, things that open and close, toys that involve turning knobs and dials, and peek-a-boo games.

At this age, children enjoy blocks, but be sure to get blocks that are large and have no sharp corners. Just a few blocks will suffice; too many will be confusing. Blocks that are covered with soft fabric and light, foam-filled vinyl blocks are ideal.

Sorting toys teach children about color and size, and enhance manual dexterity, but make sure they are unbreakable and that pieces are too large to be swallowed.

Riding toys are dangerous for children who can't yet walk. But once your child can walk, she will enjoy them. Make sure that she can climb on and off the toy easily, that she can maneuver it alone, and that there are no sharp edges.

Push/pull toys are great for kids who are already walking, too. Make sure the ends of the handles are covered with large safety balls and that all the parts are unbreakable.

*Eighteen to twenty-four months*—Children at this age are talking and are interested in learning about size and placement.

Large blocks in a variety of shapes will interest children at this age. Start out with a small set and move on to a large set as the child's interest develops. Avoid blocks with sharp edges. Blocks that come in canisters are easiest for a child to put away when he is done playing with them. Blocks are a good investment; they hold children's interest for a long time. They are usually appropriate from the age of eighteen months to eight years.

Telephone toys give children an opportunity to engage in an adult activity, and children like the noise they make. Some of these toys even talk. Those that come shaped like cartoon characters help maintain interest. Be sure that bell parts cannot be removed and swallowed.

Shape-recognition toys that require children to fit pieces in appropriately shaped holes help develop hand-eye coordination, matching skills, and shape recognition. However, if there are too many pieces, the child will be frustrated. Watch for pieces of "swallowable" size and holes that can pinch or trap fingers.

Action toys, like a push/pull bus that has removable people in it, are very popular with children at this age, as are push/pull train sets that have removable parts and accessories. Make sure that all parts are "swallow-proof."

Pounding toys teach hand-eye coordination and enhance gross and fine motor skills. If there's a hammer involved, it should be very soft, so the child isn't injured by it.

Riding toys come in two types: those the child moves by pushing with her feet and those with pedals; the latter are more difficult for children to use. All riding toys should be stable and easy to mount. They are usually appropriate from eighteen to thirty-six months. Always supervise your child when she is using a riding toy outdoors, particularly near sidewalks or streets.

Activity toys are those that children either crawl or climb on or use to develop manual dexterity. Climbing toys should have railings and other safety features. Toys that enhance dexterity should be suited to your child's abilities; they should be challenging but not frustrating.

*Two to three years*—At this point, children are more creative. They employ make-believe and fantasy in their play. Their attention spans are longer. They enjoy doing adult-like things, and realistic toys will stimulate hours of creative play. Toys that require movement as well as those that involve dexterity are enjoyed by this age group.

Talking toys and dolls are very appealing. Make sure the dolls speak their phrases clearly and that the pull ring is securely attached.

Toy dashboards are popular, too. The more features the dashboard has, the more interest the child will have in it. Just make sure it's easy to use. Avoid toys with knobs or decals that can be easily pulled off.

Trucks are good toys for indoors and outdoors, especially for the sandbox. Trucks that have moving parts are especially appealing, but be sure there are no sharp edges and that the metal is rust-proof. The wheels should be securely attached, and the truck should be stable and maneuverable.

Push or wind-up trains are popular. Your child should be able to easily place the train on its tracks, though the tracks will usually need to be assembled by an adult. Make sure wind-up mechanisms are easy to use, and avoid toys with sharp edges.

Toy kitchens and realistic tool toys should be durable. Make sure these toys are manageable for your child, or they won't sustain interest. Also be sure that large items are stable and won't fall on your child while he is playing with them. Tool benches should provide a variety of activities without being overwhelming.

Puzzles can be an excellent purchase. They strengthen hand-eye coordination, matching skills, and shape recognition, and will sustain interest if they are matched to your child's level. Pieces should not be so small as to encourage your child to pop them in his mouth.

Play scenes provide a child with the opportunity to use her imagination. These toys will have more appeal if the scenes are familiar, so a city child will probably enjoy a toy parking garage more than a farm scene. They should be easy to assemble, have storage for individual pieces, and have moving features. Also, be sure your child isn't overwhelmed by a multitude of pieces.

Occupation toys, like a doctor's kit, inspire creative play. Your child will appreciate the toy if he is familiar with the occupation it represents.

For a more detailed discussion of the role of toys in learning, see Chapter 11.

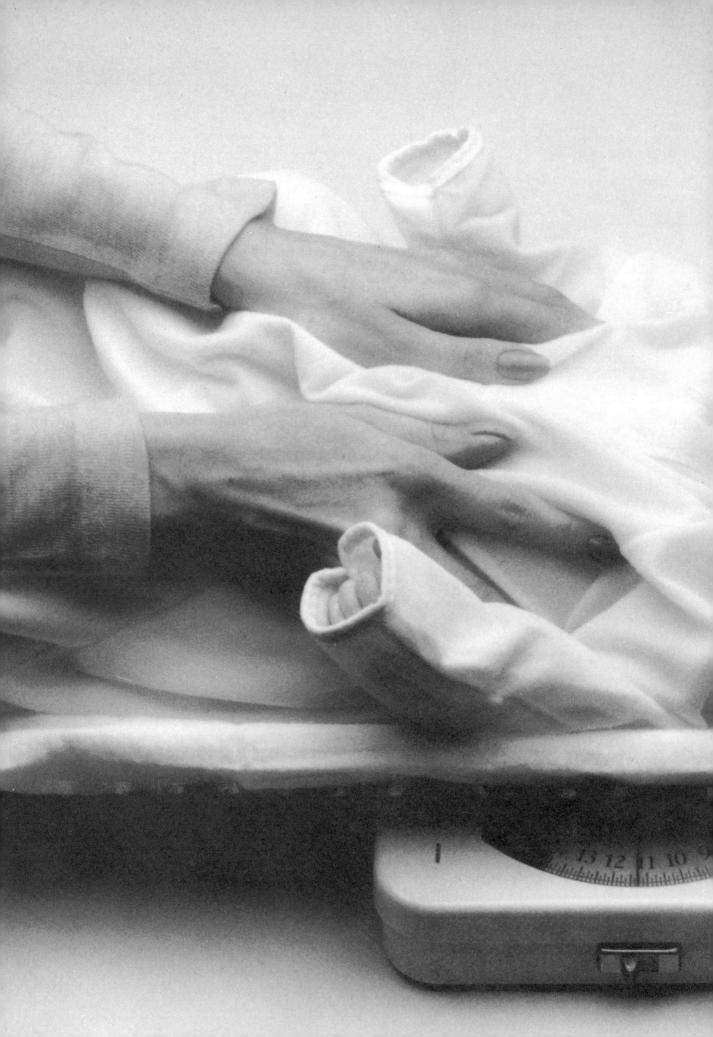

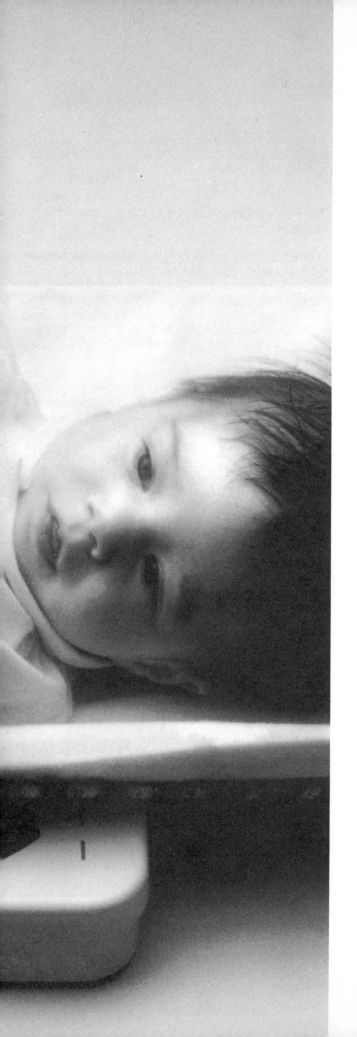

# Chapter 5:
# The Birthing Process

## Preparing for the Birth of Your Baby

As you enter the last three months of pregnancy, you may find yourself thinking more and more about the upcoming birth. Your large size and your baby's movements are constant reminders that you will become a mother soon.

You may find yourself wanting to slow down a bit, preferring quiet evenings at home, slow walks, midday rests with your feet up, and a generally slower pace to your life. The twenty-four-hour-a-day job of making a baby becomes tiring toward the end of pregnancy. When you add to that a job, child care, a social life, and the fact that you might be sleeping more lightly than usual, it is not surprising that you may want to simplify your life and take it easier from now until after the baby is born.

As you slow down and contemplate the upcoming birth and baby, you may be surprised to learn that your body has not slowed down at all. It is working at full speed, preparing for the birth. The baby is growing very rapidly, from about two to three pounds at the end of the twenty-eighth week to about six and a half to nine pounds at the end of the fortieth week. Many changes take place in your body to support such rapid growth. In this chapter we will examine these changes and the birth process itself. We will describe the newborn baby, what she looks like, what she can do, and her immediate care. In addition, we will discuss the first few weeks after birth—the immediate care of the mother and the emotional adjustments to new parenthood.

## The Third Trimester

All your baby's major systems were formed in the first trimester. The organs and skeleton took shape, and your baby took on a tiny but complete human form. During the second trimester, your baby began to move noticeably, gained the ability to see and hear, and began reacting to outside stimuli—that is, sounds outside your body, light and dark, and your eating and activity patterns. Your baby began turning somersaults, sucked his thumb, hiccuped perceptibly, and generally made you aware of his presence. The third trimester (the last three months of pregnancy) might be best thought of as a time when the final touches are put on your baby in his journey toward life outside your body.

### Nutritional Requirements

As your baby grows in size, her nutritional requirements increase. For example, she requires about one-third more protein in these last months of pregnancy, because every cell in the human body has protein as a primary ingredient, and with each passing day she has more cells. In addition, because the bones are growing and becoming strong, the need for calcium, which is important to bone strength, increases by about two-thirds during the last three months of pregnancy. The baby's absorption of iron also dramatically increases.

As you can see, with these increased nutritional requirements, it is very desirable that you eat well to supply your baby's nutritional needs as well as your own. It is a good idea to reassess your nutritional intake during this last trimester, to see if you are getting the recommended foods in each of the food groups. See Chapter 2 for further information on a good diet during pregnancy.

### The Baby's Development in the Last Trimester

As your baby grows, he also becomes stronger. All that exercise in the uterus pays off. The amniotic fluid serves as a wonderful medium for the baby to exercise in; its buoyancy allows him to move around freely. The muscles develop, and the baby becomes more and more physically capable.

He also gains a layer of fat, which will help him maintain his body temperature after birth. Also helping the baby maintain body temperature is the maturing of the adrenal glands, which make adrenalin (also called epinephrine). Adrenalin, secreted when the baby is chilled, mobilizes energy to warm him up.

Another major area of development in the last three months is the maturing of the baby's lungs. Of course, while your baby is in the uterus, he does not need to use his lungs for breathing. In fact, they are full of fluid. Oxygen is breathed in by you and is carried to the placenta and through the umbilical cord into the baby's body. But toward the end of pregnancy, the lungs gain the ability to perform the breathing functions. Within seconds after birth, the baby takes his first breath, which is usually followed by a good bellow or two. It is with this first breath that his lungs become inflated, and they will not stop functioning for as long as he lives. So this dramatic first breath of life is being prepared for in the last trimester of pregnancy.

### The Placenta

The placenta is a complex organ that develops along with the baby. Here the exchange of nutrients, oxygen, carbon dioxide, and waste products between mother and baby takes place. The mother sends to the placenta via her bloodstream all the nutrients and other substances that the baby needs to grow and develop. The baby sends waste products and his own hormones to the placenta for the mother to take up and either dispose of or use.

The placenta also is an endocrine gland. It produces hormones that maintain the pregnancy. By the midpoint of pregnancy, the placenta has taken over many of the functions of the ovaries, producing many of the same hormones, including progesterone. Progesterone causes relaxation of involuntary muscles, including the uterus. It is present in large quantities throughout most of pregnancy, and keeps the uterus from contracting very much. But during the last few weeks of pregnancy, the amount of progesterone produced by the placenta decreases. This is associated with stronger contractions of the uterus.

Many women report that they are aware of stronger contractions of the uterus in late pregnancy. You may wonder if this is true for you. How can you tell whether your uterus is contracting, or whether your baby is simply moving? The best way to tell is to press your hand in several places around the uterus when you feel any strange sensations in the area. If the sensation is caused by the baby's moving, you will feel firmness only in one area and softness in other areas of the uterus. The firmness may be the baby's back, and the strange sensation may be caused by the baby's stretching and pressing his back against your abdomen. If it is a contraction, your entire uterus will be very firm.

The structure of the placenta changes as it ages. For example, the membrane separating the mother's circulation from the baby's becomes more open to the exchange of some substances, allowing the baby to extract from the mother's blood supply some beneficial substances. For example, we all have immunoglobulins and antibodies circulating in our bodies, which protect us from many illnesses. During late pregnancy, you are able to pass some of these to your baby, giving him protection against some illnesses that lasts for months after birth. This protection continues for as long as you breast-feed your child, because these same immunoglobulins and antibodies also pass into breast milk.

## Changes in the Mother

What about the mother? What changes do you experience in preparation for the birth? The changes that come with pregnancy affect not only the baby, the uterus, and the placenta, but also the mother's entire body, her mind, and her emotions.

For example, your breasts began changing as soon as you became pregnant. You may have noticed some breast changes (for example, tenderness, tingling sensations, and feelings of heaviness) very early, even before you knew you were pregnant. These changes indicate that your body is beginning to get ready for breast-feeding. By late pregnancy, you may notice more veins in your breasts, indicating the increased blood supply in the area. You may also notice that your breasts are somewhat larger than they were before, and the areolae (the circles around your nipples) may have darkened. Inside the breasts, the milk-producing glands have grown larger. They even begin producing a type of milk called colostrum, which enables you to breast-feed whenever the baby is born.

Other parts of your body also change in preparation for the birth. For example, the ligaments begin to soften. This is particularly helpful in the pelvis, through which the baby passes during birth. Flexible ligaments allow the pelvis to enlarge somewhat, making more room for the baby. These changes sometimes cause shooting pains in your hips, stiffness in the lower part of your back, or soreness in the front joint of your pelvis (symphysis pubis) and the sacroiliac joints. Although inconvenient now, these changes really are a benefit during the birth process.

Like many women, you may experience heartburn and constipation, partly due to slowing of digestion and partly due to the size of the uterus, which is crowding your stomach and intestines and causing you to burp up acid and to have trouble moving your bowels. You can prevent or reduce heartburn by eating smaller amounts of food at a time and by not eating right before going to bed. Constipation can be helped with regular exercise, drinking plenty of fluids, and eating vegetables and fruits. Discuss with your doctor the use of antacids for heartburn and laxatives for constipation during pregnancy. Despite these discomforts, there are benefits. Your body is able to absorb more nutrients from your digestive tract because of this slowing of digestion.

Your uterus undergoes vast changes in the last trimester of pregnancy. Obviously, it becomes much larger. It must accommodate the growing baby, the placenta (which weighs about one-sixth of the baby's weight), and about one quart of amniotic fluid. As your uterus stretches around the growing baby inside, it becomes more "irritable" and sensitive. If you sneeze or bump your abdomen, your uterus often contracts immediately afterward. It is very sensitive to sudden pressure. Sometimes, while you are resting, your uterus will spontaneously contract several times in a rhythm. More than one woman has wondered if she is in labor when this kind of contraction pattern occurs. These contractions, called Braxton Hicks contractions, are an indication that the uterus has become more sensitive to the circulating oxytocin.

While Braxton Hicks contractions are not labor, they probably are causing changes in your cervix that prepare it for labor. These changes include ripening (softening), effacement (thinning), and some dilation (opening) of the cervix prior to the onset of labor. Although you are probably unaware of it, the cervix, which is usually quite firm and thick, becomes soft and thin before labor begins. A ripe, thin cervix opens up much more easily than an unripe, thick cervix. The amount of ripening and thinning can be determined only with a vaginal exam. Effacement is measured as a percentage. For example, if your cervix is twenty-five percent effaced, it is twenty-five percent thinner than usual. (The cervix is approximately two centimeters long. Twenty-five percent effaced means that one and a half centimeters remains.)

Your cervix opens slightly before you go into labor. This is referred to as dilation, and is measured during a vaginal exam by feeling the circular rim of the cervix and estimating (in centimeters) the diameter of the opening. Many women will be one or two centimeters dilated before they are aware of any signs of labor. During labor your cervix will continue dilating to about ten centimeters (a circle about four inches across).

This preliminary work of the uterus in preparation for labor is thought to be controlled by the changing hormone production in the placenta, the baby, and the mother.

### Practical Matters in the Third Trimester

As you wind down toward the birth of your baby, you will want to be conscientious about your diet and rest needs. This is the time to take childbirth-preparation classes; to prepare your birth plan; to make the decisions on employment, child care, infant feeding, and health care for your baby; and to prepare the baby's space and equipment. If they have not already done so, this is when most people take a good look at their financial situation, and figure out the impact the birth of the baby will have. There may be a loss of income for at least a while, extra bills associated with the birth, other expenses associated with the baby's equipment, and more. Try to prepare yourself for these financial changes as much as possible so that you are not caught in a financial bind be-

cause of the birth of your child. See Chapter 4 for useful budgeting information.

If your income is low, you may qualify for federal or state programs; there are also organizations that can assist you with food, health care, free or low-cost baby clothing and equipment, and other help. This is a good time to look into these matters if you have not already. If you have health insurance, find out exactly what it does and does not cover.

Pack your bag a few weeks before your due date (see the accompanying list of items) and place on top of it a list of any last-minute items to add just before leaving.

### Suggested Packing List

**For mother in labor:**
- Toothbrush and toothpaste

- Massage oil (not lotion) or powder (cornstarch is best)

- Lip cream or gloss

- Rolling pin or massage aids

- Hot-water bottle and frozen camper's ice (for comfort)

- Juice or ice pops (if not supplied by hospital)

- Music tapes and a tape recorder (battery-operated)

- Home-birth supplies ordered by your midwife

**For partner:**
- Food/snacks

- Breath mints or toothbrush

- Camera and film (very fast film allows you to avoid disturbing flash)

- Watch with second hand for timing contractions

**For baby:**
- Warm hat (may be provided in hospital) to put on soon after birth. For home birth, have several soft, warm blankets.

- Clothing and four or five diapers and pins (not needed for hospital stay, but to go home)

- Outside clothing (warm blanket, hat, booties, as required by weather)

- Car seat

**For mother after birth:**
- Nursing bras (two or three)

- Gowns, slippers, and robe (these are provided by the hospital, but you may prefer your own)

- Personal hygiene items, cosmetics, and shower cap

- Phone numbers of people to call

- Money (small change)

- Sanitary napkins and belt (provided by hospital)

- Reading and/or writing materials (birth announcements) and address book

- Clothes to wear home (should be stretchy or larger than your pre-pregnant size)

## Labor and Birth

The changes taking place in your body, placenta, and baby during the last three months of pregnancy accelerate at the end, culminating in labor. As the placenta ages and gradually loses its ability to maintain the pregnancy, the baby becomes strong and capable enough to survive outside the mother's body; the uterus begins to let go and expel the baby; and the mother becomes ready to give birth and to feed and nurture her baby. Labor consists of rhythmic uterine contractions, which open the cervix and press the baby down through the birth canal and out of your body. The uterus is a big, strong, hollow muscle; when it contracts, it tightens and hardens. This may happen anywhere from twenty-five to three hundred times during labor, which may take anywhere from a few hours to more than a day. The process involves not only your uterus, but your entire body and mind; all your energy is devoted toward the one goal of giving birth to your baby.

How will you know when you are in labor? As basic as this question is, it is one of the most diffi-cult to answer. It usually takes hours or even days to figure out whether your sensations are labor or something else (prelabor, or false labor). This is because labor does not begin suddenly. It evolves gradually. At some point, you or your doctor will recognize that these sensations are true labor, meaning that they are accompanied by increasing dilation of the cervix. In this section we will describe the signs and sensations of labor to help you recognize it. We will also describe the birth process, the emotions that accompany labor, and how your partner can help you the most.

The signs of labor may be divided into subtle signs, preliminary signs, and absolutely clear signs.

If you are within a week or two of your due date, you generally may wait until you have an *absolutely clear* sign of labor before going to the hospital, although your doctor may ask you to let him or her know if your bag of waters (amniotic sac surrounding the baby) seems to be leaking. If your pregnancy has been complicated by diabetes, high blood pressure, or other medical conditions, or if you have twins or a breech fetus, your doctor may advise you to go to the hospital with the onset of *preliminary* signs. If you are several weeks before your due date, you should notify your doctor if you have any preliminary signs, because they could indicate early or premature labor. Premature labor can often be stopped if treatment is begun early enough.

To determine whether your contractions are progressing (that is, becoming longer, stronger, and closer together), you need to time them. On a sheet of paper, list the times when contractions begin, and how long they last. Time them in this way for an hour or two. If they are not progressing, stop for a while until they seem different, then try timing again.

You should call your doctor or your hospital's labor and delivery ward to tell them you are in labor or to ask for advice. Be sure to report the status of your bag of waters; whether you have had a bloody discharge (called bloody show, which you will continue to pass throughout labor); how long and how many minutes apart your contractions are; and how strong or painful they feel to you.

### Labor

Labor varies from woman to woman; even in the same woman each labor is different. Some labors

# THE BIRTHING PROCESS

## Signs and Symptoms of Labor*

| Subtle Signs or Symptoms | Comment |
|---|---|
| 1. Vague backache that may cause restlessness | Different from the posture-related backache commonly experienced during pregnancy, this may be caused by early contractions. |
| 2. Several soft bowel movements accompanied by flu-like "sick" feelings | Probably related to increase in circulating prostaglandins, which ripen your cervix while causing other symptoms. |
| 3. "The nesting urge" (an unusual burst of energy resulting in great activity) | Helps ensure that you will have strength and energy to handle labor. You should try to avoid exhausting activity. |

| Preliminary Signs or Symptoms | |
|---|---|
| 4. Bloody show (passage of blood-tinged mucus from the vagina) | Associated with thinning of the cervix. May occur days before other signs or not until after progressing labor contractions have begun. |
| 5. Small break of the bag of waters (amniotic sac surrounding the baby), causing leakage of fluid. No contractions. | May not be associated with spontaneous labor, although cervical ripening may hasten after a membrane rupture. Occurs in ten to twelve percent of labors. Leaking occurs when you change position, laugh, sneeze, etc., and may continue off and on for hours. |
| 6. Continuing nonprogressing contractions ("false" labor, or prodromal labor). The contractions stay the same over time. | Accomplishes softening and thinning of the cervix, although dilation does not occur until later. Should not be perceived as unproductive. |

| Absolutely Clear Signs or Symptoms | |
|---|---|
| 7. Progressing contractions (those that become longer, stronger, and closer together with the passage of time) | Are dilating the cervix by the time the contractions are averaging one minute long and five minutes apart, and feel painful or "very strong" to the woman. May be felt in the abdomen, the back, or both. |
| 8. Breaking of the bag of waters with pop, gush, or leak, followed by progressing contractions | Labor usually speeds up after the bag of waters breaks. |

*Note that all women do not experience all of these signs; the most important ones are the last two. The others are more like warning signs that labor is coming soon.

are very fast, lasting only a few hours; some are average in length (about fifteen or sixteen hours for first-time mothers and seven or eight hours for women who have had babies before); some are very long, lasting a day or two. Some start slowly and then speed up unexpectedly; others start rapidly and then slow down. The amount of pain and fatigue varies also. It is best not to have definite expectations, but to prepare yourself for the wide range of possibilities.

Many factors play a part in how long and hard your labor will be. You can influence some of those factors, but not others.

## The Stages of Labor

Labor is described as having three stages: the first stage, from the onset of progressing labor contractions until the cervix is completely dilated; the second stage, from complete dilation of the cervix until the baby is born; and the third stage, from the birth of the baby until the placenta is expelled.

A fourth stage, from the delivery of the placenta until the mother's medical condition is stable and safe, is also frequently mentioned.

## The First Stage

The first stage is almost always the longest (two to twenty-four or more hours), usually starting slowly and then speeding up when the dilation of the cervix reaches about four or five centimeters. Your contractions may not be clear and strong at first, but they will become longer, stronger, and closer together with time.

Much of your time in the first stage may be spent trying to figure out if you are in labor or not. It may be exciting and fun for you, or it may be a little scary. After all, this is the moment you've been waiting for, learning about, preparing for, and dreaming of!

It is a mistake to become preoccupied with labor. If you can be distracted from your contractions, it is unlikely that you are in very advanced labor. (On rare occasions, women have been unaware of labor until the baby was about to be born! In these cases, there really is no way to prevent a hectic scene unless a woman has had such a birth previously. Then she should watch carefully for *any* sign of labor—subtle, preliminary, or absolutely clear—and call her doctor immediately.)

As labor progresses, there is no longer any question whether you are in labor. It quickens its pace, and the contractions usually become painful. Once certain that you are in labor, go to the hospital or birthing center (or if the birth is to be at home, await your care-giver's arrival). Of course, if you have any concerns or a medical problem, feel free to go to the hospital. Be sure to take your bag and have needed items on hand.

You may become serious and quiet, focused on only one thing—your labor. Jokes are not funny; world events lose their importance. You need sup-

---

### Factors Influencing Labor

**Factors you cannot control:**
- Size and shape of your pelvis

- Size and shape of baby's head and shoulders

- Baby's station, presentation, and position*

- The condition of your cervix when contractions begin

- The power of your contractions

- The amount of rest you have between contractions

- Some aspects of your general health and your baby's well-being

**Factors you can control, to some extent:**
- Your emotional state and attitude toward birth (anxiety, fear, and tension versus optimism, confidence, and relaxation)

- Presence of helpful, caring, partner(s)

- Knowledge of what to expect

- An environment and professional staff that help you feel secure, well cared for

- Good care of yourself (including good nourishment and good health habits)

*Station* refers to how low the baby is in the pelvis. *Presentation* refers to which part of the baby's body will come first (usually it is the head, but on occasion it may be the buttocks, the feet, or even a shoulder). *Position* refers to the location—on the left or the right side of the mother—and the orientation—anterior (toward the mother's front), posterior (toward the mother's back), or transverse (lying crosswise)—of a given part of the baby, specifically, the occiput (back of the head), brow, chin, shoulder, or sacrum (the bone at the lower end of the spinal column). For example, if a baby's position is *left occipitoanterior*, the back of his head is on the left, pointing toward his mother's front.

---

port, encouragement, help, and comforting gestures from your partner, doctor, and nurse.

You will probably have emotional ups and downs throughout labor. You may feel discouraged and may weep from time to time, but if you accept labor as it comes and understand what is happening and what to expect, you will be able to recover from these down periods and go on.

### Arrival at the Hospital

On arrival, your first stop is usually the admitting office, where you are asked to read and sign forms and indicate how you will pay for your hospital stay. However, since hospital procedures vary considerably, prior to going into labor it is a good idea to check with your hospital regarding their admitting policies—especially their procedures for late-night and weekend admissions.

From there you go to the maternity ward, where a doctor or nurse greets you, does a quick health

# COMMON OBSTETRIC PROCEDURES

| PROCEDURE | DESCRIPTION | PURPOSE(S) |
|---|---|---|
| **Enema in early labor** * | Spout attached to bag of watery solution is gently inserted into anus. Solution empties into intestine. You hold it in, then expel it into toilet or bedpan. | To empty your bowels |
| **Intravenous fluids** * | Bag containing special liquids hangs by bed. Tube from it is inserted into vein in hand or arm. | To ensure that you remain hydrated without drinking fluids<br><br>To provide a route to administer medication |
| **Fetal scalp blood sampling** | Blood sample is drawn from baby's scalp during labor. Tested for oxygen and carbon dioxide levels and other factors. Takes two to thirty minutes to get results. | To confirm whether fetal distress observed on monitor is real<br><br>To help decide if a cesarean is necessary |

* Hospitals and doctors vary on this. For some, it is optional; others believe every woman or baby should have it. You will need to investigate the policies in your area.

check on you, assesses your contractions and the baby's condition, and does a vaginal exam to establish how far along you are in labor.

From then on, hospitals vary widely in their routine care for labor. The following chart describes common procedures. Feel free to discuss these procedures in advance with your doctor and express your preferences.

Besides the routines described in the chart, your nurse or doctor periodically takes your temperature and blood pressure and, if an electronic fetal monitor is not being used, listens to your baby's heartbeat and feels your abdomen during contractions to determine how labor is progressing. He or she also stays close by, offering encouragement, comforting you, and answering questions.

| INDICATED OR DESIRABLE IF: | OPTIONAL IF ALL IS NORMAL | NOT NECESSARY OR DESIRABLE IF: | PROCEDURE |
|---|---|---|---|
| You are constipated, and it is slowing labor | Yes* | You have emptied your bowels early in labor<br><br>You do not mind passing some feces during late labor | **Enema in early labor*** |
| Labor is very long<br><br>You have continuing nausea and vomiting<br><br>You were given regional anesthesia<br><br>You received oxytocin to speed labor | Yes* | Labor is not prolonged<br><br>You can drink and hold down fluids* | **Intravenous fluids*** |
| Interpretation of monitor tracing is unclear<br><br>There is strong desire to avoid cesarean section | Yes | Baby's heart rate seems normal<br><br>Doctor feels there is no time to wait for results<br><br>Hospital does not have facilities to perform lab work<br><br>Mother has infection and use of procedure would increase chances of baby's catching it | **Fetal scalp blood sampling** |

continued

# THE BIRTHING PROCESS

## COMMON OBSTETRIC PROCEDURES continued

| PROCEDURE | DESCRIPTION | PURPOSE(S) |
|---|---|---|
| **Electronic fetal monitoring (external or internal) *** | External: Two belts around your waist. One contains ultrasound device to detect baby's heartbeat. Other contains device to detect contractions. Both connected to machine that records baby's heart rate and contraction strength.<br><br>Internal: Two devices placed into uterus via vagina. One is attached to baby's scalp and detects pulse; other picks up contractions.<br><br>Internal method is more accurate than external. | To provide continuous recording of fetal heart tones and the contraction pattern |
| **Artificial rupture of membranes (breaking the bag of waters)** | On vaginal exam, doctor inserts long "amnihook" and painlessly breaks bag of waters. Gush of fluid follows. | To speed labor<br><br>To check amniotic fluid for meconium, infection, or bleeding<br><br>To apply internal electronic fetal monitor |
| **Pain medications** | Injections containing drugs given into skin, muscle, or intravenous tube. Also, medications can be injected into area of spine or pelvic floor to decrease pain and cause numbing. | To reduce labor pain<br><br>To enhance sleep or relaxation |
| **Vaginal exams** | Doctor or nurse washes hands, puts on sterile glove, and inserts two fingers into vagina to feel cervix and baby's head. | To determine labor progress (dilation and thinning of cervix, descent of baby) |

\* Hospitals and doctors vary on this. For some, it is optional; others believe every woman or baby should have it. You will need to investigate the policies in your area.

| INDICATED OR DESIRABLE IF: | OPTIONAL IF ALL IS NORMAL | NOT NECESSARY OR DESIRABLE IF: | PROCEDURE |
|---|---|---|---|
| You received oxytocin<br><br>A nurse or midwife cannot be with you continuously<br><br>There are doubts about the baby's condition*<br><br>(Many obstetricians feel that all laboring women should be monitored) | Yes* | (Highly controversial) | **Electronic fetal monitoring (external or internal) *** |
| Labor is prolonged<br><br>Fetal distress is suspected<br><br>Internal electronic fetal monitoring is to be used | Yes | Labor progress is normal<br><br>Fetal heart rate appears to be reassuring | **Artificial rupture of membranes (breaking the bag of waters)** |
| Painful procedures need to be done<br><br>Labor progress is slowed by mother's anxiety<br><br>You want them | Yes | You do not want them<br><br>You are coping well using alternatives to pain medication<br><br>Labor progress is normal | **Pain medications** |
| Labor is prolonged<br><br>Decisions are about to be made on interventions or medications | To some degree | Vaginal examinations are necessary to determine the progress of labor. However, an excessive number of vaginal exams during labor is undesirable because bacteria may be introduced into the uterine cavity, which may lead to infection. | **Vaginal exams** |

continued

# THE BIRTHING PROCESS

## COMMON OBSTETRIC PROCEDURES continued

| PROCEDURE | DESCRIPTION | PURPOSE(S) |
|---|---|---|
| **Intravenous oxytocin** | Oxytocin (a hormone causing uterine contractions) is given in the same way as intravenous fluids. Amount given is precisely controlled with special infusion pump. | To contract the uterus to start or speed up labor<br><br>To contract the uterus after the birth |
| **Restriction to bed** | Mother kept in bed, sometimes in only one position. | To lower blood pressure<br><br>To provide rest<br><br>To slow labor contractions |
| **Vacuum extraction** | A suction device is placed on baby's head. Doctor pulls on it during second-stage contractions to assist or speed birth. | To speed delivery when necessary |
| **Use of forceps** | Two steel instruments (spoon-shaped at one end, with long handles) are placed in vagina on either side of baby's head and locked together. Doctor pulls during second-stage contractions to assist or speed difficult birth.<br><br>(Doctor's preference usually dictates choice between forceps and vacuum extractor.) | To speed delivery when necessary |

| INDICATED OR DESIRABLE IF: | OPTIONAL IF ALL IS NORMAL | NOT NECESSARY OR DESIRABLE IF: | PROCEDURE |
|---|---|---|---|
| You are well beyond your due date<br><br>Inadequate contractions have caused slowing of labor<br><br>There is excessive postpartum bleeding | Yes | Labor is normal or extremely intense<br><br>Pregnancy is not yet at term<br><br>Placental delivery is normal<br><br>Uterus is contracting well | **Intravenous oxytocin** |
| Blood pressure is elevated<br><br>Premature labor is threatened<br><br>A particular position benefits the fetus who is thought to be distressed | Yes | Labor is normal<br><br>Fetus is normal | **Restriction to bed** |
| Medications have reduced your pushing effectiveness<br><br>The baby's size or position is slowing the delivery<br><br>Fetal distress is suspected | Not used in normal cases | Baby's descent is normal, and there is no fetal distress | **Vacuum extraction** |
| Same as above | Not used in normal cases | Baby's descent is normal, or use of vacuum extractor is successful<br><br>Baby is high in the birth canal | **Use of forceps** |

continued

## COMMON OBSTETRIC PROCEDURES continued

| PROCEDURE | DESCRIPTION | PURPOSE(S) |
|---|---|---|
| **Episiotomy** * | Surgical cut between vagina and anus, done shortly before delivery. Done with or without anesthesia. | To enlarge vaginal opening to speed delivery or take pressure off baby's head<br><br>To try to avoid a tear of the perineal tissues* |
| **Cesarean section** | Surgical incision in abdomen and uterus to remove baby. Done with patient under anesthesia. | To deliver the baby without completing labor:<br><br>If vaginal birth is dangerous or impossible;<br><br>If there are emergency problems for mother and baby |

* Hospitals and doctors vary on this. For some, it is optional; others believe every woman or baby should have it. You will need to investigate the policies in your area.

| INDICATED OR DESIRABLE IF: | OPTIONAL IF ALL IS NORMAL | NOT NECESSARY OR DESIRABLE IF: | PROCEDURE |
|---|---|---|---|
| Fetus is in distress | Yes* | Progress in delivery is good | **Episiotomy \*** |
| Perineum is rigid and unable to stretch | | Your perineum will stretch | |
| You or your doctor wants to prevent a tear | | Your fetus is doing well | |
| | | You want to avoid an episiotomy | |
| Hemorrhage is present | Not used in normal cases | Labor progress is normal, and the fetus is not in distress | **Cesarean section** |
| True fetal distress is suspected | | Problems can be solved with less risky procedures | |
| Cord prolapse is suspected | | | |
| Labor has failed to progress | | | |
| Position or size of baby will make delivery hazardous | | | |
| Presentation is breech | | | |
| This is a multiple birth | | | |
| You have a certain illness (for example, active herpes infection or cardiac disease) that would make vaginal delivery hazardous | | | |
| A difficult forceps delivery is the alternative | | | |
| There is a placenta previa | | | |

continued

### COMMON OBSTETRIC PROCEDURES continued

| PROCEDURE | DESCRIPTION | PURPOSE(S) |
|---|---|---|
| **Suctioning of newborn's breathing passages** | Tip of rubber suction device is placed in each nostril and then in mouth to suck mucus and fluid from airway. Done as head appears or immediately after birth. A longer tube may be inserted via nostril down into windpipe to remove deeper secretions. | To clear the airway<br><br>To remove the liquids and meconium that might impair breathing |
| **Baby placed in warming unit** | Baby placed in special bed with heater above. Thermostat taped to baby's skin turns up heat if baby cools. | To maintain or increase baby's body temperature |
| **Eye care with antibiotic ointment or silver nitrate drops** | Medication placed in each eye of baby within first hour of life | To prevent infection and blindness due to gonococcal and chlamydial organisms sometimes present in vagina |
| **Bottle feeding of water, glucose water, or formula** | A substitute for breast-feeding | To "wash out" jaundice*<br><br>To provide calories and liquid before milk comes in*<br><br>To check baby's ability to swallow*<br><br>To feed baby if you are unwilling or unable |

*Hospitals and doctors vary on this. For some, it is optional; others believe every woman or baby should have it. You will need to investigate the policies in your area.

| INDICATED OR DESIRABLE IF: | OPTIONAL IF ALL IS NORMAL | NOT NECESSARY OR DESIRABLE IF: | PROCEDURE |
|---|---|---|---|
| Baby passed meconium into amniotic fluid before birth<br><br>Baby is not breathing well<br><br>Baby cannot cough or sneeze to rid airway of secretions<br><br>Baby has excess of secretions in nose and throat | Yes, though most babies are suctioned with bulb | Baby is breathing well<br><br>There were no signs during labor that baby might develop problems | **Suctioning of newborn's breathing passages** |
| Baby's body temperature drops<br><br>Observation in nursery is deemed advisable<br><br>Baby is premature | Yes | Baby can be placed skin-to-skin with mother and covered with hat and warm blanket<br><br>Parents want time with normal baby | **Baby placed in warming unit** |
| Infection is present<br><br>(State and provincial laws require it) | No, all states and provinces require it | | **Eye care with antibiotic ointment or silver nitrate drops** |
| You do not wish to or cannot breast-feed<br><br>Your baby has phenylketonuria (an inability to tolerate the protein in breast milk) or other rare problem in digesting breast milk | Yes | You wish to establish breast-feeding<br><br>You wish to avoid nipple confusion between breast and bottle for your baby | **Bottle feeding of water, glucose water, or formula** |

continued

## COMMON OBSTETRIC PROCEDURES continued

| PROCEDURE | DESCRIPTION | PURPOSE(S) |
| --- | --- | --- |
| **Limited time with baby** | Baby is taken to nursery and cared for by nurses, except at certain times spent with mother. | To let you rest<br><br>To observe a sick or premature baby |
| **Circumcision** | Skin is separated from end of penis and removed with surgical knife or tied to special plastic "bell" device (foreskin will drop off within days). Usually done without anesthesia. | To remove the foreskin from a baby boy's penis |

\* Hospitals and doctors vary on this. For some, it is optional; others believe every woman or baby should have it. You will need to investigate the policies in your area.

### Mother's Activities During Labor

Once settled in at the hospital, you will find a routine for handling contractions, perhaps based on what you learned in childbirth classes. For example, the following is a routine that many women learn and use successfully with their contractions:

1. Greet the contraction with a long sigh. As you breathe out, release all bodily tension.

2. At the same time, focus your attention in some way (for example, focus on your partner's face or on a picture or object of your choice; close your eyes and "see" your cervix opening as your uterus contracts; "see" a peaceful, relaxing place and picture yourself there; focus on music of your choice, or the soothing voice of your partner; or focus on the feel of your partner holding or stroking you).

3. Breathe slowly and easily.

4. Maintain relaxation throughout the contraction. Stay limp. It may help if you focus on one part of your body with each breath out. Try to release tension in that part as you breathe out. Then focus on another part with the next breath.

You can follow this routine with every contraction and in any position—lying down, sitting, standing, on hands and knees. You can do it in the tub or shower, in bed, in the car, in a chair, in the hospital corridor, or in your room. You can lean on your partner, the wall, or your bed.

These techniques are often effective in keeping pain within manageable limits for part or all of your labor. Women who use them generally need less pain medication than others. Indeed, some women do not need to use any pain medication when using these techniques.

Some women learn several types, or levels, of breathing to use progressively during labor. Besides the slow pattern just described, they may learn a lighter, faster, but still relaxing pattern and other variations.

Besides using a routine for each contraction, you should try to change position every twenty or thirty minutes, go to the bathroom every hour or so,

| INDICATED OR DESIRABLE IF: | OPTIONAL IF ALL IS NORMAL | NOT NECESSARY OR DESIRABLE IF: | PROCEDURE |
|---|---|---|---|
| Baby needs observation or special care<br><br>You are unable to care for your baby | Yes | You wish more time to become acquainted with your baby and to become skilled in baby care and feeding | **Limited time with baby** |
| Religious or cultural beliefs require it<br><br>You prefer the appearance and ease in cleaning of the circumcised penis* | Yes* | You wish to avoid the pain and risk of the surgery<br><br>You prefer the appearance of the uncircumcised penis*<br><br>Your child's penis is abnormal in structure<br><br>The baby is ill | **Circumcision** |

and sip liquids or suck on ice after every contraction. These measures may be comforting.

You may find that hot packs on the lower portion of your abdomen, your groin, and your perineum (external genital-rectal area); cold packs on the lower part of your back; and a cool, moist washcloth rubbed over your face and neck will all feel wonderful. Being touched and rubbed, especially in tense, sore areas, such as the shoulders and the lower part of the back, helps a lot. If you feel a bit out of control, it helps if your partner holds you tightly, or gently but firmly holds your head in his hands.

During intense periods, like the "transition" phase (from about seven to ten centimeters of cervical dilation), you may feel almost out of control. You may feel that your body is running away with you, and that you are being swept along in a tide of intense sensations. Fighting these sensations is pointless.

However, you may feel an urge to push but be told that you are not yet fully dilated. It is important that—for the time being—you resist the urge. Push-

ing too soon could injure the cervix and perineal tissues and may lead to heavy bleeding. What helps the most is knowing that there is nothing wrong. Let it happen—accept that your body is in charge, and don't try to stay "in control." Let your loved ones help you, moan and complain if you want to, and know that it will not last long.

### The Second Stage

The second stage ranges in length from fifteen minutes to three or more hours. The baby is born during the second stage.

When your cervix is fully dilated, the intense, out-of-control feelings may subside. The contractions often space out somewhat, and you may even get a short break from contractions (this is more likely with first-time mothers). It is always wonderful news when you are told that your cervix is fully dilated and you can begin pushing whenever you feel like it.

During the second stage, you may behave differently than in the first stage. You may find yourself

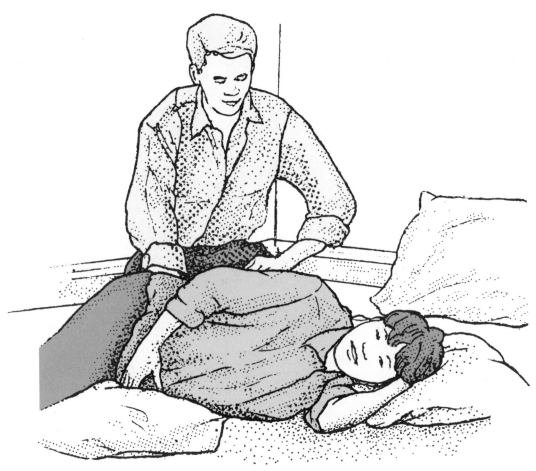

*Relaxation techniques and the support of your partner are important elements of a successful labor.*

holding your breath or slowly letting it out, while bearing down (something like, but much more than, what you do when having a bowel movement) and releasing your pelvic floor (relaxing the muscles in the area around your vagina). This last is most important, because tensing the pelvic floor is actually fighting against the birth of your baby—and it hurts much more than letting go.

You will probably notice a real change in your contractions in the second stage. Most contractions will contain a reflex need to strain or grunt, called an "urge to push," which comes and goes three to five times per contraction. With each urge to push, the combination of the uterine contraction and your bearing-down effort pushes the baby closer to the outside. It is hard work and it hurts, but it is also an exciting time, with lots of cheering and praise for your efforts. Most women find they have the strength to keep pushing.

The best way to push is to push only when your body makes it happen—only when the urge to

push comes. That way you won't hold your breath so long that you or the baby gets too little oxygen. The following is a routine many women use during second-stage contractions:

1. Greet the contraction with a long breath, and curl your body forward whether you are reclining, lying on your side, squatting, or even sitting on a toilet or a birthing chair.

2. Breathe as you did during first-stage contractions.

3. When you feel the reflex urge to push (it is unmistakable), follow it by grunting or holding your breath and bearing down. You will need reminders to relax your pelvic floor. The urge to push will go away after a few seconds. Then breathe again until the urge returns. Repeat until the contraction ends.

4. Relax or change position between contractions.

*Positions for the Second Stage*

Unless the baby is coming fast, you will have time to change positions. Many childbirth educators encourage women to learn to squat comfortably before labor because this is such a helpful position for the second stage. When you squat, you are giving the baby more room to come down through your pelvis than in other positions. Sitting on the toilet may help if you have trouble relaxing your pelvic floor.

Lying on your side is a good position if the baby is coming fast, if you have painful hemorrhoids, or if you must lie down for some reason. Resting on your hands and knees may help if the baby is large or is having a slowing of the heartbeat during contractions. Semi-sitting is a good position because you can see your doctor and the baby as he comes out. It is also a convenient position for your doctor.

Lying on the back with the legs up in stirrups (the lithotomy position) used to be the way all women gave birth. Most women disliked the position. Their objections to it, plus the fact that it sometimes caused slowing of the baby's heartbeat and other problems for the mother, finally led to its being discontinued as a routine position by most midwives and many physicians. It is still used, however, particularly with anesthetized births and deliveries assisted with forceps or vacuum extraction (see the "Common Obstetric Procedures" chart).

You might use several positions during the second stage, ending with semi-sitting or lying on your side for the actual birth. Discuss positions for the second stage with your doctor in advance.

## The Moment of Birth

As the baby's head emerges, you will know. You will feel a stretching or burning sensation in your vagina. This is an exciting, intense time. You know the baby is almost here and may be tempted to push as hard as you can to get him out quickly. That would be a mistake, however, because a sudden push could make the baby come out too quickly and damage your perineum (causing tearing). It is important for you not to push hard at this time. Let your uterus do the work alone. You should breathe rapidly and lightly (pant as animals do during birth), so the baby can emerge gradually. Your doctor will give instructions and help the baby out slowly. You will soon be holding your baby in your arms.

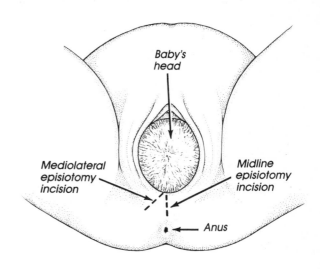

An episiotomy is done to make childbirth easier and to avoid tearing of tissues. The most common type of episiotomy is a midline incision from the midpoint of the vaginal opening directly toward the anus. Some doctors, however, prefer an incision at an angle, called mediolateral episiotomy.

After the head is born, the baby turns to one side, and a shoulder and the whole body are born. And what a sense of relief you feel! Labor is over (or nearly so). You have a baby. It may take a while for it all to sink in. In the meantime, you may be holding your baby and watching as a nurse or doctor examines him and cares for him.

## The Third Stage

Your job is not quite finished. The placenta still needs to be expelled. The third stage usually lasts from five to thirty minutes. The nurse or doctor will keep a hand on your abdomen to determine when the placenta separates from the wall of your uterus. Then you will be asked to push it out. You may feel some cramps, but there is usually very slight discomfort.

## The Fourth Stage

Immediately after birth, while you are holding and admiring your new baby, your doctor focuses on your well-being. The condition of your uterus and vagina is of major concern. It is important that your uterus remain contracted after birth, which keeps it from bleeding as much as when it is relaxed. Most women lose about one cup of blood at the time of birth. While this may seem like a lot, remember that among the many other changes of pregnancy, your blood supply greatly increased. That excess blood is no longer needed; you will lose some of it at the time of birth and will continue to lose some over a period of several weeks (this discharge is called *lochia*). Your doctor watches the amount of blood lost immediately after birth and, if necessary, takes measures to reduce the blood loss. These may include massaging your uterus vigorously, asking you to lightly stimulate your nipples, or giving you an injection of a medication (Methergine [methylergonovine] or Pitocin [oxytocin]) that will cause your uterus to contract.

Your doctor will also check your vagina to see if you need any stitches. If an episiotomy was performed (see the "Common Obstetric Procedures" chart), you will definitely need stitches. Some tearing of the vagina or perineum may also have occurred when the baby was born. Although the idea of tearing sounds rather unpleasant, be assured that the tears (or cuts) are usually not serious, and will usually heal rapidly. If necessary, your doctor will begin stitching within a few minutes after birth. You will be given a local anesthetic for pain relief if you have not already had one.

## Natural Versus Medicated Childbirth

Before leaving the subject of birth and going on to the newborn, we should discuss an important choice that was mentioned in Chapter 3: the choice between natural childbirth and medicated childbirth. Your preparation and decision-making and the course of your labor will differ depending on which you prefer.

Having read the previous discussion of labor, you now have some sense of the physical and emotional events of normal spontaneous labor. It is concern about or fear of labor pain that influences many women to choose to use pain-relieving medications in labor. The following discussion of labor pain and medications for birth may help you decide which you wish to attempt.

### The Use of Pain Medications or Anesthesia in Childbirth

Pain medications have been used in childbirth for centuries. Alcohol, opium, and other drugs have been used, though how extensively is not known.

When using pain medications, you make a trade-off. In return for relief of pain and tension and possible speeding up of labor, you accept the possibility of side effects on labor progress, your mental or physical well-being, or on your baby. You should balance the advantages and disadvantages as they apply in your situation before using or not using a particular medication.

What are the kinds of medications available, how do they work, and what are their risks and benefits? This section provides an overview that will assist you in discussing the subject with your doctor and making a decision on your preferences.

First of all, the choice of natural versus medicated childbirth really exists only as long as the labor remains normal. Some interventions are painful or stressful and increase the need for pain medications. If, however, you or your baby *requires* intervention (such as induction of labor, use of forceps, or a cesarean section) for medical reasons, you will need pain medication.

*Medications for Early Labor*
Because the medications that provide the greatest pain relief also tend to interfere with early labor progress, they cannot be used too early, unless you want to stop labor. There are medications available if a very prolonged and exhausting prelabor or early labor has caused excessive anxiety and worry. Sedatives or barbiturates (sleeping pills or medications) may help you rest. These are given in pill form or by injection. They may temporarily halt your labor while relaxing you or allowing you some sleep. These drugs reach your baby, who cannot easily excrete them, so it is important not to receive large doses. Because babies born with such drugs still in their bodies may have problems breathing or sucking, your doctor will probably use only small doses and will try to be sure that they have worn off before birth.

Tranquilizers are also used in long prelabors to reduce muscle tension and anxiety. Some also help if you have severe nausea and vomiting. Depending on the drug chosen, you may feel dizzy and confused, your mouth may feel dry, and your blood pressure could be altered. These drugs also cross the placenta to the baby and may have effects on fetal heart rate and newborn muscle tone, suckling, and attentiveness.

Morphine, a narcotic, may be used in an attempt to stop a long, nonprogressing labor. While it may cause you nausea, dizziness, and confusion, it also may do just what you need—put you to sleep and stop labor temporarily. Narcotics tend to linger in the baby and can have some effects on behavior and breathing after birth. The greater the amount of the drug given, the greater the effects on the baby.

*Medications for Established Labor*

Once your labor is well established, it is less likely that drugs can slow it for more than a short time. More effective pain-relieving drugs may then be used. Also called analgesics (pain-relieving drugs), they are given by injection under your skin, into your muscle, or into an intravenous line. Demerol (meperidine) is the narcotic analgesic most widely used in obstetrics. Its effects are similar to those of morphine and may be associated with a speeding up of labor in some circumstances. If anxiety, tension, and pain are great enough to actually slow labor, a narcotic or tranquilizer may reduce anxiety and allow labor to speed up again. These drugs reduce your pain, though you are still aware of the peaks of your contractions. They also help you sleep or relax between contractions. You may feel nauseated shortly after receiving them, and may not like the dizzy, confused feeling. The pain relief lasts for an hour or so, after which another dose may be given. The drug does accumulate in the baby's body, however, and larger total doses may have more noticeable effects on your baby's behavior. If your doctor sees that you will give birth when the narcotic effects on the baby will be at their greatest, she may give you (or your baby after birth) a drug called a narcotic antagonist, to reverse the effects of the narcotic.

*Regional Anesthesia*

*Analgesia* means relief of pain; *anesthesia* means loss of sensation. There are ways of injecting certain drugs in particular areas of the body to cause a loss of all sensation (numbness) in a limited area. Local anesthetic agents (like Novocain [procaine], used by your dentist) are used in this way. Agents such as lidocaine and Marcaine (bupivacaine) are used in obstetrics.

Depending on where they are injected, they cause varying amounts of pain relief. For example, a spinal or saddle block creates a rather large area of total numbness. An injection of anesthetic is made in the lower part of the back, and the medicine enters the spinal fluid. The anesthetic is heavy and stays low in the spine. You might become numb from your ribs down to your toes (spinal block) or from your buttocks and lower part of the abdomen down your inner thighs (saddle block). The amount of numbness is determined by how low the injection is given and how low the medicine remains in the body. You can have a "spinal headache" after a spinal anesthetic; this is very painful, can last for days, and usually requires that you lie down much of the time.

Epidural and caudal blocks differ from spinal blocks, since they are given with the same anesthetic agents but in slightly different places. The main difference is that they are not given into the spinal fluid. The medicine is placed low in the back, just outside the canal where the spinal fluid is (therefore, you will not get a spinal headache). Although trickier to give than a spinal block, anesthesiologists prefer them for labor because they are not as likely to stop labor and the actual area of anesthesia can be better controlled (especially with the epidural).

The main difference between the caudal and the epidural is in where they are given: the caudal is given at the top of the separation of your buttocks; the epidural, a few inches higher. As a result, the area of numbness with the epidural tends not to extend as far down into your birth canal and legs as with the caudal. You can push better and move your legs better with an epidural than with a caudal.

Both spinals and epidurals are also used for cesarean births, allowing the mother to remain awake and alert to greet her baby.

Pain relief with these forms of regional anesthesia can be excellent; in fact, many women report total relief of pain. This welcome relief comes with no effects on your mental capacity. You do not become groggy or sleepy.

Because spinals can stop labor at a critical time, they tend to be used for very late labor and for cesarean births.

Forceps-assisted deliveries tend to be more common after regional anesthesia because women cannot push as well when anesthetized. Anesthesia can be "light" or "heavy"; women can push better (and feel more) if the anesthesia is light.

Another drawback to regional anesthesia is the possibility of a sudden drop in blood pressure soon after receiving the anesthetic. This sudden drop can temporarily reduce the amount of oxygen available to the baby. Since this side effect is well known, measures are taken to prevent it (a large amount of intravenous fluid is given to rapidly increase blood volume, which decreases the chance of low blood pressure), identify it as soon as it happens (blood pressure is checked constantly while the anesthetic takes effect), and treat it, if necessary, with drugs to raise blood pressure.

### Local Anesthesia

Three types of local anesthesia may be used for childbirth: the paracervical block, the pudendal block, and local infiltration of the perineum.

The paracervical block is given during the late first stage. Two injections of local anesthetic drugs are made into the cervix and bring pain relief during contractions. Although this form of anesthesia rarely causes problems for the mother, it frequently causes sudden drops in the fetal heart rate and noticeable effects on the baby's muscle tone and reactivity after birth.

Although the amount of pain relief provided by a paracervical block is far less than with the regional blocks, a significantly greater amount of the anesthetic agent is used—thus, there are more serious side effects. For these reasons, this form of block has been discontinued in many areas of the country.

The pudendal block causes anesthesia in the birth canal, and is given in the second stage. Local anesthetic agents are injected into each side of the vaginal wall. Again, a larger amount of medication is used than for an epidural, but the incidence of drops in fetal heart rate appears not as serious as with the paracervical block. It can be used for forceps delivery or pain in the second stage. Most doctors also give a pudendal block before an episiotomy is performed.

Local infiltration of the perineum consists of several injections to numb the area of skin and muscle between the vagina and the anus. It is most commonly used after natural childbirth if stitches are needed. It can also be given in the second stage before an episiotomy is performed. Side effects of a local block appear to be slight.

### General Anesthesia

General anesthesia means a loss of consciousness along with pain relief. In other words, a woman is put to sleep, and wakes up after the anesthetic has worn off. Nowadays, general anesthesia is uncommonly used—and is generally reserved for emergency situations.

General anesthetics are usually gases, which are inhaled. They cause a total loss of awareness. Nitrous oxide, Trilene (trichloroethylene), and Penthrane (methoxyflurane) are examples of such inhalation agents. Sometimes these are used along with sedatives that cause drowsiness. The sedatives might be injected into your vein.

One reason that general anesthetics are used less often today is that they have profound side effects. The mother's breathing may slow down or stop; her blood pressure may drop and cause her heart rate to change. General anesthetics may also stop contractions of the uterus and cause excessive bleeding after birth. The baby is also affected. Babies often have breathing difficulties, sucking difficulties, and poor muscle tone after general anesthetics have been used.

## The Newborn

At first sight, your newborn may not be quite what you had expected. For the first half-minute or so, his skin may be bluish-gray, and he may appear lifeless. That may be a shock if you are not expecting it, but this is the color of all babies in the uterus. As your baby begins breathing and more oxygen enters his body, his color will turn pinker or ruddier—first the head and body, then the arms and legs, and last the feet and hands.

Your baby will be soaking wet, streaked with blood, and smeared with *vernix*, a white, sticky substance. Some babies have a great deal of vernix all over their bodies, and some have small amounts only in the creases and folds. Vernix is almost like a hand cream, in that it protects the baby's skin while he is floating in amniotic fluid.

His face may be swollen, and he may have long fingernails. You may also be surprised by the size of your baby's genitals. Both little girls and little boys have very large, red genitals. The size and color subside in a few days, when their genitals take on a more normal appearance.

## Immediate Care

Even though most babies do not really need it, care-givers routinely suction babies' noses and

## Apgar Scoring

| Sign | No Points | One Point | Two Points |
|---|---|---|---|
| Heartbeat | None | Slow (below one hundred beats per minute) | One hundred beats per minute or more |
| Breathing | None | Slow, irregular breathing; weak cry | Good, strong cry |
| Muscle tone | Limp | Some flexion (bending up) of arms and legs | Active movement |
| Reflex irritability (reaction when suctioned) | No reaction | Grimace | Cough or sneeze |
| Skin color | Blue-gray, pale | Normal skin color, except bluish hands and feet | Normal skin color all over |

mouths very soon after birth to remove excess amniotic fluid and mucus. In fact, sometimes they begin suctioning when only the baby's head is out. It is done with a rubber bulb syringe or with a little jar and tube called a mucus trap. The mucus trap is used if the baby's airway seems to be very congested or if the baby was under stress during labor and breathing problems are anticipated at the time of birth.

Your baby's umbilical cord will be clamped in two places close to his abdomen. Then the cord will be cut between the two clamps. Sometimes the father cuts the cord. Otherwise, the doctor does it. Even though there is a spurt of blood when the cord is cut, neither you nor your baby will feel it at all, since there are no nerves in the umbilical cord. Then your baby will be either placed on your abdomen or taken to a special warm bed in a corner of the room for an examination and other care. If he is placed on your abdomen, you will feel the warm wet baby on your now-soft belly. Many women find this a very pleasant sensation.

Your baby is dried off by rubbing briskly with soft towels to keep him from getting a chill (a major concern of your doctor). Your baby will be wrapped in a warm blanket or two, and his head will be covered. In fact, it is a very good idea to have a warm little hat to place on the baby's head as soon as possible after the birth because the baby's head is such a large part of his body that a lot of heat can be lost through it.

### The Apgar Score

Your baby will be given the Apgar test. This test (named for Dr. Virginia Apgar, the pediatrician who devised it) is used to assess whether your baby needs extra medical care right away. See the above chart for a description of the items checked on the Apgar test. Babies with breathing problems or nervous system problems may need extra care. The Apgar score is determined twice—one minute after birth and again five minutes after birth—and gives your doctor an idea of whether these problems exist. Usually, scores of between seven and ten are signs that your baby is in good condition. If his scores are below seven, your baby may be taken to the nursery for observation and care. Be sure to ask about your baby's Apgar scores.

Within the first hour after birth, most babies receive a medication in their eyes. This might be erythromycin or tetracycline (both antibiotics) or silver nitrate. As required by law in all states and provinces, these medications are given to prevent infections of the eye, which could result in blindness. On rare occasions, a mother may have organisms in her vagina which, if picked up by the baby during birth, could cause eye infections. *Gonococcus* and *Chlamydia* are two common organisms that can cause serious problems. Because we do not have laboratory tests that are one hundred percent accurate in discovering whether a woman has these organisms, laws exist to protect babies who might be infected unexpectedly. Many parents prefer the antibiotic ointments over silver nitrate, since they do not burn or irritate babies' eyes as silver nitrate does. Your baby's vision will be blurry until the ointment is absorbed.

This immediate care can be done with your baby in your arms or very close by. Once these procedures are completed, you may spend some uninterrupted time with your baby. Although your nurse or midwife will be observing the baby and periodically checking your temperature, your blood pressure, and the condition of your uterus, she should try to stay in the background and disturb you as little as possible. This is the time when you and your partner can become acquainted with the baby and start the first feeding, if you plan to breast-feed. Most parents describe this as a wonderful time. Usually the baby is alert and calm, very interested in your faces and voices and in the new sounds he is hearing. When held close to your breast, your baby will begin nuzzling and licking, and then will take the nipple in his mouth and begin to suckle.

Even after a long, tiring labor, you and your baby will probably be wide awake and interested in each other. After spending one or several hours together, both you and the baby will probably doze off, possibly very soundly.

## Examination of the Baby

Besides the Apgar score, which is determined right after birth, a more thorough physical examination of the baby will be done a few hours later. The newborn exam is a thorough check of all the baby's systems. A midwife, family physician, pediatrician, or nurse practitioner may carry out this exam. You may ask that it be done in your presence, so that you can learn more about your baby. From head to toe, the examiner checks such things as the fontanels ("soft spots" at the top and back of the head); the eyes, ears, nose, mouth, and throat; the ability to suck and swallow; the size of the head; the weight and length; the breathing pattern; the size of the liver and spleen; the heart tones and sounds of the lungs; the genitals; the hip joints; the overall appearance of the baby; and the baby's reflexes. The baby's ability to pass urine and move his bowels is also noted. Some babies are further assessed for their actual gestational age; there is a test called the Dubowitz examination that helps determine whether your baby was born early, on time, or late.

In the hospital, babies receive identification bracelets, sometimes on both wrist and ankle, and mothers receive a matching wrist bracelet; this is to prevent mixing up of babies in the nursery. Footprints and handprints are also taken. Immediately after the umbilical cord is cut, a sample of blood is taken from the cord, labeled, and stored, in case it is needed later for blood-typing or other laboratory tests. The baby's temperature, feeding patterns, activity levels, breathing and heart rate patterns, and urination and bowel movement patterns are observed for the next several days. If at home, the parents make these observations after being instructed by their care-giver. In the hospital, nurses usually make these observations.

Within an hour or so after birth, your baby will receive vitamin K to help prevent bleeding problems. Vitamin K helps in the clotting of blood; since babies do not have vitamin K in their systems for the first few days after birth, it is considered an important preventive treatment. Vitamin K can be given by injection in the thigh or by mouth. At present, most doctors prefer to give it by injection.

Your baby will receive a number of laboratory tests. The skin is also examined for any marks or other important signs. A sample of blood is drawn from the heel of each newborn at least once within the first few days after birth. The one test given to all newborns is a test for phenylketonuria (PKU). PKU is an inherited disorder that can be very serious if not detected very soon after birth. A baby with PKU cannot properly process protein and needs a special diet that is low in phenylalanine, the component of protein that isn't handled well. If PKU is detected and the baby receives this special diet, she will grow up normally. If it is not detected and treated, however, PKU can cause mental retardation. Because of the seriousness of PKU, all states and Canadian provinces require that all babies be tested for it. The same blood sample is checked for another condition, congenital hypothyroidism. Some people do not make enough thyroid hormones for normal development. If this condition is discovered early, a baby can be treated and grow up without any problems.

Blood is frequently drawn from newborns for other purposes. If your baby appears to be developing jaundice (indicated by yellowing of the skin and the whites of the eyes), your doctor may draw some blood to analyze its bilirubin level. Bilirubin, a yellow substance, forms when red blood cells break down; the presence of excessive amounts gives a yellow tinge to the baby's skin. If the biliru-

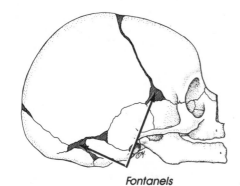

Fontanels

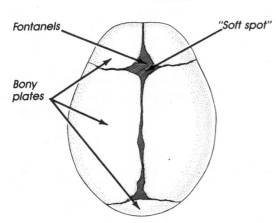

Fontanels

"Soft spot"

Bony plates

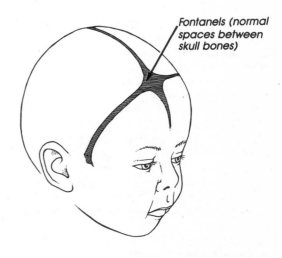

*Normal newborn skull*

Fontanels (normal spaces between skull bones)

Fontanels are the gaps between the bony plates of an infant's skull. Fontanels permit the head to adapt without injury to being squeezed during birth, and after birth they allow room for the brain to grow. Eventually, the bones meet and knit together.

bin reaches a certain level, your doctor may feel it is appropriate to treat the baby to lessen the jaundice. While jaundice in a newborn is rarely a serious condition, it is important to keep track of bilirubin levels in jaundiced babies and to determine the cause. The usual treatment, phototherapy, involves keeping the baby in a brightly lit bassinet, except for feedings. On rare occasions, a blood transfusion is done.

Blood glucose (a form of sugar) levels are also checked in some babies—those who are very large or very small, those whose mothers have diabetes, and those with other possible problems.

### Urination and Bowel Movements

Many babies urinate within minutes after birth. This is an important milestone and is recorded in your baby's medical chart when it happens.

The first bowel movements of a newborn baby are called *meconium,* which forms in the intestine long before birth. In fact, some babies pass some meconium while still in the uterus. It mixes with the amniotic fluid. While this is usually harmless, when your doctor spots meconium in your amniotic fluid during labor, he or she will be concerned that the baby not inhale it deeply with the first breaths after birth. If meconium is breathed deep into the lungs, it can cause breathing problems. If meconium is present, deep suctioning with the mucus trap is done before the baby breathes.

Many parents are unprepared for their babies' strange bowel movements. Your baby will have a meconium bowel movement within a few hours after birth. Meconium is black and sticky and difficult to clean off. Some parents think ahead and rub olive oil on their new baby's bottom before it happens. It is then much easier to clean off.

As the baby begins to feed, the bowel movements become runny and greenish-brown. Once the colostrum has changed to milk, a breast-fed baby's bowel movements become yellow and liquid and nearly odorless. Breast-fed babies normally move their bowels anywhere from once a week to once each feeding. Formula-fed babies move their bowels less frequently, and their bowel movements are dark, firm, and strong smelling.

131

## Circumcision

If your baby is a boy, you will decide whether to have him circumcised or not. (See Chapter 8 and the "Common Obstetric Procedures" chart in this chapter for a description of circumcision.) In hospitals it is usually done on the second day of life, and parents do need to use special care in diaper changes and keeping the area clean for a week or two after surgery. If you decide not to circumcise, there is no special care of the penis. The one important thing to remember is that at birth the foreskin of the penis is usually not separate from the end of the penis, as it is in an older uncircumcised boy. Therefore, you should *not* try to pull the foreskin back. To do so could cause tearing of the skin and scarring, which could be a real problem later in life. The best care for an uncircumcised penis is to leave it alone except to wash and rinse it whenever the baby has a bath.

Some researchers conclude that there are significant health benefits to both the circumcised male and his future spouse—other investigators disagree. Although most men and boys in the United States are circumcised, the practice of nonreligious circumcision remains controversial.

## Care of the Cord

Usually shortly after the cord is cut, your doctor will apply a special substance called triple dye or some other antiseptic agent to it. This may make the cord appear blue. The clamp that was left on the cord at birth is removed on about the second day. For one to three weeks afterwards, your baby will have a black dry stump of cord where the belly button will be. The stump will gradually dry up and fall off. In the meantime, you will probably be taught how to keep the cord clean. The best way to do that is to take a cotton swab, dip it in rubbing alcohol, and gently wipe it around the base of the cord each day.

## Other Considerations

Other matters become very important in the first few days after birth. During the time when you and your baby can become acquainted with and accustomed to each other, you have many choices. For example, it is for you to decide how much time you want to spend with your baby. Studies have shown that being together from birth seems to improve the parent-infant relationship. "Bonding" (a strong attachment between parent and child) is enhanced by more contact. The only reason your time together might have to be limited is illness in either mother or baby. Hospital routines should not keep you apart. You also will decide how you're going to feed your baby—breast or bottle. There are many other matters. See Chapter 3 ("The Newborn Care Plan").

## Postpartum Care of the Mother

Planning for postpartum care of the mother should begin long before the baby is born. Make plans for the first few weeks after birth so that you will not be overwhelmed. For example, try to arrange for some help with household tasks, meal preparation, and grocery shopping for a couple of weeks after the baby is born. Your husband may be able to take some time from work and spend it with the family. The three of you together can slow down and take your time, not worrying about housework, meetings, deadlines, and so on, but just taking a slow, easy pace to rest after the birth, become used to the baby, and meet his needs. A period of time like this, lasting one to three weeks, can get a new family off to a wonderful start. Try to take the pressure off yourself and enjoy this time together.

The baby's grandmother or another relative or friend might also be available to visit and help out with the day-to-day tasks. This person might also be able to offer you advice and pointers on baby care and feeding. Some people hire household help, baby nurses for a few weeks, or teenagers to come in and do some housework each day after school. The important thing is to have some help so that you won't become too tired trying to maintain life as usual along with recovering from childbirth and taking care of a new baby.

Many women find it useful to prepare meals in advance. If you have a freezer that can hold some casseroles or other dishes, take advantage of it. Planning two weeks of meals in advance makes it easier later on. You can do much of the shopping for those meals ahead of time, so that all you need for the first couple of weeks is fresh produce and perishables. With some planning, you will not have to worry about meals when you are tired or preoccupied with the baby.

This kind of advance preparation will make your first couple of weeks much easier, and enable you to rest, which should be your number one concern at this time, along with caring for the baby.

## Physical Changes

In your first few days after birth, you may seem to be preoccupied with basic body functions—urination, bowel movements, vaginal discharge, establishment of breast-feeding or drying up of the milk supply (depending on how you choose to feed your baby), and nourishment. At times, it seems as though every opening in your body has something coming out or coming in.

It is true that the birth process does alter many of your body functions. For example, your uterus has undergone a tremendous change in the hours of labor and birth. Now it is much smaller than it was right before you began labor. The process of involution (the return of your uterus to almost its pre-pregnancy size and shape) continues for a matter of weeks. Your uterus continues to contract after birth, and gradually gets smaller. At the end of a few weeks, your uterus will be about the size of a large pear.

As stated earlier, if the uterus remains contracted after birth, your blood loss will be minimal. It is not unusual, however, for your uterus to relax from time to time, especially if this is not your first baby. When you press the lower part of your abdomen, you should be able to feel your uterus, which should be the size and shape of a large grapefruit. If you cannot find your uterus, it is because it has relaxed. In that case, you should help it to contract. Putting your baby to breast and allowing him to suckle or simply nuzzle at your breast will often cause your uterus to contract. This is the most pleasant way, and has the added benefit of helping establish your milk supply.

You also can massage your uterus to make it contract. Simply place the side of one hand just above your pubic bone and press it in. With your other hand slightly cupped, massage in a circular direction over your lower abdomen—ask your doctor or nurse to show you how. You will feel your uterus gradually tighten up under your massaging hand. You may need to massage very firmly in order to get this result. It may even hurt, but it is so important that your uterus remain firm that you must disregard the discomfort of the massage. If your uterus or lower abdomen becomes extremely painful, notify your doctor or nurse immediately. Check your uterus frequently and massage it whenever necessary in the first two or three days. After that, it usually stays contracted very well.

Lochia (the bloody vaginal discharge that occurs for several weeks after childbirth) is similar to a menstrual period. It begins as a heavy red flow and gradually decreases in amount and turns browner and lighter over time. This discharge comes from the lining of the uterus, which had been thick and rich with blood supply. Since it is no longer needed to house the baby, your body will gradually get rid of it. Sometimes overactivity causes the lochia to revert to a heavy, bright red flow; if it does, you should call your doctor for advice. You will probably be told to take it easier and to avoid overexertion. If this extra bleeding is accompanied by pain or a fever, your doctor should definitely see you and evaluate your problem.

Afterpains are contractions of the uterus that occur while you breast-feed and at other times. They are sudden and can be quite painful. They may be spontaneous or may be caused by stimulation of the nipples, which results in oxytocin release. (As you may remember, oxytocin causes the uterus to contract.) While these afterpains are uncomfortable, especially for women who have had more than one child, they are effective in bringing your uterus back to its pre-pregnant state. Afterpains usually last only a few days. Remember to use relaxation and breathing techniques to help you if they are severe.

### The Perineum

Your perineum may be sore and swollen for a few days after birth, due to stretching of the birth canal or to the episiotomy or tearing that might have occurred. It helps to put an ice pack on your perineum off and on for the first twenty-four hours or so after delivery to reduce swelling and discomfort from stitches. The area is sensitive to touch, so after going to the bathroom, rather than wiping your perineum, squirt the area with some warm water from a bottle, then pat it dry with a clean, soft tissue.

Sitting in about four inches of either very warm or very cold clean water in a tub is also very soothing. You can take such sitz baths several times a day for twenty to thirty minutes. Keep the water clean; don't bathe in this water. Showers are better than baths for the first few weeks after birth because soapy, dirty water could contaminate the healing areas of your perineum.

For some women, hemorrhoids (swollen, painful blood vessels at the anus) may be a problem. The sitz baths may help, as may gently patting the area with cotton pads or tissues soaked in witch hazel. Hemorrhoids tend to improve with time, but if you have a lot of trouble, see your doctor.

When your perineum is sensitive and sore, straining for a bowel movement is painful and a little scary, because you may worry about putting too much stress on your stitches. It is important to have a bowel movement within three days or so after delivery. Make a point of eating high-fiber foods, such as bran and raw vegetables and fruits. Also, drink plenty of fluids, including prune juice. These foods and liquids will help prevent constipation. If you are unable to move your bowels, you may need a laxative. For that, contact your doctor.

At first, you may be surprised at the amount of urine you pass. Whereas in late pregnancy the baby crowded your bladder, requiring that you empty it frequently, now it may seem that your bladder can hold a tremendous amount of urine. Urinating is one way your body rids itself of all the excess fluid it carried during the pregnancy. Occasionally, the urethra (the tube from your bladder to the outside) is swollen after childbirth, causing trouble with urination. Your doctor can help with that.

*The Breasts*
Whether you choose to breast-feed or not, your breasts will begin making and secreting milk. At first, they make colostrum, the perfect food for a new baby. Within two or three days, the colostrum changes to milk. Sometimes, when the milk "comes in," your breasts become very engorged (full to the point of discomfort). If you are breast-feeding, the best way to prevent excessive engorgement is to let your baby nurse frequently. If your baby is a sleepy or lazy nurser, you may relieve engorgement by expressing (forcing out) milk from your breasts, either by hand or with a breast pump.

If you have decided not to breast-feed, efforts will be made to prevent milk production. Cold packs, a well-fitting bra, or medication may be used to slow down or prevent milk production. Usually within a few days, milk production stops.

There is more information on feeding your baby in Chapter 9.

## Emotional Changes

Just as your body undergoes a tremendous adjustment after the birth of a baby, so does your emotional state. There is the impact of a huge role change on your lifestyle. Suddenly you are a par-

ent, with twenty-four-hour-a-day responsibilities to a dependent, helpless baby. The role is a new one; it is tiring and a bit puzzling at times. Combine that with the fact that you are already tired and are undergoing sudden changes in hormone production, and you have a situation of emotional stress. To top it all off, there is the tremendous commitment you feel for your tiny baby. Intense emotions, sometimes highs and sometimes lows, are to be expected at this time. You may find that you cry easily, both from happiness and from sadness and frustration.

Your time is not your own now. Your baby's needs often do not come at convenient times. It is not possible to make plans and expect to stick to them. The women who cope best at this time are those who can accept the realities of the early postpartum period. They place high priority on caring for the baby and getting rest. They also are supported in this by their husbands and other loved ones. Getting help and avoiding heavy demands on yourself are two of the most important gifts you can give to your baby and yourself. Chapter 7 contains further discussion of the adjustments to new parenthood.

The postpartum period represents a gradual return to a more normal lifestyle. Your body recovers from childbirth and adjusts to the new demands of parenthood, including interrupted sleep, feeding schedules, and a constant awareness of the needs of the baby. Thus begins a new phase in the growth and development of all family members.

## A Word to Fathers

Before leaving this subject, it is important to direct a message to those who are closest to the mother and baby. Your role as the mother's companion through pregnancy, labor, and parenthood is unique in its importance because:

- You know her better than the professional staff and almost anyone else.

- You love and care for her more than anyone else.

- Along with the baby's mother, your love and concern for the baby exceed those of anyone else.

Even if you are not an expert on childbirth or parenting, your contribution is of supreme importance. Helping the new mother through a stressful, intense, and possibly exhausting life experience is a generous gesture of caring that she will not forget. It is also the thrill of a lifetime for both of you!

How can you help? Depending on your relationship with her and your personal feelings, find from the following list those things you can and want to do.

*During Pregnancy:*

- Take an active role in the pregnancy. Recognize that pregnancy brings fatigue and anxiety; do your normal share of household chores—and then some.

- Encourage and support lifestyle changes she is trying to make, such as improving nutrition, stopping smoking and alcohol or drug use, and exercising more.

- Take an interest and an active role in decision-making. Attend prenatal appointments and discuss both your concerns.

- Attend childbirth classes and participate. Be sure you learn what you need to know. Read and become knowledgeable.

*During Labor:*

- Stay with her unless you and she really do not want that. (If you will not be with her, be sure someone else is.)

- Help her to be comfortable. Rub or press tense, sore places; wipe her brow with a moist cloth; give her drinks or ice; help her change position and walk; apply cold or hot packs.

- Help her get questions answered.

- If you are worried and wondering if everything is all right, rather than telling her how worried you are, ask the doctor or nurse. If you express anxiety or worry to your partner, she may become unnecessarily anxious.

- Try to express calm through your voice and touch.

- Remind her to change positions, use the shower for pain relief, rest, and take it easy between contractions.

- Help her focus, relax, and breathe by talking her through contractions and encouraging and praising her in between.

- During the second stage, help her into positions she will use (it's hard to move very much at this time!). Encourage her as she pushes, especially to relax the muscles of her pelvic floor, to let the baby come out.

- Take care of yourself. Eat and drink. Nap (in the labor room, if you can) if there is someone who can relieve you.

*After the Baby Is Born:*

- Try to be patient. Life with a new baby is hectic and tiring for everyone. Remember that learning to breast-feed and care for a baby comes gradually. You may be surprised at how a baby can disrupt your lifestyle. You may feel that no one else could possibly be having as hard a time as you are. Not so. Almost everyone has a hard time at first.

- Recognize and support your partner's need for rest. Assume your baby care and household responsibilities as just that—your responsibilities. Don't act as if you are doing your partner a favor. After all, the baby is your child too. Try to avoid making extra demands.

- If you find the stress is getting you down, try to vent it somewhere other than at home. Talk about it with your parents, friends, co-workers, childbirth classmates, or your childbirth educator.

- Keep in mind that this is not a permanent state. The baby brings huge changes and makes great demands, but soon begins giving a lot back by smiling, responding to your cuddling, settling into a predictable schedule, lighting up when you walk into the room, loving bath time, suckling like a pro, and more.

In short, the childbearing year, with all its excitement and anticipation, is also surprisingly demanding. Your support and understanding enable both of you to cope with the difficulties and gain rewards of satisfaction and fulfillment. This time is one of growth for all family members.

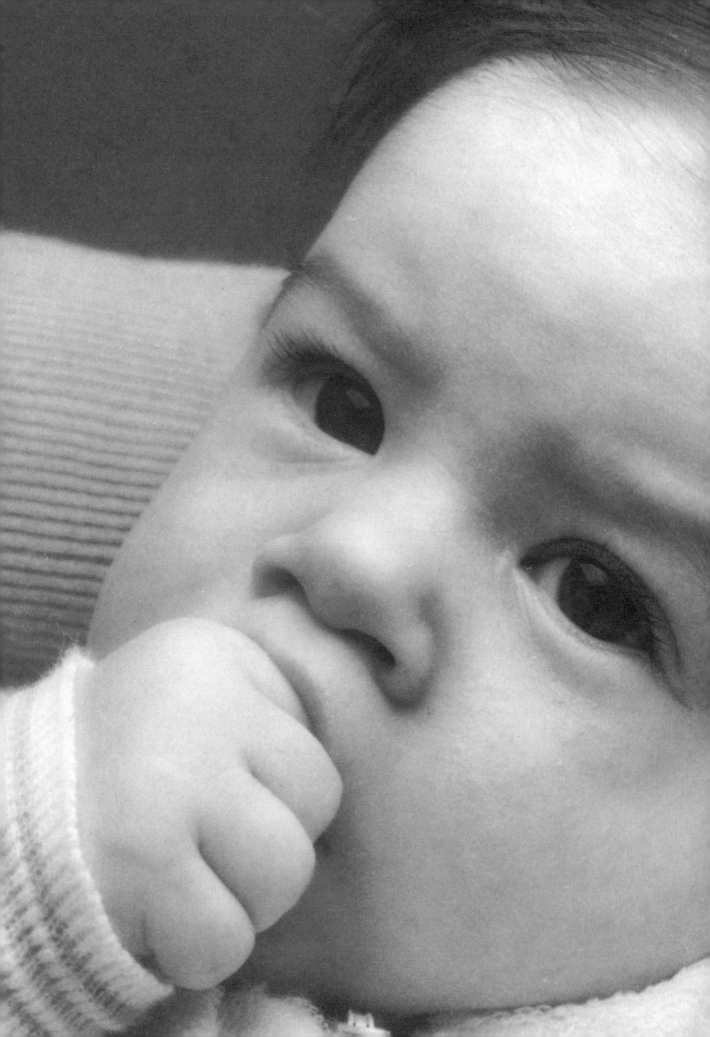

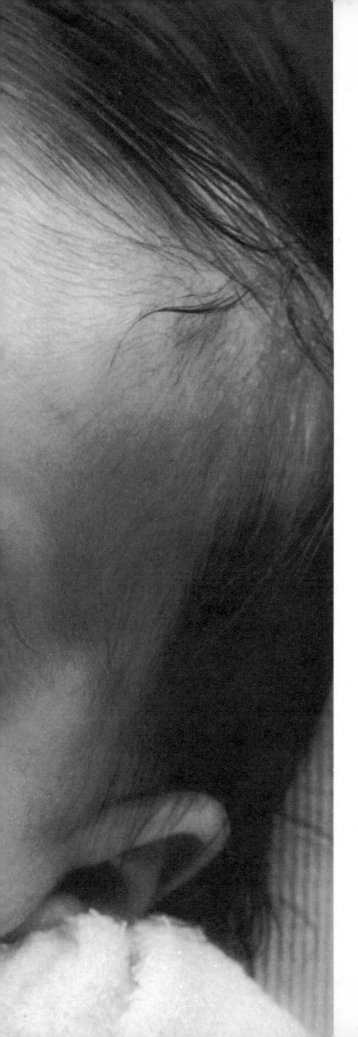

# Chapter 6: Complications of Pregnancy and Birth

## When Complications Arise

It is the hope and dream of all parents to experience a normal pregnancy and to take home a healthy child. But, although the majority of pregnancies and deliveries are uneventful, some involve complications that range from minor to life-threatening—for the mother, for the baby, or for both.

Complications of pregnancy may develop gradually or suddenly and without warning. One objective of prenatal care is the prompt diagnosis and treatment of these complications before they worsen.

In this chapter, we will describe the most common complications of pregnancy, their causes and symptoms, and how they are treated.

# COMPLICATIONS OF PREGNANCY AND BIRTH

## Older Mothers

By medical tradition, an "older" mother is defined as a woman pregnant at the age of thirty-five or older. In recent years, there has been a trend for women to put off childbearing until their thirties and to have additional children in their thirties. In 1983, for instance, there were nearly 625,000 children born to women aged thirty to thirty-four; nearly 180,000 born to women aged thirty-five to thirty-nine; nearly 26,000 born to women aged forty to forty-four; and nearly 1,200 born to women aged forty-five to forty-nine.

Though most older women will experience successful pregnancies and deliver healthy babies, a variety of problems may be encountered.

### Infertility

The inability to become pregnant—called infertility—is more common in older women. Because women begin to ovulate less frequently at age thirty, the number of opportunities to achieve fertilization decreases as each year goes by. For example, the average woman at age thirty will ovulate thirteen times a year; by the time she has reached forty, she may ovulate only five or six times a year.

Older women are also more likely to have problems with their genital organs, which may prevent pregnancy from occurring. Extensive endometriosis and uterine fibroids may make it impossible to become pregnant.

### Chronic Illness

As we become older, we are more likely to develop chronic illnesses, for example, high blood pressure, diabetes, and glandular disorders, such as an underactive thyroid gland (hypothyroidism). Though these illnesses may not be serious or life-threatening to the nonpregnant woman, they may become more serious or even uncontrollable during pregnancy. Furthermore, certain chronic illnesses of the mother are associated with an increased risk of miscarriage and stillbirth.

### Birth Defects

Older mothers are also at greater risk of having babies with severe birth defects caused by abnormalities of the baby's chromosomes.

Chromosomes are structures contained within all cells of the body, including the egg and the sperm. These chromosomes contain the genetic information that is passed on from parent to baby. Normally, the sperm and the egg each contain twenty-three chromosomes. When the sperm and the egg join, the resulting cell, which will develop to form the baby, will contain the normal chromosome number of forty-six.

In some cases, the egg may contain twenty-four chromosomes instead of the normal twenty-three. If this egg combines with a normal sperm containing twenty-three chromosomes, the resulting fertilized egg will contain forty-seven chromosomes—an abnormal number. The baby that results from this fertilized egg will then contain forty-seven chromosomes in all the cells in its body.

In many cases, a fetus with an abnormal chromosome number will miscarry, accounting somewhat for the higher miscarriage rate in older women. Those pregnancies that continue normally will involve a fetus with any one of a number of physical abnormalities.

The most common condition associated with an abnormal chromosome number is Down syndrome, also called *mongolism*. In this condition, the babies are mentally retarded and may have serious abnormalities of the heart and digestive system. Children with Down syndrome have a characteristic facial appearance, with slanted eyes, heavy eyebrows, and a large, thick tongue.

Though Down syndrome babies may be born to mothers of any age, they occur more commonly in older mothers. At the age of twenty, a mother has one chance in 1,667 of having a child with Down syndrome; at the age of thirty-five, she has one chance in 370; at age forty, she has one chance in 109.

### Treatment

The prenatal care of an older woman is generally like that of a woman in any other age group. If the woman has a history of high blood pressure, diabetes, or other chronic disorders, prenatal office visits may be more frequent than usual, especially during the last two months of pregnancy.

Mothers thirty-five years of age and older will be offered amniocentesis—a test to determine the presence of chromosome abnormalities in the fetus. Amniocentesis is performed between the sixteenth and the eighteenth weeks of pregnancy. After an area of skin on the mother's abdomen has been anesthetized, the doctor inserts a long, hollow needle through the mother's abdominal wall into the uterus. (Prior to the doctor's inserting the needle, an ultrasound study will be performed to determine the exact location of both the fetus and the placenta.) With the needle in the amniotic sac surrounding the baby, the doctor draws off into a syringe about two tablespoons of amniotic fluid. This fluid contains cells that have fallen off the skin of the fetus. After these cells have been grown on a special culture plate and examined under a microscope, the fetal chromosomes can be analyzed to see if there is an abnormal number. If an abnormality is discovered, the mother will be given the option of terminating the pregnancy.

### Labor and Delivery

Most older mothers experience normal labor and delivery. However, certain problems are more common in this age group, for example, placental abruption and pre-eclampsia (a severe condition associated with high blood pressure that may lead to convulsions). For these reasons, the rate of cesarean section is somewhat higher in older mothers.

## Teenage Mothers

Over the last two decades, the number of births to teenage mothers has continued to increase; in one recent year, about ten thousand babies were born to American teenagers under the age of fifteen, and nearly a half million babies to teenagers aged fifteen through nineteen. Because teenagers often do not use contraceptives, the pregnancy rate in this age group is higher than in adult women, who are more likely to use some form of contraceptive.

Unfortunately, nearly two-thirds of all teenage pregnancies are unintended. Though teenagers represent only about eighteen percent of sexually active females, they account for nearly forty-five percent of births to unmarried mothers.

Few unwed teenagers give up children for adoption or care by others. For this reason, the mothers often must drop out of school and cannot hold full-time employment. They must suddenly assume the responsibility for raising a child before they are ready, either emotionally or financially.

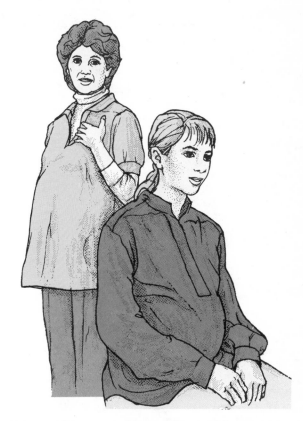

*Older and teenage mothers require special care during pregnancy.*

### Risks

Compared to mothers in older age groups, teenage mothers are at greater risk of having medical complications. Because the teenage mother is more likely to receive little or no prenatal care, she often becomes anemic and is more likely to develop pre-eclampsia. Vitamin deficiencies are more common, and the teenage mother's weight gain is likely to be inadequate. Since the teenage mother herself is still growing, she needs to eat properly not only for her own continued growth, but also for normal growth of the fetus.

Pelvic bones do not reach their maximum size until about the age of eighteen; therefore, the pelvis of the teenage mother may not have grown enough to allow vaginal delivery of a normal-sized baby. For this reason, the incidence of cesarean section is higher in teenage mothers—a baby that can be delivered vaginally when the mother is twenty years old is often too large to have been delivered vaginally when that mother was fourteen.

Babies born to teenage mothers are twice as likely to die in the first year of life as babies born to mothers over the age of twenty. Since the teenage mother is less likely to eat correctly during pregnancy, her baby often has a low birth weight (under five and a half pounds), making it more likely that the baby will become ill.

## Treatment

The teenage mother should be encouraged to seek prenatal care early in pregnancy, eat a nutritious diet, take prescribed vitamins and iron supplements, and engage in healthy physical activity. Though a supportive family can help the teenage mother cope with her new responsibilities, social service agencies may be needed to help her find ways to finish school and seek employment.

## The "Due Date"

The average length of pregnancy is forty weeks, or 280 days, from the first day of the last normal menstrual period. The "due date," or expected date of delivery, for a pregnancy is calculated simply by adding nine months and seven days to the first day of a woman's last normal menstrual period. For example, if the first day of the last menstrual period was January 1, the expected date of delivery is nine months and seven days later—on October 8. In reality, the majority of women do not actually give birth on the due date. About eighty percent of babies are born within ten days of the due date—either ten days before or ten days after. A pregnancy in which delivery occurs during this time period—that is, between thirty-eight and forty-two weeks of pregnancy—is called "full term."

A delivery that occurs many days before the due date is called a preterm delivery, and a delivery that occurs significantly after the due date is called a postterm delivery.

## Preterm Delivery

A preterm, or premature, delivery is defined as the birth of a baby between the twentieth and the thirty-sixth week of pregnancy. A baby born during this time period is called premature. About eight to ten percent of deliveries in the United States are classified as premature.

## Causes

A preterm delivery occurs because the mother goes into labor too early. Though in most cases there is no clear reason, abnormally early labor is often associated with the following conditions: multiple pregnancy, such as twins or triplets; an abnormally shaped uterus that may crowd the fetus; placenta previa; placental abruption; high fever in the mother; untreated diseases of the thyroid gland in the mother; other severe diseases in the mother, such as high blood pressure, diabetes, and kidney disease; and severe infections in the mother, such as kidney infection. Contrary to popular belief, severe emotional trauma and physical injury, such as might result from a fall, are uncommon causes of premature labor. If a mother has premature labor in one pregnancy, she has a twenty-five percent chance of its recurring in the next pregnancy.

## Complications

The major complication of preterm delivery is the birth of a baby that is unable to survive outside the mother's body. Though the baby's organs may all be correctly formed, his lungs may not be developed enough to allow him to breathe adequately. Recent advances in the care of premature infants have allowed babies as small as one and a half pounds at birth to survive and grow up normally. Despite these significant medical advances, prematurity remains the leading cause of death in the newborn.

## Treatment

If a woman suspects that she is in labor before the thirty-seventh week of pregnancy, she should call her doctor and go to the hospital immediately. The doctor will then check the cervix to determine if it has dilated (opened). An electronic monitor may also be used to detect uterine contractions.

Several different drugs may be used to stop the uterine contractions of premature labor. These drugs are initially given intravenously, and some may be given orally once contractions have stopped. Once it has been determined that contractions have stopped, the woman will remain in the hospital for two to three days to make certain that contractions do not start again. Once she goes home, the doctor will generally advise her to restrict physical activity and refrain from sexual intercourse, and to rest in bed as much as possible.

Drugs used to stop labor are successful only if the cervix has not dilated more than four centimeters (one and a half inches). If the cervix has dilated any more, most attempts to stop labor fail and the baby will be delivered prematurely. This is why it is important to report to the hospital immediately if premature labor is suspected.

## Postterm Pregnancy

A postterm, or postdate, pregnancy occurs when the baby has not been delivered by the end of the forty-second week of pregnancy. In the United States, about eight percent of deliveries are postterm.

### Cause
The cause of postterm pregnancy is not known. In most cases, however, it is believed that the mother misstated the exact date of her last menstrual period and the pregnancy was not postterm after all. If a woman has had one postterm pregnancy, she has a greater than average chance of this happening again in subsequent pregnancies.

### Complications
Postterm pregnancy poses no health risk to the mother. However, as the placenta continues to age beyond the forty-second week of pregnancy, its ability to transmit oxygen and nutrients to the fetus may begin to decline. In some cases, this reduction in the transmission of oxygen and nutrients may be severe enough to cause the death of the fetus. When the baby is born, it commonly has a characteristic postterm appearance: wrinkled, cracking, peeling skin; long nails; abundant hair; and little fat tissue beneath the skin. The postterm baby often passes fecal material called meconium into the amniotic fluid before delivery. If the baby sucks meconium into his lungs at the time of delivery, severe pneumonia may result.

### Treatment
The usual treatment for postterm pregnancy is to start labor by administering the drug oxytocin intravenously. Oxytocin stimulates uterine contractions similar to those of normal labor. A fetal monitor is generally used to detect any abnormalities of the fetal heartbeat. Most women with an induced labor will experience a normal labor and delivery.

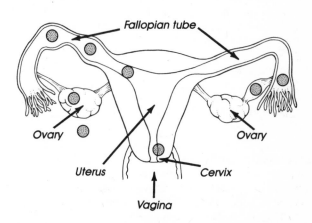

*An ectopic pregnancy is one in which the fertilized egg develops outside the uterus, most often in the fallopian tubes, but also in the ovary, on the cervix, or attached to another organ in the abdominal cavity.*

## Ectopic Pregnancy

Ectopic (out of place) pregnancy occurs when the fertilized egg develops outside the uterus. The most common location of ectopic pregnancy is in one of the fallopian tubes (structures that extend about four and a half inches from the ovaries to the uterus and through which the egg travels from the ovary to the uterus). An ectopic pregnancy that occurs in a fallopian tube is called a tubal pregnancy. On rare occasions, the pregnancy starts to develop in the ovary, on the cervix, or attached to the surface of a nearby organ.

One of every one hundred to 150 pregnancies is ectopic, with the majority occurring in a fallopian tube.

### Causes
The usual cause of ectopic pregnancy is an obstruction or narrowing of a fallopian tube that prevents the fertilized egg from passing through the tube into the uterus. This obstruction or narrowing is usually the result of inflammation and scarring from a previous pelvic infection caused by gonorrhea or Chlamydia infection. Tubal infections caused by numerous other bacteria can also occur after miscarriage, after childbirth, or during the use of an IUD (intrauterine contraceptive device). If these infections are severe, blockage or narrowing of the tube may result.

Other less common causes of tubal obstruction or blockage include abdominal infections, such as appendicitis; pelvic tumors; and scar tissue formation after abdominal surgery.

## Complications

An ectopic pregnancy may be fatal unless it is promptly treated. The danger with a tubal pregnancy is that it will not be detected until it has ruptured (broken through) the tube enclosing it, leading to profuse bleeding into the abdomen. Ectopic pregnancies located in other areas, such as the ovary and cervix, can invade nearby blood vessels and cause massive bleeding. In earlier years, ectopic pregnancy was catastrophic, often leading to death. Today, with the advent of safe blood transfusions and better diagnostic methods allowing early diagnosis, death resulting from ectopic pregnancy is uncommon.

## Symptoms

Symptoms of ectopic pregnancy usually appear two to four weeks after a woman has missed her menstrual period. Irregular spotting of blood from the vagina is one of the earliest symptoms. This is frequently followed by sharp, continuous pains on one side of the lower abdomen. If the ectopic pregnancy ruptures, the woman will usually experience sudden, sharp, severe pain in the lower abdomen accompanied by rapid heartbeat and backache and, in some cases, fainting. Sometimes, even up to the point of rupture, the woman may experience no unusual symptoms.

## Diagnosis

During a pelvic examination, the doctor may discover a tender swelling on one side of the pelvis. Movement of the uterus or ovaries during this exam may cause pain. When an ectopic pregnancy is suspected, the woman is usually hospitalized immediately. Ultrasound scans of the pelvic structures may in some cases reveal the location of the ectopic pregnancy. Blood that has leaked from the ectopic pregnancy into the abdominal cavity may be detected by inserting a hollow needle through the wall of the vagina beneath the cervix and drawing off blood. The diagnosis of ectopic pregnancy is confirmed by inserting a laparoscope (a lighted, tube-like instrument) into the abdominal cavity through a small incision made below the navel. This allows the doctor to look directly at the pelvic organs and precisely locate the ectopic pregnancy.

## Treatment

Treatment for ectopic pregnancy is the surgical removal of the embryo. When the pregnancy is in a fallopian tube, the entire tube and sometimes the ovary must be removed to stop bleeding. However, it is sometimes possible to remove the affected portions and reconstruct the tube so that it will function normally in the future.

A woman who has had one ectopic pregnancy has a fifteen percent chance of having a second one. This does not mean that she should not try to become pregnant again, but when she does try, she should be especially watchful for symptoms of ectopic pregnancy, and she should see her doctor immediately so that the location of the pregnancy may be determined.

# Stillbirth

The death of the fetus at some time between the twentieth week of pregnancy and birth is called stillbirth—in medical terms, an intrauterine fetal demise. This tragic outcome of pregnancy is uncommon today because of better prenatal care and improved methods of diagnosing and treating abnormal pregnancies.

## Causes

The primary cause of stillbirth is interruption of the normal flow of oxygen and nutrients from the mother to the fetus via the placenta and the umbilical cord. Conditions that may adversely affect the placenta and cause stillbirth include toxemia, chronic high blood pressure, diabetes, placenta previa, and placental abruption. Less commonly, a problem with the umbilical cord, such as twisting or breakage of a blood vessel, may cut off the flow of blood to the fetus and lead to stillbirth. Certain abnormalities of the fetus—including erythroblastosis; severe abnormalities of the heart, kidneys, and nervous system; and even fetal heart attack—may lead to stillbirth. It is extremely rare for an injury to the mother to cause stillbirth.

## Complications

The death of the fetus within the uterus usually does not jeopardize the mother's health. The body generally has no reaction to fetal death except for loss of weight. Uncommonly, death of the fetus may cause abnormalities of the mother's blood clotting system, but only after the fetus has been dead for several weeks.

### Diagnosis

Fetal death is usually brought to the doctor's attention by the woman's reporting that she has not felt the fetus move for a day or two. This absence of fetal movement is significant only in the last few months of pregnancy; before this, failure to note fetal movement for a day or two is normal. If careful examination by the doctor fails to detect a heartbeat, confirmation of the diagnosis of stillbirth is sought with either an electronic heartbeat monitor or ultrasound.

### Treatment

Spontaneous labor may begin any time from a few hours to up to sixty days after the death of the fetus. When labor does occur, it is usually normal. Today, most doctors choose to induce labor and deliver the fetus as soon as possible after the diagnosis of fetal death. This is accomplished by administering the drug oxytocin intravenously.

## Miscarriage

A miscarriage (in medical terms, a spontaneous abortion) is the expulsion from the uterus of the fetus and placenta before the beginning of the twentieth week of pregnancy. At that point, the fetus is not developed enough to survive outside the uterus on its own. (After the twentieth week of pregnancy and before the thirty-sixth week of pregnancy, expulsion of the fetus and placenta is considered a premature delivery.) Most miscarriages occur within the first fourteen weeks of pregnancy.

It is impossible to know the exact number of miscarriages that occur during the first month of pregnancy, before a woman realizes she is pregnant. The only indication may be a slightly late menstrual period with a heavier than normal flow. However, about fifteen percent of known pregnancies end in miscarriage.

### Types

There are different categories of miscarriages. A *threatened miscarriage* is experienced by about one of every five pregnant women when they bleed vaginally during the first three months; although it may indicate that a spontaneous abortion will eventually occur, it is often no more than a threat, and the pregnancy will continue normally. An *inevitable miscarriage* occurs when the woman begins to bleed and the cervix di-

lates; it is then only a matter of time before the contents of the uterus are expelled. A *missed miscarriage* occurs when the fetus dies and the placenta stops growing; this may occur several days to weeks before the contents of the uterus are naturally expelled. An *incomplete miscarriage* occurs when only part of the uterine contents has been expelled; a *complete miscarriage* occurs when all of the uterine contents have been naturally expelled.

### Causes

The reason that a miscarriage occurs is not always known, but in many cases it is believed that a fetus aborts because it is not developing normally. Several factors can contribute to abnormal fetal development, including abnormalities in the father's sperm; abnormalities in the egg; disease in the mother, most notably rubella (German measles), severe heart or kidney disease, diabetes, or thyroid disease; abnormalities in the uterus; the mother's use of certain drugs; and the mother's exposure to toxic substances or certain environmental pollutants. Contrary to popular belief, severe emotional trauma or stress, automobile accidents, and simply falling rarely, if ever, cause miscarriage.

The expulsion of the fetus because of an abnormality is thought to be a chance event, usually not due to a defect in either parent. Of women who miscarry once, most (eighty percent) have a successful subsequent pregnancy.

Although it is uncommon, some women miscarry three or more times in a row; they are called *habitual aborters*. When this occurs, the physician will conduct a thorough evaluation of both the woman and her partner to determine the cause, if any. Frequently, a chromosome abnormality in one parent or an abnormality of the uterus is found. If an abnormality of the uterus is the cause of miscarriage, corrective surgery may be performed and a successful pregnancy often results. Unfortunately, if the cause of miscarriage is a chromosome abnormality in either parent, nothing further can be done.

### Complications

Miscarriage is rarely a life-threatening condition for the mother, especially when diagnosed and treated promptly. Though blood loss may occur, it is generally not enough to cause serious problems.

# COMPLICATIONS OF PREGNANCY AND BIRTH

## Symptoms

The symptoms of miscarriage are vaginal bleeding (from a few drops to a heavy flow) and uterine cramps (either dull and constant or sharp and intermittent) felt in the lower part of the abdomen or back. The bleeding can start suddenly or follow a brownish discharge. A solid clot of blood or tissue may pass from the vagina. If possible, this should be saved for the doctor, who may be able to examine it and determine the cause of the bleeding.

A pregnant woman who starts bleeding or experiences abdominal pain should contact her doctor **immediately**.

## Treatment

If a threatened miscarriage is diagnosed, the doctor generally directs the woman to rest in bed, avoid heavy lifting and pushing, and abstain from sexual intercourse. Though it is traditional for doctors to give this advice, many physicians feel that there is little that can be done to stop or avert a miscarriage.

After an inevitable, incomplete, or missed miscarriage, any tissue remaining in the uterus will cause continued bleeding and possibly infection. To remove any retained tissue, the doctor will perform a D & C (dilatation and curettage). This is a surgical procedure in which the cervix is dilated using tapered metal dilators and the contents of the uterus are scraped out using a sharp instrument called a curette.

## Multiple Births

Twins occur once in eighty-eight births; triplets once in about 7,700 births; and quadruplets once in about 680,000 births. Other denominations of multiple births occur quite rarely. Multiple births occur more commonly in older women; women who have had at least one previous pregnancy; women who have a family history of multiple pregnancy on the mother's side of the family; and women who have taken fertility drugs to stimulate ovulation (the expulsion of an egg from the ovary).

## Types

There are two types of twins. One type starts from a single egg, which divides in two very early after fertilization. Because a single egg is fertilized by a single sperm before this division, the two off-spring will be of the same sex and alike in skin, hair, and eye color and in general appearance. They are identical twins.

An extremely rare form of identical twinning is called conjoined, or Siamese, twinning. In these unfortunate cases, the twins are attached to each other at the head, chest, abdomen, or back. Surgical separation of Siamese twins may be successful, but often results in the death of one or both babies.

The other type of twinning is the result of fertilization of two eggs by two different sperm. Twins of this type—called fraternal twins—may be of the same sex or of opposite sexes and will bear no greater resemblance to each other than any other brothers and sisters. Most twins that result from the use of "fertility drugs" are of this type.

Approximately one-third of twins are identical, and two-thirds are fraternal.

One or more eggs may be involved in other forms of multiple pregnancy. For example, quadruplets may result from one, two, three, or four eggs.

## Causes

In most cases of multiple birth, the cause is unknown. Why certain families have many sets of twins is also not understood. Fertility drugs used to stimulate ovulation are often associated with multiple births—sometimes up to seven or eight fetuses.

## Diagnosis

Doctor and patient alike will often suspect multiple pregnancy when the woman's uterus grows more rapidly than would be expected with one baby. This suspicion is confirmed if the doctor hears two separate fetal heartbeats or if an ultrasound scan shows two or more fetuses.

## Complications

The major complication of multiple pregnancy is premature labor, with the delivery of small, premature babies that are not yet ready to live outside the mother's body. In general, the more fetuses a woman is carrying, the earlier in pregnancy she is likely to go into labor. Other complications that may affect the mother are anemia and pre-eclampsia.

### Treatment During Pregnancy

The doctor's special care of a woman with a multiple pregnancy is aimed at preventing premature labor and detecting and treating anemia and pre-eclampsia. When multiple pregnancy is diagnosed, the woman is advised to avoid strenuous activity and rest in bed as much as possible. She may even be admitted to the hospital a few weeks before the expected delivery date. Prenatal visits will be more frequent than usual (at least once a week) so that the doctor will be able to detect the early stages of anemia and pre-eclampsia.

### Labor and Delivery

Most of the time, the labor of a woman with a multiple pregnancy will be normal. However, the positions of the twins in the uterus are quite variable: the first baby may be head first and the second breech (buttocks or legs first), the first baby breech and the second head first, both babies breech, and so on. If both babies are head first, doctors will usually allow a vaginal delivery. When the babies are in other positions, however, a cesarean section is usually performed to ensure a safe delivery of both babies. Because of the serious problems that may be encountered in the vaginal delivery of other types of multiple pregnancies, most pregnancies involving three or more babies are delivered by cesarean section.

## Abnormal Bleeding in Late Pregnancy

From the time of the last normal menstrual period to the time of labor, a pregnant woman should not experience any bleeding from the vagina. During the first half of pregnancy, the most serious causes of bleeding are miscarriage and ectopic pregnancy; during the last half of pregnancy, the most serious causes are placenta previa and placental abruption.

## Placenta Previa

In placenta previa, the placenta is located low in the uterine cavity, partially or completely covering the opening of the cervix. As the lower portion of the uterus stretches and dilates during the latter weeks of pregnancy, portions of the placenta may be torn from their attachment to the wall of the uterus. This leads to variable amounts of bleeding, ranging from light to profuse.

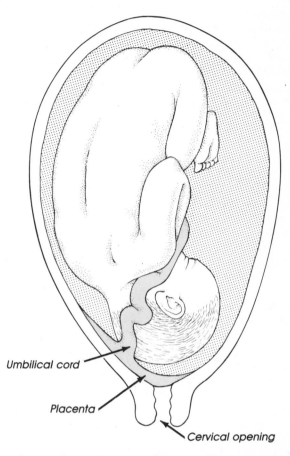

Umbilical cord

Placenta

Cervical opening

*The embryo usually attaches itself in the upper part of the uterine wall, but sometimes implantation takes place in a lower location. As the placenta grows, it can partially or completely cover the opening of the uterus, thus interfering with a normal delivery.*

### Causes

The exact cause of placenta previa is unknown. It occurs in about one of every two hundred pregnancies and is more common in women who have had previous pregnancies.

### Symptoms

The major symptom of placenta previa is painless vaginal bleeding. This bleeding may begin as early as the twenty-fourth to twenty-sixth weeks of pregnancy, though it is more common during the last four or five weeks. The blood is usually bright red, indicating that the bleeding is fresh. This bleeding occurs without any previous injury (for example, from a fall). In some cases, the blood flow is light (referred to as spotting). Abdominal pain or cramping generally does not accompany the bleeding unless the woman is in labor.

# COMPLICATIONS OF PREGNANCY AND BIRTH

### Diagnosis

Any vaginal bleeding during pregnancy is abnormal and should be reported to the doctor immediately. An ultrasound scan of the mother's abdomen will be performed to locate the placenta. In most cases of placenta previa, the ultrasound scan will show the placenta covering part or all of the opening of the cervix.

### Complications

Bleeding from a placenta previa may be extremely heavy, leading to severe blood loss from the mother. This bleeding stops only after the baby has been delivered and the placenta has been removed. Unless treatment is rapid in the case of heavy bleeding, death of both the mother and the baby may result.

### Treatment

Since the placenta covers part or all of the opening of the cervix, a normal vaginal delivery cannot be attempted since extreme hemorrhage will occur. For this reason, babies of most mothers with placenta previa are delivered by cesarean section.

Once placenta previa has been diagnosed, the doctor will decide the best treatment—either delayed or active. Delayed treatment involves admitting the woman to the hospital, keeping her on bed rest, and closely monitoring her for any recurrence of bleeding. The purpose of delayed treatment is to give the fetus time to mature so that it can survive outside the mother's body. Once the maturity of the fetus has been established, delivery will be by cesarean section. In the case of active treatment, the baby is delivered by cesarean section as soon as possible.

The degree of vaginal bleeding will usually dictate the type of treatment. If vaginal bleeding is slight and the fetus is not yet mature, delayed treatment is generally chosen. If vaginal bleeding is heavy, a cesarean section is performed immediately to save the life of the mother and the baby, even if the baby is premature.

## Placental Abruption

After delivery of a baby, the uterus will begin to contract, causing the placenta to separate from its wall and be pushed into the vagina. In the case of placental abruption, the placenta begins to separate from the uterine wall before the delivery of the baby. This potentially serious condition occurs to some degree in about one of every fifty to one hundred pregnancies.

### Causes

The exact cause of placental abruption is unknown. However, a number of conditions are commonly associated with placental abruption, including high blood pressure in the mother, severe trauma to the mother's abdomen, and advanced age of the mother.

### Symptoms

The major symptoms of placental abruption are vaginal bleeding and strong, continuous pain over the uterus and sometimes across the back. Bleeding may be as slight as a tablespoon or extremely heavy. In some cases, there is no visible bleeding and the only symptom is pain. If blood loss is great, the woman will experience rapid heartbeat, difficulty breathing, fainting, and even shock.

### Diagnosis

The diagnosis of placental abruption is made on the basis of the woman's history and the doctor's findings of blood in the vagina and a tender, painful uterus. There are no specific tests that can be used to diagnose placental abruption. In most cases, even the ultrasound scan will be normal.

### Complications

Bleeding associated with a placental abruption may be extremely heavy, leading to death of both the mother and the fetus. Even if the mother does not bleed heavily, the placenta may separate from the wall of the uterus to an extent that the fetus is not receiving a sufficient oxygen supply to survive. In some cases, the mother's blood may fail to clot normally, leading to even more profuse vaginal bleeding.

### Treatment

Like the treatment of placenta previa, the treatment of placental abruption may be either delayed or active. If vaginal bleeding is slight or has stopped and the fetus remains unharmed, the mother will be admitted to the hospital for observation until all signs of placental abruption have stopped. If, on the other hand, vaginal bleeding is heavy or if the fetus is showing signs of lack of oxygen, delivery must occur quickly. A mother who is already in labor will be monitored closely and may expect to give birth vaginally if she and the fetus remain stable. In the case of heavy bleeding, a cesarean section is performed immediately. Before or after delivery, the mother may require blood transfusion if she experiences severe blood loss.

## Cesarean Section

Cesarean section is the delivery of a baby by cutting through the abdominal wall and uterus and removing the baby through these incisions. About fifteen to twenty percent of births in the United States are by cesarean section.

### Reasons
Cesarean section is performed when delivery of the baby is necessary and when a natural vaginal delivery would cause injury to either the mother or the baby. Some of the specific reasons for a cesarean section include the following:

- To save the baby's life when problems with the placenta or the umbilical cord are cutting off the blood supply to the baby; this may be detected by abnormal heart rate patterns on a fetal monitor

- To deliver the baby if the mother fails to give birth after a long labor, usually because the baby is too big to pass through the pelvis

- To prevent infection of the baby by dangerous bacteria in the surrounding amniotic fluid, or by a dangerous vaginal or cervical infection

- To prevent injury to the baby during a breech birth, when the baby would emerge through the vagina buttocks or feet first rather than head first; many obstetricians believe that all breech births in first-time mothers and all premature breech births should be done by cesarean delivery

- To treat disease of the mother or baby that can be treated better if birth occurs as soon as possible

- To prevent the chance of rupture of the uterus during labor if the mother has already had a cesarean section with a previous birth

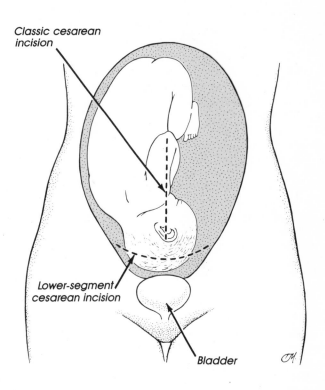

A cesarean section is the delivery of a baby by cutting through the abdomen and uterus and removing the baby through these incisions. The two types of cesareans are the classic and the lower-segment; the incisions for each are shown here.

- To deliver multiple pregnancies involving three or more fetuses

### Types
Two types of cesarean section are performed:

- In the classic cesarean section, a vertical cut is made directly down the center of the uterus in its thick upper section. The incision on the skin is also made vertically and extends from the navel to the pubic bone. This operation is generally used only if the baby is lying in an abnormal position or if the placenta is in an abnormally low position in the cavity of the uterus. With this type of cesarean section, there is more bleeding than with other methods, it is more difficult to repair the incision, and the uterus is more likely to rupture during a future pregnancy. For these reasons, the classic cesarean section is seldom used today unless there are specific reasons for its use.

# COMPLICATIONS OF PREGNANCY AND BIRTH

- The lower-segment cesarean section is the more commonly performed operation. Here, the incision is made in the lower, thinner portion of the uterus. The incision made on the skin may be either vertical down the middle of the abdomen or smile-shaped (the "bikini" incision) near the lower part of the abdomen.

### Risks

To minimize risks of a cesarean section, the operation should be performed only by a skilled obstetrician, accompanied by an anesthesiologist to administer anesthesia to the mother and a pediatrician to take care of the baby after birth.

Risks of a cesarean section include possible infection, excessive bleeding, and dangerous blood clots that may enter the blood circulation. Further, the operation may be inconvenient for the mother, requiring her to stay in the hospital for five to seven days instead of going home with the baby three days after a vaginal delivery. She may not be able to see the baby for a number of hours after delivery if she has undergone general anesthesia. Breast-feeding may also be difficult at first if the mother is being given strong medications to relieve pain, which may keep her asleep for long periods of time. There is pain from the operative incision, and the mother's activity is restricted once she arrives home. It takes up to six weeks for complete healing of the incision. However, all these inconveniences are small if the result is a healthy mother and a healthy baby.

Today, cesarean section is an extremely safe operation because of improved antibiotics and better anesthesia.

### Effects on Parents

In the past, women undergoing cesarean section have been separated from their husbands during surgery, and as a result have often expressed negative feelings of isolation and inadequacy for having failed to accomplish a vaginal delivery. To assist these parents and prevent this from happening to others, many childbirth instructors are providing couples with more information about cesarean section. In many hospitals, husbands are allowed to remain with their wives during the operation. Generally, allowing fathers in the operating room has not caused problems, and women who have undergone cesarean section with their husbands at their sides have shared and enjoyed the birth experience in a far more positive way.

### Vaginal Birth After Cesarean Section

In the past, a firm rule in obstetrics was "once a section, always a section." More recently, obstetricians have found that many women with a previous cesarean section can have a safe vaginal delivery in a subsequent pregnancy. To minimize the risks of rupture of the uterine scar during labor, certain criteria must be met: the previous cesarean section must have been only the lower-segment type; the mother must have had only one previous cesarean section; the mother's pelvis must be of normal size; the baby must be in the head-first position; and the indication for the previous cesarean section must not exist with the present pregnancy.

## Birth Defects

All expectant parents dream of having normal, healthy children. Unfortunately, sometimes this does not happen. Although most babies are born normal and whole, about three percent are born with some form of abnormality. Fortunately, about half of these imperfect babies have only minor defects that can be easily corrected, leaving no trace. In the other half, however, the defect may be severe and life-threatening.

### Types

Birth defects, also called congenital anomalies, can affect nearly every organ of the baby's body. In some cases, these defects are visible on the surface of the body; in other cases, the defects involve internal organs, such as the heart or intestines. Another type of defect, called an inborn error of metabolism, is not visible but rather is an abnormality of the chemical system of the body in which normal chemical reactions in certain organs cannot occur.

The following is a list of the most common serious birth defects:

- *Head and face*—Hydrocephalus (an abnormally large head due to accumulation of fluid), microcephaly (an abnormally small head), cleft lip and cleft palate (an abnormal opening in the lip and the roof of the mouth)

- *Heart*—Congenital heart disease (a variety of different defects in the valves and walls of the heart)

- *Lungs*—Absence of one lung, abnormal lung development

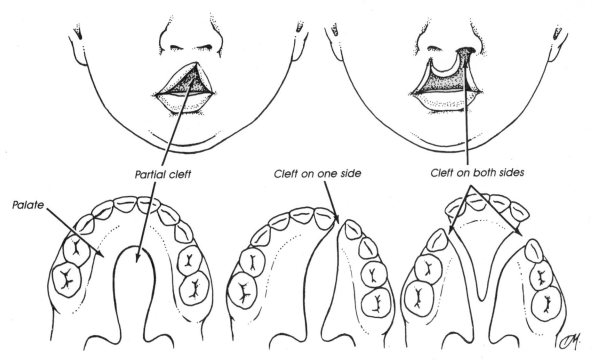

Partial cleft    Cleft on one side    Cleft on both sides

Palate

*Cleft lip or cleft palate is a split running through all or part of the upper structure of the mouth. In its most severe form, the cleft may divide the palate into three parts, resulting in a split on either side of the nose and leaving a middle section of upper jaw and gum dangling, as shown on the right.*

- *Stomach and intestines*—Abnormal blockage

- *Abdominal wall*—An opening through the navel or a large defect that causes the intestines to protrude

- *Kidneys*—Absence of one or both kidneys, large cysts in the kidneys, developmental abnormalities of the kidneys (such as variations in structure)

- *Back*—Spina bifida (an abnormal opening in the backbone in which nerves are contained in a thin, sac-like structure)

- *Arms and legs*—Absence of fingers or toes, fused fingers or toes, total absence of an arm or leg, clubfoot (an abnormal inward turning of the foot)

## Causes

Little is known about the cause of most congenital anomalies. Heredity plays a role in some cases; some families have several members with similar abnormalities. Certain drugs, environmental pollutants, toxins, and high doses of radiation are known to cause specific abnormalities. Cer-

tain infections in the mother—the most important of these is German measles (rubella)—may cause multiple severe abnormalities. In most cases, however, the exact reason for the abnormality is not known and probably derives from a disturbance in the normal organ development of the fetus.

## Diagnosis

The ability to detect congenital abnormalities before birth is a relatively recent medical achievement. In addition to allowing some couples to terminate an abnormal pregnancy, it has enabled others who may be at risk of having abnormal offspring to continue a pregnancy knowing that the fetus is normal.

During the first prenatal visit, the doctor will obtain a thorough history of both parents, including age, race, ethnic background, and previous abnormal conditions in the family. This information will be used to determine if testing for an abnormal fetus will be necessary. The following tests may be used to detect specific abnormalities:

- *Ultrasonography*—This test uses sound waves to produce pictures of the internal organs and the external surface of the fetus; abnormalities

*Talipes equinovarus*

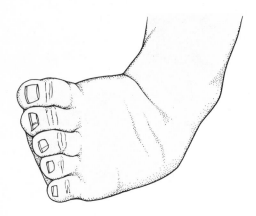

*Metatarsus varus*

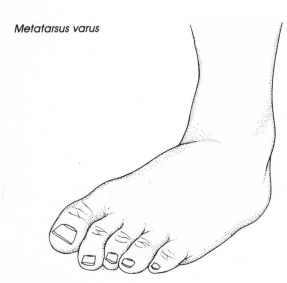

The most frequent form of clubfoot is talipes equinovarus, *in which the foot points down and turns in with the front of the foot curling toward the heel. Related to clubfoot is* metatarsus varus, *in which the front of the foot turns inward. The condition is often called "pigeon toe."*

that may be detected include hydrocephalus, microcephaly, spina bifida, tumors, heart defects, intestinal blockage, and absence of an arm or leg.

- *Fetoscopy*—This test uses a thin telescopic instrument to look directly at the fetus while it is still in the uterus. This is done by making a small incision on the mother's abdomen and gently passing the instrument through the wall of the uterus. Abnormalities that may be detected include defects involving the face, spinal cord, and extremities.

- *Blood tests*—Certain chemical tests performed on the mother's blood may detect possible fetal abnormalities.

- *Amniocentesis*—This test involves drawing off fluid from the amniotic sac surrounding the baby and then analyzing either the cells or chemicals contained in the fluid. This test will detect chromosome abnormalities, spina bifida, and nearly one hundred chemical disorders in the fetus.

## Treatment

Once an abnormality of the fetus has been detected, the parents will need to make a decision regarding either terminating or continuing the pregnancy. However, many birth abnormalities that were very serious a few decades ago can be wholly cured today by the many remarkable advances in medical and surgical care. Many heart defects, intestinal obstructions, and abnormalities of the abdominal wall can be corrected surgically, and those children born with them can expect to lead normal and healthy lives. A pediatrician and a surgeon will be helpful to the parents in describing the extent of the fetal abnormality and the chances of correcting it. Research is now being conducted that may enable surgical correction of certain types of congenital abnormalities while the fetus is still in the uterus.

## Future Pregnancies

Fortunately, in most cases, birth defects do not repeat themselves in future pregnancies. For parents with one abnormal child, there is an average risk of less than five percent of having another child with the same abnormality. If, however, the defect is thought to be inherited from one parent, there may be a specific pattern of this abnormality repeating itself. Before the parents of an abnormal child plan another pregnancy, it is best that they meet with a doctor skilled in genetics and fetal abnormalities to discuss the risks of abnormalities appearing again. For additional information about genetic disorders, see Chapter 8.

## Impact on the Parents

The birth of a physically abnormal child is an unexpected event that often produces feelings of shock, disbelief, sadness, and even anger in the parents. All members of the family will in some way be affected by the birth. A mutual support system between the father and the mother is of great importance in resolving this crisis. Gradually, the parents will resolve their grief and become as closely attached to this child as they would to any other.

## Rh Incompatibility

Approximately eighty-seven percent of white persons and ninety-three percent of black persons are born with a substance on their blood cells known as the *Rh factor,* so called because a similar substance is found on the blood cells of rhesus monkeys. Individuals who have this factor on their blood cells are called Rh-positive; those without it are called Rh-negative. The presence of the Rh factor is inherited from one's parents.

Problems can occur in the fetus if the mother is Rh-negative and the fetus is Rh-positive. Normally, some fetal blood will escape from the placenta and enter the mother's blood. If both the mother and fetus are Rh-positive, this leakage of fetal blood will cause no problems. However, since this fetal blood containing the Rh factor is a "foreign" substance to a mother who is Rh-negative, the mother's body will form antibodies against the Rh factor. Antibodies are normally formed in the body in response to foreign substances—usually bacteria and viruses that may be harmful. These antibodies act by destroying the foreign substance, thus protecting the body against their harmful effects. A person who forms antibodies against a substance is called "sensitized" to that substance.

If the mother forms these antibodies against Rh-positive blood, the antibodies will cross from the mother into the fetus and start destroying fetal blood cells. This leads to a serious condition in the fetus called *erythroblastosis,* which may lead to anemia, heart failure, and even stillbirth.

When an Rh-negative mother becomes sensitized, it is usually at the time of the birth of her first Rh-positive baby. This baby is generally unaffected. However, the mother will keep her antibodies against Rh-positive blood for life. If she has another pregnancy with an Rh-positive fetus, this fetus may be affected.

About twenty years ago, a substance was developed that could protect a mother from becoming sensitized to Rh-positive blood. This substance, called human anti-Rh immune globulin, is injected into the mother shortly after the delivery of an Rh-positive baby and destroys any Rh-positive blood cells that may have entered her blood. After a mother has received this injection, she will not become sensitized and will not have to worry about erythroblastosis developing in her next baby.

During early pregnancy, the doctor will perform a blood test to determine if the mother has Rh-positive or Rh-negative blood. If the mother is Rh-negative and her baby is found at birth to be Rh-positive, the mother will be given an injection of human anti-Rh immune globulin within two days.

## Medical Problems of Pregnancy

The majority of women enter pregnancy healthy and remain so until delivery of the baby. Aside from a variety of minor problems—for example, backache, morning sickness, and constipation—the woman generally tolerates the many physical and chemical changes in her body that result from pregnancy.

In some cases, however, either the mother enters pregnancy with a medical problem or a problem develops during pregnancy. Some of these conditions will affect only the mother, while others may affect both mother and baby.

### Toxemia of Pregnancy

Toxemia of pregnancy is a severe condition that sometimes occurs in the latter weeks of pregnancy. It is characterized by high blood pressure; swelling of the hands, feet, and face; and an excessive amount of protein in the urine. If the condition is allowed to worsen, the mother may experience convulsions and coma, and the baby may be stillborn. The term *toxemia* is actually a misnomer from the days when it was thought that the condition was caused by toxic (poisonous) substances in the blood. The illness is more accurately called *pre-eclampsia* before the convulsive stage and *eclampsia* afterward.

#### Causes
The causes of pre-eclampsia and eclampsia are not clearly understood. They tend to develop more often in mothers from lower socioeconomic groups and in mothers at the extremes of childbearing age—that is, teenagers and women over the age of thirty-five. One theory proposes that certain dietary deficiencies may be the cause of some cases. Also, there is the possibility that some forms of pre-eclampsia and eclampsia are the result of deficiency of blood flow in the uterus.

# COMPLICATIONS OF PREGNANCY AND BIRTH

## Symptoms

The symptoms of toxemia of pregnancy (which may lead to death if not treated) are divided into three stages, each progressively more serious:

1. *Mild pre-eclampsia symptoms* include edema (puffiness under the skin due to fluid accumulation in the body tissues, often noted around the ankles), mild elevation of blood pressure, and the presence of small amounts of protein in the urine.

2. *Severe pre-eclampsia symptoms* include extreme edema, extreme elevation of blood pressure, the presence of large amounts of protein in the urine, headache, dizziness, double vision, nausea, vomiting, and severe pain in the right upper portion of the abdomen.

3. *Eclampsia symptoms* include convulsions and coma.

## Treatment

Pre-eclampsia and eclampsia cannot be completely cured until the pregnancy is over. Until that time, treatment includes the control of high blood pressure and the intravenous administration of drugs to prevent convulsions. Drugs may also be given to stimulate the production of urine. In some severe cases, early delivery of the baby is needed to ensure the survival of the mother.

## Prevention

There is no known preventive for toxemia of pregnancy. Though the restriction of salt in the diet may help to reduce swelling, it will not prevent the onset of high blood pressure or the appearance of protein in the urine. During prenatal visits, the doctor will routinely check the woman's weight, blood pressure, and urine. If toxemia is detected early, complications for the mother and baby may be reduced.

## Heart Disease

Although the incidence of heart disease of women in their childbearing years has declined dramatically in recent years, it still remains one of the major causes of death in pregnant women. Most women with known heart disease withstand pregnancy without any problems. However, in some cases in which the heart muscle or valves are seriously diseased, the added strain that is normally placed on the heart during pregnancy may lead to heart failure and even death. For this reason, any woman who knows that she has a heart problem should check with her doctor before attempting to become pregnant.

## Kidney Disease

The most common disease of the kidneys during pregnancy is *pyelonephritis,* which is a bacterial infection of the kidney. This can occur when an infection of the bladder allows bacteria to travel up to the kidneys. Symptoms of pyelonephritis include fever, severe low back pain, and chills. It is important to treat pyelonephritis quickly because it may cause a pregnant woman to go into premature labor. For this reason, all instances of severe low back pain and fever should be reported to the doctor immediately.

Women who have severe kidney disease before pregnancy can have many serious problems during pregnancy. Extremely high blood pressure and kidney failure (inability to produce urine) are life-threatening complications for both the mother and the fetus. Some women with severe kidney disease may be advised not to become pregnant. Consult your doctor if you have any questions.

## Diabetes

Before the discovery of insulin for the treatment of diabetes, women with this disease rarely became pregnant; when they did, pregnancy was often fatal to both mother and baby. Today, a diabetic woman can expect to become pregnant and, in most cases, deliver a healthy, normal baby.

Even though medical care of the diabetic woman has improved greatly in the last decade, a variety of serious problems may be associated with pregnancy, including an increased chance of pre-eclampsia, stillbirth, and abnormally small babies. For these reasons, the diabetic woman should expect more frequent prenatal office visits and more laboratory testing. It will also be important for her to maintain a strict diet, exercise appropriately, and take her insulin at all the prescribed times.

Another form of diabetes, called gestational, or pregnancy-induced, diabetes, affects women only during pregnancy. In this disorder, women who were not diabetic before pregnancy display signs of diabetes only when they are pregnant. During routine prenatal office visits, the pregnant woman's urine is always tested for the presence of sugar (urine should normally contain no sugar). If sugar appears in the urine, the doctor will generally do a blood test to see if the woman's blood sugar level is abnormally high. Women with pregnancy-induced diabetes are generally treated only with a special diet that restricts their intake of sugar and carbohydrates. Insulin is rarely necessary to bring the blood sugar level down to normal. Since women with pregnancy-induced diabetes also are at a greater risk for pre-eclampsia and stillbirth, they can expect to have more frequent prenatal visits.

## Digestive System Problems

The most common digestive system problem affecting pregnant women is called *hyperemesis gravidarum.* In this condition, the woman suffers from excessive or abnormal vomiting. This type of vomiting is more severe than that caused by normal "morning sickness," which usually clears up on its own within a few months. In hyperemesis gravidarum, the vomiting leads to starvation, loss of water in the body, and an imbalance in bodily fluids.

Symptoms of hyperemesis gravidarum include loss of weight and dehydration. The condition is most often treated in the hospital through the use of anti-vomiting drugs and intravenous feeding to correct the possible malnutrition, dehydration, and imbalance of bodily fluids. A pregnant woman should not attempt to treat herself with drugs for vomiting without first consulting her doctor.

## Lung Disease

Lung disease is uncommon in pregnant women with the exception of occasional bouts of cough and congestion associated with the flu or a cold. The most serious lung disease to affect a pregnant woman is asthma. In women who have only mild asthma attacks before pregnancy, their asthma may stay the same, improve, or worsen. In women with severe asthma before pregnancy, symptoms usually worsen during pregnancy. Severe asthmatics are also more likely to have premature labor and small babies. Before a woman with severe asthma attempts to become pregnant, she should check with her doctor.

## Liver Disease

There are no diseases of the liver strictly associated with pregnancy. However, those that may develop may be more difficult to treat during pregnancy, and preexisting liver disorders may be exacerbated by the pregnancy. Viral hepatitis (an inflammation of the liver), for example, is often more severe if it develops during pregnancy. If a woman knows that she has liver disease, it is best that she check with her doctor before attempting to become pregnant.

## Nervous System Disease

The most common nervous system problem in a pregnant woman is headache, generally caused by tension, migraine, or an infection of the sinuses or throat. Simple measures, such as lying down in a quiet room and applying ice packs over the forehead, will cure most simple headaches. However, since headache may be a symptom of high blood pressure associated with pre-eclampsia, all severe or persistent headaches should be reported to the doctor immediately.

Numbness and tingling of the fingers, thighs, and toes are quite common in pregnancy and usually result from retention of water and swelling.

Epilepsy is the most serious nervous system problem that can affect a pregnant woman. About one-half of women with epilepsy will become worse during pregnancy. Furthermore, certain drugs that are commonly used to treat epilepsy may cause birth defects in the baby. Before a woman with epilepsy attempts to become pregnant, it is best that she check with her doctor.

## Skin Disease

Several types of skin changes are common in pregnant women and result from the normal hormonal changes of pregnancy. Darkening of the skin is common, especially on the face, abdomen, vulva, and thighs and around the nipples. As pregnancy progresses, the palms of the hands often become red, and small "spider veins" may develop on the arms and face. "Stretch marks" on the skin of the lower part of the abdomen usually develop late in pregnancy. There are several types of skin diseases that occur only in pregnancy. These appear as numerous small, raised bumps that are usually extremely itchy. Though rarely serious, any unusual skin changes or itching should be reported to your doctor.

## Infectious Diseases

Though most common infectious diseases, such as colds and the flu, will have no effect on pregnancy, some diseases that may be caught from others may have very serious effects on the baby.

The herpes virus is responsible for frequent, painful ulcers that may occur in the genital areas of both men and women. This virus is sexually transmitted and is spread by direct contact between the genital organs of a man and a woman. Though this infection rarely causes serious problems in the woman, the newborn baby may become seriously infected and die if it comes into contact with an open herpes ulcer during delivery. For this reason, cesarean section is performed if a woman has a herpes ulcer in the genital region when she is in labor. If a woman knows that she has had herpes, it is important that she tell her doctor, since he or she will then carefully examine the genital area during prenatal visits.

Syphilis is another sexually transmitted disease that may seriously affect the baby. If a mother has an active syphilis infection during pregnancy, the bacteria may enter the baby's bloodstream and cause a variety of abnormalities, including malformations of the heart, eyes, bones, and mouth. As a part of the routine blood testing of the mother during the first prenatal visit, a blood test to detect the presence of syphilis is usually performed. If a pregnant woman thinks that she may have caught syphilis during pregnancy, she should tell her doctor immediately.

Rubella (German measles) is a common infectious disease that usually affects children. The rash and fever of rubella usually pass within a few days, and complete recovery from the infection is the rule. Rubella infection during pregnancy, however, may have many serious effects on the baby, especially if the infection develops early in pregnancy when the organs of the fetus are just beginning to form. Complications in the baby may include microcephaly (abnormally small head), mental retardation, seizures, defects in the eyes, heart malformations, and deafness. If a pregnant woman suspects that she may have come into contact with someone with rubella, she should report it to her doctor immediately, even if a rash or

fever has not yet appeared. The doctor may then perform blood tests to determine if the woman has actually caught rubella. Since rubella infection in pregnancy is serious, a woman who is considering becoming pregnant should be tested to see if she is immune to rubella. Usually, if a person has had rubella at one time in her life, she will never get the infection again. If a woman is not immune, most doctors advise that she obtain a rubella vaccination before becoming pregnant.

Toxoplasmosis is another infection that may have serious effects on the baby. The mother may become infected with the toxoplasmosis organism if she eats infected raw meat or if she is in close contact with cats infected with toxoplasmosis. Babies born to infected mothers may have many serious birth defects, including microcephaly, seizures, and disorders of the brain, liver, blood, lungs,and kidneys. To avoid infection with toxoplasmosis, the pregnant woman should always cook meat thoroughly and avoid contact with cat litterboxes.

## Abnormalities of Labor

Labor is defined as the process by which the uterus rhythmically contracts and expels the baby and placenta. Labor is a progressive process that generally does not stop until the baby and placenta have been delivered.

For a woman pregnant with her first child, the average length of time from the beginning of labor to the delivery of the baby is about fourteen hours; for a woman with at least one previous delivery, it is about eight hours.

During a woman's labor, the doctor will examine the cervix periodically (about every two hours) to determine how far it has dilated (widened). Before labor begins, the cervix will be dilated by only about one-half to one centimeter (there are 2.54 centimeters per inch). When the cervix is "fully dilated," it has reached ten centimeters in diameter. At this point, the baby's head has enough room to move into the vagina and be delivered.

The nurse or doctor will also check the baby's heartbeat during labor. Sometimes a special stethoscope called a *fetoscope* may be used. More commonly today, an electronic fetal monitor will be used. With this device, a special microphone is placed on the mother's abdomen above the uterus and secured with a strap. This microphone is connected to the fetal monitor, which will amplify the sound of the heartbeat and record the heart rate on a moving strip of paper. The baby's heart rate during labor is normally in the range of 110 to 160 beats per minute.

Another function of the fetal monitor is to record the mother's labor contractions. A special pressure-sensing device is secured to the abdomen with a strap and then connected to the monitor. Each time a labor contraction occurs, it will show up on the monitor paper as a short wave. By watching the monitor, the doctor can tell how frequently the mother is having contractions.

### Slow Labor

Some women may experience an abnormally slow labor, which is usually caused by mild or infrequent contractions. The doctor will detect this by looking at the fetal monitor and noting that the cervix is dilating slowly. The usual treatment of slow labor is to give the drug oxytocin intravenously. Oxytocin speeds up labor contractions and causes them to become stronger.

### Failure to Progress

In some cases, the mother may have been in labor for many hours without giving birth. The doctor's examination will usually show that either the cervix has stopped dilating or the baby is still high up in the mother's pelvis. In medical terms, this problem is called "failure to progress."

Failure to progress is usually caused by one of two problems: either the baby is too large to fit through the mother's pelvic bones or the mother's pelvic bones are too small to allow the delivery of even a normal-sized baby. To help diagnose this problem, the doctor may obtain x-ray films of the mother's pelvis to determine if it is large enough to allow delivery.

Since in many cases of failure to progress the baby cannot fit through the pelvis, cesarean section will be necessary to ensure a safe delivery.

### Prolapse of the Umbilical Cord

The umbilical cord is the attachment between the fetus and the placenta. It literally forms the lifeline of the fetus through which it obtains oxygen and nutrients from the mother. During labor, a portion of the umbilical cord may prolapse (fall down) into the vagina before the baby is delivered. If this occurs, the umbilical cord may become compressed between the fetal head and the walls of the mother's pelvis, thereby cutting off the blood supply to the fetus. Unless a vaginal delivery is expected to occur immediately, cesarean section must be performed to save the baby's life.

### Abnormalities of the Fetal Heart Rate

During labor, the fetal heart rate is normally steady. In some situations, however, there may be a decrease, or deceleration, of the heart rate during uterine contractions. Compression of the fetal head against the wall of the mother's pelvis may give a particular pattern of deceleration that is quite normal, especially during the latter parts of labor. Serious causes of fetal heart rate deceleration include problems with the placenta and a compressed or pinched-off umbilical cord. Since these decelerations may mean that the fetus is not getting enough oxygen, immediate delivery of the baby—usually by cesarean section—is necessary.

### Hemorrhage

Excessive bleeding or hemorrhage is a serious complication of labor and is usually caused by either placenta previa or placental abruption. Immediate cesarean section is usually necessary to save the life of both the mother and baby.

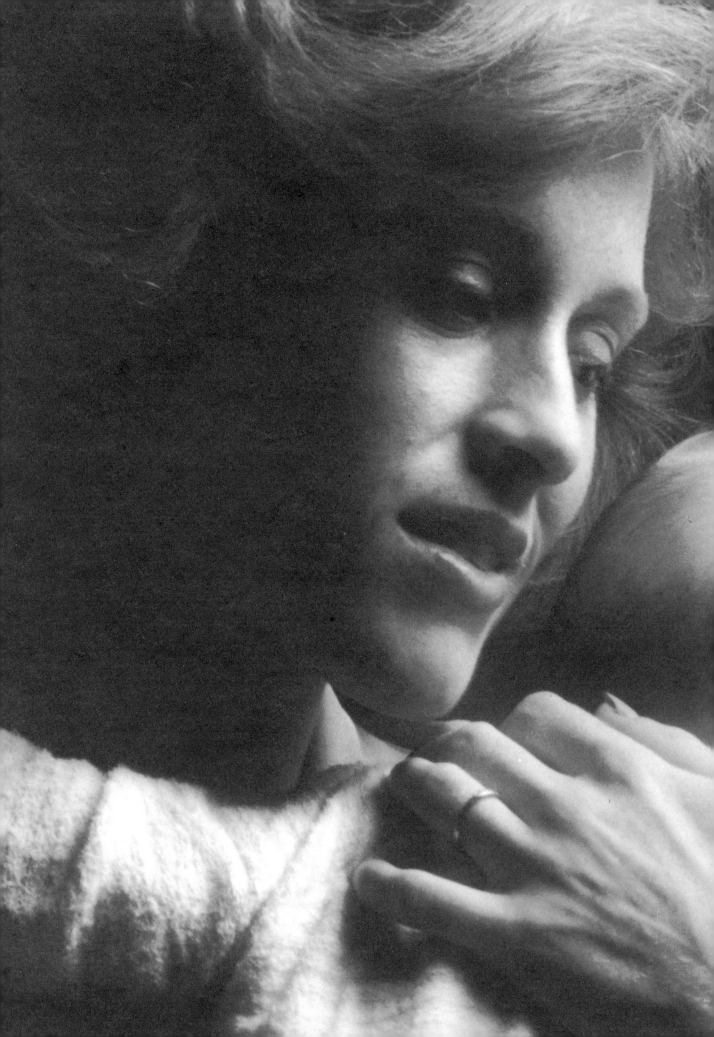

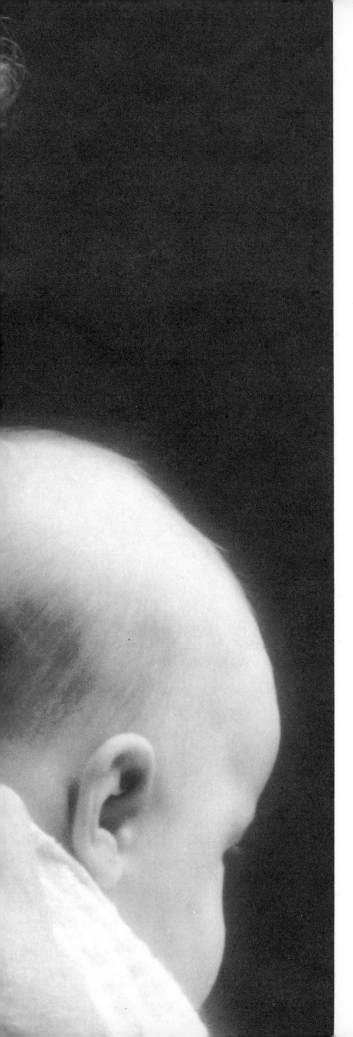

# Chapter 7: Adjusting to Your New Baby

## Coping With the Post-Delivery Blues

Beginning the day you bring your new baby home, your life will undergo more changes, and more drastic changes, than it probably ever has under any other circumstances. As your baby's life begins, a new life begins for you, too. Your responsibilities are increased instantly and dramatically, your spousal relationship begins to undergo certain changes, and your relationships with family members and perhaps even friends are apt to change also. Your child is your child forever, and life will never be the same for you again.

Pregnancy, labor, and delivery are hard work and have required tremendous effort on your part. Ideally, you might take things easy for several weeks, as you would try to do after any such strenuous experience, but few parents today can enjoy that luxury. Recovering from the physical stress in-

# ADJUSTING TO YOUR NEW BABY

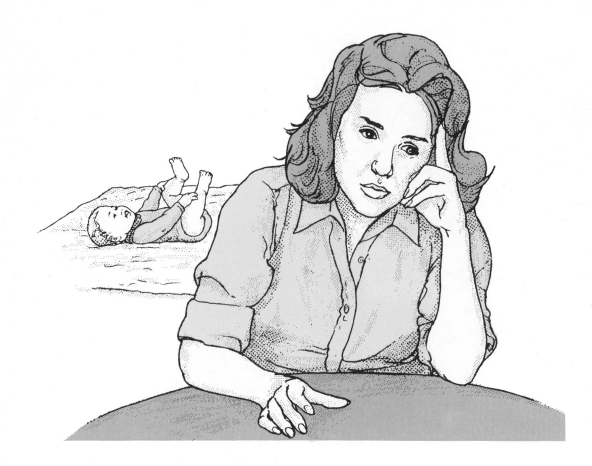

*Postpartum depression–the "blues"–affects some new mothers.*

volved in giving birth, dealing with unfamiliar emotional changes, and making adjustments necessary to meet the new demands being made on you may take several weeks, or even several months.

## Why You Have the Blues

Many women report that after giving birth they enjoy a feeling of euphoria they have never before experienced. This sense of well-being, of having accomplished a miracle, carries them through those first difficult weeks of fatigue and apprehension about their skill in caring for the new baby. Others—about fifty percent—are not so fortunate. For reasons medical experts have not been able to agree upon, you may find yourself suffering from *postpartum depression*—more simply, the blues—beginning a few days or even a few weeks after the birth of your baby. (Strangely, and for reasons no one can explain, these feelings seem to occur more frequently after the birth

of a second child.) Most likely, the blues result from a combination of psychological, sociological, and physiological conditions.

Some authorities say that the blues are caused by a drop in the level of maternal hormones. Others believe they can be the result of an unusually taxing birth with prolonged, difficult labor. Still others blame the mother-infant separation that occurs in the hospital. Many mothers say the cause is simply the total exhaustion that results from too little sleep and too much responsibility, plus the fact that a woman may be attempting to emulate the Supermom standards she has read and heard about—the standards that say any intelligent, healthy woman can do everything, handle everything. Doctors think that other factors that may make one woman, rather than another, susceptible to postpartum depression may be an unhappy childhood, perhaps including mental or physical abuse; a history of depression and difficulties in managing stress; an unwanted baby, or one whose birth was expected to solve a couple's

158

marital problems; a premature birth, or an ill baby.

Whatever the cause, when the pleasant experiences of being waited upon and cared for in the hospital and of being the center of attention among admiring friends and relatives are over, you may feel let-down, frightened, and very much alone. Waves of sadness can sweep over you unexpectedly, and you may have frequent crying jags. Other symptoms might include a distressing lack of energy, anxiety attacks, headaches, insomnia, confusion, worry about your physical appearance and attractiveness, and a totally negative attitude toward your husband. You may feel as if you are actually in mourning for your lost self, the confident and carefree self you used to be.

## Helping To Prevent the Blues

Fortunately, doctors today accept the fact that the blues are real, not just a figment of a woman's imagination, as some of their earlier counterparts used to insist. Even though doctors can't explain the condition to their satisfaction and are unable to offer much in the way of concrete help, they take a woman's suffering seriously, offering sympathy and counsel. They assure their patients that there is no reason to be embarrassed, ashamed, or alarmed because they cannot seem to cope with their new responsibilities, and that they are not alone in suffering from depression. Many of them discuss the blues with their patients before delivery and suggest ways to avoid the condition. Prepare yourself for the fact that not everything will be perfect; anticipate some mood swings. Consider requesting rooming-in for your baby if your hospital offers such arrangements. Plan to have the best help you possibly can for the first few weeks, and try to cut down on social obligations or avoid them altogether for a time. Doctors can also assure their patients that for almost all women the blues are short-lived. As new mothers acquire confidence in their new roles as parents and regain their strength, most will find that their approach to life falls into a sensible perspective. They will return to their former selves.

For a few, though, the blues are more profound. They last for two weeks or more, interfering persistently with sleep and affecting appetite. The mother is mired in hopeless depression and may find herself wishing that the baby had never been born or even that she could die. In some cases, but not all, such an extreme reaction may be an indication that serious and unacknowledged psychological problems existed before the birth and were heightened by it. Professional help is needed; the obstetrician or family doctor will probably be able to recommend a therapist.

## Related Feelings

First-time parents usually learn a few surprising things about themselves, finding, for example, that they have more physical stamina or more natural parenting ability than they thought they had. They also may find that they are neither as patient nor as perfect in their new jobs as they had expected to be. Sometimes accompanying the mother's postpartum blues and perhaps contributing to them is her feeling that she is a "bad" mother, unnatural and heartless, because she does not feel instant, overwhelming love for this new little creature who is so completely dependent upon her. This feeling is as perfectly normal as the blues and should be accepted matter-of-factly, with the attitude that "this, too, shall pass." Love at first sight is not a common occurrence, in spite of its frequency in romantic novels. Deep, lifetime love almost always develops slowly, over a period of time, and the unique bond of love a parent feels for a child is the deepest and longest-lasting of all. Love will come; believe in it and let it grow at its own pace.

Another feeling that contributes to depression is that of total incompetence and inability to properly care for this tiny, helpless, incessantly demanding human being. Expectant parents rarely are ignorant of babies' habits today. You very probably were aware that besides sleeping a great deal, your baby would require feeding from six to ten times in a twenty-four-hour period and a change of diapers several times a day, and that he or she might spend some time each day crying. Now that you are on call every minute of the day and night, you find that these things aren't as simple as you were led to expect. The baby sleeps at the wrong times, for shorter periods than you expected and perhaps more often and longer during the day than at night. You worry about the amount of covers to use in the baby's crib, the temperature in the room, and the household noise that may wake the baby. Feedings are sometimes tense as you struggle with the unfamiliar routines of breast- or bottle-feeding and wonder if the baby is taking enough or too much milk or formula. Dressing the baby and changing diapers are not the smoothly orchestrated operations you imagined them to be, even with cleverly constructed infant clothing and fitted disposables that need no pins. And the baby's crying is more frequent, more distressing, and less explainable than you thought it would be. In short, you feel totally inept, and you cannot imagine ever being anything *but* inept at this job of baby care. Remember this: Competence will come, as surely as it has in everything else you have learned during your life. Infants can't judge the quality of their care, and by the time yours is old enough to know whether you are an expert, you will be one.

## Curing the Blues

To accommodate your physical tiredness and the baby's constant demands on you, you may have to review what is most important to you and make some changes in your lifestyle. If you are a perfectionist who has always insisted that things be done the "right" way, you may find that you must relax your exacting standards a bit. If you suffer from inertia, it may be necessary for you to grit your teeth and force yourself to arrange for the rest, moderate exercise, and proper nutrition that are so essential for you and often so difficult to achieve. Realize that when you look your best, you are more apt to feel in control. Don't allow yourself to skimp on good hygiene habits because you are too busy or too tired. Dress completely every morning, do your hair and use whatever cosmetics you usually do. This is not the time to make demands on your strength and energy by beginning a reducing diet, however anxious you may be to get your figure back to normal.

Above all, don't try to bottle up your feelings in hopes they will go away if you ignore them. Talk about them with your spouse, your doctor, your mother, or a friend who has suffered them already. Be in touch, if only by phone, until life settles down.

Every parent should get away from the routine of house and a new baby on a regular basis, and this escape is even more important if you are suffering from post-delivery depression. Even a brisk walk around the block will help, when your spouse or someone else can care for the baby, but an entire afternoon or evening out occasionally will do even more for you. You need not feel guilty about going out for a few hours, as long as a reliable babysitter is in charge.

## First Babysitters

Finding that just-right, reliable person to whom you will entrust the care of your precious baby may be something of a challenge, and you will be glad if you began your search before the baby was born. Many mothers feel most comfortable leaving their new babies with grandmothers or other relatives, but family members are not always available. And while you know and trust them, they may be critical or make you feel as if you are imposing on them. Later, you will probably look into the availability of teenage sitters in your neighborhood (you'll find that it's wonderful when you can find a family with two or more young people who like to babysit, so that when one is not available, another may be). Until your baby is a little older, you will probably prefer someone more experienced—perhaps a woman who has had a baby herself—unless you can locate a mature teenager who has a certificate from a good babysitting course. Check with such local agencies as the YWCA, Girl Scout Council, Camp Fire Girls office, and the park or recreation department; if any have offered courses, they probably keep lists of dependable, qualified sitters. Other possibilities are a college home economics department or a hospital school of nursing. A good idea when you have a young, new sitter is to arrange for a get-acquainted visit before you leave him or her alone with your baby. You might wish to have such a young person come in on a regular basis to help you with the baby.

You may not be ready yet to accept the responsibility of caring for others' babies as well as your own, so you may not now consider making reciprocal baby care arrangements with a friend or neighbor or joining a babysitting co-op, but you may find that there's a capable neighborhood woman who wants to earn a little money. Agencies that supply trained and bonded adult sitters are listed in the Yellow Pages, but their fees are higher than those charged by individual sitters.

Your sitter has the heavy responsibility of caring for your child, but you have a responsibility to the sitter, also. You should be as reliable as you expect him or her to be, returning home when you say you will and paying fairly and promptly. Always leave a phone number where at least one of the parents can be reached in case of an emergency. It's a good idea to leave other emergency numbers as well, such as those of a nearby neighbor and of the police and fire departments. Don't make your sitter guess what's to be done; leave careful instructions about feeding and caring for the baby and tell the sitter where to find diapers, bedding, and other supplies. If you have pets, give instructions about them, too. It's also a good idea to have basic information about your house available, such as the locations of fuse boxes or circuit breakers, flashlights and fire extinguishers, and how the smoke detector and burglar alarm work.

### Information to Give a Babysitter

- Address and phone number of your location.

- Doctor's name and phone number.

- Emergency room phone number.

- Police department phone number.

- Poison control center phone number.

- Fire department phone number.

- Phone number of neighbor and/or relative.

- Time you will return.

- Locations of:

  ___ Phone

  ___ Exits

  ___ Bathrooms

  ___ Food and baby supplies

  ___ Medication

  ___ Fire extinguishers

  ___ First aid supplies

- Timing of feedings, medication, bedtime.

## New Relationships Between Mother and Father

The period immediately after the birth of the first child can be one of the most difficult in the best of marriages. It seems to the parents that there's no time for fun anymore, no place in their lives for the pleasures they used to enjoy. Impossible now are an impromptu meal at a favorite restaurant, a movie on the spur of the moment, or even a quiet evening at home with a well-prepared and nicely served dinner, followed by a few hours of uninter-rupted talk or reading. The new parents are too tired for love. Worse, even after the recommended time of abstinence from sexual activity has passed, some women find themselves so preoc-cupied with their new roles as mothers that sex holds no interest for them. They are still out of touch with their former physical desires. Others say that the process of bonding with their infants makes strong or passionate feelings for anyone else, including their husbands, impossible. Such a woman finds it possible to willingly give herself only to her baby.

The demands of the baby drain the energy and dull the perceptions of both parents, leaving them too fatigued to consider each other's feelings, de-sires, and needs. They're apt to be cranky and short-tempered with each other, quick to take offense and to feel slighted. Unconsciously, the father may resent the baby for taking so much of his wife's at-tention and energy, and the mother in turn resents his resentment. Their expectations of each other are too high. Their self-images may be undergoing a change in which, temporarily, they no longer per-ceive themselves as persons but only as parents, caretakers, and suppliers to this new baby, and im-portant only as they relate to him or her.

Those who have had time to get adjusted to each other and to being married before having their child are perhaps the most likely to sail smoothly through the early weeks of their baby's life and survive without scars. Others who are quite young and have not known each other for long, or who are divided by religious or cultural differ-ences, may be better off waiting a few years be-fore having a baby.

Every couple will be wise, on the days when nothing seems to be going right and life has lost its charm, to remember their reasons for getting mar-ried in the first place: They loved each other, de-sired each other's companionship, and wanted to share both the everyday aspects and the exciting parts of their lives with each other. They enjoyed being together, either because of the comfort-able pleasures of similar tastes and backgrounds or the stimulations and attractions of different ones. All that is still the same. They must recognize the source of whatever problems they have—and the main problem is not the baby but their own fa-tigue, confusing emotions, and inexperience—and somehow take advantage of short respites to concentrate their thoughts and feelings on each other as they used to do. Praise and appreciation are important; the at-home woman's efforts at her new job of child care are as commendable as were her achievements in the outside world of work, and the man's provisions for his family and his cheerful and consistent support of his wife are praiseworthy. Both need the comfort of touch—a warm hug or caress can change the whole complexion of a stressful, exhausting day. New mothers and fathers need "mothering" occasionally, and they can provide it for each other.

## Parent Support Groups

New parents should begin again to share outside interests as soon as they possibly can. Because of their mutual absorption in their infant, many couples choose to become involved in parent support groups. As they take a break from home responsibilities and enjoy the company of others, they are learning the skills of parenting. Local service organizations such as the YWCA sometimes offer seminars or workshops at little or no cost. Parents who have taken childbirth education courses together often continue to meet on an informal basis after their babies are born, to reinforce friendships begun and to trade tips. Still others form their own groups and meet informally with friends and neighbors. Later, some parents join one or another of the well-known, professionally organized groups such as Parent Effectiveness Training (PET) or Systematic Training for Effective Parenting (STEP). These organizations offer classes for a fee. Often, when the courses are over, some or all of the parents continue to meet, both for socializing and for sharing with one another what they are learning about their growing children.

## Including the Father

A young father may find himself feeling left out and useless as his wife goes about the business of being the main care-giver for their baby. He's also apt to be undergoing the emotional upheaval that his change of role brings on, even though he thought he was well prepared for the readjustments he would have to make in his life. He may be worried about finances, especially if the couple will now be dependent upon only one salary instead of two. He may be apprehensive about his increased responsibilities and the changes he already sees in his relationship with his wife. And he may actually be jealous of the bond that is so clearly being formed between mother and child, especially if the baby is being breast-fed. He is being called upon to do household chores and to relieve his wife by taking over

the baby occasionally when she is exhausted, but it seems to him that he is only doing more work and not getting the fun and joy he had expected the new baby to bring.

It's wise for him to acknowledge these feelings, to realize that they are no more abnormal than his wife's preoccupation with the baby, and to bring them out in the open to be discussed. The mother's attitude is the key to the solution of his problems. She should recognize his uncertainty about his fathering ability, and be careful not to deride his initial efforts. She should treat him as her partner, not as her assistant, in their new joint venture of parenthood. Besides expressing her appreciation for his help with some of the household drudgery, she can find ways to include him in the satisfying aspects of baby care as well. A father can bathe a baby and rock a contented one as well as one who is crying and in need of soothing; he can feed a bottle-fed baby. If his wife is breast-feeding, he can get the baby up and bring him or her to the bed or to a comfortable chair to be nursed. Some parents like to give their babies one or more "relief bottles" a day of either formula or the mother's expressed breast milk. (See Chapter 9 for information on storing and freezing of breast milk.) While the main reason for this simply may be to allow the father the pleasure of feeding the baby, a side benefit is that the baby will become accustomed to the occasional bottle that will be necessary if the mother will be absent at some feeding times because of her return to work or for other reasons.

## A New Dimension to the Marriage Relationship

The parents of this wonderful new human being will never again return to their old relationship, even when the child has grown and left home and they are alone again as they were at the beginning of their marriage. They will move on to a new relationship—a broader, more satisfying one. They are no longer a couple; they have become a family. The baby has added a new dimension to their marriage and a new reason for each of them to exist. Even if they have initial problems in adjusting to the changes, even if they feel out of touch with each other for a short time, their common love for and enchantment with their child will bring them together again. No one in the world cares as much about their baby as they do; no one else can share their particular, unique experience of parenthood.

## New Responsibilities of Parents

Perhaps the most difficult part of the responsibility of caring for a new baby is being on call constantly, twenty-four hours a day, 168 hours a week, with never a moment off. No other job requires such dedication as that of parenting. Babies don't eat, sleep, or cry on schedule. You will be called upon to feed or comfort your infant at any and every hour of the day or night, whether you are asleep, or ill, or occupied with a project of the utmost importance. In short, you will be required to adjust your lifestyle to accommodate the total dependency of your baby. This shift in the focus of your life may be traumatic for you at first, especially if you have been particularly independent and unencumbered.

### Supplying the Basics

The primary responsibilities of parents are to provide their children with food, clothing, and shelter—the basic requirements of human life. In principle, all but the most poverty-stricken of new parents can accept those responsibilities with few qualms, because they are the ones they fulfill for themselves. It's the day-to-day details of supplying them that may make you feel insecure and far from confident in caring for your infant. You may feel, as some parents do, that while your childbirth education courses have prepared you very well for actually producing a baby, you've not had adequate preparation for caring for your child. The all-important questions of *what, how, when, how often,* and *why* have not been answered to your complete satisfaction. In truth, they cannot be, because every baby, and every set of parents, is unique. Every family is different from every other, and every individual in every family is different from all the others. Some routines and procedures simply have to be tried out and perhaps discarded before you are comfortable in handling even the most ordinary of your responsibilities to your infant. You may wonder if the trial and error method of mastering a skill is a suitable approach for the serious work of rearing a human being.

In searching for knowledge about how to care for their babies, many parents are apt to be intimidated by "experts," who may include the baby's grandparents and next-door neighbors as well as pediatricians and psychologists, and to accept as truth any scrap of advice they are given, whether or not it "feels" right to them or has been substantiated in their experience. Of course there are times when nothing can be substituted for the knowledgeable orders and advice of experts in the professional fields of medicine, nutrition, and child psychology. But it is important for you, as a new parent, to learn to trust yourself. Remember that there is no one right way to do most things involved in child care. You can read, you can take classes, you can question your doctor closely, you can listen to your friends and relatives, but ultimately you must make your own decisions about what is best for your own unique child. And because you know that child better than anyone else in the world, you are far more likely than others to make the best decisions.

Remember, as you make those decisions, to enjoy your baby as you learn to care for him. Try to look at parenting not as a series of problems to be overcome or even, in the positive language of public relations, as challenges to be met. For a little while, at least, let the rest of the world go by as you give yourself up to this new life you have created; appreciate the miracle of every day.

### Feeding Your Baby

Feeding the baby, either by bottle or by breast, takes a great deal of time and energy. (Details concerning both breast- and bottle-feeding are covered in Chapter 9.) But whichever method you choose, you will find that feeding time is a time of closeness. You are giving the baby life-giving nourishment and thus meeting the child's most basic physical need. At the same time, you are fulfilling a deep psychological need for love and attention. As you provide food, you are holding and cuddling the baby, and he is getting to know your touch and your voice. A bond that will never be severed is developing between you.

### Helping Your Baby Sleep

You cannot force a child to sleep; you cannot teach a child to sleep. Neither you nor your baby can control her sleep cycles. Provided the baby gets enough to eat, is not in pain, and is not interrupted constantly, she will get as much sleep as is needed. The need varies widely: one infant may require as many as twenty or twenty-one hours a day; another, only eleven hours. The actual amount of time is not important, except to a parent; a baby who sleeps very little can be as strong and healthy as one who sleeps a great deal. On average, your newborn will have about eight sleep periods a day. Some periods may last as long as two to four hours; others will be catnaps that last for only minutes.

You can intellectually assimilate all these facts about sleeping, and you can realize that your baby's sleep habits are not an indication of your parenting abilities or the baby's "goodness." Still, you feel responsible for helping her get whatever amount of sleep is necessary in any way you can. You will probably find that your baby doesn't fall asleep instantly upon being put into the crib; in fact, wakefulness, perhaps accompanied by crying, may last as long as a half hour. Put your baby down when she is full and has been thoroughly burped. A warm bath and a massage with a light lotion, a period of cuddling or a ride in the carriage in the fresh air may encourage sleep. And the room need not be darkened, unless your baby is confusing night and day and you are having trouble changing a sleep pattern started in the hospital, where the nursery is bright and bustling with activity all day and all night. A room temperature of about 70° will be most comfortable for the baby, who should be clothed in a loose sleep sack (a covering blanket is not then necessary), a comfortable gown, or a sleep suit.

Do not worry about eliminating all household noise; the baby will become accustomed to the ordinary sounds very quickly. In fact, babies often find certain sounds soothing and go to sleep more quickly if those sounds are present. The intrauterine sounds the baby is used to are simulated in various crib toys and devices, including a rather expensive teddy bear with a tape cassette. You can reproduce very similar sounds at little cost by taping a running dishwasher or washing machine with your own tape recorder. Other sounds babies sometimes find soothing are the running of the vacuum cleaner, the "white noise" produced by a radio station that's off the air, a ticking clock, or soft music.

A ride in the carriage is only one way to supply the motion that sometimes helps babies sleep. Windup or cradle swings serve the same purpose, and you can rock the baby or walk the floor or dance around the room with her in your arms. You can even lull the baby to sleep by gently jiggling the bed, especially effective if it's a water bed.

Vary your newborn's sleeping positions. Lying on the stomach will provide a pressure that may bring up troublesome air bubbles, but you may find that your baby prefers to lie on one side or the other, or on her back. Don't worry if the baby is comfortable in only one position at first and her head flattens a bit. It will regain its normal shape in a short time. Babies often seem to like the feeling of being lightly swaddled. To do this, lay the baby diagonally on a small cotton receiving blanket. Fold one side of the blanket loosely over the baby, turn up the bottom corner, and then fold the other side over. Your baby is snugly enclosed in an "envelope" that will keep her warm and secure. When you pick the baby up, you can let the top corner rest on her head, like a hood, if you wish. Babies also like to be in small spaces. Try placing your baby in a corner of the crib, touching the bumper on one side and a rolled blanket on the other. Putting the baby down on the same small, soft blanket every time, perhaps one on which you've put a drop or two of your own perfume or cologne, may help induce sleep. (And that little coverlet may become your child's all-important security blanket, to be treasured and slept with for several years, so consider changing off between two identical ones in order to have one available while the other is in the laundry.)

Parents eagerly anticipate their baby's sleeping through the night, but an eight-hour sleeping period probably will not be something your baby achieves until she is several months old. Someone will very likely advise you to give the baby cereal at the last, late-night feeding as a way to induce a longer sleeping period. Don't do it. Your baby's doctor will tell you when your baby is developed enough (immune system, swallowing mechanism, etc.) to handle solid foods.

A pacifier may help put your baby to sleep. The La Leche League discourages the use of pacifiers on the grounds that they may diminish a baby's need to suck and therefore make her a less efficient nurser. Some parents disapprove of them, too, probably because they find distasteful the not-uncommon sight of a toddler whose sucking needs have long since been outgrown walking around with a pacifier stuck in her mouth like a plug. In fact, some find the sucking that is one of a baby's instinctual needs somewhat difficult to understand at all. They may feel that extra-nutritional sucking indicates that something is lacking in the emotional development of their child, and that therefore they are "bad" parents.

Nothing could be further from the truth. Newborns need to suck; it is their most satisfying form of gratification. The benefits of a pacifier can be seen when a baby's need to suck goes beyond her need to eat. Infants may awaken a short time after a feeding and indicate what seems to be hunger by trying to put their hands in their mouths or crying, when what they really need is simply to suck. Thumb-sucking would be a good substitute if infants could manage to find these natural, flesh-and-blood pacifiers when they want them. Since a tiny baby rarely can put thumb to mouth at will, a pacifier meets her need to suck and eliminates unnecessary feedings that inconvenience you and may upset the baby's digestion.

Another possible benefit of pacifiers has been discovered in using them with premature babies. Those who were induced to accept pacifiers in the hospital were found to develop sucking muscles sooner than those who did not take them, and thus were able to be taken off intravenous feedings and fed by mouth sooner.

If you give your baby a pacifier in bed, do take it away when she is asleep, to avoid the baby's becoming dependent upon it to stay asleep. And never, *never* tie it on a string around the baby's neck. It could cause strangulation. After six months or so, the need for extra sucking will disappear. If you dislike the pacifier you can probably arrange for it to disappear about the same time.

### Helping Your Baby Stop Crying

Another of your major responsibilities will be to comfort your baby when she is crying. Crying is especially distressing to new parents, who assume something must be dreadfully wrong. However, it is perfectly normal for babies to cry. It gives them a certain amount of exercise, and it is, after all, their only way of letting you know that they need something. The difficulty is to figure out what those needs are. In a newborn, there are only a few things a cry will signify, if the baby is not ill or in pain: hunger, the need for a diaper change (within a few weeks, the baby will become used to the feeling of wetness and a wet diaper will not bother him), and the need to be held and comforted. Infants have a characteristic fussy-sounding cry that often seems to reach a peak when they are about six weeks old and tapers off at about three months.

Babies are individuals. Each will tell you in special ways what he needs from you. Many experienced mothers say they can tell the reasons for their babies' crying, saying, for example, that the hunger cry is rhythmic and repetitive, the pain cry is loud and shrill, and the ill cry is continuous,

whiny, and nasal. (The distinctive cry that indicates a baby has colic, and the other typical distress symptoms of and aids for that frustrating nondisease, are discussed in Chapter 8.) As the baby grows, he will find more reasons to complain by means of crying: boredom, frustration, loneliness, fear, overstimulation, and, sometimes, the overtiredness that prevents sleep. As you get to know your own child better, you will learn to interpret the reasons for crying.

Occasionally, a baby will cry because he is in pain. One traditional cause for pain is the prick of an open safety pin, largely avoided now by the use of specially designed diaper pins and eliminated completely by the use of disposable diapers that need no pins. Another cause for pain is a raveled thread from the baby's clothes wrapped tightly enough around a finger or toe to cut off circulation. A baby crying because of sickness will usually have other symptoms of illness, such as a fever, diarrhea, or a runny nose. An earache is indicated by the baby's pulling on, or attempting to pull on, his ear. Generally, a healthy baby will have a strong, loud cry. If your baby's cry becomes abnormally weak, consult your doctor right away.

Sometimes, especially if postpartum depression has you in its grip, you and your baby can get into a joint crying cycle. When the baby cries, you get anxious and nervous. The more the baby cries, the worse you feel, and nothing you do seems to help quiet the baby. The baby senses your feelings; your anxiety in turn makes the baby anxious and uncomfortable; and the child expresses these feelings by crying even more. You dissolve in tears yourself, and neither of you can seem to stop. One way to help both of you calm down is to take a warm bath together. The skin contact and the warm, liquid environment are soothing and may be all you need. However, if you find yourself getting into these cycles with any regularity, talk with an experienced parent or your doctor.

You'll find that some of the things you can do to help your baby stop crying are the same as those you do to help him go to sleep. Most of these are based on warmth, rhythmic sound, and gentle, repetitive motion. These three great comforts can be ideally combined when you cuddle your baby closely as you sing softly to him and you rock together in a cozy, padded rocking chair. This will also soothe and rest you, and you will probably find it a more reasonable solution than letting your baby "cry it out," as some will likely advise you to do to teach him who is "in charge." Picking up your infant when he cries does *not* spoil the baby, whatever you may hear from others. Remember, too, to let your baby know that crying is not the only way to get you to show your concern and love. Pick up and cuddle your baby sometimes when he is awake and not crying.

## "Women's Work"

"A woman's place is in the House . . . and in the Senate" is a popular saying that has grown out of the women's movement in recent years. Besides expressing a woman's right to work at any job she is qualified for, it connotes the choices women have today. The luckiest of career women who become mothers are those who can ask three questions: "Should I go back to work or be an at-home mother for a few months or years?" "If I decide to go back to work, when is the best time—how long should I wait?" "Should I return to my old job or type of work, or should I move on to something different?" Unfortunately, not every woman has these options; economic necessity frequently forces a mother's return to her old job the day after whatever maternity leave she is entitled to has ended.

If you are one of the lucky ones who can make choices, and you choose to stay home, you may find yourself having second thoughts about your decision after a few weeks of uninterrupted baby care. On the bad days when everything goes wrong, you may feel hemmed in, trapped, and angry. You may be jealous of your spouse, who escapes every day to the adult world. And if you go back to work, whether because you want to or because you must, you probably will not be entirely satisfied either. First, you'll need to come to terms with the daily separation from your baby, then with the fact that you will almost surely miss some "firsts"—the first time she smiles, or turns over, or says "Mama." In addition, you may be bothered by another problem common to working women. One who does not feel pressure and guilt as she tries to satisfy her responsibilities as a wife, mother, and worker is indeed a rarity, even if she is able to stay home for several months, or even years, after the baby's birth. As some have put it, she takes on three full-time jobs and tries to do all three part-time. A fragmented feeling of being too much needed, of being pulled in several directions at once, simply seems to go with the territory of being a working mother.

Of course many mothers go back to work very soon after their babies are born and neither they nor their babies suffer. Most are gone from home for eight to ten hours a day. A few manage to work at home, to work part-time, or to have the advantage of working under the flexible-hours provisions that some forward-looking companies now offer, but every arrangement has its disadvantages.

However, many of those mothers and most medical professionals recommend that you wait, if you can, until your baby is four to six months old before you return to work, for several reasons. One, of course, is the matter of your health, both physical and mental. Your recovery will probably be complete by that time and your baby's sleeping habits are likely to have become fairly well established. Proper rest, nutrition, and exercise remain essential for you, even though time for them becomes more scarce. And along with the roles of worker, spouse, and parent, you should devote at least some time and attention to your own needs.

## Day Care

It's almost certain that every parent trying to find a good day care situation has thought of the sexual abuse that's been reported in the media. How do you know you're leaving your child in a safe place, and what are the different options?

Breast-feeding can be a problem of convenience, though for some working women who are adaptable and willing to experiment, it is possible to have the best of both worlds—working and nursing. Your success will depend upon your working conditions, your day care arrangements, your milk supply and other factors. The tiniest of babies can be incredibly flexible, and you may be able to nurse the baby in the evenings and on the weekends when you are at home and have your care-giver feed the baby bottles of formula or your expressed breast milk. Your breast milk can be safely stored by refrigerating it for up to twenty-four hours or freezing it for two weeks. An occasional woman is lucky enough to find as a care-giver a nursing mother who will feed her infant charge as well as her own baby.

First, consider your child's needs. Some centers may expect your child to play quietly all day; others may provide a preschool atmosphere with structured activities. Consider how many children will be together during the day; large groups may not work well for a shy, easily "lost" child. The point here is that the "ideal" day care situation will be different for each child. One one-year-old may be ready for a structured preschool-type day care center, while another may be much happier staying with a neighbor.

Consider *your* needs. What hours will you need care, and what location would be most convenient? And don't forget to consider how much you can afford.

The most difficult problem in leaving a baby only a few weeks old is that of finding adequate care for him or her while you are gone. Most new mothers who return to work leave their babies with trusted and competent relatives. If you do not have family members who can supply this care, you may have trouble finding a sitter or day care center that will accept responsibility for such a young baby, and charges will probably be higher than they would be for an older baby.

## Out-of-Home Care

*Day Care Centers.* While day care centers often have long waiting lists, they offer good hours and shift workers, so they can remain open from very early in the morning until evening.

Your child will have playmates, and you will likely meet other working parents, making the day care center the hub of a sort of extended family. If this community aspect appeals to you, you'll want to find out whether the center does anything to encourage communication between parents.

If you're considering a day care center, the workers should be well trained and well paid. A poorly trained, dissatisfied worker is probably not going to have the skills or the patience to deal well with both the demands of the children and her own frustrations; abuse or neglect could result. Questions you should ask include: How much employee turnover is there? Do the workers seem happy? Do they seem to respect each other?

Day care centers may be privately owned or operated by nonprofit groups such as parents' cooperatives (which allow parents' active involvement), educational institutions (sometimes to provide training for students), or municipalities. A licensed center is governed by regulations concerning things like the ratio of care-givers to children. You can receive a copy of the exact regulations in your state from the human services agency that monitors the licensing. When you

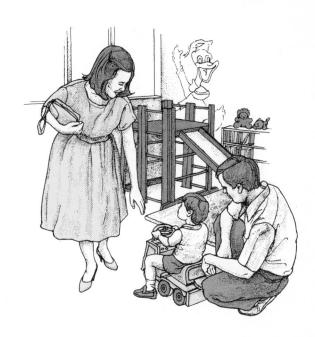

*Investigate your day care options thoroughly before making a decision.*

have a choice, choose a licensed center or care provider. In some states, in-home care-givers must also be licensed.

*Family Day Care.* Day care in a private home, or family day care, provides a home atmosphere and personalized attention. Typically, a mother of a child takes several others into her home during the day. This is usually less expensive than having a sitter in your home, and if the care-giver is really able to be with several children and still be sensitive to each child's needs, the situation is a good one. Your child will develop skills by being with other children in a homey atmosphere, but won't be exposed to different workers, as she would be in a day care center.

If you're considering family day care, meet the person in the setting where your child would be cared for. Gear your questions to find out about the care-giver's priorities, interests, strengths, and experience with children. Give him or her pertinent information about your child's needs (medical history, diet, interests, idiosyncrasies) and your expectations. Obtain references—the names of other families whose children stay with him or her—and check them out.

*General Considerations.* If you're considering family day care or a day care center, gather information about each placement you are considering so that you can compare hours of operation, vacancies, fees, adult-to-child ratios, and general philosophies about child care. If the center is handling very small babies, the adult-to-child ratio should ideally be three to one, but no more than four to one. If the children are between two and five years old, there should be one adult to five children.

Arrange to visit the most attractive options. Bring your child and go at a busy time. This way, you can check your child's response to the care-giver and also watch the care-giver's style of interaction with other children.

- Is the care-giver sensitive to the needs of children of different ages (especially at mealtime)?

- How does the care-giver respond to a crisis?

- If you're there early in the day, how does the care-giver respond to an upset child being left by his parents?

- Does the care-giver take the time to allow the parents to express concerns?

- Is the child given enough attention to ease the pain of separation?

- Are children sensitively helped to make the transition from one activity to the next?

- When you talk to the care-giver, do you feel as though you would be a member of the "team," or do you feel defensive? It's essential for you to feel that the care-giver respects your relationship with your child and your feelings.

Look at the overall cleanliness of the center or home—let your instincts give you a reading on its feel. Does the physical environment seem safe, or are there detergents or medicines within easy reach, or such dangers as uncovered light sockets? What kinds of toys are provided? Are they safe? Do they allow for creative play and skill-building? Licensed day care facilities should be able to provide you with a written program description. If you still have questions after your visit, make a phone call or a follow-up visit.

Many parents are reluctant to expose a very young baby to the risk of infection outside the home, and to take the chance of having an outsider bring disease into the house. Such fears are understandable, but should not be allowed to un-

realistically limit your baby's contact with people and the outside world. Germs are inevitable—you will bring them into your house yourself, and into contact with your baby. You naturally will not knowingly expose your baby to someone who is suffering from a terrible cold or other communicable ailment; you can and should watch for such situations in your baby's day care environment, and elsewhere. This sort of reasonable caution (which includes regular visits to the pediatrician and a regular program of immunizations and inoculations) should assure that your baby will enjoy normal health.

Once your child is placed in out-of-home day care, the only way to be sure that he is safe is to make unannounced visits during the day. If there are rules against this, *question* the rules.

## In-Home Care

*Nanny/Mother's Helper.* This essentially means you pay a sitter to stay in your home with your child. For a small baby, this may be the easiest option, since only one environment is involved. This is also the most *expensive* option, and doesn't always pan out as the best one, since in-home care-givers often burn out and have been known to put the child in front of the television and carry on with their normal routine. Finding a person who has an emotional reason for wanting to take care of someone else's child may help; financial motivation alone does not guarantee superior care.

If you're hiring a mother's helper, you should have a sense that she respects your child and understands his needs—and yours. Is she willing to structure a nap into the afternoon so that your child is not cranky when you get home? If your child is rested, you can spend some quality time with him. Most important, what do your instincts tell you about this person? Do you think you can have a cooperative relationship with her? Check references. Once you've hired a candidate, find some reason to go home unannounced during the day in order to get a sense of what's happening. Does your sitter run out the door as soon as you arrive home, or is she able to tell you what your child did that day, giving you a sense that she is involved and concerned?

## Adjusting to Day Care

Once you've made a day care choice, whatever it is, finalize all arrangements in writing. If you are hiring a care-giver, you will need to draft a letter that covers your agreement with that person with regard to hours, salary, responsibilities, sick leave, and vacation. A licensed day care center will have forms available.

You'll need to explain all of this to your child—what's going on, where you'll be going, who will be taking care of her, and that yes, you'll be coming back for her. You may need to stay with her for a while the first few days; decrease the amount of time each day. Allow a reasonable amount of time for your child to become accustomed to the arrangement. If you child seems upset at the end of the day after a reasonable settling-in period, you'll need to find out why. Stay in touch with the care-giver(s) on a weekly basis. Try to maintain a collaborative, supportive relationship. Work together to solve any problems that may arise.

## New Roles for Fathers

Family life has undergone many changes in recent decades, and the responsibilities once assigned specifically to one or the other of a pair of parents have shifted and become somewhat blurred. There are more single parents today, and more never-married parents. Many of them shoulder total responsibility for their families. When both parents work outside the home, they learn to share responsibilities for housework and child care as they share the responsibility of breadwinning. Nearly one million men in the United States today are raising their children alone. It is no longer cause for eyebrows to be raised and gossips to gather when a divorced father is awarded sole custody of his children. And joint-custody provisions in divorce—described as "equal opportunity in parenting"—have now been adopted by a majority of states. Some men take on the role of househusband, assuming the major part of the nurturing of their children, while their wives' careers provide family financial support.

Still, the traditional nuclear family survives, and in many homes the familiar structure of the mother as full-time homemaker and the father as financial provider continues. It used to be customary for the at-home mother to be almost entirely in charge of the house and the children. Today, however, we find fathers taking more interest, helping more often with household chores, and involving themselves more fully in the lives of their children than their own fathers did. They are no longer strict and unapproachable beings who

are seen by the children for only a few minutes a day and who demand peace and quiet when they are home. Their relationships with their children are personal and openly loving; they talk about feelings, they show that they care.

There are also other, more public indications today that men no longer measure their worth only by their achievements outside their homes, as their fathers did before them. Both child-care literature and advertising now direct information to "parents," instead of only to mothers; childbirth education courses require the participation of fathers. Parental leave of absence, extended to males in Sweden in 1979, is becoming more common among companies in this country, and federal legislation may soon guarantee men as well as women eighteen weeks of unpaid parental leave from their jobs in any two-year period, offering protection for both the employees' jobs and their benefits during their absences.

Men usually are not able to choose between their children and their work, as some women can, and many have not had the role model of a nurturing father to emulate. However, a father today is apt to involve himself as much as he possibly can from the very beginning of his wife's pregnancy, sharing the important decisions about the doctor she will see, the birthing environment, and the hospital at which the baby will be born. He may accompany his wife on some of her visits to the obstetrician. He participates in childbirth classes, in which he learns to coach his wife during the birth of their child, and then supports and aids her throughout her labor and delivery. Various studies have indicated that delivery times are shorter, anesthetics are used less frequently, mothers and babies are calmer, and infants' feeding problems are less likely when fathers are present in delivery rooms. After their babies are born, fathers often accompany their wives on visits to the pediatrician, if their work hours allow, and some take their babies for checkups alone.

In the early weeks of the new baby's life especially, a father can share household responsibilities, being sufficiently supportive and perceptive to see what needs to be done and pitching in to do it. By exercising some control over the number of visitors and the time they are allowed to stay, taking over household errands, and performing routine tasks, such as getting some meals and cleaning up after them, doing the laundry, and running the vacuum cleaner, he can help provide the serenity and order that will give the family's home life a semblance of normality in a time of

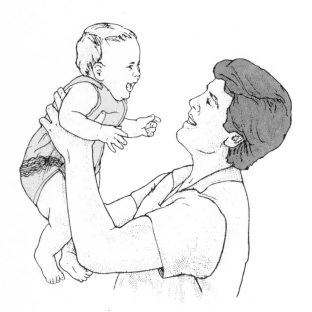

*Modern fathers are actively involved with their babies, and with the responsibilities of baby care.*

stress. However inexperienced he is in child care, he can learn within a very short time to be skilled at and to enjoy changing, bathing, and comforting the baby, and, if not feeding her, performing the important after-feeding task of burping.

Though you will find your child reacting to her father differently as the child grows—your eighteen-month-old, for example, will enjoy roughhousing with Daddy, but when in trouble will very likely turn only to Mommy—the effect of a close, nurturing relationship with a male figure is good for both boys and girls. The popularity of Fred Rogers for nearly twenty years on public television's *Mister Rogers' Neighborhood* indicates how enthusiastically children react to the caring presence of men in their lives.

Besides lending a hand around the house and accepting some of the responsibility for the care of his child, the new father often takes the traditionally male responsibilities very seriously. He may feel the financial burden of a third member of the family very strongly, especially if the mother's income has been important and she does not plan to return to work in the near future. And he may envy his wife her opportunity to stay home with the baby as much as she envies his being able to get out every day.

Men who participate as fully as they can in the births of their babies and who continue to share the responsibilities of home and children find the

rewards great. Their lives take on a new dimension; their marriages are strengthened and become more meaningful. Fathers can "mother," too, and those who choose to accept that responsibility are today the norm, not the exception. Reports of surveys bulge with statistics. Here are just a few: Eighty-five percent of fathers are present during their wives' labor; fifty percent during delivery. Ninety-six percent help with baby and child care; eighty percent do not refuse to change diapers.

## Holding and Handling the Baby

For a new parent who has had no experience with infants, either within his or her own family or during the course of a babysitting career, simply picking up and holding a baby is a little scary, dressing one is frightening, and bathing one is downright terrifying. Luckily, infants aren't able to squirm about much, so you don't have to worry right away about yours twisting out of your arms or escaping from your grip on the changing table. And babies are tough; they don't break under the stress of normal handling. (Don't worry about emotional fragility, either. Your baby's psyche won't be damaged for life if you are cross, in a hurry, or preoccupied once in a while.)

It will be necessary to support your baby's head with one hand for about three months when you pick him up and to hold the baby against your shoulder so his head won't fall backward when you carry him. It used to be common to swaddle babies loosely in receiving blankets, and some parents like to enclose their infants' arms and legs this way until they are used to holding and carrying them. (See page 164 for directions on swaddling.) You'll soon find yourself going smoothly through the tasks that involve moving and handling your baby and subconsciously avoiding the sudden movements and loud noises that frighten or startle babies.

### The Importance of Touching

This statement bears repeating: Picking up and holding your baby will not spoil him. The importance of touch to an infant cannot be overstressed, a fact now recognized to be part of the bonding process encouraged by doctors. It is even said that mothers who are separated from their newborn infants during the first hour after birth are somewhat less confident about their intuitive mothering skills than those who go through the bonding process. Your baby's skin is his or her most well-developed sensory organ immediately after birth, and the largest organ of the body. Its stimulation can have a profound effect on the baby's behavior. Your gentle, confident, and firm touch will calm your baby, as well as assure him of your love.

## Diapering and Dressing Your Baby

You'll probably feel a little awkward and clumsy the first few times you diaper and dress your baby, but with a little practice, you'll be handling him with ease and confidence. Use a waist-high table of some kind, even for a tiny baby, so you won't have backaches. An old dresser with a pad on top will do, but modern changing tables have built-in safety straps to hold your baby when he is old enough to squirm and resist you. If you use disposables, diapering is almost automatic: Lay the baby on the diaper, fold the front half of the diaper up over the baby and fasten it with the convenient, attached tapes. (Those tapes sometimes tear; instead of throwing a diaper away, mend it with masking tape.) To keep wetness from soaking into outer clothing, use disposables with elasticized legs and turn the plastic top of the diaper to the inside. A cloth diaper can be given a figure-eight twist at the crotch, for both double thickness and a tighter fit. Pin the back of the diaper over the front, slipping one or two fingers between the cloth and the baby's skin to keep the pin from sticking the baby. Use a pincushion or a bar of soap to hold diaper pins (do not use ordinary safety pins, and keep them out of baby's reach). *Never* hold pins in your mouth. Whichever kind of diaper you use, lay an extra one over your baby boy to avoid being squirted as you change him.

The kinds of clothing you choose for your baby will reflect your own taste and inclinations. Some parents are willing to spend the extra time necessary to iron natural-fiber, woven-fabric outfits because they like the look of a dressed-up baby; others opt for simpler knit clothing that needs little care. Whichever kind of clothing you prefer, look for garments that will be easy for you to put on and take off the baby—those with few, if any, buttons, necklines with openings large enough to slip easily over the baby's head, and sturdy crotch fastenings that make diaper-changing easier.

## Bathing Your Baby

Most infants come home from the hospital with a remnant of the umbilical cord still attached to the belly button, or *umbilicus.* Until this falls off, give your baby only sponge baths. Clean the navel area twice a day or so with a cotton swab dipped in antiseptic. Do this gently but thoroughly, making sure to get to the base of the cord stump. Watch for yellow matter, a sort of "weeping" that may develop, and for redness. These are signs of possible infection—notify your baby's doctor if they persist. Keeping the top edge of the baby's diaper folded down below the navel will help to keep the area dry. When the cord falls off, usually within about ten days to two weeks after the baby's birth, it is not unusual for a few drops of blood to be left on the navel. No bandage, binding, or tape is required. If the umbilicus doesn't dry up within a few days after the cord comes off, an *umbilical granuloma* may be present. This is a little nubbin of tissue in the umbilicus at the junction of the old cord and the new skin. Your doctor can remedy the situation easily at the baby's first checkup. If there is much bleeding or a foul odor coming from the cord, consult your doctor earlier for instructions about any special care needed.

For a sponge bath, you'll need a warm, draft-free room, a basin of lukewarm water, and two big towels—one to bathe the baby on, and one to wrap him in after the bath. If your baby cries when totally undressed, give the bath in stages, removing only part of the clothing at one time. Many babies love the feeling of being totally naked, though, and enjoy waving their arms and legs about freely. Your don't really need soap for a newborn; some parents don't use it for several months. If you can't bring yourself to skip it altogether, use very little, because soap will dry your baby's delicate skin. Ordinary scented soap may trigger an allergic reaction, and it will disguise the wonderful "baby smell" that lets everyone in the house know there's an infant present.

Infants do not need to be bathed every day. The diaper area is of course cleaned frequently, and two or three full baths a week are sufficient. Many babies are bathed daily, though, because bath time can be so much fun for both parents and baby, once the initial apprehension wears off. Fathers often opt for this pleasant activity simply because it's so enjoyable. You'll want to set up and follow a regular routine for bathing, at least until you're well-accustomed to the procedure. At the outset, though, remember: NEVER LEAVE YOUR BABY ALONE IN THE WATER FOR ANY REASON! No matter how much or how little water is in the tub, or how quickly you will return, the bath is *never* a safe place for an unattended baby or small child. Do not even turn your back. Your child requires CON-

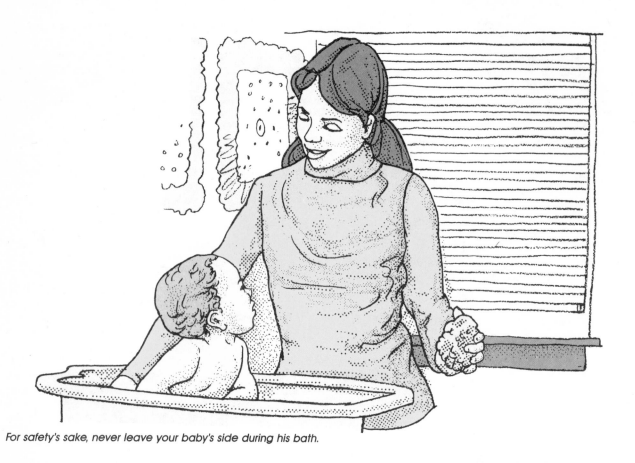

*For safety's sake, never leave your baby's side during his bath.*

STANT, SECOND-TO-SECOND SUPERVISION! Now, here's a bath procedure you might follow:

1. Be sure the room where you will bathe your baby is warm and not drafty. Lay out everything you will need, including the clean clothes in which you will dress the baby when the bath is finished. Consider unplugging the telephone; you will *not* interrupt the bath to answer it if it rings.

2. Put a portable tub or basin on a table or countertop at a comfortable height. Or bathe the baby right in the kitchen sink, being careful to run cold water last so the baby won't be burned if her skin touches the faucet.

3. Unless you use a specially contoured tub designed to keep the baby from slipping, line the tub or sink with a towel.

4. Put only a couple of inches of lukewarm water in the tub or sink, until you get used to bathing the baby. She will enjoy deeper water in which to move about when you are a bit more confident. Remember that water that seems comfortably warm to your hand will be too hot for your baby. It should register about 90° to 100° on a bath thermometer or feel pleasantly warm on the sensitive skin on the inside of your elbow.

5. Ease the baby gently into the tub. Using a soft cloth, wash the baby's face with plain water. The baby's face will not be really dirty, and soap in the eyes will only hurt the baby and make the rest of the bath miserable for both parent and infant. You might like to wear a pair of old, white cotton gloves, which will serve as a washcloth and reduce the chances of a slippery baby escaping your hands. Hold the baby with a "football grip," with your hand and wrist supporting her head and neck. Sing and talk as you go along, to entertain the baby and to reassure both of you.

continued

continued

6. Wash the baby's abdomen and back, arms and legs, and genitalia and rectal area carefully, using a little mild baby soap if you wish. Pay special attention to skin folds and creases. If your baby boy has not been circumcised, gently pull back the foreskin and wash the tip of the penis, then carefully pull the skin over it again.

7. Using soap, especially if the baby has cradle cap (a condition more thoroughly discussed on pages 225 to 226 and below), rub the baby's scalp gently but vigorously with the cloth or your gloved fingers. Still holding the baby like a football, tip her head backward slightly and rinse the soap off, being careful not to get any suds in the baby's eyes.

8. Take the baby from the tub and quickly pat her dry. If you pin a large, soft towel around your neck before you start the bath, it will be available to wrap up the baby warmly as well as keep you dry during the bath.

9. Use cotton swabs to clean crevices in and behind the baby's *outer* ears, but never use them to clean the ear canal, nose, or any other body opening.

10. Be sparing in the use of any powders or oils after the baby's bath. If you do use powder, shake it into your hand first, away from the baby's face, so she will not inhale it and draw it into the lungs. Be aware also that powder can build up in skin creases and cause rashes.

Most babies love being immersed in warm bathwater, almost from their first baths. Later, it's common for them to be afraid of the water. Enjoy the bath while you can and try not to hurry it; it's really playtime, a time for your baby to relax her muscles and make little swimming motions with the arms and legs, enjoying the buoyancy the water provides. Occasionally a baby will not care for the bath at first though, and will scream loudly to let you know that she is too hungry to wait, that the water is either too warm or too cold, or that her sense of security simply is threatened by being put into the water alone. A happy solution may be to bathe together. Run water in the big tub, a little cooler than you usually have it, and, holding the baby closely in your arms, ease down into it. Enjoy the skin-to-skin contact. Mothers can nurse the baby if he or she wishes it.

## Coping With Cradle Cap

Cradle cap *(seborrheic dermatitis)* is a skin condition in which yellowish, scaly, or crusty patches, made up largely of oil and dead skin cells, appear on the scalp. The condition is most common in infants, but it is seen occasionally in children through age five. Some temporary loss of hair may even occur. While the patches most often appear on the scalp, they may extend onto the forehead. They may also appear in the skin fold behind the baby's ears, on the ears themselves, and in the diaper area. The most typical location is over the soft spot *(anterior fontanel)* on top of the baby's head.

Cradle cap is quite common and not difficult to treat. Mild cases can usually be cleared up by daily shampooing, using regular baby soap on a wet, rough facecloth wrapped around your hand. Soften the crusts first by massaging a small amount of baby oil into the baby's scalp and letting it remain there overnight. Rub the baby's head vigorously during both the washing and the drying; don't worry about the soft spots; you won't hurt them. Gently comb the baby's scalp, whether or not he has hair.

If regular shampooing doesn't work, you can use a special shampoo that contains coal tar or salicylic acid. Your doctor or pharmacist can recommend one. Ointments containing sulfur, salicylic acid, or coal tar can be used for especially difficult cases. Be especially careful to keep medicated shampoos and ointments out of your baby's eyes, and stop using them if the scalp or skin becomes irritated or red. If the cradle cap doesn't respond to treatment, see your doctor, who can determine if a yeast infection or allergic skin reaction may be causing the problem.

## Diaper Rash

When you are bathing or changing your baby, you are likely to see signs of diaper rash; almost all babies have it at one time or another. Diaper rashes may be caused by moisture, urine, or irritating chemicals in diapers, whether cloth or disposable. These rashes can usually be identified by their appearance, their location, and other typical symptoms of different types of rashes.

*Simple diaper rashes* are red, slightly rough, and scaly. The rash may appear over the whole area touched by the diaper. The skin may be irritated by chemicals used in laundering cloth diapers—detergent, bleach, whitener, water softener, or soap. Plastic or rubber pants worn over cloth diapers sometimes affect the skin. The skin may also react to the chemicals used in manufacturing disposable diapers.

*Ammonia rash* is a form of diaper rash caused by the urine itself. The skin is literally burned by the ammonia that is formed when urine is decomposed by normal bacteria on the skin. Not surprisingly, ammonia rash is worse after the child has been asleep for a long period of time without a diaper change. It is identified by an ammonia smell, noticeable when you change the diaper.

Besides these two basic diaper rashes, a variety of other rashes may appear in the diaper area, including those caused by an allergy to a food or drug, by a skin infection, or by a contagious disease, such as chicken pox or measles.

If your baby develops a rash in the diaper area, look for the signs that indicate these different types of rashes. The appearance and location of the rash, an ammonia odor, or a rash elsewhere on the body are all clues. Asking yourself a few pertinent questions can help you and your doctor find the cause of the rash. For example, have you recently switched from cloth to disposable diapers, or changed brands of disposables? Have you made any changes in your laundry products? Has the baby been given any new food (a change in formula, perhaps, or the addition of cereal to a feeding) or medication?

To treat simple diaper rash or ammonia rash, keep your baby as dry as possible, changing diapers frequently, even if they are only slightly wet, and avoiding any airtight coverings. If you favor cloth diapers, use double diapers during the daytime, triple diapers at night. Put a pad under the baby and let him lie undiapered sometimes, if possible. Wash the diaper area with plain water each time you change your baby, and apply a protective cream or ointment such as petroleum jelly, zinc oxide, or vitamin A & D ointment, or an ointment combining zinc oxide, cod liver oil, petrolatum, and lanolin. Use only one type of ointment at a time, unless your doctor has instructed you to use more than one. Do not dust the baby's

skin with cornstarch, a remedy that used to be recommended; it has been found to encourage the growth of fungi. Try a different brand of laundry soap on cloth diapers and do not use fabric softener with every wash load, because your baby may be sensitive to buildup of the product. Give cloth diapers a try if you are using disposables, or switch brands; and try disposables if you are using cloth diapers. Cut down on the use of powders and oils for your baby, and be sure that any you use are mild and nonallergenic. If you are using colored toilet tissue to clean your baby's genital area, switch to plain white.

An allergic rash from foods or drugs is more likely to occur in an older baby who is eating several different kinds of foods or perhaps taking some medication than in one who is fed only on breast milk or formula. The treatment is to stop giving any new foods, beverages, or medicines started within the past month, and then to give the child just one of these items each week. If one causes the rash to return, the culprit has been found and can be eliminated permanently. Remember to consult your doctor before starting or stopping medication.

Treat a rash caused by an infection or contagious disease by washing the diaper area with soap and water and frequently applying an antibiotic ointment, such as bacitracin or neomycin. If your baby has any other symptoms of illness, such as fever or loss of appetite, if the diaper rash is spreading or severe, or if it gets worse after two days of home treatment, see your doctor. He or she may identify the rash by its appearance or may culture or scrape the rash to identify bacteria or fungi. The doctor may prescribe a medicated ointment.

## Adjusting to Your Baby's Schedule

A generation or so ago, young mothers were told to put their new babies on a strict four-hour feeding schedule and to leave them in their cribs between feedings. We know better now. Babies don't tell time with clocks; they're governed solely by their needs to be fed, changed, and comforted. They are far too young to be "trained" or "taught" to adapt to the schedule you might prefer to set up, and for about the first three months of your new baby's life, you will both be better off if you adjust to his schedule, haphazard as it may be. This isn't easy. Day and night may blend for you into an endless round of feedings, diaper changes, laundry, and rocking or pacing the floor with a crying infant. It may seem that all the good care you gave yourself when you were pregnant—the adequate rest, the nutritious diet, the healthful exercise, the mental stimulation, and the social activity—is impossible to maintain. But this is the worst possible time for your life to be chaotic and disorganized, and for you to be operating in a state of exhaustion. You need to be at your best to care for your new baby properly and to appreciate and love him as you were so sure you would when you were waiting for the birth.

## Coping With Loss of Sleep

Interrupted sleep at night is perhaps the most difficult change to which you have to become accustomed. Sharing night duty with your spouse will help. A father can handle a bottle-fed baby very well, and can give a bottle of expressed milk to a breast-fed baby. Many fathers look forward to and enjoy the quiet times alone with their infants. At the very least, a father can deliver the baby, changed and ready for nursing, to a breast-feeding mother in her bed. Sometimes the best way to share the night wakings is to alternate feedings, but at other times a whole night of sleep for one parent while the other takes over completely is better. A grandmother or another person who has come to help can assume responsibility for a night now and then, too, even if your agreement is that she will do the housework and you will care for the baby.

However you arrange things, though, the fact remains that you are not getting enough sleep, and you're not getting it in the time period you're used to. You need every nap you can possibly take to make up for some of the lost night hours and to restore your energy. You may feel you should catch up on the housework or the laundry when the baby sleeps, but you should resist this temptation. You need to sleep, or at least rest, whenever your baby sleeps, whatever the time of day. Go to bed, or settle into a comfortable chair with your feet up. Close your eyes, breathe deeply to release the tension you feel, and clear your mind of every thought except peace and relaxation.

Try to ignore the clock at night; it doesn't matter to the baby whether it's 2 A.M. or 4 A.M., and it won't do you any good to know. And don't keep track of the number of hours of sleep you get; knowing it was only three, and divided at that, won't make you less tired. Reward yourself with small luxuries or conveniences to make night feeding more

pleasant; a thermos of hot cocoa, a good book to read, an old movie on television, soothing music on radio or tape. Remind yourself often that sleep experts say you do not need to replace lost sleep hour for hour. What you need is deep sleep (technically called REM [rapid eye movement] sleep)—this is the stage at which you dream, and which you will slip into easily when you are very tired. Remember too that this period in your life will come to an end, and that during those long, wakeful nights you are not alone. Thousands of other parents are struggling with exhaustion as they feed or comfort their babies in the middle of the night, just as you are doing.

## The Family Bed, Pro and Con

Parents in many foreign countries sleep with their babies routinely, and not always because of a lack of space. In Asia and Central America, for example, parents' concepts of nurturing make it incomprehensible to them that anyone would expect a child to sleep alone in a bed, not to mention in a room alone. This practice has been frowned upon, to put it lightly, in this country since at least the beginning of the twentieth century, but it seems to have become more common in recent years. One reason may be the ever-increasing interest in breast-feeding. The simplest and most convenient way to nurse a baby is to lie comfortably in bed with her and to fall asleep together when the feeding is over. Today even medical people who have disapproved most adamantly of parents and babies sleeping together have begun to reevaluate their convictions, and some have swung around completely.

One of the main worries parents have had about sleeping with infants is that they will roll over and smother or injure their babies. That's not at all likely. First, you will have a mind-set that assures your care about avoiding this, however deep your sleep. And second, your baby will surely wake up and cry if you begin to hurt her.

Some of the worries of pediatricians and psychotherapists have been that a child may become "addicted" to sleeping with the parents, may be frightened by seeing the parents in the act of sexual intercourse, or may be overstimulated by the intimate body contact with adults. Parents who advocate the family bed say that children almost always want their own beds by the preschool years, if not before, and that they themselves have been able to move the children out easily whenever they've wanted to give up the practice. They ensure their sexual privacy by making love during the baby's deepest sleep periods or by simply moving to another place in the house. And they insist that the bodily closeness and touching that sleeping together offers brings a feeling of security and comfort to a child, not harm. In addition, they say that both parents and infant sleep better in the same bed. The baby does not always fully awaken if she is not hungry, and may go back to sleep easily. And the parents can stay comfortably in bed and at rest, if not asleep, while the baby is awake.

The family bed question is obviously a very personal one that parents must settle for themselves. If they disagree about the wisdom of sleeping with their children, or if either is deprived of needed sleep because the child is present, they would be foolish to consider adopting the family bed. Some parents who are only lukewarm about having an infant sleep with them work out compromises of some sort. They may take the baby into their bed for only the first few difficult weeks, or they may carry the baby back to the crib when she has fallen asleep. Later, they may limit access to their bed to the kids on weekend mornings or to a sick or frightened child in the middle of the night.

## Modifying Your Expectations

One of the first decisions you may have to make in order to adjust your own life to your baby's schedule is to modify your expectations of yourself, especially if you are something of a perfectionist. The Supermom who runs a home with consummate efficiency, serves three gourmet meals at the same hours every day, gives skilled care to a brand-new infant, and is always perfectly groomed is a myth. Trying to make that myth a reality has caused many a mother serious trouble.

If you are a new parent who does not have a full-time housekeeper, an immaculate house must take second place to a lovingly cared-for baby and to parents rested enough to handle their daily responsibilities. A quick pickup every day will keep your home tidy enough to be comfortable. Heavier household jobs can be postponed or skimmed over until there's more time, or can be delegated to someone else. The best helper will probably be the baby's father, if his work schedule allows or if he can arrange for leave or vacation, because it gives him a chance to get to know his child in an everyday, unhurried fashion, as he goes about the housekeeping chores. If this is not possible, try to arrange for some extra help, either by hiring someone to come in for a few hours a day or a week, or by accepting offers of friends and family members to clean and do laundry.

Cut down your expectations of the way family meals should be prepared and served, too, but do not skimp on nutrition. You need a well-balanced diet of wholesome foods to supply the energy your new responsibility requires, but you can do without fanciness and formality. Enjoy the casseroles and baked goods thoughtful people supply and don't feel guilty about occasionally bringing in a fast-food meal. When you must cook, choose simple basic foods that can be prepared quickly and easily.

## Time-Savers for New Parents

Many of the ways you can save time center around good organization. Of course, definite scheduling of your time is impossible now; you can't be sure exactly when or how often your baby is going to need you. Every plan you make that involves other people or a specific time must be expendable or have an alternative. This way, you can shift gears at a moment's notice when your baby requires an extra feeding or when some other normal but unanticipated incident takes place. At the very least, you'll want to consistently allow yourself more time than you think you'll need for everything. Experienced parents have found many ways to save themselves time and confusion as they go about the business of life with a new baby. Here are some of their ideas:

- Keep shopping lists, lists of chores that must absolutely be done, and lists of thank-you notes to be written for baby presents. By writing everything down, you free yourself of having to remember details at a time when you are most apt to be forgetful and preoccupied.

- At night, do as much as you can to get ready for the next day. Set the table for breakfast, lay out clothes for yourself and the baby, pick up the newspaper. Any nuisance chores and decisions you can handle ahead of time will make the day start that much better.

- Cut down on time-consuming trips around town by banking by mail and shopping by phone or through catalogs whenever you can. Try to do several errands whenever you are out, and plan them so that you waste the least possible amount of time driving around.

- Practice doing two things at the same time: for example, make out a grocery list or do your stretching exercises while you talk on the phone; fold the laundry as you watch television; or clean the bathroom while the tub fills.

- Above all, *do not rush.* "Haste makes waste" is a cliché, but it is as true today as it was when it was first uttered by someone who knew that the faster he or she tried to do something, the more likely it was that there would be an accident.

## Your Social Life

One thing you do not have to do is uphold your former standards of hospitality for friends and relatives who drop in to see your new baby, unexpectedly or by appointment. It's not necessary for you to provide refreshments or even to offer a cup of coffee. Let visitors see the baby (asleep or awake), chat with them for a few moments, and let them go on their way. Discourage their handling and passing the baby around. Refuse to let anyone who has a cold or other illness into the same room as the baby. The parents among your visitors will understand all this perfectly, and if others do not, don't worry. Your baby's health and well-being, and your own, are of primary importance right now.

You may find, during the first months of your baby's life, that every aspect of your social life changes. If you've always loved to entertain at home, you'll probably find it more enjoyable to save time and energy by meeting friends at a restaurant for dinner—and it will be good for you to get out of the house occasionally. If you are accustomed to going out a great deal, rarely spending a weekend evening at home, you may now prefer to spend quiet evenings by the fire.

This certainly does not mean that you must—or should—give up seeing friends and going out altogether or never do the things you enjoy. It only means that your priorities will probably change when you have an infant in your household, and that you're not required to continue any old habits that you've outgrown or that you wish to put aside for a time.

## Time for Yourself

As you reorganize your life to adjust to having a baby, do not forget your own requirement for some time for yourself, however difficult it may be to schedule. You need private time to be a person in your own right and not only a parent, a homemaker, a spouse, and perhaps an employee. You need the time to build and maintain the self-esteem that makes you effective in all those roles and effective at being yourself. You need time to exercise, to groom yourself, to read or work on a hobby . . . or to look at sky or water and let your mind wander. Finding this time will probably never be easy for you again, but it will continue to be very important that you do find it. Always look on it not as a luxury or a reward, but as an obligation to yourself. You won't always be able to have the hour or more that would do you the most good and be the most enjoyable, but you'll find that even a few minutes snatched from a busy day will refresh you.

If you are an early riser, at your best in the morning, you may enjoy a few minutes of peace and privacy over a cup of coffee before the rest of the family is awake. Your baby's daytime naps may give you some precious time. Even later, when you may not feel the need to sleep every time your baby does, nap time should be for *you*, not for housework. Evening is a wonderful time for a leisurely bath, even for a good read in a warm tub.

And evening is probably also the best time for a quiet hour or two for spouses. As important as it is for each to have some solitary time, it is equally necessary for a married couple to spend at least some time together, alone.

## Reactions of the Rest of the Family

As expectant parents, you perhaps thought that the baby soon to be born would be all yours, alone. Not quite so, as you've probably found out. If you have other children, they share proprietorship with you; they are, after all, of the same generation as their new sibling. When they all get older, you may have the feeling, as some parents do, that it's "them against us." Your own two sets of parents, and perhaps your grandparents as well, have a vested interest in your child; they are his ancestors. They probably feel qualified, and perhaps duty-bound, to advise you about every aspect of the care of your baby. Many other people will also speak to you of "our baby" and offer advice. Anyone who knows you and cares about you felt like a participant throughout the pregnancy and will continue to do so during the rearing of your child, including aunts, uncles, and cousins; old and new friends; neighbors; colleagues at work; and probably the checkout clerk at the supermarket and the teller at the bank. You even share your baby with your pet, whose function in life now is to be the companion and protector of the child.

## Preparing Your Children for the New Baby

Ideally, you'd tell your toddler or preschooler that you're expecting a baby only a short time before your due date, because with his or her undeveloped concept of time, six months or more is too long to wait. However, you don't want the child to hear the news from someone else, so you'll probably share it about the time you're telling everyone. For a young child, try to tie the coming birth to something other than a specific date: "about the time of your own birthday" or "when the leaves on the trees are getting green." An older child who can handle the time lag can be told earlier, and a teenager can be told very soon after you know for sure yourself. Being first to know, even before Grandma, will give this older child the adult status that builds self-esteem. Just don't tell a child of any age until you're ready for the whole world to know. That kind of secret is impossible to keep.

The ages of your children will also determine to a large extent how you answer the questions about reproduction that will inevitably follow your announcement. The most important thing to remember is to give a child only the amount of information he or she actually asks for and can handle. A toddler, for example, probably wants only to know and can take in no more than that "the baby is growing in a special place inside Mommy and will come out when it's big enough." A bright preschooler or a school-age child is likely to insist on knowing all the details of the baby's life "in there." If you have a preteen or a teenager, your pregnancy gives you a golden opportunity to pass on something of your value system as you candidly discuss human sexuality, reproduction, and family life. With children of any age, use the correct terminology for body parts and functions. Any shyness or embarrassment you may feel about speaking frankly will wear off with repetition, and you will be doing your child a favor, because he or she won't have to relearn the words. You may find it helpful to draw upon the vast number of excellent books available for parents and children on the subject of reproduction (and, for little kids, about what it's like to have a baby brother or sister), many of which are designed to be read together. Your librarian or bookstore clerk can lead you to the best of what's available. Be

willing to answer questions whenever they're asked. With young children, don't be surprised if you must repeat your answers several times.

Your children's questions won't all be about where babies come from. Children are naturally self-centered, and yours will want to know how this baby will affect their lives. Once a young child accepts the fact that a real baby will definitely join the family as another child for Mommy and Daddy to love, he or she will begin to worry about being "deposed," supplanted in your affections and perhaps even in your home. The more imaginative the child, the more horrible may be the fears. Talking about the baby in terms of the child—saying, "*You* will be a big sister," instead of "The baby will love you," for example—and speaking of the baby as *ours,* not *mine,* will help. If a baby coming means that the child will move to a big bed or another bedroom, make the change well ahead of time, so that it will be interpreted as growing up, not being pushed out. Don't try to break your child of the pacifier habit just before the baby is due, and don't send him or her off to nursery school just then, both for the same reason. Do be more generous than ever with your hugs and kisses and the special time you spend with your child each day. Bedtime is a wonderful time for a leisurely, loving cuddle that will reassure your child of your love.

Once their questions have been answered, older kids may disappoint you a little in their reactions to the coming baby. School, outside activities, and friends keep them busy and make them independent, and they don't expect a baby to make much difference in their lives. They may enjoy being allowed the privilege of sitting in on your discussions about what to name the baby, but you'll want it understood that their choices will not necessarily be final. You may find preteens or teenagers showing signs of embarrassment about your pregnancy; kids that age don't always like to have the results of their "old" parents' continuing sexuality displayed for all the world to see. You may be able to make them feel better by pointing out examples of other teens with infant siblings among friends and relatives. Be careful not to turn them off by telling them how much help they will be able to give you in caring for the baby.

Kids of any age may enjoy helping you go through the baby clothes ("Did I *really* wear that?"), set up the bassinet, and arrange the articles on the changing table. If a child really wants to—and *only* if that's the case—you might consider taking him or her to the doctor with you a

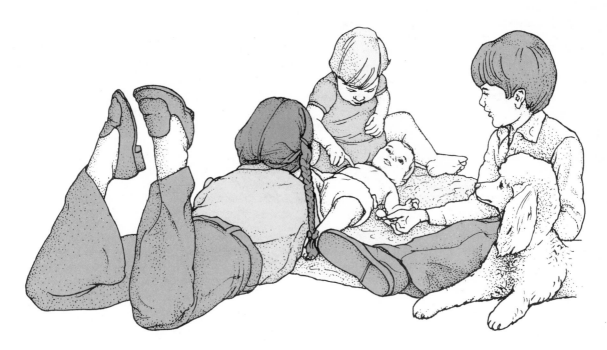

*The new baby's siblings will be eager to become acquainted with her.*

time or two, to hear the baby's heartbeat. And if you can occasionally bring a baby into the house as a guest or babysitting charge, both you and your child can get a little practice in seeing how things will be when your own baby arrives.

## Bringing the Baby Home

Even if your young child has visited you and the baby in the hospital, the baby's homecoming may be a bit traumatic. What had been talked about and thought about as an event to come has become reality—the future is here, and the baby is a real, live creature. There are three schools of thought concerning the best way to bring your new baby into the house. Some parents feel that a toddler or preschooler should be away from home, perhaps visiting Grandma, and should be brought back only after mother and infant are well settled. Others think a young child should definitely be part of the reception committee. They advise that the mother have someone other than herself carry the baby into the house and that she devote herself to the older child exclusively for a short time after coming home. And still others say the child should accompany the father to the hospital to pick up mother and infant. The method you feel is right for your family is the one you should choose.

Is it wise to come home bearing gifts for your older child? Some parents like to give the older child one large present to celebrate the birth of the new brother or sister, choosing one that will emphasize his or her maturity, such as a new game or some "big kid" art materials. You may also want to have a supply of small gifts to hand out when visitors bring presents to the baby only. It's best not to overdo the gifts, though, either before or after the baby arrives. Even toddlers recognize bribery when they see it, and the message you send is an apology for bringing home an interloper.

## Helping Siblings Adjust to the Baby

Your children will react to the actual presence of the baby in different ways, depending upon their ages and personalities. However well prepared they are, they will at first almost surely be surprised and most likely disappointed. The baby is neither the playmate your toddler or preschooler secretly expected, in spite of your warnings to the contrary, nor the smiling, gurgling, picture-perfect infant your older child probably visualized. Even the baby's sex may be disappointing, and the fact that he or she does nothing but eat, sleep, and cry—and monopolize your attention—surely will be.

# ADJUSTING TO YOUR NEW BABY

Your main enemy at home will be *time*, especially if you have a toddler or preschooler; there'll never be enough of it. Many mothers feel guilty of neglecting the older child, because the infant takes so much time. Psychologists tell us that underlying that guilt is anger at being torn between the two children. One way to help yourself feel better and to make your older child feel wanted is to include him or her in every possible part of the care of the baby. Even a two-year-old can fetch a diaper from upstairs, perch on a stool beside you at the dressing table, or help you pat the baby dry after a bath. Little kids can sort the baby's laundry, help you gently pat up a burp after a feeding, and "entertain" the baby with nursery songs and finger plays.

Let your child hold the baby on a pillow, in a big chair, when you are close. If you're bottle-feeding, let him or her hold the bottle for a few minutes, and demonstrate the way to gently pat the baby's cheek to see the baby's head turn. Warn the child about the *anterior fontanel* (the soft, boneless spot at the top of the head), but don't be unduly alarmed if he or she touches it; it's protected by a firm membrane. Do be sure to supervise very carefully any "help" or playing with the baby. Be sure your child understands that he or she must never try to pick up or carry the baby. Avoid any possibility of harm to either child by putting the baby in the crib or in an infant seat inside the playpen if you have to leave the room.

Feeding time may be difficult, especially if you are nursing the baby—a time when your toddler or preschooler feels left out and is apt to show displeasure with you by getting into trouble. The feedings that come when your older child is napping or has gone to bed for the night, or when someone else is in the house to provide distraction, will be the ones during which you can devote your attention entirely to the baby, providing the eye contact that is important. When your older child is present during feedings, settle yourselves on the sofa and cuddle him or her with your free arm as you read or watch television together. Or sit comfortably on the floor, with your back braced against a piece of furniture, and watch or help while the child works with puzzles, games, or coloring projects. The baby won't suffer; your touch and the sound of your voice will be soothing.

What if your older child wants to try nursing again? It won't hurt, if you are agreeable to the idea. The chances are that one quick try will be enough. The child won't like the taste of your milk and probably won't be able to suck properly.

Wanting to go back to nursing is only one of several signs of regression you might expect, and they won't necessarily show up immediately after the baby arrives. A return to baby habits concerning toilet training, eating, sleeping, talking, or dressing may be more a sign of stress than of jealousy. Whatever the cause, your child is trying to get your attention by competing with the baby on the baby's own level. The best way to handle regressive behavior is to go along with it patiently and without showing anger or disappointment; it will pass. Be generous with praise for any mature behavior, and reward it with grown-up privileges, such as staying up a bit later than usual or going on an important errand with Daddy.

## Dealing With Jealousy

Real jealousy will almost surely rear its ugly head sooner or later among children younger than school-age. Busy and independent older ones will probably take the new arrival in stride, suffering little, if at all, from feelings of rejection. Very likely they will be proud to have a baby in the family. They will look upon the infant as a sort of live plaything to be loved and cuddled and shown off to their friends. The best ways to help the little ones through their feelings of displacement and rejection are to show them your love in every way you can and to spend as much time alone with them as you possibly can.

Your toddler is too unsophisticated to be anything but up-front about his or her feelings; life with the interloper who makes so much noise and takes all Mommy's time is unbearable. He or she will likely ask you to take the baby back and will be frankly envious of the attention the baby is getting. You may be able to cheer up the child a little by stressing how lucky the baby is to have such a fine big brother or sister and by letting him or her help you care for and entertain the baby. This child isn't old enough yet to have developed much feeling about right and wrong, and pinching, hitting, or sitting on the baby won't seem a crime to him or her. You'll need to watch the child closely and lay down a no-nonsense law that the baby *must not* be hurt. This may be one of the rare times you choose to use strong discipline.

By the age of three, your child understands that deliberately hurting the baby is wrong. Do, however, watch the pats and squeezes and hugs; they may be a bit too hard. This child may be so angry about the baby's appearance that he or she won't talk to you, won't cooperate in any way. Or, he or she may be afraid to displease you by showing the anger. The child may be excessively "good" or fake exaggerated and unfelt love for the baby. You can admit to this child that yes, the baby can be a nuisance, bothering you when you two are reading or playing. Be careful not to give the idea that there's any solution other than the baby's ultimate growing up into a reasonable child.

Your preschooler will probably try to take your attention away from the baby by showing off his or her feats of strength and skill and cleverness. The child feels rejected and cannot understand what you see in this infant who can't do anything interesting or worthwhile. A little girl may be particularly jealous of Mommy, a boy of Daddy, and each may try to take over the other parent. Feelings are strong, and you will do well to acknowledge them and encourage the child to talk about them.

## Grandparents and Other Doting Adults

Willing and able grandmothers, aunts, and cousins—once almost universally available to give generously of their time, material wealth, and advice to new parents—have now become rare. Today they're apt to live far away across the country or to be fully occupied with their own leisure or business commitments. A grandmother who does live near you and wants to be involved in the care of your baby can be a help or a hindrance, depending upon her common sense and personality and upon your own attitude toward her interest. If she is critical of your efforts at housekeeping or baby care, plays the martyr, or refuses to consider the possibility that any way but hers is the right way to do anything, you won't be overjoyed to see her coming. But if she gives advice only when she is asked for it, accepts you as you are, and is willing to help you in the ways *you* choose, she can be the best thing that's happened to you—and to your child, as well. If you treasure memories of a special relationship with a grandparent, you want your child to have that same experience, one that can develop only between individuals separated by a generation. Your baby's grandfather, too, will have a special interest in your baby—his descendant. Accept his involvement in your baby's life and encourage him to develop that privileged relationship that exists between a man and his grandchild. He may not be as actively involved with your baby as the baby's grandmother, but his feelings may be just as strong.

Your first experience in sharing your child with a grandmother may be immediately upon your ar-

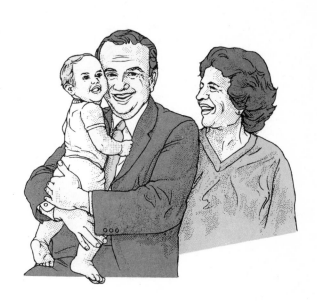

*Grandparents have a special relationship with a new baby.*

rival home from the hospital, when she comes to give you a hand during the first days or weeks. Don't be surprised if she prefers to do the cooking and cleaning and leaves the care of the baby to you. If she hasn't been around a newborn for some time, she may be hesitant to test her long-forgotten skills. You perhaps prefer that arrangement anyway, but don't be resentful if she does want to do some things for the baby. You'll have your chance later, when she has left.

It's possible that as you and Grandma talk about your baby, a difference of opinion between the two generations will arise. The problem will be one of conflicting information. Grandma may have to make many mental adjustments before she can accept and approve of your enthusiasm for some practices that were considered old-fashioned and outdated when she herself was a young woman. Giving birth without anesthesia, for example; options such as birthing rooms, overnight hospitalization, and home births; and today's emphasis-on breast-feeding. She may find a young father's total involvement in birth and child care inappropriate, because her husband left all that to her—and rightly so, according to her upbringing. You may find that you and she disagree about the use of pacifiers, about having a rigid schedule for feeding and bathing the baby, about whether to use cloth diapers or disposables. If Grandma is inflexible, you may dread the years ahead, anticipating continuous conflict about everything from nutrition to discipline.

# ADJUSTING TO YOUR NEW BABY

However, those of the older generation who have raised families have a great deal to offer. Not every piece of advice Grandma will give you is based on a myth or an old wives' tale; her years of experience taught her much that you can probably make use of. And many older relatives are willing to learn from new-generation mothers that, for example, a baby who is picked up every time he or she cries does not become spoiled and demanding, or that an immaculate house is not important to a baby's health and welfare or a family's happiness.

## Dealing With Unwanted Advice

With goodwill and a sincere desire for communication, you may very well be able to take the best that your parents and other older relatives have to offer and tactfully teach them the best of what you know, without lowering your standards or sacrificing your values. First, use the many available resources to back up your opinions. We all tend to believe what we read, and women of the older generation held doctors and other experts in high regard, so show Grandma the passages in books and magazines that reinforce your opinions. Quote your pediatrician to her. Share with her the literature you have from organizations such as the La Leche League and the National Childbirth Education Association. Tell her what you've learned from people whose opinion she respects—your neighbor, whose children she always admires, or your sister or sister-in-law. Sometimes simply stalling is a good technique. Thank her for her advice, and say and do nothing more about the matter. Or "forget" to try her method, or tell her you'll probably "start soon." With good humor and consideration, you can probably work things out with Grandma so you at least approach the ideal relationship, in which you are working together for the benefit of your child and in which the child is more important to both of you than each other's opinions about child care are. Bear in mind that the ultimate benefits of your rapport with Grandma will go to your child, whose relationship with her is priceless.

The bottom line, in dealing with Grandma or anyone else, is that *you* are the parent, an intelligent and well-informed person, and you have the right to determine what is best for your child and to raise him or her as you see fit. In the end, if you have to, you can remind these people that they chose their ways and you will choose yours. Of course, all this is easier with acquaintances or strangers, who will perhaps surprise you with their audacity in telling you what to do or in asking you impertinent questions about the way you are caring for your child. You do not need to justify your actions to such people; you can avoid confrontations by simply thanking them politely for their interest and going on your way.

Do be sure that you are actually being criticized before you react. Remember that the more insecure we are, the more we tend to infer criticism when none was intended, and that we all sometimes overreact to situations in which our children are concerned. There are few issues important enough to force confrontations with relatives or close friends.

## The Family Pet

No, your cat will not suffocate your infant in the crib. The myth that says it will dates back to the days of witchcraft, when infant mortality was high and standards of hygiene were low. Someone always seemed to remember seeing a cat in the crib of a baby who subsequently died. The underfed animal was probably attracted to the crib by the smell of milk. A cat, or any other animal, for that matter, is incapable of forming a complete seal around a baby's mouth and nose and so could not possibly suffocate him or her.

However, it is wise to consider the possible reactions of your dog or cat to a new baby. If you have no other children and have had your pet for some time, it is probably accustomed to being "the baby," a valued and well-loved member of the household, and may very well be jealous of a rival for your attention. The animal will most likely adjust quickly and learn to love the baby as much as it does you. You can ensure this acceptance by preparing the pet for the baby, much as you have prepared an older child. First, consider obedience training for a dog that will not obey your commands to sit, stay, and be quiet, or that cannot be kept from jumping up on people or furniture. If your dog or cat is not accustomed to children, try to arrange for it to spend some time with a baby occasionally. Speed up the process of your pet becoming acquainted with your baby by bringing home from the hospital something the baby has used so the dog or cat will get used to the unfamiliar scent. Some parents put a cloth diaper or a small blanket in the hospital bassinet with the baby to pick up this odor. And when you get home from the hospital with the baby, try to spend a few minutes alone with the pet to assure it of your love, just as you would an older child.

Of course, you don't want even the most loving of dogs or cats in your infant's crib. If you have not been able to train your dog to stay off beds and other furniture, or if your cat shows an interest in leaping into the crib to investigate the new arrival, block the door of the baby's room with the gate you will later use to keep your child from tumbling down the stairs or otherwise getting into dangerous trouble. This will allow you to see into the room, but will keep the pet out.

The possibility that your dog or cat will not adjust to having a baby in the house and will have to be banished is probably remote, but the chances that the baby will be allergic to your pet may not be. About one child in five develops allergies to one or another substance. Pollen, food, or dust may be responsible—even the bacteria that survives in your water bed—anything that can be touched, eaten, or breathed, including the tiny particles of dog or cat hair or skin (called *dander*) that are suspended in the air of your house. A tendency toward allergies is often inherited, but the specific allergies do not always take the same form in one family member as in another. For example, you yourself may be sensitive to certain foods or to a plant that blooms at a certain season of the year, but not to animals. Your child may inherit your tendency to allergies, but react, at least in infancy, only to animals.

The symptoms of allergy to animal hair are similar to those of the hay fever caused by pollens of trees, grass, and other plants. You may at first confuse them with the symptoms of a cold: itchy, runny eyes and nose, a general stuffiness of the head, an ear infection, or perhaps even a little wheeziness in breathing. If you suspect that an allergy to your pet is causing the baby's discomfort, see your doctor. Until something is done, the symptoms will increase and can cause sleeplessness, loss of appetite, inflammation of the eyes, ears, sinuses, throat, and bronchial tubes, and perhaps even a full-blown asthma attack. Unfortunately, your only solution will be to get the animal out of the house. Allergies do change as people grow older, and at some time in the future your child may outgrow this one and be able to enjoy the benefits of having a dog or cat.

Do be aware that pests, such as fleas, and even some illnesses can be transmitted from pets to children. Keep your pet clean and insect-free. Wash your hands carefully after handling or cleaning up after your pet. Ask your veterinarian's advice if your dog or cat is sick or if there are animal illnesses prevalent in your community.

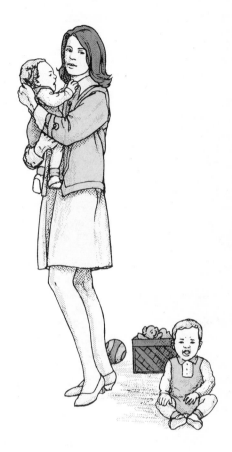

*Twins present special pleasures–and problems.*

## A Word About Twins

Parents of twins or larger sets of multiples report feeling either exaltation or resentment; some feel blessed, others feel as if they have been unfairly afflicted. There's no denying that caring for twins is extremely difficult for the first few months. Later, say some parents, twins become easier than two children who are merely close in age. They can be treated alike as far as daily care goes, and they amuse and teach each other. They may learn to dress or feed themselves rather early, if the one waiting gets impatient as you tend the other.

The names you choose for your multiples will reflect your personal tastes. Some parents like names that rhyme, like Ronald and Donald; others like those that begin with the same letter, like Sandra, Susan, and Steven. Still others prefer to use names that are not at all similar, like Elizabeth and Christopher. Do be careful not to give your multiples (or any child) names that are hard to pronounce or so unusual or fanciful that they will hate them. Naming one child after one of the parents or another relative may be considered a sign of favoritism later.

The thing that will probably be of the most help to you with your infant twins will be to get them on approximately the same schedule of eating and sleeping. Of course this is easier said than done, but putting them down at the same time and occasionally even waking one for a feeding may help. Feeding on demand will probably be impossible, but you will be tempted sometimes to prop a bottle for one baby while you hold the other to feed. This practice is discouraged as a general rule, but if you have two ravenous babies and will be present to carefully watch the one with the propped bottle, no harm will be done.

You will soon learn which times of the day are most difficult, with both babies awake, fussy, and hungry. One of these times is apt to be late in the afternoon, when you yourself are worn out and badly in need of a rest. Adjust whatever schedule you are trying to establish so that you have as little as possible to do at these times, and try to arrange for some help for yourself. If your husband or another relative or friend can't be with you, try to get a teenager to come in for an hour or so to assist you, under your supervision.

Be aware that while you might never let a single baby cry for more than a moment or two, there will be times when one of your twins will have to cry until you have time to attend to his or her wants. Babies are surprisingly adaptable, and even screaming for a quarter of an hour will not hurt your twins. Bath time will probably be one of these times. Do not try to bathe two infants at the same time; possibilities for injury to a baby, not to mention tension and stress for a parent, are more than double when both are wet and wriggling. Indeed, bath time may be the one time at which it is most helpful and practical to have two caregivers present to split up the tasks of bathing, drying, and dressing the babies.

One common problem with multiples is keeping track of such routine things as which has been fed or bathed, which has had a bowel movement, which has slept for several hours. The solution is simple: Write down everything. Some mothers of multiples find it convenient to hang a chart at the foot of each baby's crib to record such important events. If you have trouble telling one identical twin from another, paint a finger- or toenail of one with nail polish or leave the hospital bracelet on one.

Right from the beginning, become conscious of treating your twins as individuals, not as a "matched set." Of course they are adorable together, but dress them differently sometimes, and take at least some pictures of each of them individually. Sing and talk to one, then to the other, and use their names when you talk to them or about them. Try to avoid complaining to others about how much work your babies are and using the old clichés about "double trouble." Your twins won't understand you right now, but one day they will, and if they learn to think of themselves as problems who cause their parents nothing but drudgery, their self-esteem will be damaged and they may live up to the negative description.

## As Your Twins Grow

Learn to save your strength as you care for your twins (or any baby) by lifting them as seldom as possible and, when you do lift them, by using the muscles in your legs instead of those in your back. When they can crawl or walk, save steps by letting them come to you for playing and loving as you sit on the floor. Child-proof your home very carefully (see pages 267 to 273 for information on child-proofing); two inquisitive little people will find more than twice as many things to get into as one.

It's wise to prepare yourself for strong jealousy of your twins among other children, both older and younger. Twins receive a great deal of admiration and attention from outsiders, they take more of their parents' time, and they are often so devoted to each other that they shun other children. On the other hand, many twins wish they were singletons. They tire of always having to contend with a sibling of the same age who receives the same treatment.

That is one reason you will continue to treat your twins as individuals. Provide two birthday cakes. Don't always dress them alike. Encourage them to have different interests. Don't use nicknames that mark them as twins ("Pete" and "Re-peat," for example) and try to discourage others from doing so.

Make a point of not worrying about your twins' development in comparison with that of other children their age. If they were born prematurely, think of them in terms of their gestational age—their expected birth date—rather than their chronological age. They may be so content with each other's company that they aren't in a hurry to move from one stage to another. Twins often develop their own special language, which only they can speak and understand; discourage this by speaking to one twin at a time and waiting for him or her to answer.

## Seeking Support

Your doctor may know if your community is served by a branch of the Mothers of Twins Club, Inc. If there is not a branch near you, or if you would like more information, write the national club at 12404 Princess Jeanne NE, Albuquerque, NM 87112. Joining this group while you are pregnant may be the best thing you can do for yourself and your babies. After coming home from the hospital, you'll receive the moral support of others in your situation, and possibly some physical support as well. Club meetings offer speakers, workshops, and clothing and equipment exchanges, as well as social benefits. The national group publishes a quarterly newsletter and other helpful and informative literature.

The Center for the Study of Multiple Birth (333 E. Superior Street, Suite 476, Chicago IL 60611) provides information for parents, serves as a clearinghouse for information on twin research, and operates a bookstore. If you live in Canada, you can obtain information about twins by writing to Parents of Multiple Births Association of Canada, 283 7th Avenue South, Lethbridge, Alberta, Canada T1J 1H6.

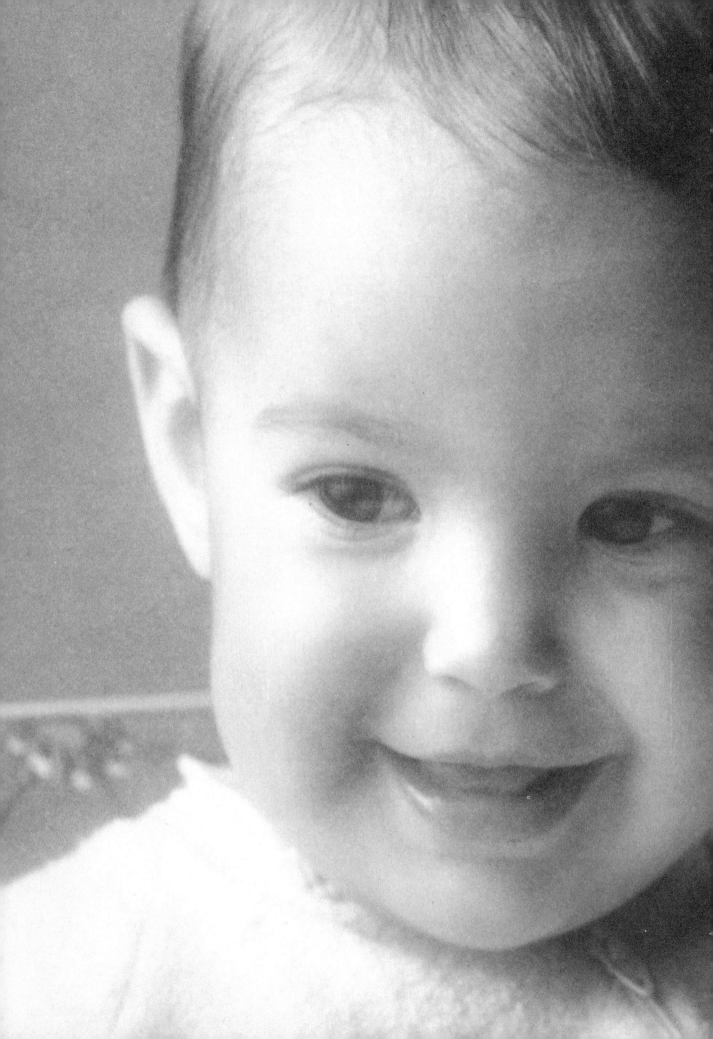

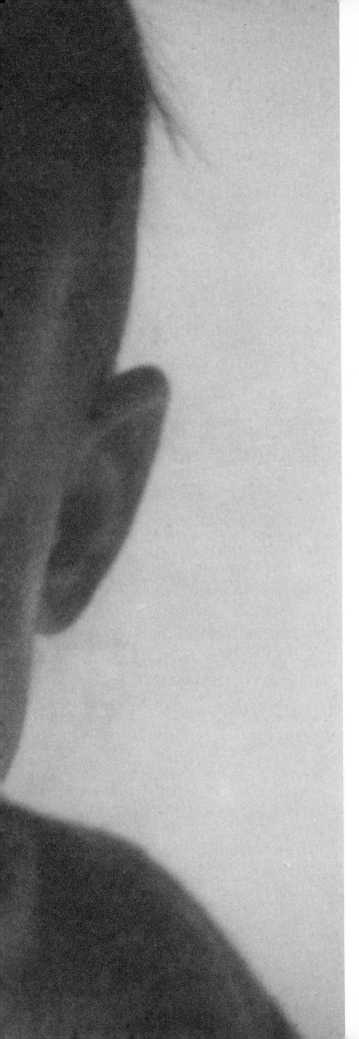

# Chapter 8: Health and Well-Being of Mother and Baby

## Fitness for New Mothers

The postpartum period is an exhilarating, exhausting, rewarding, tearful time of discovery. Often thought of as just six weeks of recovery until you are "back to normal," the postpartum period actually extends a full three months. At the end of this twelve-month cycle, the physical and psychological aspects of the new mother—body and mind—have reached a new level of adjustment. Your physical appearance, feelings, and attitudes are a direct reflection of your efforts. Your rewards can be great.

You will probably never be your "old self" or "back to normal" again. Your body underwent an enormous effort to grow and give birth to (and perhaps now feed) your new baby. But you can be on your way to a new and better self!

### Rest and Relaxation

This may sound like a contradiction for the post-partum period—a time that is often associated with sleepless nights, baby blues, tears, and fatigue. Babies get hungry around the clock at two- to four-hour intervals—more often if they are breast-fed, because human milk is digested faster and more easily than cow's milk. So most mothers (and many fathers) find that they get only two to three hours' sleep at one time, if that! Ongoing sleep disturbances—for days, weeks, or even months at a time—can leave you feeling cross, irritable, and depressed. When you are this tired, even little problems become difficult to solve, and it is hard to make decisions about even the smallest things. In the extreme, especially for those individuals who require more sleep than others, disorientation and confusion set in.

Yet it can be a time to tune into your body and use part of the natural scheduling of your day to release the tension. If friends or family offer help after the birth, let them take over the cooking, grocery shopping, and housework. (Have them cook a little extra each time and freeze it in boilable bags. With a bit of planning and thought, you might not have to cook for a week or more after your help has left!) Your help should mother you, while *you* mother the baby. Continuing the relaxation techniques learned in your prepared childbirth classes is extremely important. There is less uninterrupted time for yourself, so make the most of the time you *do* have. During feedings, take a few deep breaths and clear your mind—just enjoy this quiet time and free your body of tension. (If you're nursing, be sure you have a glass of water or juice nearby to sip, since you may get thirsty.) As soon as you lay the baby down for a nap, lie down yourself; walk directly from the baby to your own bed or couch. Resist any temptation to clean up or catch up on chores or calls; otherwise, before you know it, the baby will be up again and you won't have a chance to relax.

The postpartum period is a time to reset priorities and decide what is *really* important to you personally. You'll find that six months from now you won't remember how clean your house was or if dinner was on time, but you will remember if you were tired and frazzled or peaceful and rested, enjoying this special time.

Rest and relaxation are the complement of a fitness program—you must have both to rejuvenate your strength and vitality.

### Getting Started Again

Body conditioning and toning exercises should be started in bed, the day of delivery. The sooner you start, the sooner your body will respond with firm, toned muscles, especially pelvic floor and abdominal muscles. Follow the exercises as they are shown in "Exercises for Immediately After a Vaginal Delivery" or "Exercises for Immediately After a Cesarean Delivery," depending on the type of delivery you had. Unless you experienced multiple complications and find yourself extremely fatigued, you can begin performing these movements as suggested.

Once you get home, don't wait to exercise until the baby is asleep. Just lay out two blankets—one for each of you—and begin. The baby will enjoy the movement, the music, and your smiles. If baby tires, she'll drop off to sleep, whether there is music on or not. Get moving—don't wait or waste precious hours or days!

If your physician says not to exercise for six weeks or more after delivery, show her the list of exercises you want to do. Do not just ask to "exercise"—be specific. These exercises are so gentle and safe that she will probably give her consent. If, however, your physician feels that even these exercises are inappropriate for you just yet, of course follow her advice.

## Exercises for Immediately After a Vaginal Delivery

Begin the day of delivery, while in bed. Do them on the floor once home.

### Head Curl-Up

*Begin with five to ten twice daily; move toward twenty.*

1. Lie on back, with knees bent and feet close to buttocks. Press back down. Inhale slowly and deeply.

2. Exhale slowly; at the same time lift up *just the head*. Hold as you complete the outward breath.

3. Relax.

4. Repeat for a total of five times.

continued

*Note: Do this as many times during the day as you can. Then progress to Head and Shoulders Curl-Up.*

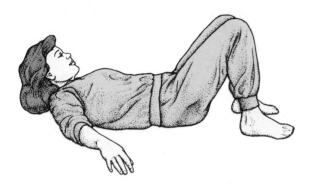

**Step 2**

## Head and Shoulders Curl-Up

*Begin with five twice daily; move toward twenty.*

1. Lie on the bed or floor, with knees bent and feet close to buttocks. Press the back down and inhale slowly and deeply.

2. Exhale slowly; at the same time, lift head and then shoulders. Hold as you complete the outward breath. Perform slowly with control (no jerky movements). Head should stay in line with the spine; do not throw head forward! The "lift" comes from the shoulders and should be *straight up,* about six inches *maximum,* face toward ceiling.

3. Relax, return to starting position, and repeat.

## Pelvic Floor Squeeze

*Do sixty or more each day, in sets of three or four.*

1. Sit or stand comfortably (you can do this exercise in most positions). The farther the legs are apart, the more challenging.

2. Thinking about the vagina and perineum, tighten the pelvic floor as if to lift the internal organs or to stop urination in midstream. Hold as tightly as possible for a slow count of three (gradually work up to a count of ten). Be sure to breathe.

3. Relax completely.

*Note: Because these muscles fatigue easily, repeat in sets of three or four squeezes throughout the day anytime, anywhere. Concentrate on the sensations of tension and lifting, relaxing and lowering within the pelvis.*

## Pelvic Tilt

*Begin with ten a day and work toward twenty.*

1. Lie on back, with knees bent and heels close to buttocks.

2. Inhale and press back to the floor. Hold for a slow count of five (working toward ten). Concentrate on pressing the back to the floor by using your abdominals—do not push with the feet. For an extra benefit, squeeze your buttock muscles *and* the pelvic floor.

3. Relax, then repeat.

*Note: This is a wonderful stretch that will help relieve a tired or achy back.*

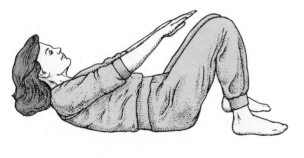

**Step 2**

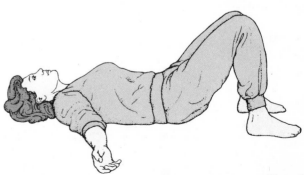

**Step 2**

## Bend and Straighten Legs

*Start with ten a day; progress to twenty. Start with Variation A. Using comfort as your guide, progress through Variations B and C to Variation D as quickly as possible.*

### Variation A
1. Lie on back with both legs bent, feet flat on bed or floor.

2. Slowly straighten the right leg and bend back to place.

3. Repeat with opposite leg.

### Variation B
1. Lie on back with one leg bent and the other leg straight.

2. Slide the bent leg out straight and then back to a bent-knee position.

3. Repeat with the straight leg, returning to a straight-leg position.

### Variation C
1. Lie on back with one leg bent and the other leg straight.

2. Bend one leg as you straighten the other. (Both moving at the same time, slowly, in opposition.)

### Variation D
1. Lie on back with both legs bent.

2. Move legs down and up at the same time.

## Exercises for Immediately After a Cesarean Delivery

Begin the day of delivery (as soon as you return from the recovery room). Do them in bed. Perform them until you are up on a regular basis.

### Deep Breathing

*Five times every hour that you are awake.*

Breathe slowly and deeply to expand the upper, middle, and lower portions of your chest.

## Huffing

*Two or three times every hour that you are awake.*

This is especially important if you had general (gas) anesthesia. In response to the anesthetic, the lungs produce mucus, which, if not removed, can clog the small air sacs and breathing tubes of the lungs. "Huffing" should be used instead of coughing.

Here's how: A huff is a quick outward breath. It is like saying "ha"—a short, quick breath, with force, from the abdominal muscles. The outward breath must be done quickly. Otherwise, the force is not sufficient to dislodge any mucus. Spit out the mucus you cough up; don't swallow it.

If huffing doesn't bring up any mucus and you still hear a "rattle" in the chest, try Deep Breathing again to loosen it.

With huffing, the abdominal wall is pulled in instead of out; therefore, huffing is more comfortable than Deep Breathing. Still, you may want to support the abdominal wall with your hands or a pillow. Be reassured that the stitches will *not* be pulled out.

## Foot Exercises

*Five times every hour that you are awake.*

1. Do five ankle circles to the right and five ankle circles to the left. Make them slow and big. Repeat with the other ankle.

2. Slowly point and flex the foot. Repeat with the other foot.

## Pelvic Floor Squeeze

*Twenty a day, moving toward sixty, in sets of three or four. Begin when the catheter is removed.*

1. Lie or sit (later you will be able to stand) comfortably with the legs apart. (The farther the legs are apart, the more challenging.)

2. Thinking about the vagina and perineum, tighten the pelvic floor as if to lift the internal organs or to stop urination in midstream. Hold as tightly as possible for a slow count of three (gradually work up to a count of ten). Be sure to breathe.

3. Relax completely.

*Note: Because these muscles fatigue easily, repeat in sets of three or four squeezes throughout the day anytime, anywhere. Concentrate on the sensations of tension and lifting, relaxing and lowering within the pelvis.*

## Leg Squeeze

*Three times every hour you are awake.*

1. Lie on back with one leg bent and the other leg straight with foot flexed.

2. Slowly press the straight leg to the bed and tighten all the muscles in that leg, gently pulling the toes toward the face.

3. Repeat with the opposite leg.

4. With both legs straight and ankles crossed, tighten all the muscles in your legs—press knees down, tighten thigh muscles, squeeze the buttock muscles. Hold while you slowly count to five (don't hold your breath!).

5. Release.

6. Repeat.

*Hint: If needed, prop yourself up on pillows.*

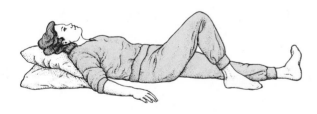

**Step 2**

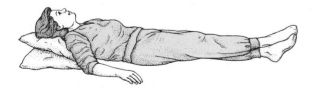

**Step 4**

## Pelvic Tilt

*Three to five times every hour you are awake.*

1. Lie on back, with knees bent and heels close to buttocks.

2. Inhale and press your back to the bed. Hold for a slow count of five (working toward ten). Concentrate on pressing the back to the bed by using your abdominals—do not push with the feet. For an extra benefit, squeeze your buttock muscles *and* the pelvic floor.

3. Relax, then repeat.

*Note: Slow, controlled movements are the key to success with this exercise. In the beginning, abdominal pain will let you do only a third or a half of this movement. That's fine—listen to your body. Improving pelvic circulation is important—do the best you can with this movement. As your body heals more and more each day, hold the tilt longer and longer. Remember to breathe. Add a Pelvic Floor Squeeze, too.*

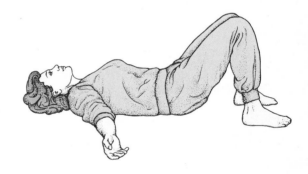

**Step 2**

## Add on Third Day

### Bend and Straighten Legs

*Repeat Variation A three to five times, twice a day. Using comfort as your guide, progress through Variations B and C to Variation D as soon as possible.*

**Variation A**
1. Lie on back with both legs bent, feet flat on the bed.

continued

2. Slowly straighten the right leg and bend back to place.

3. Repeat with opposite leg.

### Variation B

1. Lie on back with one leg bent and the other leg straight.

2. Slide the bent leg out straight and then back to a bent-knee position.

3. Repeat with the straight leg, returning to a straight-leg position.

### Variation C

1. Lie on back with one leg bent and the other leg straight.

2. Bend one leg as you straighten the other. (Both legs are moving at the same time, slowly, in opposition.)

### Variation D

1. Lie on back with both legs bent.

2. Move both legs down and up at the same time.

## Add on Seventh Day

### Head-Up Lift

*Three to five times twice a day. Add more as comfort guides you.*

1. Lie flat on back with no pillows, knees bent.

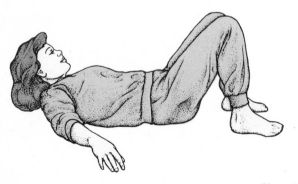

**Step 2**

2. Press back down (Pelvic Tilt). Inhale slowly and lift *just the head*. Hold for a count of three.

3. Lower head and relax.

*Note: Using comfort as your guide, progress to lifting head and shoulders on exhalation. Concentrate on lifting head and shoulders as a unit toward ceiling, just an inch or two off floor. Do not thrust head forward on the lift.*

## The Pelvic Floor

When thinking of exercise after delivery, most new mothers think of a flat abdomen as the first priority. Actually, the pelvic floor should receive prime attention, with the abdominal muscles coming in second. Strong pelvic floor muscles ensure good support of internal organs and sphincter control (urethra, rectum, and vagina). They also ensure pleasurable sensations during sexual intercourse for both the woman and her partner.

After vaginal delivery, the pelvic floor may be bruised, swollen, and tender. After a cesarean section, it may be lax, with loss of tone or elasticity from the weight of the baby and months of slug-

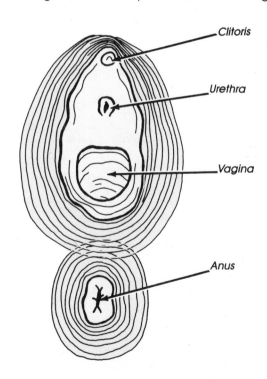

*Structure of the female pelvic floor. The muscles form a figure eight around the three openings in the pelvic floor.*

gish circulation. Initial attempts at tightening or "lifting up" the muscles of the pelvic floor immediately after delivery are often accompanied by surprise—you feel little or nothing! Many times, muscles have been torn or cut and nerves have been damaged. It's no wonder there is little sensation. Perhaps, too, the structure of the pelvic floor was surgically repaired. Exercise can improve all these situations by (1) alleviating discomfort (although it is uncomfortable at first to even gently squeeze those muscles) and (2) improving circulation to the area, which will increase the oxygen supply, remove waste products, decrease swelling, and promote the prompt return of urine control.

If you neglect this important area, the muscles will remain stretched and loose. They will become further weakened as you resume your usual schedule. The sooner you start after delivery, the faster the muscles will respond. Waiting will only result in more time and effort being necessary than would have been required if you had started immediately after delivery. You have only benefits to gain.

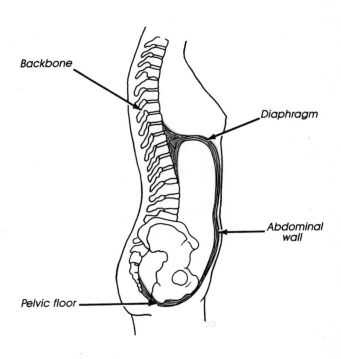

*The boundaries of the pelvic cavity.*

## The Abdominal Wall

Right after delivery, you may wonder if your stomach will ever be flat again. If you begin an exercise program early (within twenty-four hours of giving birth) and are fiercely persistent with frequent repetitions of the appropriate exercises, your stomach will indeed be flat once more.

The abdominal muscles we feel and notice most often are the rectus muscles (see illustrations on page 194). They are long, slender muscles located along the center of the abdominal wall. They run vertically from the end of the sternum (breastbone) and the lower ribs to the pubic bone. There are right and left rectus muscles, which are separated by a band of fibrous connective tissue about half an inch wide that is called the *linea alba*.

The *internal and external oblique muscles* lie on the sides of the rectus muscles. They cover the waist—a hard area to tighten even when you haven't had a baby. The external obliques cover the front and sides of the abdomen from the rectus muscle to the back muscles. The external obliques are attached to the ribs at the top edges and have a wide area of attachment, running from the lower eight ribs to the front surface of the pelvis and on down to the pubic bone.

The internal obliques are located directly below the external obliques. Their muscle fibers run at almost a ninety-degree angle to those of the external obliques, most of them nearly horizontal. The internal obliques run from approximately the waist area down to the pubic bone.

All this may sound unnecessarily technical when you just want to have a flat belly again, but getting to know how your body is put together will enable you to understand how the exercises work and what kinds of exercises are needed to "renovate" those muscles after delivery. Getting in touch with your body and learning to listen to it are primary steps in getting started.

The lower ends of the rectus muscles go through a slit in the deep abdominal muscles before they become attached to the pubic bone. When the rectus muscles are relaxed, as they are when you walk and move around, they follow a curved line; they become straight *only* when they contract (when you consciously and tightly hold your stomach in).

Hereditary factors come into play in the deposition of fat in the lower abdomen, even when weight is lost and body fat is at the ideal level (twenty-two to twenty-four percent for women). Even then, because the rectus muscles are

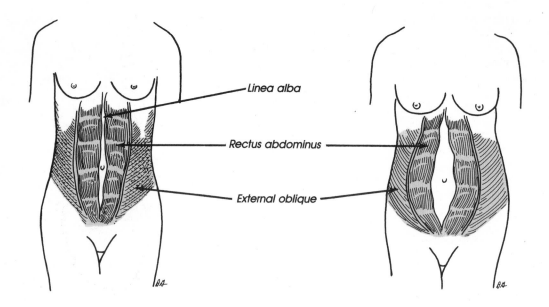

*Normal abdominal muscle alignment*                    *Stressed abdominal muscles with large diastasis*

curved and because small deposits of fat are stubbornly held in that area, most women find their "stomach" is still slightly rounded.

## Checking for Diastasis

After delivery, the abdominal muscles are always loose and soft. The abdomen looks and feels like gelatin, which can be quite a shock. It is important to check the linea alba between the rectus muscles for separation, called *diastasis*. The opening between the muscles may be slight or so large that the uterus or abdominal contents can be felt bulging through the opening.

Since there must be a good balance between back and abdominal muscles, a large diastasis will eventually cause backaches (and possibly radiating leg pain) just from moving through the normal day's activities of caring for an infant or managing a full-time job at or away from home. If no corrective attempts are made to close the opening, reestablishing muscle balance and strength, there will be little support for a subsequent pregnancy. Posture will be poor, and many aches and pains will develop, all from lack of abdominal strength.

Check for diastasis on the third or fourth day after delivery. Until this time, the area will feel too slack for you to get an indication of the state of the

abdominals. Also, you will have had a few days' worth of abdominal exercises to help improve your strength.

To check:

1.  Lie on your back, with your knees bent. Place the fingers of one hand on your abdomen covering your navel (your fingers should point toward your pubic bone). Apply firm pressure.

2.  Inhale deeply. Then exhale slowly and at the same time lift your head and neck slowly. As you lift, you'll feel each of the rectus muscles tighten and pull toward the center (toward your fingers).

3.  Check to see how many fingers will fit in the gap. One to two finger-widths is normal and to be expected; this will gradually decrease with exercise. Three to four finger-widths will require special attention from you to repair and rebalance the muscles.

Don't hesitate to ask for help from a nurse (preferably a registered nurse) or your physician if you have difficulty checking your abdominals.

## Correcting Diastasis

The following special exercise is very effective for closing a large diastasis. Raising just the head in this exercise ensures that only the rectus muscles will be activated. As they become stronger, you will be able to lift your shoulders, thus working the other abdominal muscles also. It is important to strengthen the rectus muscles first, thus ensuring their stabilization and alignment as the other muscles come into play.

Repeat this special exercise often, at least fifty times a day. To speed progress, do ten each hour you are awake. Remember to use slow, controlled movements, resting whenever you feel the need. The gap should be back to the normal half an inch within a week or so. If you do fewer repetitions than those recommended above, closing the gap will take longer.

Because the other abdominal muscles are attached to the rectus muscles and because the abdominals in general are weak and out of balance, avoid the following exercises, which will serve only to increase the diastasis: (1) those rotating the trunk of the body ("waist twists"), (2) those twisting the hips, and (3) those that cause the trunk to bend to the side ("waist or side stretches").

If you breathe out while raising your head and shoulders, the intra-abdominal pressure will not be increased (as it would be if you held your breath.) Increased intra-abdominal pressure would just increase the diastasis, which would defeat the whole purpose of the exercise and just add time to the muscle rehabilitation.

Do not let the abdominal muscles bulge. Tighten your abdomen at any time you might strain.

### Exercise for Correcting Diastasis

*Do at least fifty times a day.*

1.  Lie on your back, with knees bent. Cross your hands over the abdominal area so you will be

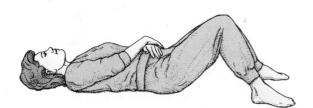

**Step 1**

able to pull the muscles toward the center of the abdomen as you slowly raise your head.

2.  Take a deep breath. As you slowly exhale, lift your head (and later your shoulders, to a forty-five-degree angle), at the same time pulling the muscles together with your hands. Return your head (and shoulders) slowly to the bed or floor.

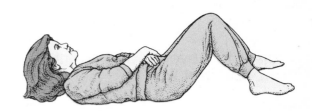

**Step 2**

## Continuing the Program

Once you have completed the appropriate exercises for after your type of delivery, gradually replace the post-delivery exercises with the ones you did during pregnancy. These exercises also work all the muscle groups that are important during the postpartum period, with no muscle or joint strain. The Pelvic Rock, which can now also be done while lying on your back with your knees bent, will improve posture and ease back strain. It is wonderful for working buttock, abdominal, and pelvic floor muscles all at the same time, and provides a great back stretch. Remember to do it slowly with control and gradually increase the time you hold the tilt.

Begin with the first eight strengthening exercises on pages 41 to 45. When you feel comfortable with these, gradually increase the repetitions, then add the remaining four exercises on pages 45 to 46. Gradually increase your repetitions with these also, letting comfort be your guide. Don't rush through them. Be sure to warm up (walk or march in place for three to five minutes) and then stretch for five minutes before beginning any floor exercise. Turn on music with a strong, regular beat. Music will help you move smoothly, make time pass quickly, and add an element of fun.

### Extra Help

The following exercises are good for a stubborn, protruding abdominal wall (a potbelly).

Because the rectus muscles are long, vertical muscles that run from the breastbone to the pubic bone, you will need to have exercises that cause action at *both* ends of them. To shape and to strengthen these muscles, at least two exercises must be performed: Reverse Sit-Ups and Reverse Trunk Twists. The Reverse Sit-Ups can be alternated with the U-Seat, or all three can be done at each session. For all these exercises, begin with five of each and gradually increase the repetitions as you get stronger. The key to success is controlled movements, with no "sling and fling" moves.

## Exercises to Develop and Maintain a Flat Abdominal Wall

### Reverse Sit-Up

*Start with five and increase gradually.*

1. Lie on back with knees bent and arms at sides, palms down.

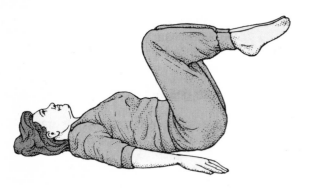

**Step 1**

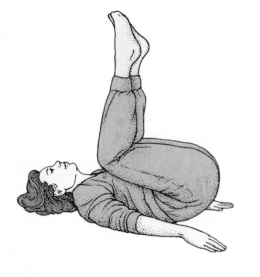

**Step 2**

2. Keeping knees bent, raise legs until knees are past level of breasts or above face. Raise buttocks toward upper body. Head and shoulders stay flat.

3. Return to starting position and repeat.

*Note: You may notice a tendency to press down or grip the floor with the hands or you may feel a strain in the neck or upper shoulders as you attempt to reach the desired height with the knees. This will disappear as you become stronger and more relaxed with the movement. (Remember to breathe during this exercise.)*

*Another hint is to start by getting only the hips off the floor; gradually you will be able to lift more and more of the hips and lower back. Notice the angle of the lower legs in relation to the upper legs in the drawing. Height is not gained by slinging or throwing the lower legs above the head. The action should be smooth and come from the abdominals.*

*This exercise works the lower fibers of the rectus muscles as well as the external obliques. To work the horizontal fibers you should also perform Reverse Trunk Twists.*

### Reverse Trunk Twist

*Start with five and increase gradually.*

1. Lie on back with arms out to sides and with legs raised ninety degrees from floor with knees bent slightly.

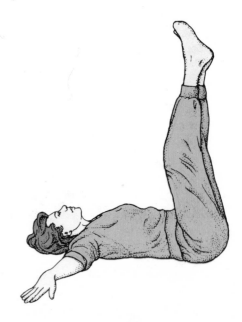

**Step 1**

2. Lower legs to right and touch floor with outside of foot. Shoulders and arms must remain on floor at all times.

3. Return to starting position and repeat, alternating sides on each repetition. (After a time, you will probably notice increased flexibility of your midsection while performing this exercise.)

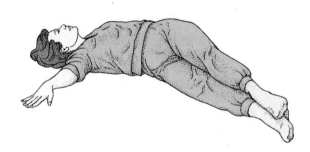

**Step 2**

**Advanced action:**

Begin with same starting position but with legs straight. Legs should remain straight as they are lowered to side. Be sure to press your back to the floor as you come toward the center each time.

*Note: If your shoulders come off the floor as you drop your legs to the side, have someone hold them down. This person should be on all fours with his or her hands on your shoulder joints (not the neck area), arms straight, and shoulders directly above yours. As flexibility and strength increase, you will not need assistance.*

*On the advanced exercise, if you have difficulty keeping the legs straight because of tight hamstring muscles, bend your knees slightly but keep the legs together. The more the knees are bent, the easier it is to do this exercise. Doing it in the straight-leg position is the most effective, so try to work up to it.*

*The Reverse Trunk Twist works all portions of the internal and external obliques, tightening the front and sides of the abdominal wall much more than any other abdominal exercise. This exercise also strengthens the spine because it uses the small muscles—both the deep and the surface muscles —that hold the bony vertebrae together and twist the spine. Strengthening these muscles will ease the typical overuse backache and may help prevent injuries that occur when quick, twisting movements are executed.*

**The U-Seat**

*Start with five and increase gradually to a maximum of twenty.*

1. Lie on back with arms behind head, knees bent, and feet on the floor.

2. At the same time, raise head and begin raising knees toward chest. As the head and knees are in motion, begin raising shoulders and buttocks off floor. Continue both actions and try to touch knees to chest. At the end of these movements, your pelvis and upper body should be off the floor. Do *not* push head and neck forward with hands—simply rest head in hands, letting the shoulders do the work.

3. Return to starting position and repeat.

*Note: Knees should be brought up quickly but smoothly, using the abdominals, to develop momentum; this action makes it easier to raise the pelvis. Think of it as two steps: (1) raise head and knees, then (2) raise shoulders and buttocks. This timing allows for proper coordination and smooth movement between pelvis and chest.*

*When performed correctly and smoothly, the U-Seat exercise maximally involves both the lower and upper portions of your abdominals.*

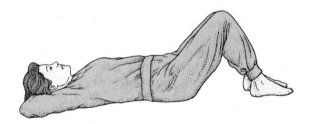

**Step 1**

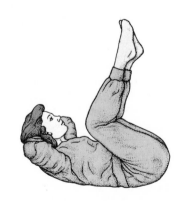

**Step 2**

## Recovery Time

Recovery time is very individualized. It depends on what kind of shape you were in before and during pregnancy, in addition to how much effort, time, and planning you are willing to now give to your body. If your abdominals were strong and if you exercised them regularly before and throughout pregnancy, one to two months—at the most, three months—should see you back to normal.

On the other hand, if your abdominals were not strong and you didn't exercise them regularly, then it will probably take between six and twelve months of regular exercise to become a better you. (These time frames assume that you are performing abdominal exercises four to six days a week.)

What if you took up regular exercise for the first time in your life *during* pregnancy? This does give you something of a head start. However, the advancing growth of the baby did not allow as adequate a workout of the abdominals as if you had also exercised before pregnancy. In this case, the return of strong, firm abdominals should take between three and six months (which is still much faster than for someone who neglected to exercise in pregnancy).

If you never put into action your resolve to restrengthen your abdominal wall, there is no telling how long the process will take. In fact, some women's abdominals never return to their original shape. The truth is that it takes action on your part to improve your figure. A slack set of abdominals will probably mean you will have a lot of backaches and fatigue.

The abdominals do forty percent of the work involved in supporting the trunk of your body as you move through your daily activities. If they are doing only ten percent, the back muscles will pick up the load—or attempt to anyway. The back muscles are responsible for sixty percent of the work of keeping the body upright and helping to lift, move, and bend. Increase that workload by ten to thirty percent and the muscles respond by fatiguing faster ("tired back") and by having painful spasms, especially in the lower back. Sometimes the lower back muscles become so tight that the angle of the normal pelvic tilt is changed. These tight muscles squeeze or press on the nerves coming off the spine in the lower back area. These nerves, in turn, divide and branch out to each leg. Pain may be felt in the lower back,

one or both buttocks, and one or both legs (upper or full length). Don't allow this kind of problem to decrease the joy of those first beautiful months with your new baby.

Other factors to consider in estimating recovery time are how much weight you gained and how much your abdominal wall expanded (partially due to the size of the baby and how you carried the child). Diet, the amount of rest you are currently getting, and the types of activities you're involved in must also be considered.

## The Role of Aerobic Exercise

Much literature has been written on the benefits of aerobic exercise. The benefits we are most concerned with here are those specifically dealing with a new mother. Those benefits are increasing stamina and endurance—the ability to do more but feel less tired—and decreasing body fat.

See Chapter 2 for important information concerning your target heart rate zone; before beginning your after delivery exercise program, refer to the chart on page 37.

### Decreasing Body Fat

After delivery and with exercise, your body will slowly begin losing some of the stored fat it laid down during pregnancy. How much you accumulated during the nine months depended on your percentage of body fat going into the pregnancy and the kinds and amounts of foods you ate during pregnancy. The leaner your body was, the less likely it is that you laid down large fat stores. Hereditary factors also come into play.

After delivery, the fat stores will gradually decrease over a period of four to six months. There are no miraculous changes that occur within the first six weeks, as many sources may lead you to believe. You may notice a difference in your body during the first two weeks after delivery, when much of the accumulated pregnancy-related fluid is lost through urination. After that, it's up to you.

Breast-feeding women initially lose weight faster than women who bottle-feed. However, because of hormonal factors in operation throughout breast-feeding, their body fat level remains slightly higher, their breast tissue weighs more, and they retain a small amount of extra fluid beneath their skin as a reserve. As a result, breast-feeding women tend to weigh about three to seven pounds more than their pre-pregnancy weight during breast-feeding, regardless of efforts at losing weight. Having taken that fact into consideration, if you still don't seem to be losing the weight that you expected to lose, take a good look at your diet and calorie intake. A diet full of excessive amounts of sweets and fats will not help you return to your pre-pregnancy weight easily. Check with your physician if planning a reducing diet while breast-feeding: many breast-feeding women can lose weight on seventeen hundred to eighteen hundred calories a day and still maintain a good milk supply; others must have two thousand calories a day to maintain an adequate milk supply. Making milk itself takes lots of energy (hence, uses up calories). Add aerobic activity for twenty to thirty minutes a day, five to six days a week, and you will lose weight.

Breast-feeding should not be seen as an impediment to recovering your pre-pregnancy figure—or as an excuse for not trying. On the other hand, don't let the fear of extra weight gain keep you from breast-feeding in the first place. The few pounds of weight that can be attributed to breast-feeding will be with you only temporarily; the benefits of breast-feeding for you and your baby will be with you forever.

Remember, it may take four to six months for body fat to start dropping. A daily nudge with aerobic exercise will start things happening. Be patient. Many answers still lie ahead of us as more and more studies are being done to help us understand the mechanisms of the body that just gave birth to new life. One thing is absolutely certain: having a new baby is not an excuse for looking or feeling out of shape.

## Increasing Stamina and Endurance

Women often say, "I already walk a lot just caring for the baby, and I'm very tired. The last thing I want to do if I have spare time is walk—I just want to sit down and relax or nap!" But walking while caring for the baby is a lot of stop and start movements, never really going very far from one place to another. What is needed is slow, steady, rhythmic movement for a period of five to fifteen minutes, uninterrupted. This kind of activity, after you get over the initial tiredness of doing it the first few times, will actually give you energy and release you from feeling tired and sluggish.

## When to Begin or Resume Aerobic Exercise

This depends on a number of factors, such as how fit you were before giving birth, whether delivery was vaginal or abdominal, whether there were any complications, how much sleep you are getting, and what your emotional reaction to the birth was. (Some women take days, weeks, or months to work through unexpected or unpleasant birth-related events. They may feel sad, angry, or depressed. Emotional factors may sometimes prevent a woman from taking hold of her situation and following through with desired action.)

General guidelines are as follows: If a woman exercised regularly for eight to twelve weeks before delivery, she can safely resume moderate aerobic exercise ten to fourteen days after an uncomplicated vaginal delivery, or approximately twenty-one days after a cesarean delivery. If a woman had a high fitness level before pregnancy and exercised regularly all through pregnancy, she will probably find it comfortable to begin short, brisk walks during the first week after a vaginal delivery, or during the second week after cesarean delivery.

Whatever aerobic activity you choose to begin with, be sure to monitor your pulse; work at about sixty percent of your SHR for the first few weeks. Do not start at a level of seventy or seventy-five percent. Remember that you have just had a baby (and, if by cesarean, major surgery as well). Remember also that you are almost certainly getting less sleep than usual. Start your exercise program at sixty percent, and work gradually to seventy-five. If you are new to exercise, take twelve weeks to make this transition. To develop stamina and endurance and to retrain your body to burn fat as fuel, you never need to work at a pulse rate higher than eighty percent of your SHR. The old "no pain, no gain" slogan is not true—pacing, regularity, and persistence are the keys to successful exercise.

The very best guideline for resuming aerobic exercise is to tune in to your body. And remember, never exercise to exhaustion. If you feel yourself tiring, slow down or stop. End your workout at the point at which you feel you could go another ten minutes. Learn to pace yourself.

This is the time to think about joining (or rejoining) an exercise class. A pregnancy/new mother class is ideal. You have the support, advice, and caring of women in your same life situation. Al-

## Walking Program

| | Warm-Up Stretch | Walk | Cool-Down Stretch |
|---|---|---|---|
| **Weeks 1 and 2** | 5–10 minutes | 5 minutes slowly<br>15 minutes briskly<br>5 minutes slowly | 5–10 minutes |
| **Weeks 3 and 4** | 5–10 minutes | 5 minutes slowly<br>30 minutes briskly<br>5 minutes slowly | 5–10 minutes |
| **Week 5 and thereafter** | 5–10 minutes | 5 minutes slowly<br>45 minutes briskly<br>5 minutes slowly | 5–10 minutes |

- Remember: Walk with your pulse in your target zone.

- Never exercise to exhaustion. End your workout at the point at which you feel you could go on for another ten minutes.

- After delivery, start at Week 1. Listen to your body—it will tell you how fast to progress.

though you may not do all the exercises in the class during your first weeks of attendance, getting out of the house, forcing yourself to be organized, being with other mothers, and being in a formal class can do wonders, beyond the benefits of the exercises themselves.

## Choosing a Baby Doctor

One of the most important decisions you'll make about your baby's health is selecting his doctor. Finding the right doctor isn't easy. There are many questions that must be asked and answered before you make the selection. It's important to find a doctor you feel comfortable with—someone whom you can talk to and who'll answer your questions to your satisfaction. The doctor's style must be right for you!

You should meet with several doctors before you have your baby. This will give you an opportunity to find out what they are like—their style, their approach, their fees, and so forth. Most doctors encourage this, and don't charge for it.

### Family Practitioner Versus Pediatrician

There are two different specialists who take care of babies—family practitioners and pediatricians. Both have completed a residency (extra

training after graduation from medical school). A family practitioner's training covers all areas of medicine, including adult medicine, pediatrics, obstetrics, and surgery. A pediatrician's residency is focused primarily on pediatrics. He has spent more time dealing with very ill children and children with special problems. A family practitioner will take care of your entire family—from the very young to the very old. Most family practitioners encourage this. They find it easier to treat an individual if they know the whole family. Family practitioners frequently are better able to deal with emotional or family problems that affect everyone in the household. A pediatrician takes care of children exclusively. Usually, they stop seeing a child when he is in his mid-teens.

Both kinds of specialists can take care of normal children equally well; however, if your child has special problems, a pediatrician may be better.

### Questions to Ask

When you go for the "get-acquainted visit" before your baby is born, you should bring with you a list of questions. The doctor's answers to your questions are important, and you should make notes. Follow up on any answers you don't understand. Be aware of the doctor's style and how he answers the questions.

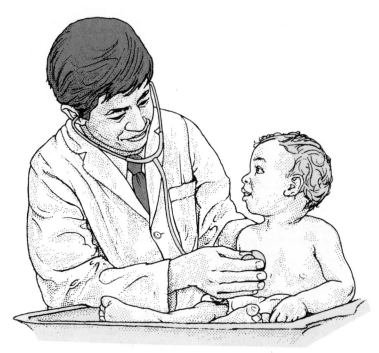

*Your baby's doctor is vital to your baby's well-being and to your peace of mind; he or she should be chosen with care.*

Here is a list of some questions you should ask:

- *What hospitals do you use?* You may want to be sure the doctor uses the hospital you prefer. Does he have a preference for a hospital far from your home? If so, find out why. Perhaps that hospital offers special services or has a different approach to taking care of children.

- *What hours is your office open?* With medicine becoming more competitive, doctors are now doing more to attract and keep patients. This includes offering evening and Saturday office hours. If a doctor's office hours are inconvenient for your family, you may want to find another doctor.

- *What services do you provide in your office?* Many doctors now provide a number of services in their offices to make things easier for you. For example, they may perform many laboratory tests there or take blood samples that need to be sent out to a laboratory for special tests. Many doctors also perform hearing and vision tests in their offices. The more done in the office, the fewer places you may have to take your child.

- *What should I do if my child is sick at night or on the weekend and I can't reach you?* Most

doctors arrange to have other physicians "cover" for them (take care of their patients) when they are not working or are out of town. Be sure the doctor has such a system. Find out who the covering doctors are because you may have to deal with them. Be wary of a doctor who tells you to take your sick child to the emergency room when he's not around.

- *How do I fit into the care of my child?* Some doctors want parents to be active participants in the medical care of their children. Other doctors want to be completely in charge and make all the decisions without input from parents. You need to know the doctor's feelings in this area. If they conflict with yours, the doctor probably isn't right for you.

- *How do you feel about patient education?* In this day of increasing medical awareness by parents, most doctors encourage parental education. However, there are some doctors who still buck this trend, believing that a little learning is a dangerous thing.

- *What are your feelings on "routine" medical care?* There is controversy about some aspects of pediatric care (for example, routine immunizations and circumcisions). Is this doctor dogmatic in his approach? Is his way the only right way? If you have strong feelings about your child's care, such an approach may lead to conflict.

- *What are your fees?* This used to be a difficult question, one that both patients and doctors avoided, but this is changing. There are large differences in what doctors charge for the same services. Get a price list for the routine things like well-baby examinations.

- *What type of training did you receive?* Any doctor should be willing to tell you about his training—medical school, residency, and any special training. Don't be impressed by a wall full of fancy diplomas. In and of themselves, they may not mean much. Almost every medical organization sends out diplomas, and many don't signify much except that the doctor paid his dues. The competence of a physician isn't measured by the number of diplomas and certificates he has. It is, however, a good idea to ask him if he is board-certified—that is, if he has demonstrated, by completion of certain requirements and passage of an examination, competency in his specialty.

After you have made your visits, talk to some of your friends. Find out whom they use and why. Ask them the questions you asked the doctors (especially about service and availability), and see if you get the same answers.

When you have all this information, you will be in a position to make an educated decision. Once you decide, let the doctor know. Find out if there's any information her office needs to know about you. If your children have records with another doctor, arrange for them to be sent.

After all this work, there's still a chance you'll decide, after a few visits, that your new doctor isn't what you expected. You should discuss this with her. Try to explain why you aren't satisfied. Maybe there's a misunderstanding that's easy to correct. Your doctor's reaction to what you say is important. If she gets mad or rude, you should look for another doctor. Don't feel obligated to stick with her if you don't agree with her on some important matter, like her approach, treatment, or fees.

When you change doctors, you should get your child's old medical records. This is easy to do. Just send a note to his former doctor asking for his records to be sent to the new doctor. Physicians will do this as a service to all patients. Most states require doctors to do this. The law says the contents of the records belong to the patient even though the actual records belong to the physician. When you send your request, be sure to sign it. Without a signature, the records can't be sent.

## Physician Extenders

Two relatively new health-care practitioners are seeing more and more children. These are nurse practitioners and physician's assistants—often collectively referred to as *physician extenders*. Nurse practitioners are registered nurses who take one or two years of further training in physical examination, diagnosis, and prescribing medicines. Many work with physicians, although a number practice by themselves. Physician's assistants graduate from a two-year program in which they learn the same skills as the nurse practitioner.

Many physicians employ a physician extender who sees patients in the office. Frequently, they see children for routine health care. They can spend more time talking with you, answering your questions, and teaching you what you need to know. Most often the charge is the same whether you see the physician extender or the doctor.

## Well-Baby Care

During your baby's first three years of life, she will see her doctor a number of times. These visits are important to make sure she is growing and developing appropriately. Her doctor will ask you a number of questions to see how things are going, and he will examine your baby, checking for normal growth and looking for problems. Routine and regular checkups are particularly important for your baby during her first three years of life. Problems found at this age, if not treated early, may have serious implications for her later in life.

The first time your baby's doctor sees her will be within twenty-four hours of her birth. The doctor will do a complete physical examination of the baby and will want to talk to you about your pregnancy, labor, and delivery. If you smoked, took any drugs (prescribed or "recreational"), or drank much alcohol, you need to tell this to the doctor. These factors may affect your baby's health and growth. The doctor will examine your baby daily while she's in the hospital and also talk to you. These visits to you are important. Not only will you find out how your baby is doing, but you will have an opportunity to ask questions. Prepare for these visits— write down your questions ahead of time Your doctor will give you advice on taking care of your new baby, such as feeding instructions and safety ideas.

One of the most important office visits is the first one. Most doctors like to see the new baby when she's two to three weeks old. During her first month, the baby will change a lot. You will have many questions and concerns about your new baby, and this visit gives you the opportunity to ask them.

Your doctor's staff will probably ask you some questions before you see the doctor. How is the baby feeding? Is she sleeping well? Are there any problems with her bowels? Are there any skin problems? These are just a few of the questions you may be asked. They will also measure the baby's weight, head circumference (the distance around her head), and body length. These measurements are important for monitoring your baby's growth. Each will be plotted on a growth chart. These charts are the best way to determine if your baby is growing well.

When you see the doctor, he will go over all this information and ask more questions if needed. Next comes the examination of your baby. Your baby should be completely undressed for this examination. The doctor will begin the examination at the top of her head and go to the tips of her toes, examining everything in between.

After examining your baby, he'll tell you his findings and if there are any problems. Rarely are there any surprises found at this visit, although occasionally a congenital abnormality (a birth defect) is found that was not apparent when the baby was in the hospital. At this age, no immunizations are given.

## Regular Office Visits

Doctors like to see infants at regular intervals to monitor their growth, development, and health. These visits are important because if any health problem is developing, it's best to find it early and treat it appropriately. Although your doctor may have a slightly different schedule of visits, most infants are seen when they are two, four, six, nine, twelve, fifteen, eighteen, twenty-four, thirty, and thirty-six months old.

At each visit, your doctor will examine your undressed baby completely. He will ask you questions about your baby's behavior and develop-

ment. He'll be looking for certain developmental milestones—things babies are usually doing at certain ages. These milestones are only guidelines, but if a baby consistently fails to reach them by certain ages, further investigation needs to be done.

## Immunizations

An important part of most well-baby visits is immunizations. They are designed to lessen the chances that your baby will come down with certain diseases. There was a time, not too long ago, when many infants died of infections. Now we can prevent many of these killers with proper immunizations. It's rare to see a child with polio, diphtheria, or pertussis (whooping cough) these days, although there's been more whooping cough recently since fewer parents are protecting their children. The number of people, both children and adults, who get rubella (German measles) has declined drastically since immunizations became common.

If immunizations are so beneficial, why has there been such an outcry against them recently, particularly the one against pertussis? There has been much publicity about some of the adverse side effects of this vaccine. These side effects may be very serious. They include severe neurologic damage and mental retardation.

There are two important perspectives from which to consider the risks of immunizations: the risk of having the vaccine and the risk of *not* having the vaccine. From the first perspective, we consider the *risk/benefit ratio*—that is, the relationship between the risk of a possible negative outcome and the benefit of the favorable outcome. For example, if one of every 100,000 children given a certain immunization died or suffered a serious side effect, that is certainly one child too many. However, if we consider that 99,999 of the 100,000 children did not die but instead developed immunity to a deadly disease, the *relative risk* for any individual child is very small indeed.

From the second perspective, we consider the *risk of no treatment*—that is, we ask whether the risk of getting the vaccine is greater than the risk of getting the disease. For example, if one of every 100,000 children who get the vaccine suffers a serious side effect, it might seem like an unnecessary risk to take. However, if one hundred of every 100,000 children who do *not* get the vaccine suffer permanent damage or even die because of the disease, then clearly the risk of no treatment is one hundred times greater than the risk of treatment.

The figures used are merely for purposes of illustration, but the principles involved are important considerations when you are deciding whether to have your baby immunized against diseases. The benefits to be reaped from immunization are great, but there is always some degree of risk. Researchers are at work on further reducing the risks involved with some vaccines. Ask your physician her opinion of currently available vaccines.

## Immunization Schedule

Over the years, a commonly accepted immunization schedule has evolved. Most doctors follow it, although there are some acceptable variations. The schedule is designed to give your child the maximum protection available as soon as possible. The reason some shots are not given earlier is that the child's own defense system hasn't matured enough to develop immunity. For example, a number of years ago, the measles-mumps-rubella vaccine was given to infants at twelve months. It was discovered that many of these infants didn't develop protection against these illnesses because their own defense systems weren't able to react to the vaccine correctly. The date was changed, and now the vaccine is much more effective.

## Immunization and Testing Schedule

2 months . . . . . . . . . . . . . . . . . . . . . . DTP and TOPV
4 months . . . . . . . . . . . . . . . . . . . . . . DTP and TOPV
6 months . . . . . . . . . . . . . . . . . . . . . . . . . . . . . . DTP
9–12 months . . . . . . . . . . . . . . . . . . . . . . . . TB test
at least 15 months . . . . . . . . . . . . . . . . . . . . MMR
18 months . . . . . . . . . . . . . . . . . . . . DTP and TOPV
2 years . . . . . . . . . . . . . . . . . . . . . HiB and TB test
4–6 years . . . . . . . . . . . . . . . . . . . DTP and TOPV

**DTP** (diphtheria-tetanus-pertussis vaccine): This immunization is given as a shot, usually in the thigh. Many children have no reaction to it. Some have swelling and redness at the injection site, as well as some fussiness.

**TOPV** (trivalent oral polio vaccine, also called· the Sabin vaccine): Your child is given a small amount of a liquid to swallow. Side effects from this vaccine are very rare.

**MMR** (measles-mumps-rubella vaccine): This vaccine is given as a shot. Your child needs only one shot to have lifelong protection from all three viruses.

**TB test** (tuberculosis test): Some doctors feel that routine tuberculosis testing is necessary and do it on all children. Other doctors feel that this testing is not needed and do it only when they believe the child is at risk of exposure to this disease.

**HiB** (*Hemophilus influenzae* type B vaccine): This relatively new vaccine protects children against developing several types of infections including one type of meningitis (infection of the coverings of the brain and spinal cord). This meningitis is more common in children two to six years old who are exposed to a number of other children, such as in day care centers, or who stay with babysitters who care for four or more children. Although this type of meningitis isn't common, if your two- to six-year-old child is in day care or with a babysitter, you should discuss the HiB vaccine with your doctor.

**Boosters:** After your child has his childhood shots, he's all set unless he is going to travel in certain foreign countries or until he turns twelve. The tetanus shot provides protection for five to ten years.

**Smallpox:** This immunization used to be routine, but it has been discontinued because the risk from the vaccine itself is greater than the risk of getting smallpox. This disease has been almost wiped out worldwide.

## The Next Two Years

As your baby grows, he will not need to be seen routinely as often as when he was an infant. Instead of every three months, most doctors see children once every six months. These visits are for the same reasons as the earlier ones—to make sure your child is growing and developing as he should and to provide you with an opportunity to ask questions. New topics will become important, although many of the old ones, such as behavior and eating, may need to be discussed again.

Your child's doctor will continue to examine your child completely at each visit. These exams may become more difficult as your baby begins to resist, not wanting a stranger to touch him. This reaction is normal as your baby grows and matures.

Doctors expect to see this resistance and actually become a little concerned if it isn't present.

You may wonder how doctors can examine a screaming child and get useful information. Surprisingly, the doctor can usually find out most of what she needs to know. Some decide not to force the issue if the child is getting extremely upset, but a fair amount can be learned from a screaming baby.

As your child grows, more emphasis is put on his behavioral growth and development. Developmental milestones are still very important. Walking, talking, toilet training, and setting limits are some of the topics you should discuss with your doctor. Safety continues to be a concern because accidents are the number one killer of young children.

## The Well-Baby Examination

Your doctor's well-baby examination consists of many different parts, each designed to help her find certain information. You may have to watch closely to see her do each part of the exam because she probably has developed her own tricks and techniques. Some doctors like to have the baby on the examination table; others prefer that a parent hold the baby. Sometimes the doctor will be talking to you while examining your baby.

Here are some of the major areas your doctor will consider and what she looks for in each category:

**General Appearance:** cleanliness, nutrition, alertness

**Skin:** color, rashes, bruises, swelling, condition of hair and nails

**Head:** shape, softness of the anterior fontanel (soft spot)

**Eyes:** redness, good movement, light reflexes (checked with an instrument called an ophthalmoscope, looking for problems with the retina)

**Ears:** irritation or infection of the ear canals or eardrums

**Nose:** congestion, discharge

**Mouth:** gums, tongue, throat, tonsils

**Neck:** swelling of the thyroid or lymph nodes, mobility

**Heart:** rate and rhythm, murmurs

**Lungs:** breathing rate, abnormal noises, air exchange

**Abdomen:** bowel sounds (normal stomach gurglings), enlarged organs or tenderness

**Genitals:** in girls—normal appearance of external genitals, redness; in boys—penis (if circumcised, check that it has healed well; if not, check that foreskin is normal), both testicles are in scrotum

**Arms and Legs:** normal movement and color, absence of swelling and discoloration

**Pulses:** equal femoral pulses (same on both sides)

**Neurologic:** tone, muscle movement and coordination, strength

## Sick-Baby Care

There's nothing scarier for a new parent than a sick baby. Your infant is fussy, is not eating well, and has a fever. Should you take her to the hospital? Should you call your doctor? Or are you overreacting? As a well-informed parent, you want to know what you should do—when to be concerned and when not to worry. You want to know when to call the doctor and what to tell him. That's what this section is all about.

### What You Need to Know

All parents need to learn to tell when their child is sick, when to seek professional help, what to do in emergencies, and how to give medicines. Once you know these facts, you will be able to make the best decisions.

One of the best ways to deal with illness is to be prepared. This includes knowing about common childhood illnesses and emergency measures, as well as having and knowing how to give the appropriate medicines. There are some general steps you should take to prepare yourself for illness or accident:

- Know the telephone numbers of your doctor, the hospital you use, the local poison control center, the fire department, and the ambulance service. These numbers should be posted near the telephone. Make sure your babysitters know where these numbers are located.

- Ask your doctor what he wants you to have on hand for emergencies and treatment of common ailments. Many doctors recommend that you have syrup of ipecac and activated charcoal on hand for poisonings. Some want their patients to keep certain common medicines on hand for late-night illnesses.

- Discuss with your doctor what you should do in an emergency. If your child eats a bottle of pills or drinks a poison, should you call your doctor, the local emergency room, or the poison control center? (Most doctors recommend that you call the poison control center first.) If your child is injured, should you call your doctor first or take your child to the emergency room? Asking these questions before an accident occurs will make things easier for both of you.

- Read about childhood illnesses and accidents. Books like this one will help you be prepared for the inevitable illnesses and injuries that befall all children.

- Take a first-aid course and learn CPR (cardiopulmonary resuscitation) and the Heimlich maneuver (for choking). Be sure the instruction pertains to both children and adults (many courses deal only with adults). Taking a class on these topics is much better than just reading about them. In the classes you have the opportunity to practice these skills on specially constructed models that are very life-like.

- Most important, in an emergency, **DON'T PANIC!** Your calmness is essential if you are going to react properly to the situation and get your child the appropriate care.

## Before You Call the Doctor

From your discussions with your doctor, you will know how she wants to deal with emergencies and after-hours calls. Keep her guidelines in mind when you think about calling her. However, if you are very concerned about your child, then call. Most childhood illnesses can be handled over the phone, and the child won't have to be seen by the doctor until morning.

Before you call your doctor, you need to gather some information and think about what information you want to get from the call. For example, if you feel your child is going to need some medicine, don't wait to call until all the local drugstores are closed. In some communities, it's next to impossible to get any medicines after the pharmacies are closed. It's better to call your doctor earlier rather than later. Also, almost all illnesses seem to get worse as the night progresses, so if your child isn't well at seven o'clock, there's little chance he'll be a lot better by ten o'clock. If you are concerned, call at seven o'clock instead of waiting until ten o'clock. If you really want your child to be seen, tell the doctor right from the beginning. It's helpful for her to know that. She will realize that all the reassurances she can give you over the phone won't help if you really want to have your child examined. However, if you just want some advice over the phone, let her know that also. It will make her job easier.

Be sure your after-hours call is really necessary. Think about what you would do if you didn't have that information until morning. Would that delay change things? Remember that doctors have families and things they like to do besides practice medicine. Out of consideration for them and their families, all nonemergency calls should wait until office hours.

Once you have decided to make the call to your doctor, there's some important information you should have on hand. By preparing for the call, it will be easier for you to let your doctor know exactly what's going on. Here are some questions you should be ready to answer when you call:

- *What are the basic data on your child?* Start with your child's name, when he was last seen by a doctor, and who that was. This will help your doctor place your child. Tell her his age and weight, what medicines he's taking, and what illnesses he's had.

- *What's wrong with your child?* This may sound like a silly question to prepare for, but all too often a parent can't answer it concisely. Think about your child's problem and be prepared to describe exactly what's going on. Things to think about include the following: What is your child eating (solids, liquids, nothing)? Is he urinating a normal amount? Is he having diarrhea? Is he acting normal? If not, what's abnormal about his actions? Is he running a fever? If so, how high is his temperature and what method did you use to take it?

- *What's happened or changed to make you decide to call the doctor now?* This is an important question for you to think about. For example, your child's temperature may have gone up a lot, or he may have suddenly begun to cry and pull at his ear, or he may have just begun to vomit violently. Or perhaps you are just concerned and want some advice. If you decide that nothing has changed or that your questions can wait, the call can probably wait until morning.

- *What do you think is ailing your child?* Often, parents know what's wrong with their child. This is particularly true if their child has had many episodes of the same illness. For example, many parents know when their child is coming down with another ear infection. Or if other members of the family have had a similar illness, there's a good chance your child is getting the same thing. Let the doctor know what you think is going on.

- *Where do you want a prescription filled?* You should decide which drugstore you want to use and make sure it's open and has a pharmacist on duty before you call. Have the phone number ready to give to your doctor.

Doctors who take care of children expect interruptions and emergencies—they go with the age group. Most have no problems with appropriate phone calls at any hour. What irritates even the most caring physician are inappropriate calls and patients who abuse their services.

## Signs and Symptoms

Whenever your child is ill, your observations of what's going on are very important. When you are assessing your child's illness, you're really looking at two different things—signs and symptoms. These terms have specific meanings to your doctor.

A *symptom* is something a patient complains about. A *sign* is something the doctor (or you) can see, measure, feel, hear, taste, or smell. So if your child complains of her ear hurting, that's a symptom; if she's pulling on her ear, that's a sign.

Signs and symptoms are indicators of illness, but they are not illnesses themselves. When your doctor treats your child, he or she may treat the signs and symptoms of the illness, the illness itself, or both. For example, aspirin or acetaminophen is frequently given to a child with a fever; either may

reduce the fever, but neither affects the underlying illness causing the fever. However, an antibiotic given to your child when he has an ear infection actually helps the body fight off the infection and, so, is treating the illness. The earache (a symptom) and the fever (a sign) will go away because the infection (the illness) is being treated.

Most of the medicines you can buy in the drugstore without a prescription treat symptoms but don't treat the illness itself. So the "cold" medicines you may buy for your child don't make the cold go away any more quickly, but they may make your child feel a little better.

There's an ongoing debate about treating signs and symptoms of common illnesses. Some doctors believe that, unless the signs and symptoms are severe, you're better off not treating them. Some of the symptoms of an illness may actually be beneficial and speed recovery (see *Fever*). Every medicine has side effects, and sometimes these can be worse than the illness itself.

## Fever

Fever in a child strikes fear in the hearts of many parents. They wonder if their child will have a seizure and develop epilepsy, or if the temperature will go high enough to "cook" their child's brain and cause permanent damage. You may be concerned about the proper way to treat your child's fever and when you should call your doctor. Fever is perhaps the most misunderstood sign in all of medicine. It's the body's normal response to infection.

Everyone has an "internal thermostat" that controls his body temperature. When an infection is present, certain chemicals are released in the body that "reset" the thermostat to a higher setting. This helps to explain the chills your child may experience when his temperature is going up. He feels cold because his body wants to be at a higher temperature. Once his fever breaks, he feels hot because his body wants to be at a lower temperature. The breaking of the fever means that his internal thermostat has been turned down to normal.

Understanding how a fever occurs helps you know how to treat the chills and sweats that often accompany an illness. When your child has the chills, it's best to add some blankets until he feels comfortable. Similarly, when he begins to sweat and feels warm, you should take off clothes or

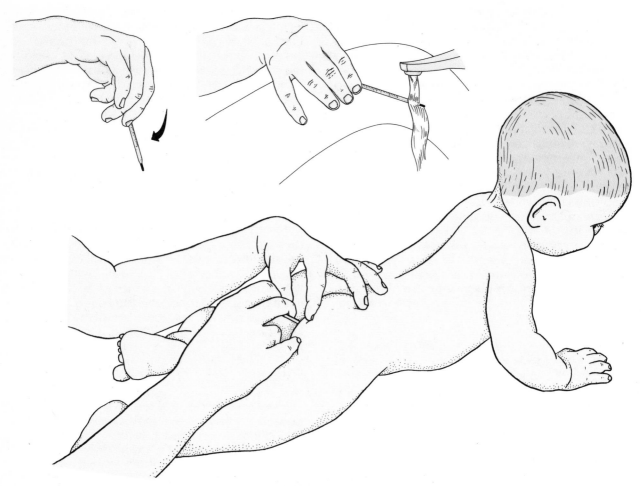

*Be sure to shake down the thermometer before each use. Separate the baby's buttocks and gently insert the thermometer. Thoroughly wash and dry the thermometer after each usage.*

blankets. Bundling him up when he feels warm is defeating what his body is trying to do.

## Taking a Temperature

It's often helpful to know your child's temperature. It is sometimes an indicator of the seriousness of the illness, although this isn't always true. A normal oral temperature is 98.6 degrees Fahrenheit. A rectal temperature is one degree higher; an axillary (armpit) temperature is one degree lower. "Normal" means average—some people run a slightly higher or lower temperature, and that is "normal" for them. Temperature also varies throughout the day; a person's temperature is usually a little higher in the afternoon and evening.

The most accurate way to take the temperature of a young child is rectally. Any thermometer

will do, although one designed for rectal use is shaped a little differently so it will go in more easily. If your child can't keep a thermometer under her tongue and can't keep her mouth closed for three minutes, it's more accurate to use a rectal thermometer.

When you are taking your child's temperature with a rectal thermometer, it's easiest if you lay your child on her stomach. Shake down the thermometer to 96 degrees or lower and lubricate it with some petroleum jelly. After separating her buttocks with the thumb and first finger of one hand, gently insert the thermometer to a depth of about one inch. Then pinch closed her buttocks. Hold the thermometer in place for three minutes to be sure you get an accurate reading.

Taking the oral temperature of a young child may be difficult. After shaking down the thermometer, put it under her tongue. She should close her mouth around the thermometer and keep her mouth shut for three minutes. Be sure she hasn't drunk anything cold within fifteen to thirty minutes before you take her temperature (if she has, the reading will be artificially low).

Axillary temperatures are not very accurate. The same applies to the temperatures taken with strips that are held against a child's forehead.

The new electronic thermometers are accurate and much easier to use than the older, glass ones. They are quicker and easier to read, and they signal you when they have reached their final reading.

### How Important Is a Fever?

Many childhood illnesses cause a fever. Most of these illnesses are caused by viruses. Unfortunately, viruses don't respond to antibiotics. There's nothing medicine has to offer to treat the vast majority of viral illnesses except symptomatic relief.

Young children are smarter than adults in many ways. One is the way they respond to illness. When they are sick, they look and act sick. They don't try to hide their illness. The way your child looks and acts is a much more accurate reflection of the seriousness of his illness than his temperature. Don't panic just because your child has a fever—see how he is acting. You should call the doctor if a child under six months old has a temperature over 101 degrees. For an older child, you should call the doctor if his temperature is over 103 degrees or if he has a temperature of 101 degrees or greater for forty-eight hours. But more important than his temperature is how he looks and acts.

### Treating a Fever

If your child's temperature is high enough to treat, or if his fever seems to be bothering him, you should go ahead and treat it. Acetaminophen is the best drug to use. Giving aspirin to a child with a viral disease has been associated with a very serious illness called Reye's syndrome. So it's best to avoid giving aspirin to young children with a fever.

Acetaminophen is sold under many different names. It also comes in different forms—liquid, syrup, and chewable tablets. Most drug doses are calculated according to the weight of the child. Your child should get between five and ten milli-

grams of acetaminophen for each kilogram (2.2 pounds) of body weight. It should be given every four to six hours. Average doses are as follows:

| | |
|---|---|
| 1–2 years old | 120 milligrams per dose |
| 2–3 years old | 160 milligrams per dose |
| 4–5 years old | 240 milligrams per dose |
| 6–8 years old | 320 milligrams per dose |
| 9–10 years old | 400 milligrams per dose |
| 11–12 years old | 480 milligrams per dose |

If you have any questions about the doses, check with your doctor or pharmacist.

Parents wonder whether they should bathe their child to bring down his temperature. Many doctors now feel that this treatment is never needed. Others may advise sponge baths if your child's fever is very high. Check with your child's doctor for her preferences. If you do sponge bathe your child, be sure to use tepid water (about 96 degrees Fahrenheit). Bathe him for no longer than fifteen to twenty minutes and no more frequently than every two hours.

Cooling by bathing lasts only for a short time. If acetaminophen isn't given in conjunction with bathing, your child's temperature will bounce right back up once he dries off. Do not use rubbing alcohol—it may actually cause more problems. Inhaled fumes may cause some damage.

### Febrile Seizures

There's nothing scarier than to see your child have a seizure. Three to five percent of all children have one at some time. Febrile seizures do not cause epilepsy or any other long-term problems.

No one knows why a fever causes certain children to have a seizure. How high your child's temperature goes seems not to be the important factor. Some children will have a seizure at 102 or 103 degrees, while others don't have seizures with a temperature of 106. It may be that the rate of rise and fall of your child's temperature is more important than how high the fever is.

If your child is having a seizure, he may first stiffen and his eyes may "roll back" in his head. His fists may clench, his elbows and knees may bend, his arms and legs may shake, and his jaws may clamp shut tightly. He may drool, hold his breath, and even turn a little blue. Frequently, a child having a seizure will lose control of his bladder and bowels. Febrile seizures last only a few minutes.

Your child may be very tired or even sleep afterward.

The most important thing to remember if your child has a febrile seizure is not to panic. You must make sure he doesn't hurt himself by hitting a hard object or falling. Don't try to pry open his jaws if they are clamped tightly shut. Turn him on his side so his saliva will drain out.

Once the seizure is finished, call his doctor right away. Although the usual cause of febrile seizures is easy to find and not a very serious illness, sometimes this isn't so. Your child needs to be evaluated by a doctor to find the source of the fever. Many children who have a febrile seizure are not admitted to the hospital.

## Infections

Infections are classified and treated according to the kind of microorganism (a living organism so small that it is invisible to the naked eye) that causes them. Infections caused by protozoa (one-celled animals) and fungi (simple plant-like organisms) are relatively uncommon in the United States, and medications are generally available to treat them once the type of infection has been identified. Viruses and bacteria are the two most common types of "germs" that cause infections.

Bacteria are one-celled microscopic organisms. They normally exist in the body by the billions. Most are harmless; in fact, some even perform useful functions, like those that normally live in the intestines and help digest food. Other bacteria cause diseases, such as diphtheria and scarlet fever. Fortunately, some bacterial diseases can be prevented by vaccination, and bacterial infections are frequently curable by drugs called antibiotics.

Viruses, the smallest known microorganisms, are responsible for diseases as prevalent and relatively harmless as the common cold and as serious as meningitis. Although there are vaccines to protect against some viral diseases (such as polio, measles, rubella, mumps, and some strains of influenza), there is as yet no medical treatment available for most viral infections. The difficulty with developing antiviral agents is that, because a virus lives and reproduces only within living cells, any treatment designed to kill the virus is also likely to harm cells. Furthermore, there are thousands of different viruses, each with different properties; an agent effective against one virus probably will not affect the others. Until effective antiviral agents are developed, viruses will continue to be responsible for most infectious illnesses.

Sometimes it's difficult to know whether a virus or a bacterium is causing an infection. Both may cause the same symptoms and may infect the same places. For example, pneumonia or a sore throat may be either bacterial or viral in origin. To make matters more confusing, sometimes both kinds of infection are present at the same time. Since, in general, bacterial infections can be treated and viral infections cannot, your physician may want to wait for the results of a culture (a technique for taking a sample from an infected area and encouraging the microorganisms in the sample to grow in the laboratory, so that they can be identified) before prescribing medication. Physicians don't like to prescribe antibiotics unless they are sure that an infection is bacterial because improper use of an antibiotic can lead to loss of its effectiveness due to the development (and possible spread) of antibiotic-resistant strains of the infecting bacteria. Also, the more often an antibiotic is used, the greater is the risk of developing an allergic reaction to it.

If a viral infection is identified, the treatment is generally only supportive, with the aim of preventing deterioration of the patient's general condition and making him as comfortable as possible until the infection has run its course. Antibiotics do not attack viruses, and although a few antiviral agents are available to combat specific infections, none is effective against the wide range of viruses involved in the most common viral illnesses. Thus, your doctor is not being difficult or unhelpful when she tells you that there is nothing she can prescribe to cure your child's cold or "flu."

## Coughs and Sneezes

A child with uncontrollable coughing makes a parent feel helpless. A chronic cough causes everyone in the family to lose sleep. And too often it seems that cough medicines just don't do any good.

Coughing is a very important reflex. It's the body's way of clearing dust and mucus from the airways. If we don't cough, or if we take medicines that suppress coughing, there's an increased risk of getting pneumonia. All the mucus, bacteria, and other material will remain in our lungs, forming a perfect place for an infection to start.

A sneeze clears out dust and other particles that may irritate the sensitive lining of the nose and sinuses. Like coughing, sneezing is a reflex that can't be controlled.

When your child coughs, she is clearing her lungs. The material she brings up has to go somewhere. Usually the coughing itself will bring the material up as far as where the trachea (the tube that carries air to the lungs) and the esophagus (the tube that carries food to the stomach) separate. If she can't spit out the mucus (which most children can't do), she will either swallow it or, more likely, gag on it. This explains why children will sometimes vomit after a coughing spell. Since they can't get rid of the mucus, they gag and vomit it out. Unfortunately, they usually vomit a lot more than just the mucus. Vomiting after coughing is not abnormal and should not cause you concern.

There are many cough medicines available in the drugstore. Some can be bought without a prescription, but the stronger ones require the approval of a doctor. There are two major drugs that effectively suppress coughing. One is dextromethorphan—the over-the-counter cough medicines that end with the letters "DM" contain dextromethorphan. The other effective cough suppressant is codeine. Cough medicines that contain codeine or one of its derivatives usually require a prescription.

You may wonder when you should try to suppress your child's cough. There are only two situations. The first is when her cough is "dry and hacking." Because it's not bringing up anything and not helping to clear out her lungs, this type of cough serves no useful purpose. The second is when the cough is so severe that it interferes with her sleep. Otherwise, it's better that she cough.

A chronic cough may be a sign of "low-grade" asthma. If your child coughs without any sign of illness and if there's a family history of allergies or asthma, it's worthwhile to discuss this with your doctor.

Coughing may last for a long time after a viral illness (sometimes up to three months) and still not necessarily be a cause for concern. If your child is acting normal and doing all the "normal kid things," you probably don't need to worry. However, if your child shows other symptoms in conjunction with coughing or just doesn't seem to be "bouncing back" to normal, it's a good idea to check with her doctor.

Remember that coughing is a sign, not an illness itself. Curing a cough alone doesn't mean that you have dealt with the underlying illness.

## Common Childhood Medical Problems

### Anemia

Anemia is not usually thought of as a childhood disease. It's something Grandma has, not your new baby. Unfortunately, this isn't true.

There are several causes of anemia. Young infants two to three months old are prone to becoming anemic because the iron they stored while in the uterus has been used up to make new red blood cells. If a child's diet does not provide him with enough iron, his body can't continue to make the red blood cells he needs. That's the most common cause. A baby may become anemic if he is bleeding internally and losing more blood than his body can make. Or his bone marrow, where the red blood cells are made, may not be functioning properly. Certain vitamin deficiencies, lead poisoning, and sickle cell disease can also cause anemia.

Usually there are no signs or symptoms when a baby is anemic. In extreme cases he may look very pale, act very tired, be short of breath, and have an abnormally fast heart rate—greater than 120 beats per minute. (Babies normally have a heart rate much faster than an adult's. The normal range for babies is 100–120 beats per minute; for adults, 60–80 beats per minute.) The best places to look for paleness are his nail beds; you might also try looking at the underside of his eyelids (carefully), and the inside of his mouth.

To determine if your infant is anemic, your doctor may perform a hematocrit, a simple test that measures the percentage of red blood cells. The test requires very little blood; generally, enough can be obtained just by sticking your baby's finger or heel. The test is done in the doctor's office, and the results are available in a few minutes. If anemia is found, your doctor may order other tests to determine why your child is anemic.

The most common cause of anemia in children is inadequate intake of iron. Your doctor may prescribe an iron supplement, additional vitamins, dietary changes, or, on rare occasions, a transfusion.

Don't give your baby more iron than your doctor recommends, though. Giving your child too much iron may cause problems; iron overdosing is one of the more common causes of poisoning among children in this country. Don't give your child an iron supplement (other than iron-fortified formula or cereal) without checking with your doctor.

## Asthma

Asthma is one of the scariest illnesses a child can have. Asthmatics may become extremely short of breath, often very suddenly. They are unable to get enough air into their lungs. Often an allergic reaction will start an episode, although many other factors may set off an attack. These include infection, physical and emotional stress, irritants in the air, and sudden changes in air temperature.

When a child has an asthma attack, the small muscles of his tracheobronchial tree (the system of tubes that carry air into and out of the lungs) tighten and narrow the diameter of these tubes. These passageways also fill up with thick mucus, which is very hard to cough up.

Asthma often runs in families. Although not everyone in the family will have asthma, many family members may have other allergy problems.

The most common and well-known symptom of asthma is wheezing. It is characterized by a high-pitched, whistling sound heard more when the child is breathing out than in. Asthma is marked by difficulty in getting air out. A saying in medicine goes, "Not everything that wheezes is asthma, and not every asthmatic wheezes." Doctors are finding that many children with mild cases of asthma rarely or never wheeze, but do have a chronic cough, shortness of breath, or raspy, rattly breathing.

The first time a child has an asthma attack, he needs medical help quickly. Either call your doctor or take your child to the emergency room. Prompt treatment is important. Depending on the severity of the attack, your child may need shots, intravenous medication, or even hospitalization. But this need not happen every time he has an attack.

Education is the key to controlling asthma. Self-care is essential to keep your child breathing clearly and to minimize hospitalizations. There are many different types of medicines used to control asthma. Once your child's first attack has been controlled, he may be given one or more asthma medicines. These include bronchodilators (aminophylline in its many forms and adrenergic drugs), inhalers, steroids, antibiotics, and others. You, your doctor, and your child (if old enough to understand) should discuss your child's asthma treatment together. You should try to identify your child's symptoms early. You and your doctor should make a treatment plan for even mild attacks, so you know what to do at home. By starting treatment early, you can control the wheezing and keep your child out of the hospital.

If an allergy is a contributing factor, consulting an allergist may be beneficial. If you know what your child is allergic to, removing those substances from his environment will lessen the probability that he will have an asthma attack.

## Birthmarks

More than half of all newborns have some type of birthmark. The most common skin blemishes are red, flat areas on the forehead, upper eyelids, upper lip, or back of the scalp and neck. These are often called "stork bites." They are not caused by trauma during birth. Although they may be extensive, they usually disappear during the baby's first year of life.

"Mongolian spots" are blue-black discolorations on the lower part of the back and the buttocks of newborns. They look like large bruises. They gradually disappear and are almost always gone by adolescence.

Strawberry hemangiomas affect ten percent of all babies. They are usually not present at birth, but appear during the first few months of life. They are red, are usually raised, and may be up to two inches across. They continue to increase in size, perhaps for a few years, and then gradually shrink and disappear by age five or six. They are an accumulation of blood vessels lying just beneath the skin. If the overlying skin is broken, they may become infected. Except for infection, they rarely require any treatment. It's generally best to leave them alone; in rare cases, surgery may be needed.

Port-wine stains are smooth, flat, and purplish. They often are quite large and may be anywhere on the body. Unfortunately, these birthmarks don't fade. Currently, there is no effective treatment for them in children younger than twelve years of age, but laser treatment is often possible in older patients.

The most common type of birthmark found in children and adults, the common mole, is not often seen in newborns. Moles tend to develop as your child grows. Most children will have ten to fifteen moles by adolescence.

## Bites

Any bite, be it animal or human, has the potential for causing serious problems. A bite may scratch, crush, cut, or puncture the skin. The bacteria that normally live in the mouth of the biter may cause an infection. Cat and human bites are the most likely to become infected. Dog bites, because of the strength of the animal's jaws, often cause crush injuries to the skin and underlying structures.

Usually, it's pretty obvious when your child has been bitten. It may be difficult to tell a claw wound from a bite; both should be treated the same. When a child bites another child, you will often see small black-and-blue areas where blood vessels broke from the pressure of the bite and bleeding occurred in the skin.

First aid is the best treatment for bites. Scrub the wound well with warm, soapy water for five to ten minutes. Then flush the wound with a large amount of warm water. Local antiseptics may be helpful, but avoid anything that stings. You must watch closely for signs of infection—redness, red streaking, pus or drainage from the wound, swelling, or increasing tenderness. If any of these signs occurs, call your doctor.

If the wound is large or deep, if it's on your child's face, or if the bleeding won't stop, call your doctor. He will want to see your child.

There's a high probability that the bite will become infected. Deep puncture wounds are particularly likely to become infected because the bacteria are forced deep into the tissue. For this reason, some doctors prescribe antibiotics right away.

Bites are one type of wound doctors frequently don't suture closed. By closing the wound, the chances of infection are increased. If the bite is on your chid's face and will leave a scar without stitches, the doctor may decide to close it.

Tetanus (lockjaw) is a serious infection that may result from an animal bite. It's caused by a bacterium that lives in soil, dust, and the intestines and intestinal wastes of animals and humans. It enters the body through a scratch, cut, or puncture wound. The DPT immunization contains an effective and safe vaccine against tetanus. If your child's tetanus shots are not up-to-date, a booster will be given.

Rabies is a serious infection that attacks the central nervous system. It's caused by a virus that's transmitted in the saliva of rabid animals, such as skunks, foxes, cattle, dogs, bats, cats, and raccoons. The decision to use anti-rabies vaccine is difficult. There are very few cases of rabies in this country, and the older vaccine caused many side effects. Newer vaccines that have fewer side effects are becoming available.

If the biting animal was a pet, try to determine when it had its shots. Don't try to catch the animal yourself, particularly if it's a wild one. Call the local authorities for assistance; the animal needs to be observed.

## Blocked Tear Ducts

Tears form in the tear glands above the eyeballs. Tears are continually produced and flow across the eyeballs and down slender ducts that connect each eye to the nose (nasolacrimal ducts). The two openings into each tear duct are pinpoint in size and can be seen at the edge of the upper and lower eyelids, near the corner of the eye next to the nose. (The existence of these ducts explains why someone who is starting to cry first has the sniffles—the tears from crying run into the nose. When the tear ducts no longer can handle the extra tears, they overflow.)

If the nasolacrimal ducts or the openings near the eyes are blocked, the tears can't flow through them. The normal tears in your child's eyes will back up and flow out the outer corners of his eyes, even when he isn't crying. Blocked openings and ducts may lead to eye infections.

If there's just excess tearing, you don't need to be concerned. Sometimes the blockage clears itself. If there are any signs of infection (pus, redness, or swelling), contact your doctor. Sometimes antibiotics are needed.

The best treatment is opening the blocked ducts. Massaging a blocked duct is often successful. Your doctor will show you this technique. If this, and time, don't work, surgery may be needed.

## Bowlegs and Knock-knees

During the time your baby spends in the uterus, his legs are curled up against his body. The first time he gets to fully stretch them is after birth. As part of his normal development, his legs "unwind." As this unwinding occurs, he will go through times when he looks bowlegged and other times when he's knock-kneed. When they first walk, most infants are very bowlegged. Usually their legs straighten out by the time they turn two years old.

The most frequent cause of true bowlegs and knock-knees used to be rickets, caused by a vitamin D deficiency. Rickets is rare today in this country. Vitamin D-enriched formula, milk, and foods have all but eliminated this once-common disease.

## Bronchitis

Bronchitis is an infection of the bronchial tubes (the air passages from the trachea [windpipe] to the lungs). It doesn't affect the lungs, although it may progress to pneumonia. It usually starts with the signs and symptoms of a cold—runny nose, cough, sneezing, and scratchy throat. Sometimes bronchitis begins without any of these preceding symptoms and signs.

Most cases of bronchitis are caused by a virus, so antibiotics don't help. If a child has asthma or other respiratory problems, she is more likely to get bronchitis.

A child with bronchitis usually has a low-grade fever, although her temperature may be normal. A dry, hacking cough and a feeling of tightness in the chest are common. She feels sick and weak, and may lose her appetite. After a few days, her cough will loosen and her breathing may become a little noisier. She has no serious problems breathing. These symptoms and signs usually resolve in a week.

The treatment of bronchitis is aimed at making your child more comfortable. If the fever bothers her, acetaminophen may be given. She should rest and drink a lot of fluids. If a child doesn't want to rest, it's next to impossible to keep her down. There's no need to keep her any quieter than she wants to be, but don't encourage vigorous activity.

Some children find that a vaporizer helps, although its value has never been proved medically. If your child feels better with a vaporizer running, there's no harm in it. If you do decide to use a vaporizer, be sure to keep it very clean. Unless vaporizers are kept clean, they can actually spread infection.

If her symptoms get worse—if her fever goes up, if she becomes extremely sluggish, if there's blood in her sputum, or if the symptoms don't begin to go away in a week—then she needs to be seen by a doctor.

## Bruises

Once your baby starts to toddle, he's bound to get many bruises on his arms and legs. A bruise is made of blood that has escaped from capillaries (tiny blood vessels) or larger vessels and seeped into the skin. The color of the bruise depends on how much blood escaped, how deep in the skin the bleeding was, and how long ago it occurred. The size of the bruise varies according to the same factors. A new bruise is usually black and blue. As it goes away, it often turns a dark yellow. A bruise of the eyeball is always bloodred.

A very deep bruise, such as from tearing a ligament or breaking a bone, may take a few days to come to the surface. Blood that has escaped from a broken blood vessel may travel and appear somewhere other than where it leaked. For example, a bruise on the forehead may cause a black eye, even though the eye wasn't hit.

The most common cause of bruising is falling or being hit. Most active children have a few bruises at all times. Children with fair complexions bruise more easily, and their bruises take longer to clear.

Sometimes a bruise appears, and there is no history of injury. These bruises, called spontaneous bruises, may be cause for concern. They appear in areas that are not likely to be hit when your child plays or falls. The first sign of certain diseases may be spontaneous bruises. These need to be seen by a doctor.

*Petechiae* are a special type of bruise. They are very small—pinhead-size to one-eighth inch in size. They are dark red or maroon and often appear in great numbers. Forceful vomiting or coughing may cause tiny capillaries to break and petechiae to appear. They are usually found on the head and neck. If they appear without any

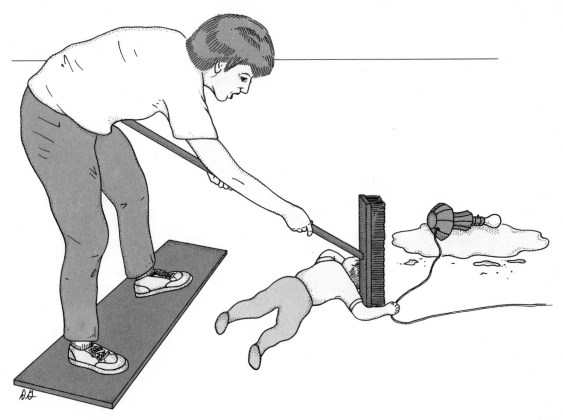

*Carefully use a nonconducting implement to separate the child from the electrical cord. Then seek immediate medical attention—**any** electrical burn needs to be seen by a doctor.*

known cause, or if your child also has a fever or extreme exhaustion, he needs to be seen by his doctor quickly.

When your child falls hard enough to cause bruising, applying cold compresses to the injured area will lessen the chance that a bruise will develop. The cold causes the blood vessels in the area to constrict, lessening the amount of bleeding. Apply the cold compresses every three to four hours while your child is awake for approximately twenty-four hours. (It takes about twenty-four hours for the blood vessels to stop leaking.) Then switch to warm compresses. Warm compresses help speed up the removal of the blood that has leaked out of the vessels into the skin.

## Burns

Burns are skin injuries caused by too much heat, certain chemicals (acids and alkalis), and electricity. The seriousness depends on the size, depth, and location of the burn. Burns are classi-fied into three categories: first degree (the least serious), second degree, and third degree (the most serious).

First-degree burns cause reddening of the skin and pain. They may blister after a few days. A sunburn is a good example of a first-degree burn. A second-degree burn reddens and blisters immediately. Third-degree burns are the deepest. Your child may not complain of any pain with a third-degree burn because it's so deep that the nerve endings have been destroyed. The skin will blister, char, or look "dead white." Usually a third-degree burn has some areas of first- and second-degree.

To lessen the damage a burn causes your child, you must know what to do and do it quickly. The first step is to get your child away from whatever is burning her. Be careful to do this without burning or electrocuting yourself. The next step is to wash off, with cool water, the burned area. If it's a large area, wrap it with wet, cool, clean cloths. Keep the coolness on the burned area for thirty minutes or until the pain lessens.

Second- and third-degree burns should be seen by a doctor. A person with severe burns may go into shock, a serious and life-threatening condition that requires *immediate* medical care and hospitalization. Burns on your child's face, hands, feet, genitals, and joint areas also need medical attention because they may leave scars that cause deformities and problems with function.

Any second- or third-degree burn is likely to get infected, so your doctor may want to prescribe an antibacterial. Tetanus is another complication of second- and third-degree burns. If your child's tetanus immunization is not up-to-date, she may need a booster.

Electrical burns cause special problems. The most common childhood electrical burn happens when a toddler chews or bites on an electrical cord. Frequently, there is only a small burn visible in the corner of her mouth. But the electricity goes deep into the skin and muscle, so she may have severely damaged tissues and muscle that you can't see. If nothing is done, the deeper tissue will die, causing serious problems. Any electrical burn needs to be seen by a doctor.

First-degree burns may be treated at home. Cover the burn with sterile, "nonstick" dressings to keep them clean. **Don't** put mud, butter, or any-

thing else on the burn without checking with your doctor. Silver sulfadiazine is the best salve for burns. It's available only by prescription. Your doctor may call your pharmacy and prescribe it without seeing your child. If a blister forms, it shouldn't be broken. Change the dressing every twenty-four to forty-eight hours, and keep the burn covered until it has completely healed. (See "Safety at Home" elsewhere in this chapter for important guidelines for burn prevention.)

## Canker Sores

Canker sores are small sores (called ulcers) found in the mouth and on the inside of the lips. Rarely is a fever or swelling of the lymph nodes in the neck present. The cause of these very painful ulcers isn't known. Canker sores, medically referred to as recurrent aphthous stomatitis, are commonly misdiagnosed as a herpes infection.

The biggest problem with canker sores is the pain, which may be so severe that your child will refuse to eat. Nothing helps the sores heal, although steroid creams and special mouthwashes may lessen the discomfort. These drugs require a doctor's prescription.

Changes in your child's diet may help lessen the pain. A bland diet, avoiding salty or acid foods, is helpful. A numbing agent may be used, although your child must be old enough to spit to avoid swallowing too much of the drug. Switching from a bottle to a cup may help. Acetaminophen often helps, although some children need a codeine preparation.

Canker sores last one to two weeks. Unfortunately, they tend to recur.

## Chicken Pox

Chicken pox is a common childhood viral infection. It's spread in the air from child to child. Symptoms appear twelve to twenty-one days after exposure to the virus. Most children develop immunity after having the disease; they generally won't get it again. Currently, no vaccine is available to prevent chicken pox, although one is being developed.

Chicken pox may begin with the signs and symptoms of a mild cold, although frequently the rash is the first sign. Each spot first looks like an insect bite. Within a few hours, the spot develops a

---

**Burns**

**Symptoms**

- Pain

- Redness

- Blistering

**Treatment**

- Get the hot substance off your child's skin.

- Apply cool compresses to the burned area immediately.

- For chemical burns, place the affected part under cool running water immediately.

- If blisters, charring of the skin, or dead white skin is present, **seek medical care.**

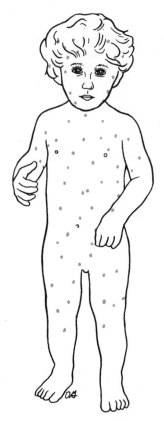

*The first symptom of chicken pox is an itchy rash that begins as small red spots on the trunk. Within hours, the spots begin spreading out from the trunk to the face, scalp, arms, and legs.*

small blister in the center. The blister eventually breaks, and a brown scab forms. The rash usually first appears on a child's trunk and moves outward. She may be getting new lesions on her arms and legs as those on her stomach and back are healing. The rash may appear anywhere—even in the mouth and on the genitals, anus, and eyelids.

The rash worsens for three or four days and then begins to go away. It may take another three or four days for the rash to heal. Your child may have no fever, or she may have a temperature. If the fever bothers her, you may give her acetaminophen, but not aspirin. A number of children have come down with Reye's syndrome, a very serious illness, after taking aspirin during a bout of chicken pox.

The rash is often extremely itchy. Even though it's difficult to prevent your child from scratching the pocks, try to stop her. Too much scratching may lead to local skin infections and permanent scarring. (It's also a good idea to cut her nails and

have her wear mittens and knee socks.) There are many nonprescription anti-itch medicines available. Don't use any that contain steroids or calamine with phenol. Your doctor or pharmacist will help you select the best medicines.

Your child is contagious from twenty-four hours before the rash appears until all the sores have scabbed over. During this period she should be kept away from anyone taking steroid medicines or immunosuppressant drugs, as well as children with immune mechanism deficiencies.

There are some rare complications from chicken pox. If your child has a high fever with headache, vomiting, and convulsions or prostration (extreme exhaustion), she may have chicken pox encephalitis (inflammation of the brain). She should be seen by her doctor right away. Also, if your child's fever is very high or if her symptoms seem to be getting worse instead of improving, contact her doctor.

If some of your child's pocks look infected, with pus and more redness than other pocks show, she may need antibiotics. The lymph nodes in the neck, armpits, groin, and back of her scalp may become very swollen and infected. If they are red and very tender, you should let her doctor know. Antibiotics may control these infections, but such drugs don't change the course of the chicken pox itself. Antibiotics don't do anything for viral illnesses.

## Choking

Choking is one of the few childhood emergencies in which your quick action may save your child's life.

Choking occurs when something in a child's mouth "goes down the wrong hole"—that is, it goes down the trachea (windpipe) rather than the esophagus (the food tube that connects the mouth to the stomach). If the trachea is blocked, air can't get into the lungs. A choking child will usually cough and try to spit out whatever he swallowed. If he can't, there will be only a few minutes before irreversible brain damage from lack of oxygen occurs.

The best treatment for choking is prevention and preparation. Prevention of choking demands that you always be aware that very young children explore with their mouths and will try to put almost anything in them. Make sure you keep any small objects out of the reach of young children. Don't let your child play with coins, loose keys, and other small things. Don't feed him small foods like peanuts, popcorn, pieces of hot dogs, ice cubes, and hard candies. Check his toys for loose parts that he may pull off and swallow, and don't let him play with very small toys. Also remember that sometimes a vomiting child will choke on his vomitus; that's why it's best to put your baby on his side when he's vomiting.

You can tell when your child is choking because he won't be able to talk or cry and he will be frantically trying to breathe. A choking child quickly becomes blue, limp, and unconscious. He may have a seizure.

Rarely does a choking child reach a doctor, hospital, or other help in time. That is why preparation for choking emergencies is so important. Your preparation for emergencies should include a first-aid course that teaches the Heimlich maneuver. This maneuver has been shown to be the best way to deal with choking. Although it is described below, it's much better to learn it in a class.

If your child is unable to breathe, you should call for some help right away. A second person can call for additional help (police, fire department, ambulance) while you deal with your child. Give your child thirty to sixty seconds to clear the obstruction on his own. If he can't get the object out, try the Heimlich maneuver (for a toddler or child) or a combination of back-blows and chest-presses (for an infant).

## Choking

### Symptoms

- Inability to breathe, speak, or cry

- Blueness of skin

### Treatment

- If you suspect your child is choking, call for help **IMMEDIATELY.**

- Give your child one minute to cough up the object.

continued

## continued

- If your child can't get the object out himself after one minute, perform the Heimlich maneuver or Back-blows/Chest-presses.

- **Don't** use mouth-to-mouth resuscitation until the object is out.

- **Don't** try to get the object out with your fingers unless *all* other attempts have failed.

## Heimlich Maneuver

1. Stand behind your child.

2. Reach around him with your arms, lock your hands together, and place them just below his breastbone.

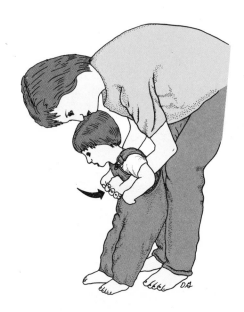

3. Then use a quick, upward motion while pulling his stomach in. You are trying to quickly squeeze the upper part of the abdomen and the lower part of the chest. This will swiftly force up the diaphragm (the large, flat muscle that separates the chest from the abdomen) so that air will be pushed out of the lungs. Ideally, the rush of air will pop the object out of the airway. Most often, trying to grab an object only pushes it in farther.

Mouth-to-mouth resuscitation is only effective if the airway is at least partially clear. If the object is still in place, you may actually force it farther down. Once the object has been removed, mouth-to-mouth resuscitation is appropriate if your child isn't breathing (for more information on mouth-to-mouth resuscitation, see *Drowning*, page 229).

### Back-blows/Chest-presses

When a baby is choking:

1. Lay the baby face down on your forearm, with your hand supporting his head. The baby's head should be lower than his chest.

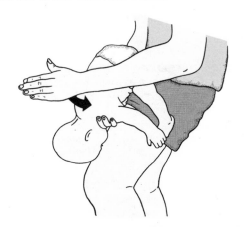

2. Using the heel of your hand, give four quick blows to the baby's back between the shoulder blades.

3. Turn the baby over. Place your free hand on the back of his head and hold him between your forearms. Turn him face up, with his head still lower than his body.

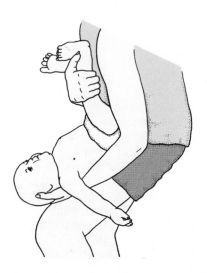

4. Put two fingertips on the baby's chest between the nipples. Press quickly and fairly hard four times.

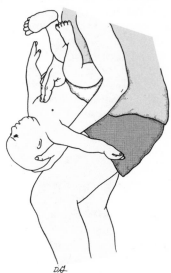

5. Repeat the cycle of four blows and four presses for as long as the baby is still choking. *Don't give up.*

6. If breathing stops, begin mouth-to-mouth resuscitation (once the airway is clear). See *Drowning*, page 229.

## Circumcision

Circumcision is the surgical removal of the foreskin of the penis (the piece of skin that covers the tip of the penis). For centuries, several religions have required circumcision. In this country most male infants are circumcised, although in many other developed countries circumcision is not common.

Many doctors now feel that circumcision rarely needs to be done for medical reasons. In rare cases, boys are born with a very small opening or no opening in the foreskin, which interferes with the passage of urine. Circumcision is therefore the curative procedure. Some people believe circumcision makes it easier to keep the penis clean. Smegma (a waxy material) forms under the foreskin and needs to be removed. Circumcision may make this easier.

Circumcision is a surgical procedure, and there is a slight chance of complications. The most common is bleeding (in about one percent of cases). On rare occasions, accidental injury to the penis occurs.

If your son has been circumcised, keep the area covered with petroleum jelly on gauze, as was done in the hospital. His penis shouldn't be submerged in water until it has healed completely. Keep the area clean, and wash it gently after each dirty diaper. If there's any bleeding (more than a few drops), you should call his doctor. If any signs of infection (pus, redness, or swelling) appear, call his doctor right away. Infection can be a serious problem if not treated immediately.

## Colic

Colic means different things to different people, physicians and laymen alike. The main characteristic is crying—not just short periods of fussiness that can be stopped by changing or feeding or cuddling—but long periods of full-blown wails of misery that defy all attempts to stop them. These bouts of crying can last for hours and often occur as if on schedule (most often in the late afternoon or early evening). Colic often begins when an infant is two to four weeks old and ends two to three months later. It is a time of great stress for all concerned.

In some babies, the crying spells seem to be related to gastrointestinal discomfort—they pull their legs up toward their chest, their abdomens are distended as if with gas, and they often pass gas. However, other babies seem to have no such digestive symptoms; their crying seems more likely related to general irritability. Both conditions have been called colic, and indeed some babies may have a combination of the two.

Because there is some disagreement about what colic is, it should not be surprising to find that there is controversy about what causes it.

The word "colic" is related to the word "colon" (the large intestine) because for centuries it has been assumed that colic arises from some gastrointestinal disorder. However, studies have shown no correlation between colic and poor weight gain or excessive vomiting, constipation, or diarrhea. Colicky babies are generally quite healthy, with no signs of nutritional problems; in fact, their weight gains are often not only normal but above normal. Nor does the problem appear to be hunger, because the crying spells often begin after a feeding, not before one. It has been suggested that bottle-feeding may be at fault (perhaps because of the assumption that breast-feeding must be better for babies in every way), but one study

showed that breast-fed infants were just as likely to have colic as bottle-fed infants. Lactose intolerance and food sensitivities and allergies have been suggested as causes of colic, but research findings have been inconclusive, and at times contradictory.

Even if those factors could be definitely related to colic, they don't seem to apply to all those infants whose colic appears to be associated with irritability rather than with any digestive distress. It may simply be that some babies, like some adults, have "difficult" temperaments, and are more tense and easily upset. Some physicians believe that transmission of anxiety, anger, or tension from parents to infants causes colic, although studies have shown that mothers of colicky infants are no more anxious or emotionally unstable than mothers of noncolicky infants. It has also been suggested that immaturity of the neonatal nervous system or exceptional sensitivity to the environment makes some babies more irritable than others.

It is possible that for some babies crying itself is the trigger for colic. A baby may begin colicky crying in response to the sound of his own crying, in much the same way that an infant is startled by his own startle reflex. Also, babies swallow air when they cry, which builds up an air bubble, just as happens in feeding. The more a baby cries, the more air he swallows, which increases the size of the air bubble and the severity of his discomfort, making him cry all the more.

Folk "wisdom" blames colic on exposing the baby to the night air or the wind or on allowing too much fresh air into his room. Other factors that have been suggested as causing colic include being the firstborn, being a boy, being of above-average intelligence, having parents who are of higher social class, and having a mother with a high educational level. None of these factors has stood up to scientific examination.

Despite all this conjecture, however, no conclusive evidence of any one factor being the cause of colic has yet been presented. As you might expect of a condition for which there is as yet no accepted definition and no firm idea of causation, there is no reliable treatment plan. Regardless of what friends, family, and self-styled experts will tell you, treatment of colic is simply a matter of making both you and your baby as comfortable as possible until the colic passes. Fortunately, there are a number of techniques that are as likely as not to be useful. There are no guarantees with any of them, but sometimes just doing something that *might* work will give you a psychological boost.

Before beginning to "treat" colic, of course, you should be certain that colic is, in fact, what your baby has. Don't jump to the conclusion that you are in for a two-month bout of colic the first time your baby cries for no apparent reason. Check for other possible causes of crying, such as pain from an open diaper pin or discomfort from being overheated, constipated, hungry, or wet. Also check for signs of illness: colic is *not* associated with fever, diarrhea, vomiting, cough, a runny nose, or reddened eyes. Your pediatrician will want to rule out more serious causes of crying before assuming that your baby has colic.

If colic is the problem and you suspect that an accumulation of gas in the abdomen is at least in part the cause of colic, you might try the following:

- Be careful not to overfeed your bottle-feeding baby. Don't urge him to finish all the formula you have prepared, because overfeeding may cause gas and stomachaches.

- Check the nipple hole. If it is too large or too small, your baby will probably swallow more air than he should.

- Be especially careful to burp your baby thoroughly after feedings to avoid the buildup of an air bubble.

- Always hold your baby for feedings. You will be more attentive to his fullness and his need to burp.

- A warm hot-water bottle on the abdominal area may relieve some discomfort. So might gentle massaging of his back.

- Your baby may be most comfortable lying on her stomach in her crib or on your lap, or being held with her abdomen resting on your forearm. You might also try gently applying pressure to her abdomen by laying her on her back on a firm surface, bringing her legs up toward her body, and pressing her thighs against her abdomen.

- If you are breast-feeding, your physician may want to rule out an allergic reaction in your baby to cow's milk in your diet. Although there is conflicting evidence on this subject, in one study colic was related to cow's milk consump-

tion by the mother in one-third of the cases. Your physician may suggest that you try totally eliminating cow's milk from your diet for four to seven days. If your baby's colicky behavior stops, try drinking some milk to see if he reacts. If cow's milk appears to be the culprit, you may then want to eliminate cow's milk (and in some cases, other dairy products) from your diet while breast-feeding. (Some form of vitamin and mineral supplementation—especially calcium—may be necessary.) In the same way, other foods suspected of causing the problem may be removed from your diet and then reintroduced to see if there is any effect. However, there seems to be no justification for stopping breast-feeding itself; in fact, it may be one of the most comforting things you can do for your baby.

- In bottle-fed babies, allergies to cow's milk and soy formulas have been suspected of causing colic. However, studies have shown that such "allergies" often end when the colic does, which is not the way true allergies behave. Furthermore, most babies are colicky only at a certain time during the day; for such babies, it is not logical to assume that the formula they drink all day long disagrees with them only in the evening, for example. Therefore, changing formula is most likely not the answer.

- A glycerine suppository may be tried on occasion to help produce a bowel movement (although you certainly would not want to do this routinely). Check with your pediatrician first.

Your physician will probably not recommend any strictly medical treatment for colic. If your baby's colicky symptoms seem to be related to irritability, the following suggestions may be helpful:

- Colicky babies, like most other babies, seem to like rhythmic movement (like riding in a car or buggy and being rocked or walked) and a feeling of closeness (such as can be achieved by swaddling or cuddling your baby, or placing her in a small, confined space, like a bassinet or a portable crib).

- Try to keep your baby's environment as peaceful and tranquil as possible. Fatigue and overstimulation may be the result of living in an environment with too much noise, too much activity, and too much emotional stress. You might want to restrict visitors until the colic has passed.

- Handle your baby as calmly and gently as possible. (But don't handle him less—he needs your comforting.)

- Colicky babies may be comforted by certain kinds of music or by continuous sounds, like the hum of a dishwasher or the vacuum cleaner.

- Allow your baby to suck at the breast, on your finger, or on a pacifier. Sucking is one way your baby can soothe herself.

We have offered some ways of helping your baby through colic, but remember that you, as parents, are also unwilling victims of this "disease." You deserve some special attention, too.

Give yourself a break if there is someone who can relieve you for a while. Go to a movie or for a long walk. Don't feel that you are abandoning your baby—when he is beside himself with the apparent anger and frustration of colic, he may not even be aware of who is with him. You, on the other hand, need to be as rested and calm as possible to deal effectively with his needs.

Derive what small comfort you can from the knowledge that you are not alone. Colic is fairly common, occurring in ten to twenty percent of babies in the United States. Be as much support as you can to your spouse, and know that you are sharing this experience not only with each other but also with thousands of other parents on any given sleepless night.

Don't let colic make you feel bad about yourself or your baby, or interfere with the development of a good relationship between you. It is perfectly natural to feel some resentment, confusion, and even anger when all your best efforts at comforting your colicky baby meet with no success. But remember that your infant is too young to be manipulative, and don't feel that you are involved in a battle of wills. Your infant is even more confused by this state of affairs than you are.

Don't blame yourself for any supposed shortcomings as a parent, either. Colic occurs in virtually every culture and at every socioeconomic level, and does not appear to be related to anything the parents are doing. Support for this observation comes from the fact that even in the same family, some babies will be colicky and others will not.

Be reassured that the colic will end soon, and that no physical or emotional problems have been found to result from it. Colic occurs most often in babies who are growing and developing well despite their apparent discomfort and who will continue to do so when they have outgrown their colic.

## Common Cold

Your baby will get more colds than any other illness. The average youngster gets eight to twelve colds a year. Some may be very mild, with only a slightly runny nose; others may be more severe, with fever and discomfort.

Colds are caused by a number of different viruses. Each time your child has a cold, he develops some immunity against that particular virus, but that protection may last for only a short while. Because colds are caused by a vast number of different viruses, it has proved difficult to develop a vaccine to prevent the common cold.

A cold is an infection of the upper respiratory tract (throat, trachea, nose, and sinuses). Also affected may be the ears (connected to the throat by the eustachian tubes), the eyes (connected to the nose by the tear ducts), and the lymph nodes of the neck (connected to the nose by lymph channels).

Colds are transmitted from person to person in small droplets that float in the air or settle on objects. If you touch an object with a cold virus on it, and then rub your eye or nose (the two most common sites of entry for cold viruses), there's a good chance you'll come down with a cold. Symptoms develop two to seven days after exposure. Children are more likely to catch a cold than adults because children haven't developed as much immunity. Having cold and wet feet, sitting in a draft, and all the other old wives' tales about how you catch a cold just aren't true.

The signs of a cold are nasal congestion, sneezing, clear nasal discharge, scratchy sore throat, and a temperature of up to 103 degrees. Generally speaking, the younger the child, the higher the fever. Other common symptoms are reddened and watery eyes, dry cough, mild tenderness and swelling of the lymph nodes in the neck, mild stuffiness in one or both ears, mild achiness, and decreased appetite and energy level.

Most colds last three to ten days, although some of the signs and symptoms may last longer. The best indicator of how your child is doing is his actions. If he's full of energy and raring to go, he's pretty much over the cold even if he still has a slight cough or runny nose.

Treatment for a cold is aimed at lessening the discomfort. There are no "required" treatments, just whatever makes your child feel better. A humidifier may help with the congestion, but if it doesn't make any difference after one or two days, there's no need to continue using it. Bed rest is not required. Keep your child as quiet as he's willing to be without a struggle. If he needs the rest, he'll get it without your telling him to lie down. If his fever bothers him, treat it (see *Fever*). Nose drops, decongestants, and antihistamines may relieve some of the symptoms, but will do nothing to shorten the course of the illness. Cough medicines may ease his cough, but are necessary only if the cough bothers him or keeps him up at night (see *Signs and Symptoms* and *Coughs and Sneezes*). Remember that every medicine has the potential for side effects, and some medicines do more harm than good. Stay away from combination medicines that promise to do everything. Don't expect miracles from cold medicines—all they may do is perhaps lessen the symptoms and signs a little.

Infants and very young children are unable to blow their noses to clear mucus from their airways. It's a good idea to have a small suction device on hand to gently remove mucus from your baby's nose and make breathing easier. (Ask your pharmacist to recommend one.)

Perhaps the most useful thing you can do about a cold is taking steps to limit its spread. Keep your sick child away from other children and elderly people. Your child may be contagious for one or two weeks—as long as he has the symptoms. A young infant should be kept away from people with colds, especially if she is not being breastfed. Bottle-fed infants are more likely to get colds because they don't have the advantage of the immunity that comes with breast milk.

If your child's cold lasts for more than two weeks and seems not to be getting any better, you should give your doctor a call. It may be something other than a cold. Any child with a cold is more susceptible to serious illnesses. Call the doctor if your child has a high fever or a fever that lasts more than three or four days; pus-like drainage from his eyes, nose, or ears; large, red lymph nodes in his neck; breathing problems; a stiff neck; severe headache; vomiting; shaking chills; or prostration (extreme exhaustion).

## Conjunctivitis

Conjunctivitis, commonly called pinkeye, is an infection of the conjunctiva (the transparent membrane that covers the eyeball and lines the inside of the eyelids).

Conjunctivitis is highly contagious. The eye discharge, objects that have touched the infected eye, and things that the infected person has touched can spread the infection. Symptoms develop one to three days after contact. There's a good chance that the conjunctivitis will spread from one eye to the other. Conjunctivitis is caused by both viruses and bacteria. It may occur alone or with an ear infection, cold, sore throat, tonsillitis, or sinusitis.

If your child has conjunctivitis, his eye (or eyes) will be red, with a yellowish discharge of pus. His eyelids may swell, and his eyeball may feel a little scratchy. Conjunctivitis causes no vision problems (except from the discharge covering the eyeball), and there's no added discomfort from bright light. (If either of those symptoms is present, your child needs to be seen by his doctor—he probably doesn't have conjunctivitis.)

There are causes of red eyes other than conjunctivitis. Allergies may cause itching and tearing, but no pain or pus. A foreign body (which is what doctors call anything from outside the body that does not belong where it is, like a grain of sand in the eye) causes pain, light sensitivity, and tearing, but no pus. The redness from a foreign body is usually in only one part of the eye.

It's usually difficult to tell if conjunctivitis is caused by a virus or a bacterium. Treating the signs and symptoms is often all that's needed in either case. Many times, conjunctivitis clears up on its own.

If your child's eyes are matted shut in the morning, a wet compress—either warm or cool, whichever feels better—will help remove the dried discharge. The same type of compress will help soothe the itch and discomfort of conjunctivitis. It's best to use paper towels for the compresses. After one use, throw the paper towels away. This helps to lessen the spread of the disease.

If your child's conjunctivitis doesn't get better in a day or so, it may be bacterial. Your doctor will prescribe antibiotic eye drops or ointment for this. Getting the drops into the eyes of a wiggling and fighting infant can be a two-person job.

## Constipation

There are many misconceptions about bowel habits. Constipation has nothing to do with how often your child has a bowel movement. The important factor is the hardness of the stool. Having six very hard movements a day is constipation; having one soft movement every three or four days isn't.

The function of the colon (large intestine) is to hold undigested and indigestible food and to absorb water from what has been eaten. If too much water is taken from the large intestine, the undigested food, which forms the stool, will become very hard and dry. This leads to constipation.

Rarely is there a physical cause for constipation. Most cases are due to two factors: inappropriate diet and poor bowel habits.

A good diet should include fiber and other sources of bulk. These materials pass through the digestive system and accumulate in the colon. There they hold onto water, which helps to keep the stool soft. A diet without enough fiber does not offer this natural softening effect.

The second common cause of constipation is poor bowel habits—a child not having a bowel movement when he feels the urge. Since the function of the colon is to absorb water, the longer the bowel contents stay in the colon, the more water will be removed. This causes the bowel movement to become too dry, making it difficult and painful to pass. So why does a child resist having a bowel movement when he needs to? Sometimes it's because his parents are putting too much pressure on him to become toilet trained. Once the stool becomes hard, bowel movements become painful, and the child becomes even more resistant to going to the bathroom. If this goes on too long, his colon may become distended and lose its normal muscle tone. The normal impulse to have a bowel movement is thus weakened, and a cycle of chronic constipation may start.

If your baby is constipated, he will draw his legs up when he has a bowel movement and cry. He may turn blue from holding his breath while pushing it out. There may be a small amount of blood in the stool because it tears the anus while coming out. The feces may be in small, very hard balls.

An older child will complain and cry when he has to have a bowel movement. He may complain of cramps and have some blood in his stool.

You may notice that he doesn't have bowel movements very often; when he does, he may stay on the toilet or potty for a long time.

Sometimes a child with severe and chronic constipation will have diarrhea. Although this may seem odd, watery fecal material seeps around the other, hardened bowel contents.

Treating a young baby with constipation may be difficult. There are some products that can be added to the formula. Extra fluids often help, so try giving your baby some water between feedings of formula. The iron in iron-supplemented formulas causes constipation in some babies, so you may want to switch to a formula without iron for a while. If this makes a difference, discuss your baby's iron needs with your doctor. Sometimes taking a rectal temperature will help stimulate a bowel movement. Glycerine suppositories often help, but they shouldn't be used without first checking with your doctor. Breast-fed babies rarely become constipated, although they may have very few bowel movements. Any constipation that lasts more than a few days in a baby should be brought to your doctor's attention.

Children who are eating regular food should be first treated with changes in their diet. Your child needs to eat more roughage. When you add the extra fiber (whole grain cereals, fruit, vegetables), your child may complain of increased gas and cramps for a few days. This often happens and doesn't mean that he can't tolerate the fiber. These symptoms often go away in a day or two. Make sure your child drinks enough fluids, like water and juices; however, some people feel too much milk may add to constipation problems.

If the constipation appears during toilet training, stop the toilet training. Your child probably isn't ready yet. It is possible that the constipation has another cause, but this is the most likely. If you have any questions, check with your doctor.

On rare occasions, a glycerine suppository or a pediatric enema may be necessary. But if you feel the need to use them more than once or twice, you should bring your child into the doctor's office. There may be other problems that need further evaluation.

## Convulsions

A convulsion is a sign of a disease—not a disease itself. Convulsions may occur with or without a fever (see *Fever*). A convulsion that occurs without a fever may be caused by any number of illnesses.

Epilepsy is the best-known cause of convulsions. It is a disorder of the brain that causes repeated attacks, or seizures. Most children with epilepsy have an area in the brain where the nerve cells "fire" (discharge energy) when they shouldn't. This may lead to a generalized and uncoordinated firing of the brain's nerve cells, causing a convulsion. Usually, no specific cause for the misfiring can be found. Some children contract epilepsy after having encephalitis (infection of the brain), meningitis (infection of the covering of the brain and spinal column), serious head trauma, and some rare illnesses.

There are many different types of epilepsy. Each is defined according to the type of seizure a child has. Some children with epilepsy have no visible seizures at all.

A *generalized convulsive seizure* is what most people think of as a seizure. The child may cry out and then suddenly lose consciousness. His body will stiffen, and he may fall to the ground. His arms and legs will thrash around wildly from muscle spasms. He may lose control of his bladder and bowels. He may drool and turn a little bluish from breath-holding. When the seizure is over, he will be very tired and may fall into a deep sleep. When he awakens, he may be confused and sleepy. Some children have an aura (warning sensation) before the seizure begins.

*Absence*, or *nonconvulsive*, *seizures* are very different—so different that most people don't recognize them as seizures. A child may simply stare into space and not respond to anything. His eyes may blink rapidly, or his eyelids may flutter. He will remain conscious, yet be unaware of what is going on around him. If not recognized as a seizure, such an attack may be mistakenly thought of as reflecting a learning disability, lack of attention, or daydreaming.

In *complex partial seizures*, the child remains conscious, but may sit motionless or make repeated or unusual movements. In *simple partial seizures*, the child is conscious and may simply feel tingling in his hands and feet. The child may also perceive bad odors, see flashing lights, or speak unintelligibly.

If your child has a convulsion, you must take steps to make sure he doesn't hurt himself. Don't try to hold him down or prevent his thrashing. You should try to direct his arms and legs so he won't hit the floor or walls and hurt himself. Don't try to pry open his mouth if it's clamped shut. Never put your fingers into the mouth of a person having a seizure—you may lose a finger. Turn your child onto his side so his saliva will drool out and not go into his lungs. If your child has a seizure, he needs to be seen by his doctor as soon as possible.

If your doctor makes a diagnosis of epilepsy, you will need to learn as much as you can about this disease. Your child may need to take his medicine every day. Your doctor will give you instructions for dealing with the seizures.

## Convulsions

### Symptoms

- Unconsciousness

- Stiffened body

- Jerking or thrashing movements

- Muscle spasm

- Loss of control of bladder or bowels

- Deep sleep after seizure

### Treatment

- Protect your child from hurting herself while having a seizure by keeping her away from sharp objects, stairs, and so forth. Guide her jerking limbs, but don't hold them down. Don't try to pry open her jaws.

- If your child is vomiting or drooling, turn her on one side so that the vomitus and saliva will drain out of her mouth.

- **Call for emergency help.**

- Have your child seen by her doctor.

## Cradle Cap

Cradle cap is a common skin problem for infants and children up to five years old. It causes your child's scalp to look yellowish and scaly with crusty patches. The patches, made of oil and dead cells, are usually confined to the scalp, although they may spread to the forehead, ears, and diaper area. Sometimes temporary hair loss occurs.

Most cases of cradle cap can be treated at home with a little baby oil. Wash your baby's hair and scalp daily with a rough facecloth. Wrap it around your hand and vigorously scrub your child's scalp. If this treatment is unsuccessful, special shampoos may be used. Before using stronger shampoos, however, check with your doctor.

## Croup and Epiglottitis

Croup is an inflammation and swelling of the larynx (voice box), usually caused by a virus. It is fairly common and is passed from child to child the same way a cold is.

A child with croup has trouble getting air in, but breathing out is not difficult. (This is the opposite of asthma, in which the child has trouble getting air out but no problems getting it in.) This extra effort to get air causes the barking or crowing sound that is associated with croup. Hoarseness and a barking cough are typical. A slight fever (temperature of less than 101 degrees) may be present.

Mild cases of croup can be treated at home. Home treatment is aimed at making it easier for your child to breathe. Some children respond well to moist, warm air made by running the shower in a closed bathroom or by running a vaporizer; other children find that makes their breathing more difficult and respond better to cool, dry air. Whichever works best for your child should be used. If things don't get better, it's best to take him to see the doctor.

Another breathing disorder, epiglottitis, is extremely dangerous. This infection of the epiglottis (the "lid" over the opening of the larynx) and surrounding tissue is caused by bacteria. A child with epiglottitis has difficulty breathing that gets worse rapidly. Drooling is common because the child has problems swallowing. The typical position of a child with epiglottitis is sitting up, hunched forward, with mouth open and tongue partially out. Usually a temperature of 103 to 105 degrees is present. Epiglottitis is life-threatening—seek medical help **immediately**.

## Cuts

Cuts and scrapes are the most common injury your child will suffer. One of the difficult decisions with cuts is whether they need to be seen by a doctor. Many cuts look bad at first, but once they have been cleaned up, there's not much to them. The first step with any cut is to stop the bleeding. The best technique is to apply pressure to the wound. It's best to put a sterile or clean cloth over the cut, but just grabbing it with your hand will do in an emergency. Keep the pressure on the cut for ten minutes *by the clock*. Don't peek to see if the bleeding has stopped. If there's a lot of bleeding, elevating the cut above your child's heart will help. This method stops bleeding in almost every case. Rarely is a tourniquet needed. A tourniquet should be used only if a limb has been partially or completely amputated. Once the bleeding has stopped, *clean the wound well* with warm, soapy water. This may restart the bleeding. If it does, use the pressure again.

Now you are in a position to decide if the cut needs medical attention. If it's just in the skin or is

## Cuts

### Symptoms

- Severe bleeding

### Treatment

- **Stop the bleeding** by applying steady pressure and elevating the injured area above your child's heart. If bleeding does not stop promptly, seek medical attention.

- Clean the wound with large amounts of clean water and soap.

- If the wound is deep, long (greater than one-half inch), or in an area where a scar is of concern, seek medical attention.

- If your child is behind on his tetanus shots, contact his doctor.

- If you are not going to see your doctor, cover the wound with a clean bandage.

an abrasion (scrape), no medical care is needed. Deep cuts, cuts that won't stop bleeding, cuts on areas that move a lot (like the knee and elbow), and facial cuts should be seen by a doctor.

If you are going to treat the cut at home, apply a nonstinging antiseptic after cleaning the cut well. Draw the edges of the wound together and apply an adhesive strip or butterfly bandage. Use the bandage to keep the edges of the cut together.

If you decide to take your child to the doctor, particularly if you think sutures (stitches) are needed, do it soon. Most doctors won't stitch a wound that's more than eight to twelve hours old. Suturing helps a wound stay clean because there's no opening to the deeper tissues. It may lessen the scarring, but not always. Stitches probably don't speed up healing unless the cut is over a joint.

If your child cuts himself, make sure his tetanus immunization is current. All wounds should be watched carefully for signs of infection. Any redness, swelling, red streaking, or discharge of pus means that infection is present. Your child needs to be seen by the doctor for this problem. (See also *Bites.*)

# Dehydration

Dehydration accompanies many illnesses, but is not an illness itself. Because of an underlying illness, a child may lose more fluid than he takes in. This may occur if he is unable or unwilling to drink water or other fluids, or if he is losing more fluid than he can replace because of vomiting, diarrhea, sweating, excessive and rapid breathing, or passing large amounts of urine. Dehydration is the number one killer of infants worldwide, although few die of it in developed countries.

The smaller the child, the more quickly he may become dehydrated. An infant may become dehydrated in twelve to twenty-four hours; older children take somewhat longer. Rarely does decreased fluid intake alone cause dehydration. It must be combined with excessive fluid loss (most often caused by diarrhea or vomiting).

You can observe most of the signs and symptoms of dehydration. One of the first is decreased urine output. (This is not true for a child with diabetes, who may urinate in large amounts.) A young child who has gone eight to twelve hours without urinating or an older child who hasn't urinated in ten to twelve hours probably is dehydrated. Other signs of dehydration include sunken eyes, dry and doughy-feeling skin, dry mouth with stringy saliva, no tears when crying, and depression (sinking in) of the soft spot in an infant's skull.

Dehydration has many different causes, and the cause must be treated for the dehydration to end. Probably the most common cause is viral gastroenteritis ("stomach flu"). Your child will usually have a lot of diarrhea and vomiting with gastroenteritis. Respiratory illnesses, such as asthma and bronchiolitis, may cause rapid breathing leading to dehydration. Fever from any of a number of illnesses may cause dehydration. Undiagnosed diabetes mellitus causes excessive urination.

Mild cases of dehydration can be treated at home. The first step is to encourage your child to drink more fluids. It's best to start with small amounts, perhaps a few teaspoonfuls at a time, of clear liquids or commercially available electrolyte solutions (such as Pedialyte) that contain the proper mix of salts and sugar (don't give plain water exclusively). Such solutions are particularly good for infants. Older children do well with diluted juice and gelatin desserts (solid or liquid). Avoid milk and milk products.

If your child can't keep these fluids down, or if the fluid loss is still greater than his intake, contact your doctor. She is the one to decide if your child needs to be hospitalized for administration of intravenous fluids. If your child does need to go into the hospital, it will usually be for only a few days, until he can keep fluids down and the fluid loss has been stopped.

# Diaper Rash

Diaper rash is the most common infant skin problem. The rash, usually confined to the diaper area, is caused by moisture, urine, stool, or irritating chemicals, usually from the diaper. If not treated promptly and appropriately, bacteria or yeast may invade the area and start an infection.

Simple diaper rashes are red, slightly rough, and scaly. They usually involve only the area covered by the diaper. The skin may be irritated by chemicals in disposable diapers or in the detergents used to launder cloth diapers. Plastic or rubber pants worn over the diapers sometimes affect the skin (and always hold the moisture in against the skin).

If your baby stays in wet diapers too long, microorganisms and moisture can irritate his sensitive skin, leaving a large, bright red rash. Often you will detect an ammonia odor when changing your baby's diapers.

Some babies are prone to getting yeast diaper rashes. The organism that causes the rash is the same one that causes vaginal yeast infections. The rash is usually found in the skin folds of a baby's thighs.

Any of the above rashes may become infected with bacteria. The rash, instead of getting better, begins to get worse. It will become darker red, with some discharge. Oral antibiotics may be necessary to clear up an infection.

Other causes of diaper rash include food and drug allergies, skin infections, and contagious diseases (chicken pox or measles).

Most diaper rashes are simple to treat at home. Make sure your baby doesn't stay in wet or soiled diapers for very long. Change his diapers frequently. If possible, let him go without diapers— letting his sore bottom be exposed to the air is best. There are many different ointments that are protective. For some babies, they help the rash clear up quickly; but for others they seem to make things worse. Avoid airtight rubber pants. They hold the urine and feces against the sore skin. If you suspect an allergic rash, stop giving your child whatever you think is the problem food.

Some rashes just don't respond to home care. If the rash is getting much worse, if your baby is extremely uncomfortable, or if you can't figure out what's going on, give your doctor a call.

## Diarrhea

Diarrhea is a sign that accompanies many different illnesses. Like constipation, diarrhea is judged by the consistency, not the frequency, of bowel movements. Any bowel movement that is partially or completely runny is a sign of diarrhea. The frequency of this type of bowel movement is a reflection of the severity of the diarrhea. Diarrhea is one of the common causes of dehydration, particularly in infants and young children. Large amounts of fluid can be lost very quickly.

There are many different causes of diarrhea. The most frequent is an intestinal viral infection, commonly called the "stomach flu." Other causes include bacterial intestinal infections, parasites, and respiratory tract infections. Food allergies and intolerances may cause diarrhea in infants. Certain drugs, particularly antibiotics, may start a bout of diarrhea.

The looseness of your child's bowel movements is the main sign. You may notice some mucus or flecks of red blood in the feces. There's no need to be concerned unless there's a lot of blood present. Your child may have cramps and fever along with loss of appetite, vomiting, and weight loss. He may have anywhere from one to twenty bowel movements a day. One or two loose bowel movements followed by a return to normal means the diarrhea is minimal and not of concern.

The first treatment for diarrhea is dietary change. A bottle-fed baby with diarrhea may be temporarily switched to clear liquids such as Pedialyte or Lytren (check with your baby's doctor). Diarrhea in a breast-fed infant can generally be treated without having to discontinue breast-feeding.

Put your older child on a clear-liquid diet. After twenty-four hours, you can start adding foods, following what's called the "BRACT" diet: Banana, Rice, Apple juice and apple sauce, Carrots (cooked), Tea and Toast. As the diarrhea improves, you can add other foods, delaying milk and milk products for five to seven days.

Don't give your child any antidiarrheal medicines. They may cause severe problems. If the diarrhea doesn't decrease within a day, call your doctor. If your child begins to show signs of dehydration or appears very ill and lethargic, he should be examined.

## Dislocations

A dislocation occurs when a bone or bones are pulled out of their proper place in a joint. In children one to three years old, the joint that is most commonly dislocated is the elbow. This injury, called Malgaigne's luxation (or "nursemaid's elbow"), is rare in children over four years old. The dislocation occurs when a child is jerked or pulled suddenly.

If your child has an elbow dislocation, she will complain of severe and sudden elbow pain. She'll refuse to move or use her arm. Most likely, she'll hold her injured arm against her side with her good arm. Any attempts to move the injured arm will cause pain and crying. She may complain of pain in her wrist even though the injury is in her elbow.

If you suspect a dislocated elbow, your child needs to be seen by her doctor. Sometimes, an x-ray film will be taken. Often, positioning of the elbow for the x-ray study corrects the dislocation. When the elbow is relocated, your child will frequently have immediate relief and will be able to use her arm and hand again.

If your child tends to have recurrent elbow dislocations, her doctor may teach you how to relocate the elbow at home.

To prevent dislocations, it is important that you never lift or pull your child by her hands or arms. The joint structures are not strong enough to support her entire body weight (plus the additional stress of your action). To carry a baby or small child, it is best to place your hands on either side of her rib cage and gently lift her.

Babies are sometimes born with joints—especially hips—that are easily dislocated. Your doctor will check for this as part of the newborn exam, and at occasional intervals during the first year. If such joints are found, your child will be referred to an orthopedist (a doctor who specializes in disorders of the bones and joints).

## Draining Ear

Normally nothing except a little wax should come out of your child's ear. Wax, which coats and protects the ear canal, is usually brown or yellowish. It's odorless and contains no blood.

Any other material coming from the ear signals potential problems. It may be a sign of a middle ear infection, a boil in the ear canal, swimmer's ear (infection of the ear canal), rupture of the eardrum from infection or trauma, a foreign object in the ear canal, or (rarely) a tumor of the middle ear or a fracture of the base of the skull. Abnormal ear discharge may be thin and watery, bloody, odorous, cheesy, green, yellow, or white.

There's not much you can or should do about abnormal ear discharge. Your child needs to be seen by a doctor. If your child has a lot of pain, acetaminophen will help. Sometimes warm compresses are soothing. Don't pack cotton in your child's ear. **Never** put anything in his ear to try to clean it out (see *Ear Infections*).

## Drowning

Drowning is one of the most common causes of accidental death in children. Particularly at risk are toddlers, teenagers, and children who suffer seizures. Generally speaking, after four to six minutes without oxygen, irreversible changes in the brain begin to occur. If the water is very cold, this critical time is increased somewhat.

Prevention is the most important step. Children have drowned in less than six inches of water, so it isn't just swimming pools that are a danger. Teaching children a respect for water is important. There are swimming classes for very young children, even toddlers. In theory they are a good idea, but there is some controversy about how much they "protect" children from water accidents. Too often, both the child and his parents believe his swimming abilities are much greater than they really are. This false confidence can be dangerous.

It's a good idea for *all* parents to learn emergency medical techniques (such as mouth-to-mouth resuscitation, the Heimlich maneuver, and cardiopulmonary resuscitation [CPR]). These skills are best acquired by taking a safety course. Contact your local hospital, Red Cross, or YMCA to find out if and when they offer such courses.

If you find a child unconscious in the water, the first step is to get him out of the water. If he's not breathing, mouth-to-mouth resuscitation is needed. (As with the Heimlich maneuver, reading a description isn't nearly as good as taking a first-aid class.) First, make sure nothing is blocking his airway; open his mouth and check. Don't worry about water in his throat or lungs; trying to get water out will only waste valuable time. Tip his head back slightly to help open his airway. For an infant or small child, cover both his mouth and nose with your mouth. For a larger child, pinch his nose shut and cover his mouth with yours. Give him four quick puffs of air, enough to cause a rise in his chest. If he has no heartbeat or pulse, begin CPR if you know how. Signal someone to get help.

### Mouth-to-Mouth Resuscitation

When you discover that your child is not breathing or is breathing with difficulty, send someone to call for medical help and immediately begin the procedure described below. If you are alone, perform the procedure for one minute before calling for help.

### 1. *Position the child*

Lay the child on his back on a firm, flat surface. (If there is evidence of head or neck injury, turn the child as a unit, supporting the head and neck.) Quickly clear the mouth of foreign material. (Don't attempt to clear the airway, however; you may push an obstructing object farther into the airway.)

### 2. *Open the airway*

Place one hand on the child's forehead and gently tilt the head back slightly. (Do not perform this maneuver if head or neck injury is suspected.) Then place two or three fingers under each side of the lower jaw (at the angle) and lift the jaw upward slightly. Maintain this position with one hand on the forehead and one supporting the chin or the back of the neck.

### 3. *Breathe for the child*

If the child is an infant, make a tight seal with your mouth over his nose and mouth. If the child is older, pinch his nose tightly with the fingers of the hand that is holding his forehead and make a tight seal with your mouth over his mouth. Blow four *gentle* breaths into the child's airway (remember that a child's lung capacity is smaller than an adult's). Stop blowing when the child's chest is expanded.

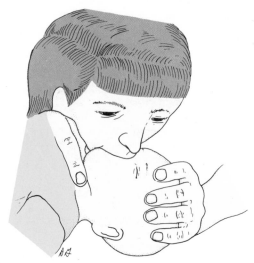

**Step 3**

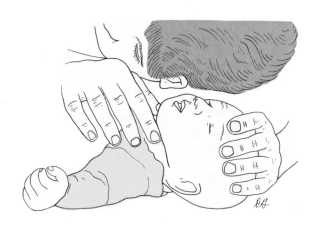

**Step 4**

### 4. *Check the airway before continuing*

Remove your mouth and turn your head so that your ear is over the child's mouth. Listen for air leaving his lungs. (If you cannot hear air leaving the lungs, recheck the positioning to make sure that the airway is open. If it appears to be open,

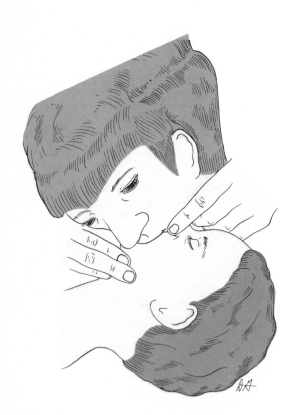

**Step 3**

there may be an obstruction beyond the visible portion of the airway. See *Choking*, page 217.) Continue breathing for the child.

5. *Check the pulse*

Check for a brachial pulse (on the inside of the upper arm between the elbow and the shoulder) in an infant or a carotid pulse (along the side of the neck) in an older child. If no pulse is present, begin cardiac compressions *if* you are trained in

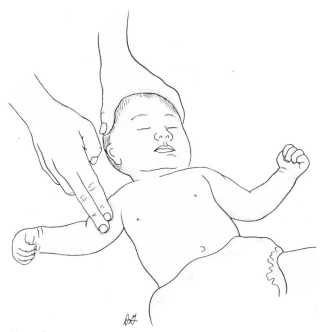

**Step 5**

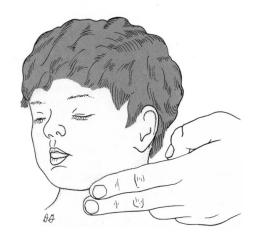

**Step 5**

cardiopulmonary resuscitation (CPR). This must be done in conjunction with artificial respiration.

6. *Continue efforts*

For an infant, the breathing rate should be about once every three seconds, or twenty times a minute; for a child, once every four seconds, or fifteen times a minute. Continue until medical help arrives or the child begins breathing on his own. (Even after apparent recovery, your child must be seen by a physician as soon as possible.)

Resuscitation efforts should be continued until the child is in a hospital. Particularly with cold-water drownings, efforts shouldn't be stopped until the child has been warmed to normal body temperature.

## Ear Infections

The ear has three different parts, each with its own function: the outer ear (comprising the visible ear and the external ear canal), which captures sounds; the middle ear, which transmits sounds inward; and the inner ear, which converts those sounds into nerve impulses that can be sent to the brain and also controls balance.

Rarely do children have inner ear problems, but if your child seems to be having trouble with balance, your doctor may suspect an inner ear disorder.

The chances are high that your child will have at least one ear infection before he is five, and it is the middle ear that is the site of most such infections. When your child has a common ear infection, called otitis media (*otitis* = ear inflammation, *media* = middle), it's the middle ear that's involved. If your child has otitis media, he will usually be fussy, may have a fever, and may pull and dig at his ears or complain of ear pain. No one knows why children get ear infections or why most children tend to outgrow them by the time they are six to eight years old. The eustachian tube equalizes the pressure in the middle ear. Some doctors think that if the eustachian tube isn't functioning properly, a vacuum occurs in the middle ear. This causes secretions to form, and an infection may set in. There are many proposed causes for eustachian tube dysfunction (abnormal function), including allergies, swollen tonsils or adenoids, and small angle of entry of the tube into the throat.

In any case, once a middle ear infection starts, your child will be very uncomfortable. He may

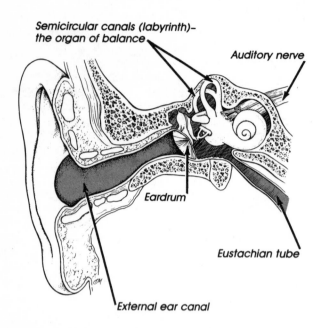

Semicircular canals (labyrinth)—
the organ of balance

Auditory nerve

Eardrum

Eustachian tube

External ear canal

*The ear is a complex and delicate structure that is responsible for the sense of hearing and for the body's sense of balance. **Never** put anything into the ear canal.*

wake up in the middle of the night screaming. The pain occurs from the increased pressure in the middle ear. The eardrum bulges and may rupture. If rupture of the eardrum occurs, the pain is often relieved because the built-up pressure has been released.

There is little you can do at home for otitis media. Sometimes acetaminophen helps. A warm compress against the ear is soothing. But the usual treatment is antibiotics. Your child needs to be seen by his doctor. Some doctors also prescribe decongestants or antihistamines to help bring down the swelling, but there is controversy about the effectiveness of these treatments.

Some children seem to be prone to getting otitis media. If your child has numerous middle ear infections, his doctor may want to prescribe an antibiotic. For children subject to severe and recurrent ear infections, surgery may be recommended to relieve the pressure, drain the region, and determine the appropriate antibiotic treatment.

Infections of the outer ear (otitis externa) are not as common in young children as otitis media. Otitis externa, commonly known as swimmer's ear, occurs when the sensitive lining of the ear canal is hurt. This can also happen when things that don't

belong in the ear are put there. Such items as cotton swabs, fingers, ends of toys, and just about anything that a child (or parent) can fit into the ear will damage the lining. Earwax helps to protect the ear canal. Otitis externa is treated with ear drops and medicine for the pain. It usually heals quickly.

## Eczema

Eczema is the most common chronic childhood skin condition. Eczema is not contagious. It seems to be inherited and runs in families that have a history of allergies and asthma. It can begin in babies two to three months old. The first phase of this disease, called infantile eczema, ends by the age of eighteen to twenty-four months. Affected children have a dry, slightly scaly, pink, itchy rash on their cheeks and scalp. Frequently, there are oval patches on the trunk. Sometimes the patches are on the backs of the elbows and the fronts of the knees.

About one-third of children with infantile eczema go on to have childhood eczema. The rash is similar, but it appears in different places. The fronts of the elbows, the backs of the knees, the neck, the wrists, and sometimes the hands and feet are affected. This phase lasts from age two until adolescence. One-third of children with childhood eczema continue to have problems as adults. Other allergic problems, such as asthma, hay fever, and eye allergies, may develop.

Eczema doesn't always follow the same pattern. Some children have nummular eczema (round, coin-like areas scattered on the body). Sometimes eczema can be confused with roundworm (see *Roundworms*). Sometimes eczema occurs in combination with seborrhea (cradle cap. See *Cradle Cap.*)

In eczema, the skin seems to be unable to hold onto moisture. The outer layer of the skin shrinks and cracks. Bacteria may enter the cracked skin and cause infections. Itching and scratching may compound the problem.

Many children with eczema also have allergies, which may make the eczema worse. If you can remove the allergen from your child's environment, the eczema will often improve, although it may take as long as a week for you to see a difference. Foods are the most common allergens, although many other common substances have been found to make eczema worse.

Treating eczema can be very frustrating. Once you think you have things under control, the irritation flares up again. The first treatment is removing anything you suspect makes it worse. Minimize the number of baths your child takes (soaking in water takes moisture out of the skin). There are special soaps and moisturizing lotions that often help the skin hold onto moisture. If you feel that certain foods aggravate your child's eczema, remove them from his diet. Once his skin has cleared up, try adding the foods, one at a time, back into his diet. Wait a week before adding another suspected food to give his skin ample time to react. This way you can play detective.

Your doctor will want to see your child if home treatment doesn't keep the eczema under reasonable control. There are many creams and lotions that can be used to treat eczema. Some are steroids and must be prescribed by a doctor. Once you know what works for your child's eczema, you will be able to handle most eczema outbreaks at home.

## Electrical Injuries

See *Burns* (page 215) and *Mouth-to-Mouth Resuscitation* (page 229).

## Encephalitis

Encephalitis is an inflammation of the brain. The causes are many, including viruses, poisons, bacteria, vaccines, and parasites. Viruses are responsible for most cases of encephalitis. Many of these viruses also cause familiar diseases, such as mumps, measles, rubella (German measles), chicken pox, herpes, mononucleosis, and influenza. The whooping cough and measles vaccines may also cause encephalitis. However, the vaccines are far less likely to cause encephalitis than are the illnesses they prevent.

Encephalitis may start with the symptoms of the common cold. A child may have no fever or a high fever (a temperature of 105 degrees). She may have a headache, be nauseated, and vomit. Often, children with encephalitis are disoriented (confused) and sleepy. Occasionally, convulsions and unconsciousness occur. The child may complain of pain when bending her neck forward; because the pain is so severe, some children refuse to bend forward. Sometimes a child with encephalitis can't sit upright without using her arms to support her in a tripod fashion.

If you suspect that your child has encephalitis, contact your physician right away. **This is a life-threatening situation.** There's nothing you can do at home. Your child needs to be in the hospital. There is no treatment to kill an invading virus, but there are many steps that can be taken to lessen your child's discomfort. If the encephalitis is caused by bacteria, intravenous antibiotics are needed.

## Eye Injuries

The eyeball is a fragile, hollow sphere not even one-eighth inch thick, within which are many complex and delicate structures. It is fairly well protected by its bony socket and the eyelids, but occasionally injuries can occur. Small objects, such as grains of sand or metallic splinters, can land on or become embedded in the surface. Sharp objects can scratch the surface or even penetrate the eye. Dull objects can jar the eye and dislodge its internal structures. Chemicals can splash into the eye to cause damage.

If your child's eyeball is injured, the pain often will cause her to involuntarily close her eyelids tightly; light may be painful. The eye must be examined to determine the seriousness of the damage. If your child cannot easily open her eye, do not attempt to force it open; any damage may be compounded. *See your doctor promptly.*

If your child can open her eye, look carefully for any of the following: blood coming from the eyeball (do not be misled by blood coming from a cut near the eye that may have run into the eye); any change in the pupil of the affected eye compared with the other eye (larger? smaller? different color?); any change in the color or position of the iris (colored part of the eye); any sign of collapse of the eyeball. Ask her if her vision is blurred. If any of these signs is present, place a soft bandage over the eye and *see your doctor promptly.* If none of these signs is present and you see a speck on the eyeball or under the lid (and the child is cooperative), you may try to remove the speck by gentle strokes with a cotton swab. If the speck does not immediately come off, stop. The object may be embedded. *See a doctor.*

The eyeball is delicate and invaluable. Be cautious about treating eye injuries yourself. Do not attempt to remove a fishhook or any other object that has penetrated the eye. If a harmful liquid or powder (acids, alkalis, caustics, gasoline) enters the eye, **immediate action is imperative. Seconds**

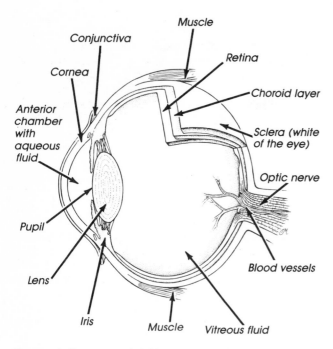

*The eye is the organ of sight.*

Labels: Conjunctiva, Muscle, Cornea, Retina, Choroid layer, Anterior chamber with aqueous fluid, Sclera (white of the eye), Optic nerve, Pupil, Lens, Blood vessels, Iris, Muscle, Vitreous fluid

bones. But if they are not correctly set, permanent deformity may result. Fractures in the growth plates (where bone growth occurs) must be treated correctly, or the bone won't grow normally.

Some fractures are easy to spot—there is a deformity of the bone. Your child will complain of a lot of pain, particularly when trying to move the broken bone. The area is very tender to touch. Redness and swelling are often seen. Other fractures are harder to detect. There may be only slight pain and tenderness. Your child may not complain all the time, just when she does certain things. If you have any doubts about the presence of a fracture, your child should be seen by her doctor.

Any time you suspect a fracture, treat it as if the bone is broken until your child sees a doctor. Keep the injured area from moving. Don't try to straighten out a deformity. Often, your child will hold the injured extremity in the most comfortable position—don't try to move it. Let your child be the guide. If you can't move your child without moving

count! Hold the eye open and flush it with large quantities of cool water. If available, put your child into a cool shower, clothes and all, and wash out her eye. Then, **immediately** take the child to your doctor for further care.

Your doctor can easily anesthetize the eye and examine it internally and externally without pain or damage. She may stain the eyeball with drops to make small injuries and foreign objects readily visible. Areas inside and outside the eye can be examined with a special microscope.

As with many childhood injuries, the best treatment is prevention. Try to keep objects that are obviously dangerous out of reach of your baby or toddler, and try to keep her away from work areas. Machine sanders, paint removers, and grindstones throw off particles. Also, some golf balls can explode and cause eye injuries if they are unwound. Carbon dioxide cartridges and spray cans can explode violently in fires.

## Fractures

Broken bones are not common in infants and young children. Their bones are fairly flexible and have a lot of give. Since children's bones are still growing, they heal much faster than adults'

---

### Fractures

#### Symptoms

- Deformity of a bone that can be felt or seen

- Pain that is worsened with movement of the bone

- Pain or tenderness when touched

- Inability to move the bone normally

- Swelling or bruising

#### Treatment

- **Splint the injured area** with a pillow, rolled-up newspaper, or whatever else is available, so your child won't move it.

- Apply an ice pack.

- Prevent your child from using or putting weight on the injured area.

- Take your child to the doctor.

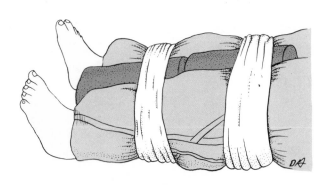

*If you suspect a fracture, immobilize the affected bone and seek medical attention.*

the injured area, it's best to call an ambulance for assistance. Ambulances have special equipment to immobilize any part of the body.

Your doctor will most likely want to get x-ray films of the injured area. That's the best way to tell if there's a fracture. Sometimes a fracture doesn't show up on an x-ray film taken shortly after the injury, and your doctor may want your child to come back for a repeat x-ray study in five to seven days. If a fracture is found, a splint or cast may be put on to immobilize the fractured bone.

## Head Lice

Even the cleanest of children can get head lice. They are tiny (smaller than fleas), grayish-white, almost transparent, six-legged creatures that live exclusively on humans. They live close to the scalp, where they bite and suck blood. Their milk-white, visible eggs (called nits) stick to hair very tightly and are about the size of a flake of dandruff. During the past few years, infestations with head lice have become common among school-age children.

Many children with head lice have no symptoms except mild itching of their scalps. Parents often learn about the problem from a note sent home from school or day care saying that some children have been found to have head lice. Sometimes a child with head lice will scratch his scalp and cause small sores. The lymph nodes at the base of his skull may become enlarged from infection caused by the scratching.

Unless your child has hundreds of head lice, they are difficult to see. It is easier to see the nits. They are attached to the bases of hair shafts. Although they resemble dandruff, they can't be easily brushed or blown away.

A case of head lice can be effectively treated at home. There are many shampoos for head lice available in the drugstore that you can buy without a prescription. Stronger medicines are available by prescription. These products come with detailed instructions, which you should follow carefully. If you don't follow the instructions, you may not kill all the lice, and the problem will recur. The shampoos may also cause side effects if not used properly.

If one family member has head lice, there's a good chance others do also. Many doctors recommend treating everyone in the family to prevent the spread of the infestation.

## Hearing Problems

Hearing can be tested in newborns, so the problem of hearing impairment can and should be caught very early in life. The most critical period for learning language is the first two years of life, and any hearing problems may severely affect this process. If a hearing impairment is not detected early, the loss of language development may never be fully recovered.

Infants at high risk for hearing impairment should be tested as soon as possible. Risk factors include a family history of inherited hearing problems, infections while in the uterus, facial or ear defects, birth weight of less than 1,500 grams, high levels of bilirubin (see *Jaundice*), and very low Apgar scores. These infants should also be tested at six months of age.

As your baby grows, you may be able to determine if she has a hearing problem. By four months of age, she should respond to a soft sound by widening her eyes, stopping her activity, and perhaps turning toward the 'sound. At six months, she should turn toward the sound. By nine months, she should be able to locate a sound coming from above her; by one year, to find the source of the sound either above or below her.

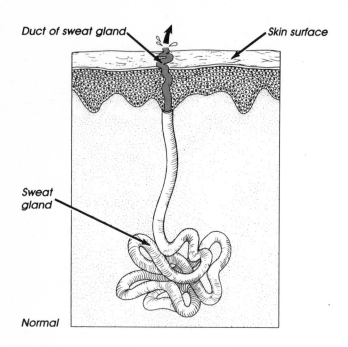

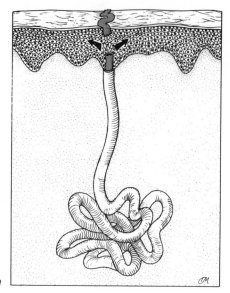

Duct of sweat gland

Skin surface

Sweat gland

Normal

Heat rash

*A sweat gland normally releases sweat through its duct onto the skin's surface. When perspiration cannot reach the skin's surface, perhaps because of folds of fat or tight clothing, heat rash results. When this happens, the sweat may break through the wall of its duct and become trapped in an internal layer of skin, causing inflammation and rash.*

The fact that your baby responds to loud noises may be misleading. Most children with a significant hearing impairment will have some hearing. They will respond to loud noises, but miss most other sounds.

If you suspect that your child has a hearing problem, speak to her doctor. Early treatment is important for her normal language development.

## Heart Murmurs

A heart murmur is an extra sound made by the heart. Normally, the blood flows through the heart smoothly and quietly. If there is any turbulence or disruption of the flow, a murmur is heard. Experts believe that at least half of all newborns have a murmur, although most are very hard to hear. Usually these murmurs do not mean that heart disease or abnormalities are present. Such murmurs are called *innocent murmurs, insignificant murmurs,* or *functional murmurs.* Most children outgrow their innocent murmurs by adolescence.

Innocent murmurs may be found when your baby is still in the hospital. During the routine examination in the nursery, your doctor will listen to your baby's heart with her stethoscope. If your doctor finds a murmur, she may want to have fur-

ther testing done to make sure there are no heart problems. These studies may include blood tests, an electrocardiogram, x-ray films, and an echocardiogram (which uses sound waves bounced off the heart to form an image).

Innocent murmurs require no treatment and don't limit your child in any way. Your baby will grow normally, and the murmur probably will disappear in time. If your doctor finds a significant murmur, your baby will most likely be referred to a pediatric cardiologist (a physician who specializes in the heart problems of children).

## Heat Rash

Heat rash is a mild skin condition caused by temporary blockage of the sweat gland openings on the skin. Heat rash, also known as prickly heat and miliaria, affects almost all babies when their skin gets too hot. Although more common during hot, humid weather, it may occur whenever children get overheated. Fair-skinned children (redheads and blonds) get heat rash more frequently than other children, and they suffer more from it.

Heat rash consists of hundreds of tiny, pinhead-sized, pink or red eruptions, or bumps, each surrounding a pore. Sometimes they resemble tiny water blisters. They may itch a lot. The rash usually appears on your child's cheeks, neck, and shoulders and in skin creases and the diaper area.

Treatment is simple—cool down your child's skin. Cool baths and proper dressing are both the treatment and the best prevention. The best rule of thumb for dressing your baby is not to put more clothes on your baby than you would wear. If it's too hot for *you* to wear a sweater, then don't put one on your child.

## Hernias

A hernia is a protrusion of tissue through the wall of a body cavity. It's similar in concept to an inner tube sticking through a hole in a tire. There are several different types of hernias.

Inguinal hernias are the most frequent. These are the common "ruptures" that occur in the groin area. An inguinal hernia may be present from birth, but usually is not noticed for a few months. The hernia begins as a bulge just above the midpoint of the crease of the groin. Over time, the bulge enlarges and moves toward the genitalia. The bulge is actually a pouch-like sac under the skin, made of peritoneum (the lining of the abdominal cavity). Some of the small intestine is in the pouch. The bulge may come and go depending on how much of the intestine is in it at any time.

Another common hernia is the umbilical hernia. A baby with this problem has a large, protruding belly button that gets bigger when he cries. This is not a true hernia because it contains no sac. An umbilical hernia appears if a baby's abdominal muscles don't completely close. The lack of closure leaves a gap. Changes in pressure in the abdominal cavity cause this weak spot to bulge. There are many old wives' tales about umbilical hernias. The best treatment is no treatment. Most go away by the time a child is five years old. Taping, belts, and other such measures don't help and may cause skin irritation.

Most hernias cause no pain and bother you more than your baby. If you can easily push the hernia down and flat, it's a "simple" hernia and needs no emergency attention unless it gets bigger or seems to cause your child discomfort. (However, as a general rule, it is best to bring any hernia to your doctor's attention.) An "incarcerated" hernia can't be pushed flat. A loop of intestine is trapped in the sac and can't get out. Such a

hernia does need treatment before it becomes "strangulated" (that is, the blood supply to the contents of the hernia is cut off), and the tissue dies. Strangulated hernias cause a lot of pain and swelling. Surgery is needed immediately to correct this situation before the tissue dies.

## Hives

Hives (urticaria) is an allergic reaction of the skin. About twenty percent of children have hives one or more times. Any area of the skin may be affected. Hives are usually caused by a reaction to foods, beverages, medicines, or something in the air. Common hive-causing substances include citrus fruits, chocolate, nuts, tomatoes, berries, spices, candies, tropical fruits and fruit juices, and artificial food flavorings. Your child may react to something she has eaten many times before without any problems.

Hives is characterized by red, itchy, raised welts ranging in size from a quarter inch to several inches across. They appear and disappear rapidly. The pattern may change within minutes. Insect bites may look like hives, but they don't change as quickly.

Home treatment is aimed at relieving the symptoms. Cool compresses offer immediate relief. Special oatmeal preparations to be added to bathwater are available in drugstores. Another useful treatment is to fill a nylon stocking with ordinary oatmeal, soak it in water, and use it as a compress against the itchy areas. Antihistamines often reduce itching. If these treatments don't work, you should call your doctor.

Hives is rarely an emergency. However, sometimes a child may experience swelling of her tongue, making breathing and swallowing difficult. If this occurs, she needs to be seen **immediately.** Injections of epinephrine (Adrenalin) help bring down the swelling quickly.

## Impetigo

Impetigo is a highly contagious infection of the outer layers of the skin. Two different kinds of bacteria, *Staphylococcus* and *Streptococcus,* cause it. They are transmitted from child to child by direct contact, that is, by touching an infected person or something that person has been using (such as clothing, towels, or toys). It takes two to five days for the signs and symptoms to appear.

Impetigo frequently appears where there has been a break in the skin (for example, from a scratch, insect bite, or scrape). First a fragile blister appears, containing thin, yellow pus. The blister breaks, leaving an open, weeping sore that increases in size. The discharge hardens into a yellow crust, or scab, that looks like hardened honey. These lesions are often described as being "honey-crusted." Impetigo spreads rapidly, often helped by the child's scratching.

Once identified, impetigo can often be treated at home—if the rash is small. Since bacteria thrive under the crusts, scrub the areas involved with soap and water. Several times a day, cover the area with a nonprescription antibiotic ointment. Keep the lesions covered to prevent further scratching. Don't reinfect your child by reusing the same washcloth. If your home treatment is working, don't stop until all the lesions have completely healed.

To prevent the spread of impetigo to other family members, keep your child's towels and washcloths separate from theirs. Wash his clothes and towels frequently. Ordinary laundering is sufficient.

If the rash doesn't improve or is spreading, your child needs to be seen by a doctor. Some children need antibiotics. Penicillin is used most often, although some bacteria are resistant to it. There are other antibiotics for these resistant bacteria. The bacteria involved can be identified only by cultures. Your doctor may decide to culture the discharge for this reason. Some infections cause kidney damage, although this is rare.

## Insect Bites and Stings

Your child may react in two different ways to insect bites and stings. If she's like most children, bites and stings are just a minor annoyance. There's itching, pain, and a little swelling. Impetigo or another infection may also develop at the site.

Some children have serious—sometimes life-threatening—allergic reactions to insect bites and stings. Bee and wasp stings are most likely to cause such serious reactions. If your child has a serious reaction, she may experience difficulty breathing because of swelling of her throat. She may suffer circulatory collapse: her blood vessels dilate (open up), and she faints.

Some specific insects cause special problems. Certain types of ticks may carry germs that cause encephalitis. Bites of the brown recluse spider often destroy tissue and cause a fever.

Flying insects usually bite exposed skin. Crawling insects bite anywhere, and often more than once in an area. Flea bites tend to be concentrated on the ankles and the lower parts of the legs of children who are walking. Bedbugs often leave three to five bites spaced an inch or two apart in a fairly straight line. Honeybees leave their stingers in the skin; bumblebees and many other stinging insects don't, so they can sting more than once. Ticks remain attached to the skin for long periods of time while they suck out blood.

You can treat most insect bites and stings at home unless your child has a severe allergic reaction. To lessen the itching and swelling around bites, apply ice as soon as possible after the sting. Calamine lotion and weak steroid creams lessen the itching and swelling. Antihistamines also help (check with your doctor first). If the bite is infected, antibiotic creams are helpful (again, check with your doctor).

---

### Insect bites and stings

**Symptoms**

- Swelling

- Itching

- Stinger left in wound

- Small, dark bumps (ticks)

- Difficulty breathing or swallowing

**Treatment**

- To relieve swelling and itching, apply an ice pack.

- Use calamine lotion or topical hydrocortisone to treat the itching.

- Nonprescription antihistamines also help to relieve the itching.

- If your child begins to experience breathing or swallowing problems, seek medical help **immediately**.

Removing ticks can be tricky. If done incorrectly, the insect's head will stay in your child's skin, increasing the likelihood of infection. There are several different ways to remove a tick. You can touch it with the tip of a hot, unlighted match; gently pull it with tweezers; or gently scrape it off.

If your child has a severe allergic reaction to insect bites and stings, there are devices for injecting epinephrine that you can keep with you for emergencies. You'll need a prescription for one. Some children with allergies are given a series of shots to desensitize them.

## Jaundice

Many newborns have yellow-tinged skin, and the whites of their eyes turn a little yellow. The underlying problem, called neonatal jaundice, occurs in sixty percent of full-term babies and up to eighty percent of premature infants. In general, jaundice occurs because the liver is not working efficiently. One of the jobs of the liver is to transform bilirubin (a yellowish-red chemical released when old blood cells are broken down) into bile, which passes into the intestines. If the liver can't handle all the bilirubin released, it accumulates in the body, and jaundice results.

Unless it becomes marked, neonatal jaundice is considered normal. It usually begins in the second or third day of life, and disappears between the fifth and tenth days. With rare exceptions, this jaundice is harmless.

Breast-fed babies are more likely to have neonatal jaundice than formula-fed infants. No one knows exactly why this happens, but many doctors believe that there's a substance in breast milk that interferes with the proper functioning of a baby's liver. Switching to formula for a day or two almost always reverses the jaundice. Extra water sometimes helps. Sunlight or special full-spectrum, fluorescent lights called "bili-lights" are used to help break down the bilirubin that accumulates in an infant's skin. Your baby's doctor will determine the most appropriate treatment.

There are two different types of neonatal jaundice. The first is the normal jaundice that most newborns have. This is called physiologic jaundice and doesn't cause any long-term problems. Nonphysiologic jaundice has the potential for causing serious and long-lasting adverse changes, including mental retardation, if not treated promptly.

The two most frequent causes of nonphysiologic jaundice are infections and erythroblastosis fetalis. Infections may destroy red blood cells and injure the liver. This combination makes it especially difficult for the liver to transform bilirubin into bile. Erythroblastosis fetalis results from incompatibility between the mother's blood and the infant's blood. The mother's blood forms antibodies (protective substances that fight off disease or anything the body interprets as an attacking organism) against her infant's blood cells. The antibodies destroy the infant's red blood cells, increasing the amount of bilirubin in the blood. Sometimes transfusions are needed to remove the mother's antibodies from the infant's blood.

Although uncommon, jaundice can also occur in older babies and children. It can have a number of causes, including infection, abnormal red blood cell metabolism, bleeding, enzyme deficiencies, obstruction of the gallbladder or gastrointestinal tract, and liver disease or abnormalities in the formation of the liver.

Any evidence of jaundice in your child should be called to the doctor's attention.

## Laryngitis

Laryngitis is an inflammation of the larynx (vocal cords). Although related to croup, it isn't associated with any breathing difficulties. It's often caused by a virus. Sometimes it occurs from overuse of the vocal cords.

The most obvious symptom of laryngitis is hoarseness. Your child may also have a dry, hacking cough and complain of a dry throat. If the laryngitis is caused by a virus, she may have a low-grade fever. There are no breathing problems.

There's nothing your doctor can prescribe to speed up the healing. Some children find that added moisture in the air from a humidifier helps. Drinking warm fluids soothes the throat. Discourage your child from talking to give her vocal cords a rest. Acetaminophen eases the discomfort. If the hoarseness persists for more than two weeks, the child should be seen by her doctor.

## Leukemia

Leukemia is a cancer of the white blood cells. It can afflict children at any age, but most fre-

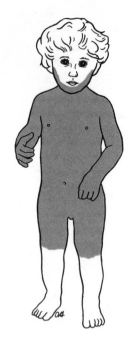

The measles rash–dark red spots that blend together as they spread–usually begins on the face, neck, and behind the ears and then spreads over the body as far as the knees.

quently occurs in children three to four years old. Although rare, leukemia is the type of cancer most frequently seen in children.

The typical signs and symptoms of leukemia are as follows: anemia, as indicated by paleness, weakness, and fatigue; bruises that appear on the body for no apparent reason and in places where you wouldn't expect to see them; swollen, red, bleeding gums; a fever; swelling of the lymph nodes without pain or redness; bone pain; frequent heavy nosebleeds; and blood in the urine and feces.

If your child's doctor suspects leukemia, he will order blood tests to look at the white cells. The diagnosis is made by examining a specimen of your child's bone marrow (the material in the center of bones).

If you are concerned that your child may have leukemia, take her to the doctor. Let the doctor know about your concerns. There are a number of other illnesses that cause many of the symptoms of leukemia. If your doctor shares your concern, he will order the necessary tests.

There are many effective drugs for leukemia. They result in long periods of remission. The sur-

vival rate for childhood leukemia has also been rising over the last few years because of newer, more effective drugs.

## Measles

Measles, medically called rubeola, is a highly contagious viral disease. It is spread from person to person in airborne droplets of moisture from an infected person's respiratory system. After exposure, it takes ten to twelve days for symptoms to develop. A child with measles is contagious during the period from five days before the rash appears through four days after the rash appears.

Measles was once a very common and often dangerous childhood disease. Since the MMR (measles-mumps-rubella) vaccination became a standard part of routine infant care, the number of cases of measles has fallen dramatically.

Most children are vaccinated when they are fifteen months old. If a child is vaccinated at a younger age, his body isn't capable of making antibodies (substances that fight infection), so the protection is very short-lived. A newborn receives temporary protection against measles from his mother, provided that she has had measles.

If your child is coming down with measles, he'll have a runny nose, reddish eyes, a cough, and fever. After three or four days, his temperature will rise, his cough will worsen, and a heavy, splotchy, red rash will appear on his neck and face. The rash will spread quickly over his trunk, arms, and legs. Once the rash has fully erupted, his fever will break, and he will soon be on the road to recovery.

If your child gets measles, the only treatment is to keep him comfortable. Acetaminophen may be given to lessen the aches and fever. A nonprescription cough suppressant may ease the cough (check with your doctor first). Keep your child away from bright lights; they may bother him, although the light will not injure his eyes.

Measles has the potential for causing serious problems. It's not the measles itself that is dangerous—it's the possible complications, such as pneumonia, ear infections, and encephalitis (inflammation of the brain). If a child with measles gets worse, complains of an earache or neck pain, has problems breathing, coughs up a lot of phlegm, or becomes lethargic, call your doctor. A complication of measles may be present.

## Meningitis

Meningitis is an infection of the meninges (the covering of the spinal cord and brain). Most often it's caused by a virus, although there are three bacterial strains that can also cause meningitis—*Meningococcus, Pneumococcus,* and *Hemophilus influenzae.* Meningitis is seldom spread by direct contact. Carriers (people who have no symptoms but harbor the organism) spread the disease. The germs responsible are transmitted in droplets in the air and inhaled into the respiratory system. Meningitis may arise as a complication of a skull fracture if the fracture extends into the nose, middle ear, or sinuses. It may also follow a respiratory tract infection or ear infection.

A child with meningitis has a moderate to high fever, headache, vomiting, exhaustion or collapse, convulsions, and a stiff neck. He will not touch his chin to his chest (with a closed mouth) because of the pain. The combination of fever and petechiae (purplish-red spots) scattered all over the body may indicate meningococcal meningitis.

Meningitis is a medical emergency. If you suspect your child has it, **contact your doctor right away.** She will want to see your child. There are many tests she will perform, but perhaps the most important is a spinal tap. Although it sounds scary—putting a needle into your child's spine—the test itself is relatively safe and is essential to make the diagnosis.

## Molluscum Contagiosum

Molluscum contagiosum is a horrible-sounding name for a relatively harmless skin problem. This viral disease has a long incubation period (the time from exposure to the appearance of symptoms) of two to seven weeks. It can be spread by direct contact.

The skin eruptions are plump, round, and slightly waxy, with a small depression in the center. They usually appear on the face, back, arms, and buttocks.

There are many different treatments for this condition. Your doctor will decide which one is best.

## Mumps

Mumps is a moderately contagious viral infection that affects the salivary glands. The measles-mumps-rubella (MMR) immunization contains an effective vaccine against mumps. In an unimmunized child, symptoms appear two to three weeks after exposure to the virus. A child with mumps is contagious from two or more days before the symptoms appear until all the symptoms are gone. A child who has the mumps develops a lifelong immunity. If your child has had the mumps or the MMR vaccine, and then has symptoms of mumps, he probably has a different infection of his salivary glands.

Mumps itself causes some discomfort, but no serious problems. However, some of the complications of mumps are very serious. They include meningitis, encephalitis, permanent deafness, and orchitis (inflammation of the testicles). It may also affect the ovaries and pancreas.

If your child has the mumps, he may have a temperature of as low as 101 degrees or as high as 105. His appetite will be decreased, and he'll have a headache. After one or two days, his salivary glands will swell, giving him a chipmunk-like appearance, and he may have some pain. The swelling lasts a week and then goes away.

There is no treatment for mumps except steps to make your child more comfortable. Acetaminophen, fluids, and rest are the mainstays of treatment. The development of abdominal pain may indicate that the ovaries or pancreas is involved. Signs of encephalitis or meningitis (see *Encephalitis* and *Meningitis*) are serious; if they are present, your child needs to see his doctor right away.

## Nosebleeds

Every child gets nosebleeds. They are usually caused by trauma—falls, hits, and fingers in the nose. Almost all the bleeding comes from rupture of small blood vessels near the tip of the septum (the tissue that divides the nose into two parts). These vessels are broken easily and bleed a lot. Allergies, dry air, sneezing, coughing, blowing the nose, and rubbing and scraping the septum may start a nosebleed. One of the most common causes of repeated nosebleeds is nose-picking.

When your child's nose begins to bleed, blood may come from both nostrils and from his mouth; he may even vomit some blood. Since both nostrils connect in the back of the nose, blood from one side may cross and come out the other side. The nose and mouth both open into the pharynx

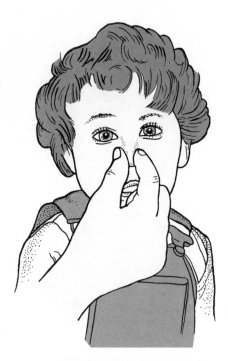

*An occasional nosebleed can be treated by sitting the child up and pinching the entire soft portion of the nose between your thumb and forefinger for ten minutes.*

(upper part of the throat), so your child may spit out nasal blood. Blood easily upsets a child's stomach, so a bloody nose may cause vomiting. The material vomited will contain blood from the nose.

Almost all nosebleeds can be treated at home. The best way to stop the bleeding is to pinch shut your child's nostrils for a full ten minutes. Checking any sooner to see if the bleeding has stopped only causes more bleeding. If pinching for ten minutes doesn't work, do it for another ten minutes. Only if two or three tries don't stop the bleeding do you need to call your doctor.

If your child has recurrent nosebleeds, you need to see if he is a nose picker. Some children pick their noses while asleep. If this is the problem, trim your child's nails very short, or have her wear mittens when she sleeps to prevent nighttime nose-picking.

Coating the septum with petroleum jelly or antibiotic cream will help to heal the raw area. Sometimes a vaporizer helps by humidifying the air.

If your child has nosebleeds and you can't find any cause, you should discuss this with your doc-

tor. There are some bleeding diseases that cause this problem.

## Pinworms

One of the most common causes of nighttime rectal itching is pinworms. These worms live in the large intestine. At night the female pinworms crawl from the anus and lay their eggs on the skin around the anus. Their movement causes the itching, which may be severe enough to awaken your child.

The best way to diagnose pinworms is to see them yourself. The worms look like thick white thread a quarter- to a half-inch long. If you suspect pinworms, the best time to check is when your child is sleeping. Spread apart her buttocks and shine a light on her bottom. If she has pinworms, you'll see them crawl toward the anus.

Children can pick up the microscopic pinworm eggs from other children or from areas contaminated with the eggs. The eggs are all around, so it's surprising more children don't have problems with pinworms. The eggs are swallowed, and hatch into larvae (the immature form of the pinworm) in the large intestine, where they mature in two to six weeks. The adult females then lay their eggs around the anus. If they are picked up there (generally by scratching) and transmitted to the mouth on the child's hands, the cycle continues.

Sometimes the egg-laying pinworms get "confused" and crawl into the wrong place. If they enter the vagina, they may cause itching there. If they enter the urethra (the tube that brings the urine from the bladder to the outside), some of the signs and symptoms of a urinary tract infection may develop.

Treating pinworms is simple. Many doctors will prescribe the medicine over the phone without seeing your child. Some doctors believe the whole family should be treated if one member has pinworms. Other physicians treat only those who have pinworms.

If your child has pinworms, you need to launder her underwear, pajamas, and bedding to kill all the eggs. Cut your child's fingernails short to lessen the chance of her picking up the eggs there when she scratches her bottom. Make sure she washes her hands frequently to lessen the chance of transferring eggs from her bottom to her mouth.

## Pneumonia

Pneumonia is an infection of one or more areas of the lungs. It's a respiratory infection like bronchitis, bronchiolitis, the common cold, and sinusitis, but each of these diseases affects a different part of the respiratory system.

There are many different germs that cause pneumonia: bacteria, including pneumococcus, streptococcus, and staphylococcus; viruses, such as influenza virus, parainfluenza virus, respiratory syncytial virus, and adenovirus; and mycoplasma, an organism considered somewhere between a bacterium and a virus.

For your child to have bacterial pneumonia, she must have been exposed to an organism that causes it. But that alone is usually not enough because many children are exposed to these organisms all the time. Her own defenses must be down, such as from a cold or other infection. (This explains why some people's colds "turn into" pneumonia and why doctors don't consider bacterial pneumonia contagious in the usual sense of the word.)

Viral pneumonia is more contagious. It takes one to seven days after exposure for the symptoms to develop. It isn't usually as serious an illness. Often, children have viral pneumonia and feel only mildly ill. This explains why viral pneumonia is often called "walking pneumonia."

A child with bacterial pneumonia will have a mild upper respiratory tract infection followed by a sudden change in her symptoms. Her temperature will quickly rise (up to 105 degrees Fahrenheit). She may have chills, a cough, rapid breathing, and sometimes pain on both sides of her chest. An infant may have flaring of her nostrils and retractions (pulling in) of the soft spaces of the chest, and may make grunting sounds when she breathes out.

Viral pneumonia begins a little differently. The symptoms appear gradually. A child will complain of a headache, fatigue, fever of variable level (a temperature of 100 to 105 degrees), a sore throat, and a severe, dry cough. Most cases of viral pneumonia are mild and often are not recognized as pneumonia, but instead are mistaken for colds. The symptoms go away in ten to fourteen days.

Your child will need to be seen by his doctor to diagnose pneumonia. After an examination, the doctor may order a chest x-ray film to look for changes in the lungs. Blood tests are frequently needed.

If your child has viral pneumonia, treat it as you would a cold. Only if his breathing becomes labored or he's not doing well is any other treatment necessary. Antibiotics don't help a patient with a viral illness.

The treatment of bacterial pneumonia is different. In the past, all children with this type of pneumonia were hospitalized. Now only the very youngest and those who are very ill are put in the hospital. Others are treated at home with antibiotics.

## Poisoning

Young children, because of their curiosity and their inexperience, are constantly at risk for poisoning. Knowing what to do (and what not to do) in an emergency can save your child's life.

It is a good idea to contact your regional poison control center *before* an emergency arises. Confirm their phone number and find out if the center is staffed with poison control specialists twenty-four hours a day. If not, try to find a center that is—and keep their phone number handy.

An equally important way to be prepared for poisoning emergencies is to stock your medicine chest with syrup of ipecac and activated charcoal (a special liquid form of charcoal). Both can be obtained without prescription from any drugstore. Syrup of ipecac is an emetic (a substance that makes one vomit). (Check the expiration date periodically to be certain of effectiveness.) Activated charcoal works by being incredibly absorbent—when swallowed, it will absorb a wide variety of substances from the stomach (including some of those poisons that should not be vomited out) and prevent them from entering the bloodstream.

The first step in preventing poisonings is to keep all medicines, cleaning substances (the most common cause of poisoning in young children), paints, and anything else you don't want your young child to eat or drink in places where he can't get to them. Many poison control centers provide information on childproofing your house; some will even send packets of "Mr. Yuk" stickers for labeling poisonous materials, so that your child will learn to identify and avoid these dangerous

## Poisoning

### Signs and symptoms

- Many times, none

- Traces of the poison on your child's mouth, face, hands, and clothes

- Rapid breathing

- Nausea and vomiting

- Overexcitement

- Unconsciousness

- Burns on lips or tongue

- Abdominal pain

### Treatment

- Get the poison away from your child, and make sure there's none left in his mouth.

- Find out what your child took, how much, and when.

- **Call your local poison control center.**
  Telephone number _____ – _____

- Keep syrup of ipecac at home, and give it if instructed to do so.

- If your child is acting abnormally (for example, if he seems uncoordinated or disoriented, or if his speech is slurred), seek medical care after talking with your poison control center.

- Do *not* wait for symptoms to occur before calling the poison control center.

It's usually easy to tell if your child has taken a poison. He may tell you, or you may see an empty bottle lying around. If your child is behaving strangely, suspect poisoning. The telltale signs of aspirin overdose are rapid breathing, ringing in the ears, nausea, overexcitement, and eventually unconsciousness. If your child drank an acid or alkaline liquid, there will usually be burns on his mouth and lips. Many liquids have a distinctive odor that may be a tip-off.

The first step in treating poisoning is to get the remaining poison away from your child. If there's any poison left in his mouth, have him spit it out. Then **call your regional poison control center right away,** before you call your doctor, the hospital, or anyone else. They will need to know your child's age and weight; what he ate or drank, how much, and when; and whether you have syrup of ipecac or activated charcoal available. They can then tell you what you should do. Treatment differs for different types of poisons. What's right for one may be wrong for another.

*Make every attempt to contact a poison control center, hospital, or doctor.* If professional help is unavailable, follow these general guidelines before taking your child to the nearest emergency room:

Don't attempt any treatment if your child is unconscious or very woozy. Concentrate your efforts on getting him to a medical facility.

Most poisons should be gotten out of a child's stomach (by vomiting) as soon as possible; however, others are better left in the stomach temporarily. As a general rule, if your child has taken a normally edible substance (such as a medication), induce vomiting with syrup of ipecac. If he has taken an acid or alkaline substance or any substance that's not normally edible (gasoline or furniture polish, for instance), do not induce vomiting—just get him to a hospital. (See the table for a list of some substances that should not be vomited.) Read the label on the bottle or container of the substance ingested; many product labels tell you if you should try to induce vomiting.

Syrup of ipecac is the best medicine for inducing vomiting. For children under one year of age, give one to two teaspoonfuls of syrup of ipecac; for children over one year of age, give three teaspoonfuls. Follow the dose immediately with one or two glasses of water. Leave for the nearest medical facility. Don't expect immediate results. It takes

substances. Put safety locks on all cupboards. Never store a dangerous substance in anything but its original container. Don't keep medications in unlabeled bottles. Use child-resistant caps on all bottles. Many drugs look and taste like candy; teach your child that medicine isn't candy, and don't present medicine or vitamins as a treat.

## Do not induce vomiting if your child has swallowed:

| | |
|---|---|
| Acids | Glue |
| Ammonia | Insect spray |
| Benzene | Kerosene |
| Bleach | Lye |
| Carbon tetrachloride | Oven cleaner |
| Cleaning fluid | Paint thinner |
| Correction fluid | Polishes |
| Dishwasher detergent | Solvents |
| Drain cleaner | Tobacco products |
| Furniture polish | Turpentine |
| Gasoline | |

five to ten minutes for ipecac to work. If you get no results, give your child more water. Don't give your child milk; it may lessen the effectiveness of the ipecac and make it more difficult to see what is in his vomitus (the material he throws up). Don't use syrup of ipecac and activated charcoal together; the charcoal will absorb the ipecac before it can work. If there are no results in twenty to thirty minutes, repeat the ipecac dose (only if the child is over a year old). Once begun, vomiting may continue for twenty to thirty minutes.

If the ipecac doesn't work, your child may need to have his stomach pumped. A flexible plastic tube will be put into his nose and down into his stomach. Although the insertion is uncomfortable, it's necessary to allow the doctor to clean out your child's stomach.

Even if you think that the danger has passed—your child seems to have vomited all the poison and to be feeling all right—take him to a medical facility as soon as you can. (Bring a sample of the poison and the vomitus, if available.) Effects of poisons are not always immediately apparent, and delayed reactions are possible.

If your child inhaled a poison (for example, carbon monoxide from car exhaust fumes or from a blocked chimney), *immediately* remove him from the vicinity of the fumes to fresh air. Then contact the emergency room or fire department.

For more information about poison prevention, and for a list of common household poisons, see "Safety at Home" later in this chapter.

## Reye's Syndrome

Reye's syndrome is a relatively rare, noncontagious disease that usually starts while a child is recovering from a viral infection. This serious disease is a type of encephalitis (inflammation of the brain). Although it affects several organs, the liver and brain suffer the most damage. The brain swells, and fatty deposits collect in the liver, kidneys, heart, and pancreas. If Reye's syndrome isn't diagnosed and treated quickly, it may cause permanent brain damage, coma, and death.

The cause of Reye's syndrome isn't known. It usually follows a viral infection. Some doctors think it's caused by a virus that has not yet been discovered. A link between Reye's syndrome and treatment of a viral disease with aspirin has been reported. Although a causal relationship hasn't been established, many doctors caution against using aspirin for any viral illness, especially chicken pox and respiratory tract infections.

Suspect Reye's syndrome if a child recovering from a viral infection suddenly starts vomiting and becomes unusually drowsy, overactive, or confused. As the disease progresses, it can cause convulsions and unconsciousness.

If you think your child has Reye's syndrome, call your doctor *immediately.* Your child needs to be seen so testing can be done to determine if he indeed has Reye's syndrome. There is no cure for Reye's syndrome. Treatment consists of supportive care to help your child withstand the disease until it has run its course.

## Roseola

Roseola proves that a high fever doesn't necessarily mean your child has a serious infection. The hallmark of roseola is a high fever (104 to 106 degrees) *without* other symptoms. The fever lasts for three or four days and is difficult to control with acetaminophen. The fever disappears abruptly; at the same time, a splotchy, red rash appears,

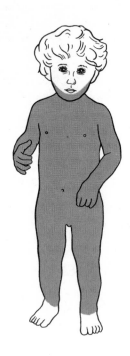

*The light pink rubella rash first appears on the face and the neck and then gradually spreads over most of the body.*

first on the trunk and then on the arms and neck as well. The rash is gone in a day or two, and the child feels perfectly normal.

Roseola is believed to be caused by a virus, although the actual virus has yet to be found. It takes seven to seventeen days from the time of exposure for the fever to appear. Roseola often occurs in epidemics. Once your child has roseola, he'll never get it again.

Contact your child's doctor so that he can confirm the diagnosis and rule out other possible causes of high fever. If your child has other signs and symptoms (such as a cough, vomiting, diarrhea, eye or ear discharge, or extreme fatigue), your child probably doesn't have roseola, and you should, again, contact the child's doctor.

## Roundworms

Roundworms (*Ascaris lumbricoides*) are, after pinworms, the second most common worm found in children. The worms live and lay their eggs in soil. Children may eat soil containing the worms or get some of the eggs under their nails and then put their hands in their mouths. The worms then grow and reproduce within the body.

If your child has a roundworm infestation, she may have no symptoms at all, or you may find an adult roundworm in her diaper one day. Some children do have abdominal pain, loss of appetite, weight loss, irritability, and short episodes of fever. In very young children, large numbers of worms may cause intestinal obstruction.

Treatment is easy and fairly effective. There are a number of different medicines your doctor may prescribe. Many infestations have no signs or symptoms, and clear up within a year unless the child ingests more eggs.

## Rubella

Rubella, commonly called German measles, is one of the milder contagious diseases for children, yet one of the most serious for pregnant women. Rubella can seriously damage the fetus of a woman who contracts it during her first three months of pregnancy. Her baby has a fifty-fifty chance of having birth defects, such as cataracts, heart problems, deafness, or mental retardation.

Rubella is caused by a virus. It's transmitted by direct contact with an infected person or by contact with articles contaminated by urine, stool, or secretions from the nose or throat of an infected person. The incubation period (the time from exposure to the appearance of symptoms) is fourteen to twenty-one days. Once your child has rubella, or is immunized, he has lifelong immunity.

If your child gets rubella, the lymph nodes in front of and behind his ears, at the base of his skull, and on both sides of his neck will swell and become tender. In a day or so, a fine or splotchy, dark-pink rash will appear on his face. The rash will spread over his entire body in twenty-four hours, last about three days, and then begin to lighten and disappear. Your child may have a low-grade fever (100 to 101 degrees) and slight redness of his throat and the whites of his eyes.

A child with rubella is contagious for a few days before the symptoms begin until four or five days after the rash appears. Infants born with rubella may be contagious for up to one year.

The signs and symptoms of rubella are fairly distinctive. Your doctor may confirm the diagnosis with tests.

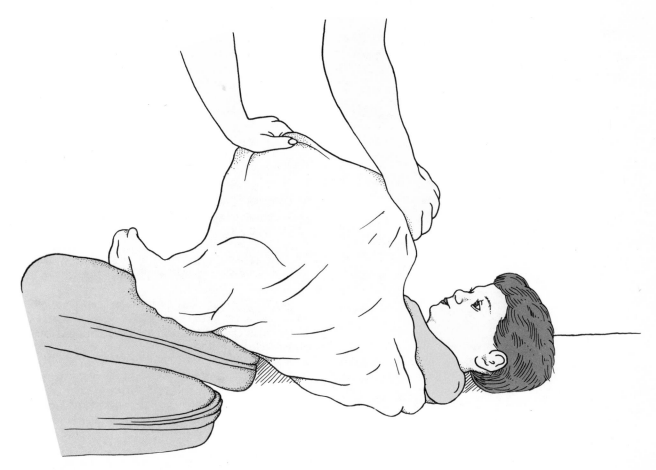

*Shock is a medical emergency. Keep the child warm and still, and call for professional help.*

If your child gets rubella, the only treatment is to keep him comfortable. Acetaminophen may be given to lessen the fever. The itching can be alleviated by applying calamine lotion or oatmeal compresses (see *Hives*) to the rash.

## Shock

Shock is the term used to describe a sudden drop in blood pressure or a collapse of the circulatory system. The amount of blood in the vessels is not enough to meet the needs of the body. Shock is extremely serious. If not treated promptly and appropriately, it is usually fatal.

There are two mechanisms behind shock. The first occurs when a child loses a great deal of blood, and there isn't enough left to meet his body's needs. The second cause is a general dilation (expansion) of his blood vessels. Blood vessels have muscles in their walls that cause them to dilate and constrict (narrow in size). If all the blood

vessels in the body open up at once, there's not enough blood to fill them. If this condition lasts very long, shock will occur. The danger of shock exists in virtually every case of serious accident, injury, burn, or poisoning. Shock can occur with almost any illness, including severe infections, wounds, broken bones, hemorrhage (severe and uncontrolled bleeding), insect stings in people who are allergic to the insect venom, excessive vomiting or diarrhea, and reactions to certain drugs.

A child in shock is weak, feels faint, has a weak and rapid pulse, and is pale. His skin is cold and clammy. He may have a cold sweat with chills. His mouth is dry, and his breathing is rapid and shallow. He may appear restless and confused. If not treated, he may lose consciousness.

**Shock is a medical emergency** requiring professional help. Call for help while beginning life-saving measures. If your child is bleeding, stop it. Make sure your child's airway is open and he is

## Shock

### Symptoms

- Weakness

- Rapid, weak pulse

- Paleness

- Cold and clammy skin

- Dry mouth

- Chills

- Rapid, shallow breathing

- Cold sweat

- Nausea

- Restlessness

- Confusion

### Treatment

- Treat cause if obvious, such as bleeding.

- **Call for emergency help.**

- Keep your child warm and still.

- **Don't** offer any food or water.

breathing. The next step is to keep your child still and lying down. If there's no head injury, elevate his feet above his head. Cover him with a light blanket to prevent heat loss. Don't give him anything to eat or drink. Try to keep your child (and yourself) as calm as possible until an ambulance arrives.

## Sore Throat

Diagnosing and treating a sore throat (medically called pharyngitis) should be fairly simple and straightforward. The doctor can both see the infected area and easily get a culture. Unfortunately, it's not so simple.

Throat soreness can be caused by many different things. The most common causes are infections of the throat, either bacterial or viral. Infections of areas near the throat, such as the tonsils and adenoids, may be responsible for throat discomfort. Inhalation of fumes, such as smoke and chemicals, will irritate the throat. Severe dryness of the air will cause the lining of the throat to lose moisture and become painful.

It's difficult to be certain an infant or toddler has a sore throat because he can't always tell you what hurts. Swollen glands in his neck, difficulty swallowing, loss of appetite, and abnormal behavior may be clues that his throat hurts. A fever may indicate a throat infection. An older child will complain that his throat hurts, it hurts to swallow, or "there's something scratching my throat."

Many parents become concerned that any sore throat is a strep throat (see *Strep Throat*). Most of the time a sore throat isn't strep, but it should be checked out to be sure.

If your child complains of throat discomfort, take a look in his throat. Redness alone doesn't mean much since many different types of infection look red. If you see white spots on his tonsils, he probably has tonsillitis (see *Tonsillitis*).

Warm liquids will help soothe the discomfort. Acetaminophen will also help alleviate the pain and treat a fever. If the symptoms are severe, your child isn't eating, or the fever continues, your child needs to be seen by his doctor. She will examine your child and try to determine the cause of the sore throat. If she feels it's strep, she will prescribe antibiotics. These drugs don't help if a virus is causing the pharyngitis.

## Stomachache

When your child complains of a stomachache, she may be referring to discomfort that arises from any of a number of different organs—the stomach, small intestine, large intestine (colon), liver, spleen, pancreas, gallbladder, kidneys, urinary bladder, or reproductive organs. Fortunately, most stomachaches are mild and pass quickly. They are usually due to one of four common causes: constipation, acute digestive tract upset (caused by viruses, bacteria, improper diet, or changes in diet), emotional stress, or urinary tract infection. Other, less frequent causes of stomach pain are appendicitis, pneumonia, infectious mononucleosis, and hepatitis (see also *Colic*).

Most parents first think of appendicitis when their child complains of stomach pain. Making this diagnosis is often difficult. There are no signs and symptoms that are specific for an inflamed appendix. Your child may complain of pain anywhere in her abdomen, although it frequently begins around the belly button and moves toward the right and down. First she'll complain of nausea, then she'll vomit. She'll have pain when she moves, particularly if she jumps or goes over bumps while riding in the car. Unfortunately, these signs and symptoms are seen with many other illnesses. If you suspect appendicitis, contact your child's doctor.

Perhaps the most common cause of abdominal pain in children is problems with their bowel movements. Although constipation may be the problem, more often your child just needs to have a bowel movement. If the pain begins around mealtime, it's even more likely she needs to go to the toilet. Her abdominal pains begin around mealtime because the introduction of food begins to make her digestive tract, from her stomach to her colon, contract and relax. If her colon is full of stool, she may experience some pain. After she has a bowel movement, the pain will disappear.

Gastroenteritis (inflammation of the stomach and small intestine) is usually accompanied by nausea, vomiting, decreased appetite, and diarrhea. Your child will appear ill. Generally, the treatment for this is dietary (see also *Diarrhea; Vomiting; Dehydration*).

The stomach is an area in which children commonly "express" their stress. Just as adults get ulcers, children may have stomach problems from too much stress. The real solution is dealing with the stress. Your child's doctor may be able to help you with this problem.

The last of the common causes, a urinary tract infection, needs to be treated by a doctor. Your child will complain of pain with urination and will feel the need to urinate frequently although she passes very little urine. The urine may be dark, cloudy, or pink to red. The presence of any of these signs and symptoms requires a visit to the doctor.

The best treatment for most acute stomachaches is sympathy and caring. Having your child lie on her stomach often helps. A warm hot-water bottle may soothe her. Have your child try to move her bowels. Do *not* give your child any laxatives or antinausea medicines without checking with her

doctor first. If the stomach pain doesn't get better within twenty-four hours, or seems to be getting worse, call your doctor.

## Strep Throat

Many parents are fearful of strep infections. They have heard that horrible things may happen to children with a strep throat. Some parents consider strep throat an emergency. Although a child with strep throat should be treated by a doctor, it is generally not an emergency situation.

Strep throat is caused by bacteria called *group A hemolytic streptococci*. These bacteria are very common: twenty-five to fifty percent of school-age children are carriers, that is, they have the bacteria in their throat all the time and are without symptoms, but can pass the bacteria on to others. Strep throat is spread from child to child by throat or nasal secretions. It takes two to five days from the time of exposure to the appearance of symptoms.

It is very difficult to diagnose strep throat just by looking at your child's throat. Even the most experienced physicians are correct only fifty percent of the time when they look at sore and red throats. Throat cultures are one way to diagnose strep throat, but this method is far from perfect. About five percent of negative cultures are really "false-negative," that is, the child really has a strep throat, although for some reason the culture is negative. Nor does a positive culture necessarily mean your child has a strep infection; she may be a carrier with a viral sore throat.

If it's so hard to diagnose strep throat, you may wonder why doctors don't treat every suspected strep throat with penicillin. Doctors don't like to prescribe antibiotics (or any drug) unless there is a specific reason. Every drug has the potential for serious side effects. Overuse of antibiotics may cause bacteria to develop resistance to them, making it more difficult to treat infections by those bacteria, and may increase the risk of allergic reaction.

There are new, rapid strep tests that take fifteen to sixty minutes to perform. They are almost as accurate as cultures, which take two days. Many doctors use these newer tests as the basis for deciding whether to treat a sore throat with antibiotics.

There are three reasons to treat any infection, including strep throat. The first is to speed up recovery. There's some controversy about how much more quickly children with strep throat improve if treated with antibiotics. Some recent studies have shown that they start to feel better twenty-four to thirty-six hours sooner than untreated children.

The second reason for treating an infection is to prevent the complications and side effects of the disease. Scarlet fever (scarlatina) develops in some children with strep throat. Other complications of strep infections include nephritis (inflammation of the kidney), rheumatic fever, and rheumatic heart disease. Although there is some controversy, current research seems to indicate that these last complications may develop whether or not the initial strep infection was treated.

The third reason for treating an infection is to lessen its spread. There is continuing debate about the effectiveness of treatment as a way to lessen the spread of strep throat. Most doctors do treat children with strep throat. But it is sometimes difficult to know if the treatment really makes a difference.

If your child has a strep throat, she may complain of a headache, sore throat, swollen lymph nodes in her neck, and perhaps abdominal pain. (The abdominal pain is from swelling of lymph nodes in her abdomen.) Her temperature may rise. If she's going to have scarlet fever, the rash will appear in twenty-four to seventy-two hours. The rash is described as sandpapery, with fine, slightly raised red spots. The rash may last from three to twenty days.

Your child's strep symptoms can be treated with acetaminophen, fluids, and rest. She should be seen by her doctor for a definitive diagnosis. If the doctor prescribes antibiotics, make sure she takes all the medicine. If, instead of getting better, she gets worse while being treated, call your doctor.

## Sunburn

A sunburn is a first-degree burn of the skin (see *Burns*). Children with fair complexions are more likely to burn, although any child, even a black baby, may get a sunburn. Too much sun, even on a cloudy day, may lead to a burn. The rays of the sun penetrate water, so a child in a swimming pool will burn.

Sunburn causes your child's skin to become red (or darkened in color), blistered, and painful. The diagnosis is usually obvious. Treating a sunburn is similar to treating any first-degree burn. Applying cool compresses to the burned area will lower your child's skin temperature and be soothing. Don't break any blisters that form. If the burn is very painful, your doctor may prescribe a silver sulfadiazine cream. This type of medication helps to lessen the pain and may help speed healing.

Prevention is the most important thing with sunburns. Your child should be exposed to the sun slowly and gradually to prevent burning. Sunscreens are effective in keeping the harmful rays of the sun away from your child's skin. They are rated with a sun-protection factor (SPF) number, ranging from 1 (provides minimal protection) to 15 (affords maximal protection).

## Swallowed Objects

Young children like to examine just about everything with their mouths. This tendency can lead to problems—poisoning, choking, and swallowing dangerous objects.

Objects placed in the mouth may find their way down one of two passageways. If something starts to go down your child's trachea (airway) toward the lungs, she will begin to choke and will need help **immediately** (see *Choking*, page 217). If the object starts to move down the esophagus (food tube) toward the stomach and gets stuck, she will probably not choke (unless the object is so large that it also presses against the trachea), but she will have problems swallowing. She may drool because she can't swallow her saliva. An object lodged in the esophagus must be removed by a doctor.

Once an object gets into your child's stomach, the immediate danger is over. Most small objects (coins, marbles, paperclips, and even sharp objects like pins and small pieces of glass) will usually pass through the digestive system without problems. Occasionally something will cause an obstruction of the digestive tract or penetrate a segment of intestine. Abdominal pain, vomiting, and fever may develop. It may be a few days after she swallowed the object before the symptoms begin. She needs to be seen by her doctor. X-ray films will be taken. Metal objects and many glass, plastic, and wooden objects may be visualized. X-ray films may also show other problems, such as increased abdominal gas or a perforation of the intestines.

## Swallowed Objects

### Symptoms

- If the object went into your child's stomach, there may be no symptoms.

- Inability to breathe or cry

- Gagging or choking

- Pain in his throat or chest

- Difficulty swallowing

- Abdominal pain

- Vomiting

### Treatment

- If your child is choking, see *Choking* (page 217).

- If your child is in pain, **seek immediate medical help.**

To be sure that the swallowed object has passed through, you should check your child's bowel movements. Each bowel movement must be passed through a sieve. If the child has been potty trained, place a basin fashioned of window screening in the toilet bowl. Then, after the child has passed a stool, wash it through the screening with hot water.

Some objects may cause stretching of your child's rectum and a little bleeding.

There are no medicines, foods, or drinks that speed up the passage of swallowed objects. Some doctors recommend eating foods that increase the size of your child's stool, such as roughage, in an attempt to ease the passage of the swallowed object.

## Swollen Glands (Swollen Lymph Nodes)

Those little lumps your child gets in her neck or under her chin when she has a cold or an ear in-

fection are often called swollen glands. Actually they are swollen lymph nodes, and not glands at all. Lymph nodes are part of the body's defense system.

Lymph nodes are found throughout the body—they are located in front of and behind the ears, at the base of the skull, under the chin, down the sides of the neck, in the armpits, in the folds of the elbows, and in the groin. There are deeper nodes in the chest and abdomen, where they can't be felt.

All lymph nodes lie along thin-walled tubes called lymph vessels. These vessels resemble and roughly follow the course of the veins. They contain lymph, a slightly sticky, thin, clear liquid similar to the watery fluid that oozes from a scrape.

Lymph nodes are important in helping the body fight infection and disease. When lymph nodes become swollen and mildly tender, it's a sign that they are fighting an illness or infection. If the infection is in just one area, like an ear infection, only the nodes in that area swell. If the infection affects the entire body, all the nodes may swell. If the nodes are swollen and tender, with red streaks, the nodes themselves have become infected.

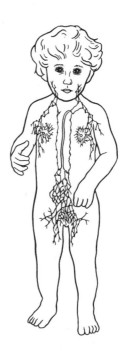

*Lymph nodes and lymph vessels are distributed throughout the body.*

Since swollen nodes are usually a sign of infection somewhere in the body, the best treatment is to find and treat that infection. Only if the nodes become infected themselves do they need treatment. If the nodes continue to enlarge, become tender, and turn red, your child's doctor, again, needs to be consulted.

Sometimes swollen nodes are the first sign of serious disease, such as lymphoma and leukemia (two types of cancer). Most swollen nodes are *not* a sign of cancer. If your child has swollen nodes without any signs of infection and the swelling doesn't go away, she should be seen by her doctor. Sometimes swollen nodes are not even painful. If they persist, these, too, should be seen by the doctor.

## Testicle, Undescended

During intra-uterine development, a boy's testicles begin their growth inside his abdomen. As he grows, they move down into his scrotum. At birth, both testicles should be in the scrotum. In one to two percent of term male babies, and in up to thirty percent of premature male babies, the testicles don't make it all the way into the scrotum before birth. In these cases, the testicles are "undescended."

An undescended testicle may be in the abdomen or the groin. Sometimes the testicle continues to migrate into the scrotum during an infant's first few months of life. Some babies have "reluctant" testicles—they move from the scrotum into the abdomen and back down again easily and frequently.

If you can't feel both of your baby's testicles during diaper changes, check them when he's in a warm bath. The heat often causes a reluctant testicle to enter the scrotum. Sometimes bending his knees toward his chest will help. If you can't feel both testicles, you should let his doctor know.

An undescended testicle left in the abdomen may become twisted, injured, or cancerous. If it's left in the abdomen too long, it won't be able to produce sperm.

If your son's testicle remains undescended, a urologist (a specialist in the urinary system) will need to examine him. Surgery is the standard cure for undescended testicles. Most often the operation is performed before the child is four years old.

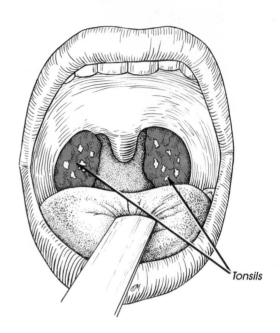

*Infected tonsils, such as these, are inflamed and display gray or yellow patches on their surface.*

## Tonsillitis

Your infant's tonsils (on both sides of her throat) and adenoids (in the back of her nose) are part of her lymphatic system. Just like the "glands" in her neck, these organs help her fight off infection. They become swollen when they have to work overtime. If her tonsils or adenoids become infected, it's called tonsillitis or adenoiditis.

An infected tonsil is red and large, and sometimes has white spots on it. Frequently you can see infected tonsils yourself quite easily. Many children have swollen tonsils that are not infected, and these rarely cause any problems.

A child with tonsillitis will complain of a sore throat and painful, difficult swallowing. A baby may have problems eating and act fussy. She may run a fever. Diagnosis can usually be made by looking at her tonsils, although sometimes a throat culture is needed. There's no way to easily see her adenoids. If the tonsils are infected, the adenoids are usually infected also.

Occasionally tonsillitis develops into a peritonsillar abscess (also called a quinsy sore throat). A large abscess forms behind a tonsil, causing intense pain and a fever of 103 to 104 degrees. The abscess may push the tonsil across the middle of the throat. A child with such an abscess will have trouble speaking and may drool. Peritonsillar abscesses need immediate treatment.

Most children with tonsillitis, adenoiditis, or both respond very well to penicillin or other antibiotics. If your child has repeated episodes of tonsillitis or strep throat, breathing problems from large tonsils, or nasal obstruction from large adenoids, or if she breathes through her mouth or snores, your doctor may consider having her tonsils and adenoids removed. In the past, it was almost routine to have a child's tonsils and adenoids removed. It is now thought that these tissues may play an important role in the function of the immune system and the defense against infections. Currently, doctors are less likely to recommend this surgery.

## Urinary Tract Infections

Your infant's urinary system consists of his kidneys, ureters (the tubes that bring the urine from the kidneys to the bladder), the urinary bladder, and the urethra (the tube that brings the urine from the bladder to the outside). Any part of this system can get infected, but the bladder is most likely to be the area of problems.

About five percent of all girls have a bladder infection (cystitis) or a kidney infection (pyelonephritis) at one time or another. Except during infancy, boys are much less likely to have a urinary tract infection (UTI) than girls. This has to do with the differences in the anatomy. It's easier for bacteria to enter a girl's urethra and migrate into the bladder or kidneys.

Any child with a UTI needs to be evaluated carefully. Over half of boys with a UTI have structural problems in their urinary systems. If such a problem isn't found and corrected, a boy will have more UTIs and is more likely to suffer permanent damage from them. Because only five percent of girls with UTIs have any structural problems, some doctors are not as quick to do extensive diagnostic testing with the first UTI in a girl. Recurrent UTIs, however, can be cause for concern and should be rigorously investigated.

A UTI may produce no symptoms at all, or may cause your child to be very ill. In infants, the signs and symptoms are often not very specific for a UTI: fever, fussiness, frequent urination, crying with urination, or cloudy or reddish urine. Older children will complain of feeling like they have to urinate all the time, yet will produce very little urine. It may

hurt or burn when they urinate; their urine may smell foul; and they may complain of back pain.

Diagnosing a UTI isn't always simple. Examination of your child's urine is the best way to determine if an infection is present. If your doctor believes your child has a UTI, he will prescribe antibiotics. Once the symptoms have cleared, he will decide if further testing is needed.

## Vision Problems

Your child learns more through her eyes than from any other sense. Proper sight is very important for normal development. Any problem, no matter how slight, may interfere. Vision problems that are ignored may be responsible for delayed learning, coordination problems, or difficulties in school.

Infants can see, although no one is sure exactly how well. At birth, infants are aware at least of light and dark; some doctors believe they can see considerably more than that. By three to five months they can distinguish colors. Depth perception begins at nine months, but doesn't fully develop until five or six years of age.

Certain eye problems can be diagnosed at birth, and examining the eyes is an important part of the newborn examination. Most newborns and infants can't control their eyes well, and their eyes may appear "crossed" now and then. If you suspect any vision problems with your child, discuss them with her doctor. Special testing is necessary to evaluate a young child's vision.

## Vomiting

Vomiting is a common problem during infancy and childhood. Most often, it's merely a nuisance, but it may be an indication of serious illness. Vomiting may interfere with your child's taking his medicines. In severe cases, it leads to dehydration.

Most infants spit up and occasionally vomit. If your infant is growing well, this vomiting shouldn't be a cause for concern. Excessive vomiting may indicate an intolerance to formula, food, or milk. Frequent vomiting during the first two months of life may indicate a narrowing of the passageway from the stomach to the small intestine (pyloric stenosis).

One of the most common causes of vomiting is coughing. Your child can't spit out the mucus he brings up from coughing. The only way he can get rid of it is to gag and perhaps vomit. Vomiting after coughing generally isn't a reason for concern.

Gastroenteritis (infection of the digestive tract) or an infection somewhere else in the body may cause vomiting. Unless the vomiting is so severe that dehydration sets in, there's little cause for concern (see *Dehydration*). Less common causes of vomiting are abnormalities of the brain (concussion, migraine, meningitis, encephalitis, tumors), poisoning, appendicitis, severe emotional distress, liver disorders, foreign bodies in the digestive system, abdominal injuries, and motion sickness.

If your older child is vomiting without any other signs or symptoms, dietary changes are the first type of treatment. Avoid solid foods, milk and milk products, and aspirin. Give your child sips of cool water and other clear liquids (such as carbonated drinks with all the bubbles stirred out, tea with sugar, and commercially available electrolyte solutions [such as Pedialyte]). Start with as little as a teaspoon every five minutes, then gradually increase to more normal amounts.

If home treatment isn't successful and the vomiting continues, contact your doctor. Sometimes children with continued vomiting need to be admitted to the hospital for administration of intravenous fluids.

## Whooping Cough

Whooping cough (pertussis) was once a rare disease in this country because of widespread immunization. Now, with more parents deciding not to immunize their children against pertussis, more cases are occurring. Whooping cough is caused by three different species of bacteria: *Bordetella pertussis* (the most common one), *Bordetella parapertussis*, and *Bordetella bronchiseptica*. The DPT (diphtheria-pertussis-tetanus) vaccine provides protection against only the first species. Contracting whooping cough caused by one species does not provide protection against the other two.

The incubation period (the time from exposure to the occurrence of symptoms) is seven to fourteen days. Whooping cough begins with a runny nose and a low-grade fever (100 to 101 degrees). The cough is initially mild, but becomes progressively worse over the next two to three weeks. The cough is worse at night than during the day and occurs in paroxysms (several coughs in a row without a break). At the end of a coughing spell, the child "whoops" (makes a strangling sound) as he sucks air into his lungs. Frequently, vomiting of thick mucus follows a whoop. The severe coughing and whooping may persist for another two to three weeks and gradually go away over the next three to six weeks.

Pertussis is very serious in infants under one year old; it can even be fatal. Newborns are not immune and do not get any protection from their mothers. All infants with whooping cough should be hospitalized.

If your child has whooping cough, there's little to do, unless the coughing and vomiting become so severe that she's getting dehydrated. A child with pertussis should be kept away from other children. Your doctor may prescribe the antibiotic erythromycin, which makes the disease less contagious and, if given soon enough, may shorten the course of the illness.

A partially or inadequately immunized child may contract a mild case of pertussis. It may be so mild as to lack most of the characteristic signs and symptoms of pertussis. If your unimmunized or partially immunized child is exposed to whooping cough, her doctor may prescribe a course of erythromycin to possibly lessen her chances of coming down with pertussis. She may also receive a booster immunization.

## Hereditary Illnesses

Happily, most children arrive in this world normal and healthy. By adulthood, children will have had their share of colds, coughs, and stomachaches. Compared with the usual childhood ailments, hereditary diseases are rare, but they do occur, and all parents should be informed about the more common ones. Genetic counseling is advisable for parents in certain high-risk groups.

### Genetic Basis of Disease

Central to any discussion of hereditary diseases is an understanding of the basis of heredity—the gene. Genes are bits of chemical information that determine all of our inborn characteristics. They are carried like beads on a necklace in structures called *chromosomes* within the nucleus of all cells.

Genes are composed of varying arrangements of molecules of *deoxyribonucleic acid (DNA)*. Each gene, by virtue of its unique DNA sequence, holds the code for a specific trait.

Except for the sex cells (eggs and sperm), each cell in the body contains forty-six chromosomes. Forty-four of the chromosomes are called *autosomes*. The two remaining chromosomes are the *sex chromosomes*.

The autosomal chromosomes are paired. For each pair, one chromosome comes from an individual's mother, the other from the father. Each gene on one chromosome is matched to a corresponding gene on the other chromosome. Thus, for every genetic trait, there are two genes, one on each chromosome.

The two genes that provide the code for a trait may not be identical. For example, if a gene pair governs eye color, one gene may code for blue eyes, the other for brown eyes. Because the gene for brown eyes is *dominant,* the eyes will be brown. The gene for blue eyes is said to be *recessive.* A person with brown eyes may also have two genes for brown eyes. For a dominant trait to be expressed, however, only one dominant gene is necessary. A person with blue eyes must have two genes for blue eyes. To express any recessive trait, a double dose of recessive genes is necessary.

Like eye color, certain illnesses are genetically determined. In some instances, the defective gene has been passed from generation to generation within a family. Parents may be aware of a family history of hereditary disease. Whether their baby develops that illness depends upon the inheritance of dominant or recessive genes.

## Autosomal Recessive Diseases

In most cases, a woman who inherits a defective recessive gene from one parent and a normal dominant gene from the other parent will not exhibit any symptoms of that illness but will be a *carrier* of that abnormal gene. However, if she has children with a man who is also a carrier, their children have a fifty percent chance of inheriting one defective gene and being nonsymptomatic carriers, and a twenty-five percent chance of inheriting two defective recessive genes and expressing the disease. (See figure 1.) This pattern is called *autosomal recessive inheritance.* The better-known of these disorders include sickle cell anemia, Tay-Sachs disease, and cystic fibrosis.

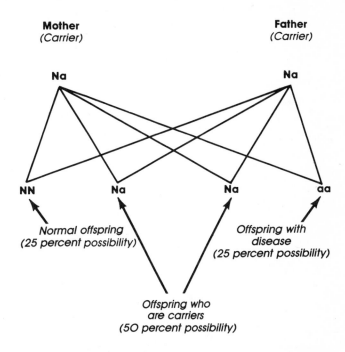

**Figure 1.**—*How autosomal recessive inheritance of disorders works. Each parent has two genes for each trait and contributes one of those genes to each offspring. If both parents are carriers, they have one normal gene* (**N**) *and one recessive abnormal gene* (**a**)*. As shown, three combinations are possible.*

### Sickle Cell Anemia

Anemia is sometimes caused by a deficiency of hemoglobin. Hemoglobin is the substance in red blood cells that carries oxygen to the other cells in the body. In sickle cell disease, the hemoglobin is abnormal. People who carry only one defective recessive gene usually have few or no symptoms of disease. People who inherited two sickle cell genes develop many problems due to the structure of their abnormal hemoglobin.

This defective hemoglobin molecule causes the normally round blood cell to sickle (assume a crescent shape). Anemia occurs because sickled red blood cells are more fragile, hence more easily destroyed. Sickled cells are also less able to bend as they squeeze through tiny blood vessels. Thus, these cells become trapped and obstruct small vessels. Episodic clogging of the vessels with sickled blood cells causes tissue damage and pain, especially in the hands, feet, joints, and abdomen. Children with sickle cell anemia are prone to more frequent infections than children without the condition.

At present, no cure for sickle cell anemia exists. Treatment includes administration of painkillers and antibiotics as necessary. With improved therapy, more children with sickle cell anemia are surviving into adulthood.

Because sickle cell anemia is most common among black persons, adults in this ethnic group are encouraged to be screened for being carriers of sickle cell anemia. Carriers can be identified by a simple blood test. Approximately one in ten black persons in the United States is a carrier. If both parents are carriers, they have a one in four chance of giving birth to a child with sickle cell disease. Sickle cell disease can be diagnosed before birth with the use of amniocentesis (see page 259 for explanation of this procedure). In many states, most newborn babies are screened for sickle cell disease at birth by a blood test.

### Tay-Sachs Disease

Tay-Sachs disease is a metabolic disorder marked by the accumulation of a type of fatty acid in the liver, spleen, and brain. It is caused by a deficiency in the enzyme that normally degrades this fatty acid. After four to six months of normal development, children with Tay-Sachs disease exhibit deterioration in their neurologic development. The disease progresses to mental retardation, blindness, and convulsions. Death usually occurs by the age of three or four. No treatment exists.

Preventive measures are available. The gene for Tay-Sachs disease is carried by one in thirty descendents of the Ashkenazim, the Jews of eastern Europe. Carriers have no symptoms of the disease and sometimes have no family history of the disease. It is recommended that all Jewish couples of eastern European descent be screened for the Tay-Sachs gene before they start their families. If both parents are carriers, diagnosis of Tay-Sachs disease in the baby can be made during pregnancy with the use of amniocentesis.

### Cystic Fibrosis

Cystic fibrosis is a serious childhood illness that causes the glands of the body to secrete abnormal sweat and mucus. The sweat glands secrete too much salt. The abnormally thick, sticky mucous secretions accumulate in and obstruct the lungs and pancreas. Since the pancreas is an important organ for digestion, these children fail to grow properly despite a healthy diet. The thick mucus in the lungs makes breathing difficult, and leads to infections. Death is usually due to respiratory failure. Although no cure exists, improved

treatment has brightened the prognosis of children with cystic fibrosis, giving them a good chance for survival into adulthood.

Cystic fibrosis is much more common in white persons of northern European extraction. In the United States, approximately five percent of white persons are carriers. One infant in every two thousand live births has cystic fibrosis. Traditionally, the disease has been diagnosed on the basis of sweat test results obtained only after the appearance of symptoms. Intensive research shows promise for much earlier diagnosis, including identification of carriers, prenatal diagnosis after amniocentesis, and postnatal diagnosis by a blood test.

### Phenylketonuria

Phenylketonuria (PKU) is a rare metabolic disorder that can cause severe mental retardation. It is caused by an inability to convert an amino acid called phenylalanine into another amino acid called tyrosine. (Amino acids are the building blocks of proteins.) At elevated levels, phenylalanine damages nerves, causing retardation.

In the United States, all newborns are screened for PKU by a blood test. Early detection and prompt treatment can prevent the mental retardation. Treatment consists of limiting a child's dietary intake of phenylalanine. If this dietary regimen is followed, children with PKU can have essentially normal development. Pregnant women who have PKU need to stick to this special diet to protect the baby's developing nervous system. New genetic research is in progress to help identify carriers of PKU and to diagnose this illness prenatally.

## Autosomal Dominant Diseases

Another category of hereditary disease is called autosomal dominant. Because the defective gene is dominant, the disease is expressed even if only one gene is defective. A normal gene cannot mask the harmful effects of an abnormal gene as it can in autosomal recessive disease. If one parent has an autosomal dominant disease, the chances are fifty percent that each child will inherit the disorder. (See figure 2.)

### Huntington's Chorea

An example of an autosomal dominant disease is Huntington's chorea, a brain disease

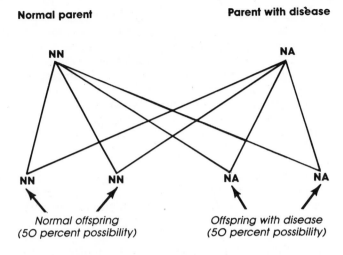

**Normal parent**          **Parent with disease**

*Normal offspring*          *Offspring with disease*
*(50 percent possibility)*  *(50 percent possibility)*

**Figure 2.**—*How autosomal dominant inheritance works. Each parent has two genes for each trait and contributes one of those genes to each offspring. A normal parent has two normal (N) genes. A parent with the disease has one normal (N) gene and one dominant abnormal (A) gene. As shown, only two combinations are possible.*

marked by abnormal body movements and mental deterioration beginning in middle age. Although a few medicines have been found to make the symptoms more tolerable, the disease is without cure.

Researchers have recently been able to identify carriers in families with Huntington's chorea by a genetic test. It is hoped that this procedure will be perfected and will also be extended toward prenatal diagnosis of babies doomed to develop this disorder.

## Sex Chromosomes and Sex Determination

As previously stated, most cells in the body have forty-six chromosomes, consisting of twenty-two pairs of autosomes and two sex chromosomes. The sex chromosomes determine whether a person is male or female. Women have two **X** chromosomes. Men have one **X** and one **Y** chromosome.

The sex cells (eggs and sperm) contain only twenty-three chromosomes—twenty-two autosomes and one sex chromosome. Each ovum (egg) contains one X chromosome. Half of a man's sperm carry an X chromosome; the other half carry a Y chromosome. During fertilization, the genetic material of the egg and sperm unite to create the full complement of forty-six chromosomes.

If the ovum is fertilized by a Y sperm, the baby will be a boy; fertilization by an X sperm results in a girl.

## X-Linked Recessive Diseases

In sex-linked inheritance, the gene responsible for the disease is located on the X chromosome. Usually, the abnormal gene is recessive. For these reasons, the resultant disorder is called an X-linked recessive disease. In a woman with such a defective gene, the effects of the abnormal gene will be masked by those of the normal gene on the other X chromosome. Although she will not have the disease herself, she will be a carrier, capable of transmitting the defective gene to her children.

In X-linked recessive disease, the Y chromosome lacks the corresponding normal gene to

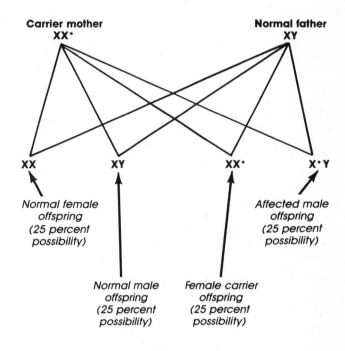

$X^* = $ abnormal recessive gene

**Figure 3.**—*How X-linked recessive inheritance works. Some diseases are caused by a defective gene found only on the sex chromosome received from the mother. A carrier mother has one female sex chromosome with a defective gene (X\*) and one normal female sex chromosome (X). A normal father has one normal female sex chromosome (X) and one male sex chromosome (Y). As shown, four combinations are possible.*

mask the harmful effects of the abnormal gene on the X chromosome. Thus, male offspring of a woman who is a carrier of an X-linked disease have a fifty percent chance of having the condition. All female offspring have a fifty percent chance of being carriers. (See figure 3.) Following are examples of X-linked recessive disorders:

### Color Blindness

In the most common form of color blindness, it is difficult to distinguish red from green hues.

### Hemophilia

In hemophilia, the blood does not clot properly. Hemophiliacs bleed excessively, even from minor cuts. The disease is managed by giving transfusions with the deficient clotting factor and with whole blood to replace blood losses. Research continues toward the accurate identification of female carriers and prenatal diagnosis of this disease.

### Duchenne Muscular Dystrophy

Muscular dystrophy refers to a group of rare diseases characterized by progressive muscular weakness. Duchenne type muscular dystrophy is the most common. Between the ages of two and six years, afflicted children develop weakness first in their legs and then in their arms and trunk. The weakness rapidly worsens. Most children die during their second decade, usually as a result of severe weakness of the muscles of respiration. The disease is without cure. Treatment includes physical therapy, braces, and, occasionally, surgery.

To date, detection of female carriers of Duchenne muscular dystrophy has not been precise. The test involves the measurement of a muscle enzyme in the blood in higher than normal amounts. The same enzyme is abnormally elevated in the fetus. Obtaining a fetal blood sample is, however, technically difficult. Because all male offspring of a mother who carries the abnormal gene have a fifty percent chance of having Duchenne muscular dystrophy, amniocentesis may be performed to determine the sex of the baby. Genetic tests are being developed for prenatal diagnosis and carrier detection of Duchenne muscular dystrophy.

## Multifactorial Genetic Diseases

Multifactorial genetic diseases are illnesses that tend to run in families. These diseases are not due simply to the inheritance of a single defective gene. Rather, a cluster of faulty genes is inherited, which predisposes the person to a disease. Given the appropriate environmental factors, the person may actually develop that disease. Examples of illnesses that run in families include such chronic adult diseases as coronary heart disease, high blood pressure, and stomach ulcers, as well as birth defects, such as cleft lip and palate and spina bifida.

In *cleft lip* (or harelip), the upper lip is divided by a vertical fissure. In *cleft palate*, the roof of the mouth is split by a longitudinal fissure. These two birth defects can occur alone or together. They are the result of incomplete fusion of the components that form the lip and mouth during fetal development.

*Spina bifida* is a failure in the closure of the bony vertebral column, with or without protrusion of the nerve tissue of the spinal cord. Paralysis below the defect often accompanies spina bifida if the spinal cord does protrude. When the spinal cord does not protrude, the vertebral defect may go unnoticed. Clues to indicate the presence of this form of spina bifida are abnormalities of the skin and tufts of hair overlying the spine in the lower part of the back. During pregnancy, spina bifida in the fetus can be diagnosed by ultrasound study and by detection of elevated levels of a substance called alpha-fetoprotein in the mother's blood and in the amniotic fluid that bathes the fetus.

## Chromosomal Abnormalities

Sometimes the structure or the number of chromosomes is not normal. Because more women are waiting until they are older to have their families, their risk of having a child with a chromosomal abnormality increases. If chromosomal abnormalities occur in the sex cells (eggs and sperm), the offspring may have physical and mental disorders.

### Down Syndrome

Formerly called mongolism, Down syndrome is a condition caused by a chromosomal abnormality. Due to the failure of the chromosomes to divide evenly during cell division, the affected person has an extra chromosome (a total of forty-seven). The presence of this extra chromosome causes a characteristic physical appearance and retarded physical and mental development.

Other ailments, such as defects in the heart and digestive system, can accompany this syndrome. Despite their handicaps, children with Down syndrome usually have pleasant dispositions and can do quite well if given special therapy.

The cause of the chromosomal abnormality leading to Down syndrome is unknown. A genetic predisposition may exist. The incidence of Down syndrome increases with increasing maternal age. The condition can be diagnosed prenatally with the use of amniocentesis. For these reasons, women who have previously given birth to a baby with a chromosomal abnormality or who are over the age of thirty-five are encouraged to undergo amniocentesis.

### Genetic Counseling

In recent years, tremendous progress has been made in the development of genetic tests to diagnose heritable diseases. You may wish to consult your physician about genetic counseling if:

- You have a family history of a hereditary disease or of mental retardation of unknown origin.

- You are a woman over the age of thirty-five.

- You have had a previous child with a chromosomal or other genetic disorder or any birth defects.

- You have had three or more miscarriages or a stillbirth.

If you have *any* concerns, ask your physician. (See Chapter 6 for additional information about complications of pregnancy and birth.) If you are considered to be at risk for passing on a hereditary disease to your children, you can receive genetic counseling. A genetic counselor will ask you about your personal and family medical history. Blood tests may be necessary to help determine whether you are a carrier of a heritable disorder. You will be advised about the chances of transmitting hereditary illness to your offspring.

If you are pregnant, the well-being of your fetus can be assessed by several procedures:

- *Ultrasonography.* High-frequency sound waves are used to produce images of the placenta and fetus. It is a painless procedure and can detect gross defects, especially of the heart, bones, brain, and spinal cord.

- *Amniocentesis.* Many genetic diseases can now be diagnosed prenatally with the use of amniocentesis. A small amount of amniotic fluid, the liquid that bathes the baby inside the uterus, is withdrawn and analyzed. Amniocentesis is usually performed between the fourteenth and eighteenth weeks of pregnancy.

- *Chorionic Villus Sampling (CVS).* This technique is still under investigation. A few fetal cells from the chorionic villus, a part of the placenta, are withdrawn and analyzed for the presence of a few select diseases. The advantage of CVS is that it can be performed earlier than amniocentesis. The disadvantage is that, currently, the risks of infection and miscarriage after the procedure appear to be higher than for amniocentesis.

- *Fetoscopy* is a procedure wherein the fetus is directly observed within the uterus by use of special lenses. During fetoscopy, fetal blood can be sampled. These procedures are currently performed only at a few medical centers for prenatal diagnosis of a limited number of serious diseases.

- *Radiography.* X-ray films are occasionally used because they can be helpful in detecting certain skeletal abnormalities.

Remember that the diseases described in this section are rare. Most expectant parents can look forward to the arrival of a healthy baby. If you are pregnant or hope to be and have any worries about the well-being of your future child, don't hesitate to address them to your doctor.

## Coping With a Sick or Dying Baby

Until two centuries ago, the death of a baby was an accepted, although tragic, risk of childbirth. Infectious diseases claimed many young lives. In mid-seventeenth century Europe, only one in four children survived to celebrate his fifth birthday. As recently as the late nineteenth century in the United States, one in five children died before the age of one. Largely due to improved hygiene, immunizations, and antibiotics, babies now die infrequently.

Although infant death is an uncommon occurrence, families sometimes have to cope with babies who have serious, chronic, and even fatal illnesses. Approximately ten percent of children in the United States suffer from illnesses that last over three months. Parents may walk an emotional tightrope between hope and despair for the long months that their child is ill.

Upon facing the diagnosis of serious illness in their infant or child, parents may at first feel nothing except shock and disbelief. Grief follows as a response to any loss. This loss may be the dissipation of their dreams of a healthy child. If the disease is expected to be fatal, parents may mourn in anticipation of the child's death. Despair, fear, anger, remorse, and loneliness are all emotions of the normal grieving reaction.

## Dealing With Guilt

Unfortunately, guilt is another emotion many parents feel when they learn that their infant is gravely ill. Parents can torment themselves with feelings of responsibility for the illness. If the baby has a hereditary disease, the feelings of self-blame may be especially overwhelming.

Self-reproach can be destructive. Negative feelings about oneself make it difficult for a parent to nurture the sick baby and the other members of the family. Guilt-ridden parents may either lavish excessive attention on the baby or turn away from her. Both responses amplify an older infant's or toddler's sense that something is wrong with her.

Parents may suffer further if communication between husband and wife is impaired. Their coping styles may be incompatible. Resentments may arise if one parent quits working to undertake the care of the sick child.

A child's illness need not inevitably impair a marriage. Couples who can turn to each other for comfort and who are able to communicate find the bonds between them greatly strengthened.

## Helping Siblings to Cope

Parents often wonder whether their other children are too young to be told about the fatal illness or death of their sibling. Most psychologists feel it is crucial that the other children be told the truth in a straightforward manner that they can understand. Children who are not informed will still know something is frightfully wrong and may invent their own fantastic explanations.

A child's ability to comprehend death and dying depends on his age and prior experience

with death (of a friend, family member, or pet). Before the age of two years, infants and toddlers are unable to grasp the concept of death. However, even very young children do react with distress to prolonged separations from loved ones.

After two years of age, given proper assistance from an adult, children are able to achieve a basic and concrete understanding of death. Still, they may have difficulty comprehending the permanence of death. Active imaginations lead to wild fantasies about where the deceased has gone. Because it is normal for children to have occasional negative feelings about their siblings, they may worry that their own thoughts or actions caused the illness. This sort of magical thinking and self-blame is especially common in children between the ages of five and eight.

A young child's response to the death of a sibling may be exasperating for parents. Using denial as a defense, he may act overtly as though nothing were wrong. Clues to inner turmoil include demanding, clinging behavior; regression to infantile behavior, such as lapses in toilet training; and increased aggression. Your warmth, understanding, and sharing of thoughts and feelings help him to grieve in a more appropriate fashion.

By eight to twelve years of age, a child's understanding of death is similar to an adult's. However, the severe illness or death of a sibling may make him overly fearful of his own mortality. (See Chapter 11 for more information about a child's understanding of death.)

## Caring for Your Baby

As the family grapples with the serious illness and perhaps imminent death of the baby, the infant must also cope with the consequences of her ill health. An infant's need to be cuddled is just as great as her requirement for food. She thrives on consistent care from her parents. A baby quickly comes to know and love these special people.

Separations, such as during hospitalizations, can be very distressing for an infant. Parents of children with chronic diseases can sometimes arrange to care for the child at home, with or without the assistance of a nurse. Should parents decide to bring their dying baby home, many communities have resources to assist them during this period (such as visiting nurses, home care nursing, and hospice care).

During necessary hospitalizations, most hospitals allow parents unrestricted visiting privileges and often provide facilities for parents to room-in with the sick infant or child. These arrangements give parents the opportunity to participate in the care of their sick baby. Caution must be exercised not to spend so much time with the ill child that the well-being of the parents and other members of the family suffers.

Things to do that can help you cope with an ill or dying baby include the following:

- Tell the physician and other hospital staff about your needs and the particular needs of your baby.

- Provide the hospitalized baby with her favorite toys and food. Display pictures of the family where she can see them. The entire family should visit the baby as often as is feasible.

- Obtain counseling with a skilled professional.

- Read about the subject. Most bookstores and libraries have many books for all age groups about coping with the illness or death of a loved one.

- Search out support groups, which exist for many types of chronic illnesses of childhood. There are also support groups to help parents adjust to the death of an infant.

- Allow siblings to visit the sick baby in the hospital.

- Attending funeral services that are brief and not morbid will help all family members to understand and accept the finality of their loss.

- Keep lines of communication open between family members. Families that can share their feelings and console each other learn that even an enormous loss can be mastered.

## Sudden Infant Death Syndrome

Although the death of any infant is tragic, the death of an infant from *sudden infant death syndrome* (SIDS) is perhaps the most traumatic. SIDS has caused the death of infants since the human race began. In biblical times, it was called *overlaying* (because it was thought that the mother had lain atop the baby in her sleep); it now is also known as *cot death* or *crib death*. Even though the causes of most diseases that have afflicted the human race eventually have been discovered, SIDS remains a mystery. It takes the life of an estimated eight thousand babies every year in the United States; based on this estimate, more than twenty babies in this country die of SIDS every day. SIDS deaths occur in families from all socioeconomic backgrounds, from all races, from all ethnic backgrounds, and from urban as well as rural areas. Autopsies have shown no consistent findings to indicate a cause of death. Although parents cannot anticipate or prevent SIDS, they need to be informed about it in case their child or the child of someone they know becomes a victim of a SIDS death.

Through the years, many theories about the cause of SIDS have been proposed, but none has been proved. Some of the more commonly investigated theories are:

- *Suffocation.* This may be the most commonly accepted theory because the baby is often found with the covers over his face and head. However, enough oxygen is usually available even under bedclothes to prevent suffocation. Furthermore, SIDS babies have been found without bedclothes, clothes, toys, or any other objects near their faces.

- *Pneumonia or some other unsuspected illness.* Although some SIDS babies have had a cold, sniffles, or other respiratory problem within days of the death, not all SIDS babies have had symptoms of these or other minor illnesses before death. Although the baby's doctor and the parents may wonder if they missed something, often no illness sufficient to cause the death is found at autopsy.

- *Allergy.* An allergy, especially to cow's milk, has been thought to cause SIDS. But babies who have been breast-fed exclusively also die of SIDS.

- *Getting too cold.* The baby may be cold when found, but this is a natural condition after death rather than the result of a lack of clothing or covering.

- *Child abuse or neglect,* or *an accidental injury.* Although it happens less frequently now, parents of SIDS babies have been accused of child abuse or neglect. These accusations were based on (a) the appearance of the baby (blood may pool at points where the body touched the bed, so the baby looks bruised), (b) the unexpectedness of the death, and (c) the lack of an apparent cause of death. These accusations make the death even more traumatic because the questioning and treatment by the authorities only increase the parents' normal guilt feelings. The parents need support at this time, not accusations. If the death was caused by abuse, neglect, or an accidental injury, evidence of this will be found at autopsy.

- *Choking.* Sometimes regurgitated food, or *vomitus,* is found in the baby's mouth or nasal passages, and the baby is thought to have choked on these substances. However, the series of events occurring at the time of death frequently includes vomiting and stooling, so these findings are most likely *results* of the death, not its cause.

- *Apnea (lack of breathing).* Many young infants have an uneven breathing pattern. Some even have periods, called *apneic episodes,* when they do not take a breath, sometimes for longer than twenty seconds. One theory is that, in some infants, the breathing apparatus is so underdeveloped that the baby does not start to breathe again after an apneic episode. Although babies with prolonged apnea may be at a greater risk for SIDS, most babies with apnea do not die of SIDS, and most SIDS babies were never observed to have prolonged apnea.

Other theories include such things as minor birth defects, botulism, nutritional deficiencies, immunizations, and lead intoxication.

The age at which SIDS most commonly occurs (two to six months of age) is a time in the baby's life when a number of events are occurring—for example, the baby may be switched from breastfeeding to bottle-feeding; the baby may be receiving immunizations; or the family may be socializing more. Researchers seeking a cause of SIDS have at various times tried to establish a connection between these and similar events and SIDS. For example, a baby may have died of SIDS shortly after a switch to cow's milk, raising the question of an allergy to cow's milk as a cause. SIDS may have occurred within days of the baby's receiving an immunization or being exposed to a person with a respiratory infection, which raised the question of immunizations or respiratory illness as a cause. But no link has been found between such ordinary events in the baby's life and SIDS.

Attempts to find a cause of SIDS are hampered by underreporting and misreporting of SIDS deaths. Only recently has SIDS been considered a separate disease entity, which means that it now can be given as an official cause of death. SIDS deaths have been, and in some instances still are, reported as caused by suffocation, pneumonia, and other ailments. In some jurisdictions, an autopsy is automatic for any death of unknown cause. In other areas, the parents must give permission for or request an autopsy. Many parents do neither, and the death may be officially listed as from another cause. Even if an autopsy is performed, there are few standardized procedures and reporting systems for SIDS, and the findings may be reported differently from one area to another. Because of this poor reporting, linking factors may be missed.

A number of factors have been associated with a higher incidence of SIDS death:

- SIDS occurs more often in boys than in girls. (However, the overall infant death rate is also higher for boys than girls.)

- SIDS occurs more often in black babies than white babies. (Black babies in general are at a greater risk of death than white babies.)

- SIDS occurs more often in families with a low income (but deaths from other causes do also).

- SIDS occurs more often in illegitimate births than in legitimate births.

- SIDS occurs more often in low-birth-weight babies than in those with higher birth weight.

- Babies from multiple births (twins or triplets) are at a greater risk of SIDS than those from single births.

- The incidence of SIDS in babies with a sibling who died of SIDS is slightly higher than the incidence of SIDS in the general population; it is even higher for the twin or triplet of a SIDS baby.

- SIDS appears to occur more often in crowded dwellings.

continued

continued

- Mothers of SIDS babies seem to have had fewer prenatal visits than other mothers; they often have no prenatal care or care only in the last three months of pregnancy.

- Mothers of SIDS babies tend to be younger than mothers of babies who die of other causes.

- Most SIDS deaths occur between November and March.

None of these risk factors has been established as a cause of SIDS and, as noted, many of these factors are also associated with a higher incidence of infant deaths from other causes.

The infant mortality rate from all causes has been declining in the United States. However, the incidence of SIDS deaths has remained about the same. For all other causes of infant deaths, the incidence is higher for younger infants and decreases as the infant becomes older. In contrast, few SIDS deaths occur in infants younger than one month old; most deaths occur when the baby is two to four months old; and the incidence of SIDS decreases dramatically after the age of six months. SIDS rarely occurs in babies one to two years old.

The first symptom of the disease is the death of the baby. The death occurs quickly and usually without being noticed. The baby apparently dies during sleep and without suffering. In the few reported instances in which a SIDS death was observed, the baby simply stopped breathing. In the most common situation, an apparently healthy baby is put to bed and is later found dead. Parents have found their baby dead while sleeping in the same room, while driving with the baby in a car seat, or even while holding the baby in their arms. In one instance, the baby's doctor had just finished a routine health examination when the baby stopped breathing. The doctor, nurse, and mother were all present, but attempts to resuscitate the baby were not successful. The autopsy revealed no cause of death except SIDS.

### Dealing With Guilt

The parents of a SIDS baby also become victims of the disease. Their grief and guilt may be over-whelming. Unlike parents whose baby was ill before dying, the parents of a SIDS baby have no warning or time to prepare emotionally for the loss of their child. Feelings of guilt and self-recrimination are normal first reactions. The parents immediately begin to wonder what they did or did not do to cause the death. *But—in the absence of risk factors—there has never been evidence that any special care, or lack of it, can prevent or contribute to a SIDS death.*

The emotional trauma experienced by the family frequently results in the family's disintegration. Rates of divorce, substance abuse, and serious psychological problems are high in SIDS families. Fathers of SIDS babies may seek excuses not to be home, such as working longer hours. They tend to internalize their grief and may have difficulty talking about the baby and his or her death. Mothers frequently wish to talk about their loss but have difficulty finding someone to talk to. They may undergo physical changes that are difficult to handle, especially if they were nursing the baby. While fathers may have a strong desire to "replace" the lost child, mothers may be less inclined to have another baby as soon as possible. In reaction to the SIDS death, both parents may become overly protective of their other or subsequent children.

The trauma suffered by other children in a SIDS family—or other care-givers, such as babysitters—may go unrecognized as everyone concentrates on the parents' loss. Yet siblings may suffer from the loss and from guilt feelings, sometimes to the extent that psychological counseling is necessary. Siblings old enough to have helped care for the baby would have established a special bond to the baby that makes their loss very real and very big. Also, they are apt to develop guilt feelings about what they might have done to cause the death, especially if they tended the baby shortly before the death. Younger siblings, who probably experienced brief periods of jealousy when they wished the baby would go away, may have difficulty coping with a feeling that they somehow caused the baby's death. In addition, young siblings may witness attempts to resuscitate the baby without understanding what is happening. They may interpret the pounding on the chest or other emergency measures as punishing the baby for having been bad. When the baby is pronounced dead, young children may believe that the parents or emergency personnel killed the baby and will kill *them* if *they* misbehave or incur their parents' displeasure in some way.

## Finding Support

Efforts should be—and in some areas of the country are being—expanded to help SIDS families. In 1972, the State of Illinois created the Sudden Infant Death Syndrome Study Commission, which is unique in its dedication to helping families. The primary concerns of this commission are to provide information about SIDS and to decrease the trauma experienced by SIDS families. The commission's activities in offering programs, counseling, and other assistance to SIDS families have served as a model for activities in other states. Some states now have SIDS projects, and all SIDS activities and counseling are available through these projects. In other states, SIDS activities and counseling are offered through state public health departments. Also, many parents of SIDS babies are active in self-help groups. Parents and others who have difficulty obtaining information about SIDS can contact the National Sudden Infant Death Syndrome Foundation, Two Metro Plaza, 8240 Professional Place, Suite 205, Landover, MD 20785 (301-459-3388; outside Maryland 1-800-221-SIDS) for more information.

## Retardation and Other Handicaps

We all want our babies to be healthy, to grow and develop to their full potential as children and adults. But sometimes a baby is not healthy.

Some children are born with genetic defects that affect one or more of the body's systems, such as muscular dystrophy (the progressive wasting away of muscles), certain mental disorders, and color blindness. Down syndrome is a genetic birth defect that often involves many of the body's systems, leading to physical problems and mental retardation.

Other children are born with genetic body chemistry disorders, such as phenylketonuria (PKU), which affects metabolism; cystic fibrosis, which affects the mucus-producing glands in the body; and Tay-Sachs disease, which leads to progressive neurological deterioration and death at an early age. Some genetic disorders, such as sickle cell anemia, hemophilia, and thalassemia, affect the ability of the blood cells to perform their natural functions.

Sometimes something happened within the cells when the fetus was forming that altered the way the baby developed in the womb. A child may have genetic defects that affect the size or shape of the body or of various organs, such as dwarfism, spina bifida (open spine), hydrocephalus (head enlarged because of fluid accumulation), clubfoot, cleft lip or palate, and some congenital heart defects.

In other cases, the baby's genes may be perfectly normal but something happened while the fetus was developing that caused damage. Perhaps the mother had rubella (German measles), which affected the baby's hearing or vision. Some babies are born too soon, before they are completely developed. Sometimes something happens in the womb or at birth that causes brain damage leading to mental retardation or cerebral palsy (which affects movement and posture).

Some children contract a serious illness, like meningitis, within their first few years that causes hearing loss or brain damage leading to disabilities. Many defects show up immediately or shortly after birth or an illness, but some problems may not be obvious until the child is several months or even several years old.

Severe handicapping conditions, when not treated, may result in stunted emotional and mental development as well as severe physical problems.

## What to Do If You Suspect a Problem

If this is your first baby, you may not wish to seem overanxious about your baby's development. Yet you may have some concerns based on what you've read about normal development or seen other babies accomplishing.

You spend many hours with your child, while your doctor spends only a few minutes at each visit. Doctors tend to look for developmental milestones and may not focus on deficiencies. If you express your concern as a general worry, your doctor may be apt to simply reassure you that the range of normal development is quite broad and that different babies develop at different rates.

When parents suspect a problem, they should write down what their concerns are. Try to think of as many examples as possible. When you take a list to your doctor, she will recognize your concern and begin thinking about specific causes for the behavior you observe. Your doctor may want to wait and see if there are changes. If she suspects a genetic or disease-related problem, she may recommend that you see a specialist at the nearest children's hospital.

If your baby's overall development seems delayed, your doctor may recommend that he be examined by a developmental pediatrician who specializes in infant development. If your doctor suspects a neurologic disorder (a problem with the functioning of the nervous system), she may refer you to a pediatric neurologist. In some cases, CT scanning (an x-ray technique that provides a computerized picture of an area of the body) may be performed. This can reveal if there are tumors or other abnormalities in the brain.

If seizure disorders are suspected, an electroencephalogram (EEG) may be performed to record the brain-wave pattern for analysis. If hearing loss is suspected, a brain-stem response study may be done by an audiologist.

An ophthalmologist may examine your child's eyes for visual function and for abnormalities. Your child may also be seen by a physical therapist, who will evaluate such things as muscle strength and control, flexibility, balance, and agility. A psychologist may assess your child's personality and intellectual functioning, while a speech pathologist may look at how your child communicates to identify factors responsible for communication disorders.

It is sometimes difficult to determine the cause of developmental delays, so parents may be asked to see a number of specialists and consent to their child's undergoing a number of tests. It may be wise for parents to select a "case manager"—a doctor or other professional who will act as liaison between parents and professionals. Often this is the family pediatrician, but it may also be a hospital social worker or other professional who can explain medical procedures and who also has experience in dealing with parents' concerns and feelings. While parents can certainly act as their own case managers, they may find it easier, especially when they are under a lot of stress, to have one person overseeing the tests.

Some procedures are invasive and potentially harmful to the child. Parents should understand why a specific test is being considered and what is involved. Do not be afraid to ask doctors to explain, and never sign consent forms without feeling sure that you understand what is to be done to your child. If you are unsure about something, wait until you have an opportunity to discuss it with your pediatrician.

## When a Diagnosis Is Confirmed

The most profound shock in a parent's life may be learning that his or her child has a handicap. All the hopes and dreams for the future of that child suddenly seem hollow and empty.

Parents often feel terribly depressed and grief-stricken. It is as if the child they knew had died and a strange child had been left in his place. Sometimes parents feel guilty and blame themselves for the handicap. They feel it is a result of something they did or did not do, or they feel they should have recognized the problem sooner. They feel they have somehow failed as parents.

Often, parents feel angry with their pediatrician or the professionals who tell them the diagnosis. They may feel that the medical profession, which they had put such faith in, has failed them. Parents may also discover they have negative feelings about handicaps in general or their child's handicap in particular.

All these feelings are normal. But they are hard to deal with and hard to live with.

As parents struggle with their own reactions of shock and disappointment, they may find that their normal support systems fail because friends and family are also struggling to cope with their feelings of concern. Parents may find themselves vulnerable to and resentful of advice and comments offered by friends, relatives, and self-styled experts. Parents often find themselves suddenly overwhelmed by information they are trying to understand and by decisions they feel must be made immediately.

Initially, parents may not be able to absorb all the information that is being given to them. They may be worried about the effect of the handicap on other children in the family and deeply concerned about their ability to relate to the handicapped child.

It may be helpful to talk to someone with experience in dealing with these emotions, someone who can help you sort out your feelings and recognize your responsibilities. Your religious leader, a psychologist, a psychiatrist, or another trained counselor may be helpful. Many parents find the greatest relief and comfort in talking to other parents who have lived through similar experiences. Parents should not try to hide or ignore their grief. In time, the pain will lessen.

For some parents, the best tonic for depression is taking action on behalf of their child, whether it is enrolling her in a therapy program or a school, talking to a specialist about prosthetic devices (an artificial limb, a wheelchair, or a hearing aid), or contacting a national organization for more information.

You will be looking at your child with new eyes, and in the beginning that can be difficult and painful. You will be establishing a new relationship with this child, different from what you may have planned and expected. But it can be a relationship that is fulfilling and rewarding as you work with your child to discover her full potential.

## Choices

A generation ago, children with severe handicaps often died of complications, if not of the handicap itself. Handicapped children were consigned to institutions, where most had little chance of developing. Handicaps were hidden away, not discussed. Today, attitudes are changing. Parents are now encouraged to keep all but the most profoundly handicapped children at home. Fewer full-time residential institutions are available, and state and local agencies provide more technical and financial support services directly to families. In most states, foster care is available for families who do not feel they can cope with the burden of a disabled child.

Technological advances in medicine have enabled doctors to surgically correct many problems that afflict children with Down syndrome, spina bifida, clubfoot, cleft lip and palate, and heart malformations so that these children can be more easily cared for at home. Many formerly fatal handicaps, such as hemophilia, can be treated with medications or blood transfusions.

Even with support services, the burdens—physical, emotional, and financial—fall heavily on families with handicapped children. Surgery or medication may not "cure" a handicapped child, although procedures that today are somewhat controversial for children, like cochlear implants, may prove to be "near-cures" of the future. Parents must take time to ask questions and become informed. One of the best sources of information will be other parents of similarly handicapped children.

If no parent-support group exists in your area, consider starting one. Names can often be provided by national organizations, medical specialists, professionals in the field, and state and local health departments. Contact with other parents, even parents in different locations, will give you a chance to discuss some problems relating to discipline at home and to relationships with peers and with family. Contact with other families will give your handicapped child an opportunity to see others like himself and give you a chance to see what other handicapped children can accomplish.

Your local library may have the names and addresses of national organizations that are concerned with specific handicaps. Medical services and assistance are provided by state and local health and welfare departments (look in the telephone pages under your state agencies). Departments of children and family services and handicapped children's services may also provide information about funding, programs, and institutions. Local service organizations, such as the Variety Clubs, Lions, Elks, Shriners, and Jaycees often provide scholarships and support hospitals and other programs that serve handicapped children.

---

### Support Organizations for Parents of Handicapped Children

- National Information Center for Handicapped Children and Youth, P. O. Box 1492, Washington, DC 20013; 703-522-3332.

- Coordinating Council for Handicapped Children, 220 S. State Street, Room 412, Chicago, IL 60604; 312-939-3513.

- National Foundation—The March of Dimes, 1275 Mamaroneck Avenue, White Plains, NY 10605; 914-428-7100.

- National Center for Education in Maternal and Child Health, 38th and R Streets NW, Washington, DC 20057; 202-625-8400.

- Self-Help Center, 1600 Dodge Avenue, Evanston, IL 60201; 312-328-0470.

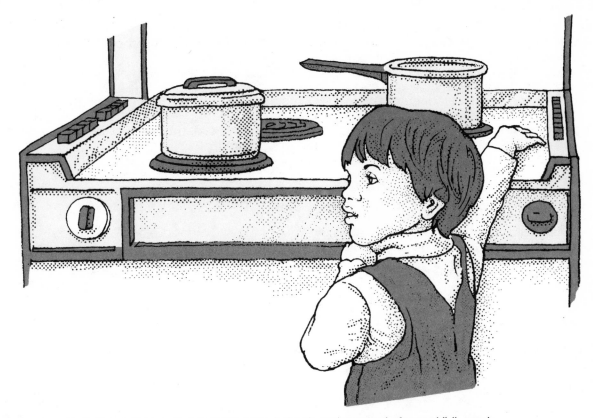

*Stovetops are potential hazards to curious toddlers—keep hot pots and pans out of your child's reach.*

See Chapter 11 for additional information about support for the handicapped.

## Safety At Home

You place your three-month-old baby on the changing table to get him ready for bed. You discover that his sleeper is wet, so you step away—just for a moment—to get a new one.

You are polishing the furniture while your nine-month-old plays quietly nearby. The phone rings. You set the bottle of polish down—just for a moment—to go answer it.

"Just for a moment" can be a moment too long. Accidents can happen in an instant. The father who steps away from the changing table doesn't expect his baby to fall. The mother who leaves an open bottle of furniture polish doesn't expect her child to drink it. But it happens.

Accidents are the leading cause of death in children. Although car accidents are the number one killer, injuries that occur around the house—burns, choking, poisoning, and falls—also cause

significant loss of life. Nonfatal injuries from these accidents are an even larger problem in terms of the number of children affected. One-third of all children each year have an injury serious enough to require medical attention, and preschool children are the most vulnerable. Children under five years old have twice as many falls as school-aged children, ten times more poisonings, and fourteen times more choking episodes.

Such statistics should alarm you. We hope they will alarm you enough to inspire you to take action. Buy recommended safety devices. Learn about high-risk situations and how to avoid them. Accidents can—and do—happen. A small investment of your time and effort can minimize the risk of accidental injury to your children.

### Burns

Burns are the third most common cause of accidental death in children, behind car accidents and drowning. However, in the one- to four-year-old age group, burns are second. In addition, preschool children have the highest number of nonfatal burns.

There are four major types of burns: burns from *house fires; scalds,* from hot liquids or inappropriately hot tap water; *contact burns,* from touching a hot surface, such as a stove or radiator; and *electrical burns,* usually from poking a finger into an outlet or biting an electrical cord. House fires cause the most deaths, and can also leave a child scarred or with brain or lung damage from smoke inhalation. Scalds cause the most nonfatal burns. Electrical burns are dangerous and can be disfiguring.

Children can be burned because of their own actions. For example, children may start a fire playing with matches, or may burn themselves by touching a hot stove. But when adult carelessness causes the injury, the damage may seem even

## Home Burn Prevention

- Reduce your water heater temperature to 120 degrees. At 130 degrees, skin is burned in only thirty seconds; at 120 degrees, burning takes ten minutes.

- Test the temperature of the bath water before putting your child into it.

- Put safety plugs into all your wall sockets.

- Don't leave an unused extension cord plugged into the wall.

- Turn the handles of pans sitting on stove tops inward, so curious hands can't grasp them.

- Don't allow your children to play with the stove.

- Keep matches and cigarette lighters out of your child's reach.

- Never place hot food or liquid on the edge of a counter.

- Don't keep gasoline or other flammable substances where a child can reach them.

- Cover or screen fireplaces and hot floor registers or radiators.

- Buy only flame-resistant or flame-retardant clothes for your child.

## Home Fire Prevention and Safety

- Don't smoke in bed.

- Extinguish all cigarettes properly.

- Don't use gasoline to boost a barbecue flame.

- Don't use or store gasoline in an enclosed basement where fumes can be ignited by sparks or pilot lights.

- Don't overload electrical circuits.

- Don't use electrical appliances near water.

- Store combustible materials safely.

- Keep matches out of your child's reach.

- Teach your child to notify the nearest adult if he or she smells smoke. Have an escape route in case exits are blocked.

- Keep the numbers of the fire department, emergency room, and your doctor near your phone.

more devastating. House fires can start when a smoker falls asleep in bed or when electrical circuits are overloaded. Children can be burned when adults use gasoline to light a barbecue.

State governments have been active in attempting to reduce the number of injuries from fire. More than half the states require smoke detectors in new housing. Most states also limit the sale of fireworks. The federal government passed a number of laws between 1953 and 1971 regulating flammable fabrics. The effectiveness of these laws is reflected in the eighty percent decrease in clothing ignition deaths between 1968 and 1979.

But there is a limit to what the government can do. The ultimate responsibility for preventing burns in your household lies with you. The combination of safety devices, appropriate storage of flammable substances, and education of your children can help prevent burns. Smoke detectors are a necessity, but they won't work without good batteries. Check the batteries regularly. Have a fire extinguisher in a handy place and know how to use it.

## Choking

Choking is the fourth most common cause of accidental death in children. However, for children under one year, it is the most common cause, ranking above even car accidents. In one recent year alone, 440 infants under a year old choked to death.

Children choke easily. Babies put everything they come upon into their mouths; it is a way of exploring. In your baby's opinion, everything must be tasted as well as looked at and touched. Unfortunately, infants are not well coordinated, and small pieces can work their way too far back into the mouth and then get stuck.

If something gets stuck, one of two things can happen. If the object is the right size, it can completely close off the child's airway, causing him to

be unable to speak or breathe. Unless removed quickly, the object can cause brain damage from lack of oxygen, or even death. If the object is sucked into one of the smaller airways, the child will cough, wheeze, and have trouble breathing. Often, such objects must be removed surgically.

Children can choke on anything small enough. Before disposable diapers, safety pins were a major hazard. Now, pieces of toys, balloons (even uninflated ones), and coins are frequent dangers. Some foods, such as hot dogs, grapes, nuts, and hard candies, as well as vitamins and baby-aspirin tablets, can cause choking.

The federal government has taken action to prevent pieces of toys from becoming the objects responsible for choking. The Consumer Product Safety Commission has mandatory safety standards, and the Toy Manufacturers of America has voluntary product standards regulating toys with small parts.

Since children choke on many things besides toys, it is your obligation to watch what your child puts in his mouth and to keep dangerous things away.

### Preventing Choking

- Examine your baby's toys and clothing for parts that could easily be pulled off and swallowed.

- Don't allow your baby to play with coins, balloons, or other items that could easily be swallowed.

- Cut or break your toddler's food into bite-size pieces.

- Avoid giving a toddler such hard, smooth foods as nuts, carrots, and hard candy. Also avoid foods that may become lodged in your child's throat, such as hot dogs, potato chips, and popcorn.

- Do not give chewable pills or vitamins to children under the age of three.

- Teach your child to chew thoroughly, and discourage talking while chewing.

- If your child does choke, don't put your finger in her mouth—you may push the object farther in.

- Learn the Heimlich maneuver, or the back-blow/chest-thrust maneuver recommended by the American Academy of Pediatrics.

## Falls

Falls are the fifth most common cause of accidental death in children. The significance of falls, though, lies in the number of nonfatal occurrences: falls are the most frequent cause of injury bringing patients into the emergency room. Toddlers have the highest incidence of falls of any age group.

Toddlers are eager to explore. They love to imitate everyone, from older siblings to television characters. But their motor skills are usually not developed enough to allow them to climb steadily and reach easily the places they want to go. Consequently, they often tumble. In addition, a small child believes that he has complete control over his world. Therefore, if he wants to climb up the bookcase, he believes that he can. But he can't anticipate consequences, such as falling off the bookcase. He isn't capable of generalizing, either. Just because he fell off a chair in the past doesn't suggest to him that he might fall off the bookcase now.

Children most often fall from common household furniture, such as beds, tables, and chairs,

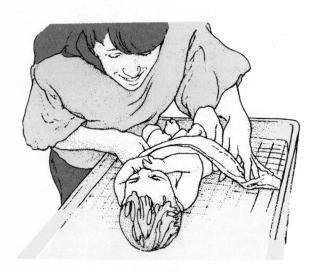

*To prevent an accidental fall, keep your baby securely tethered to the top of his changing table.*

and down stairs. Infants often fall from changing tables. Falls from high places, such as windows, balconies, and trees, are rare and usually involve older children.

What children fall from, whether it is the stairs or the table, is not as important as what they fall *onto*. In falls from the same height, landing on concrete or asphalt obviously causes much more damage than landing on a rug.

Most children are not seriously injured when they fall. Cuts, scrapes, and bumps are the most common injuries. However, sprains and fractures can occur, usually when a child falls on an arm or leg. The most critical injuries occur when a child lands on her head or neck. Concussions, skull fractures, bleeding in the head, and even death may occur. Some children are left with long-term impairment, from hyperactivity to seizures to learning problems.

Local governments play a role in limiting falls through the public building codes. For example, handrails on stairways and adequate lighting in stairwells are required. Those who design new buildings may take safety considerations into account. For instance, they may use a sand base rather than concrete for play areas.

At home, there are two ways to prevent your child from falling. The first is through the use of inexpensive gadgets. Gates on stairways are crucial. The best kind are the permanently affixed, climb-resistant mesh gates that have a straight

top edge. Gates that are not permanent can fall down the stairs with the baby. Gates with wider mesh are climbable and can pinch fingers. The widely separated slats of accordion-style gates can trap a child's head. Edge guards are also available. These attach with adhesive to the edges and corners of furniture to cushion a fall or collision, and thereby prevent injury.

The second way to protect your child is to follow some simple precautions and to teach certain ways to behave.

## Poisonings

Poisonings are the sixth most common cause of accidental death in children. Hundreds of children die of poisoning each year; one-quarter of them are under age four. More frightening, though, is the fact that two million children under age five are poisoned, fatally or not, each year.

Poisonings occur partly because children are inquisitive. Preschool children learn by exploring, and most children use their mouths to explore. That bottle of green liquid may not be dangerous

## Some common household poisons

| | | |
|---|---|---|
| After-shave | Floor wax | Mouthwash |
| Alcoholic beverages | Furniture polish | Nail polish |
| Ammonia | Gasoline | Nail polish remover |
| Anti-freeze | Glue | Oven cleaner |
| Aspirin and acetaminophen | Grease remover | Paint |
| Auto wax | Hair spray | Paint thinner |
| Baby powder | Herbicides | Perfume |
| Benzene | Houseplants (some) | Plant sprays |
| Bleach | Ink | Room deodorizer |
| Boric acid | Insecticides and pest strips | Rubbing alcohol |
| Carbon tetrachloride | Insect repellent | Rust remover |
| Charcoal-lighting fluid | Iodine | Shampoo |
| Cleaning fluid | Kerosene | Shoe polish |
| Cleaning products | Laundry products | Solvents |
| Correction fluid | Laxatives | Tobacco |
| Cosmetics | Lighter fluid | Toilet bowl cleaner |
| Deodorants | Lye | Turpentine |
| Dishwasher detergent | Medications of any kind | Vitamins |
| Drain cleaner | Mercury (from a thermometer) | Weed killer |
| Fertilizer | Motor oil | Windshield washer solution |

when it is touched or smelled, but most young children will try to taste it, too.

The real problem, though, is not so much the child's inquisitiveness, but the availability of poisons in his surroundings. Sometimes parents are just careless—they may not lock up supplies. But often, there is some other factor. The child may find a bottle of medication in a visitor's purse, or the family may be moving and products that ordinarily are out of sight have become accessible.

The most common poisonings involve cleaning supplies, such as soaps and detergents. Ingesting such products can cause a variety of symptoms, from mild vomiting and diarrhea to burns of the skin, eyes, or esophagus. Convulsions are also likely.

Plants are an easily overlooked source of poisoning. Some houseplants, such as philodendron, dumb cane, and iris, can be toxic, usually causing irritation of the mouth and sometimes vomiting

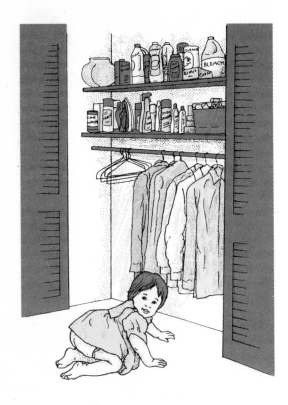

All poisons and other toxic substances must be kept beyond your baby's reach.

and diarrhea. Nontoxic plants include Boston ferns, coleus, and jade and spider plants. Poison control centers keep lists of toxic plants.

Children can overdose on vitamins. Many children take a chewable vitamin daily and so come to look at vitamins as candy. If they get hold of a bottle, they may eat every pill or tablet inside. The symptoms depend on the kind of vitamin taken. Overdoses of iron, vitamin A, and vitamin D cause the most problems.

Aspirin and acetaminophen are commonly used medications in most households. Children have taken them for fever and may therefore recognize the bottle or actually have come to like the taste. Aspirin overdose can cause a severe imbalance of bodily salts and acids, resulting in lung and brain damage, and even death. Overdoses of acetaminophen primarily affect the liver.

Over the last twenty years, there has been a seventy-five percent decline in the number of poisoning fatalities. The reason? The federal govern-

ment passed a series of laws, ranging from the 1966 Child Protection Act, which banned the sale of some hazardous household substances, to the 1970 Poison Prevention Packaging Act, which required child-resistant safety packaging. Also important in the decline of poisoning deaths was the creation in 1977 of the Consumer Product Safety Commission to deal with the safety of consumer products. As with other household accidents, though, regulation is not the whole answer.

If your child has ingested a poison, check with your doctor or poison control center before doing *anything.* They will tell you what to do. Keep a bottle of ipecac syrup in your home medicine cabinet for each child under five years of age (and check the expiration date periodically). Ipecac is used to induce vomiting and thereby empty the stomach of a child who has swallowed something toxic. However, since ipecac is not used in all cases of poisoning, *be sure to check with your doctor or poison control center first*—they will tell you whether or not to give a dose of ipecac.

Making your home a safe place doesn't require drastic remodelling, nor does it require locking your toddler away. A bit of extra vigilance and an awareness of what activities—both yours and your child's—may lead to accidents are all that is necessary. Most household injuries can be prevented—it's your responsibility.

## Poison Prevention

- Lock away all potentially dangerous substances.

- Store all products in their original containers. Bleach, for example, shouldn't be stored in an empty soft drink bottle.

- If labels have been detached, relabel bottles and cover the new label with cellophane tape.

- If interrupted while working, take any open containers with you.

- Check your house and garage every six months for proper storage of materials. This is especially important if you have a rapidly growing youngster who can get into things now that she couldn't have gotten into six months ago.

_____ continued

_continued_

- Administer medications only in adequate light after checking the label.

- Do not call medicine _candy_, and don't give the empty bottles to your child as toys.

- Keep medicine in an area that is separate from food.

- Dispose of all unused or expired medicines promptly.

- Buy medications in child-proof containers.

## Safety Away from Home

Within the confines of your home, you have some degree of control over preventing injury to your child. Locks on cabinets, caps in wall sockets, and gates on the stairs may prevent your child from getting into trouble. But once you leave home, some of that control is forfeited. No matter how carefully you drive and how good a car seat you have, you have no control over the drunk who runs a red light. No matter how carefully you supervise your child, you have no control over the psychotic who grabs her while she is out playing.

While you may not have control over other people's actions, you _can_ minimize the risk of harm to your children when they are away from home. Children spend a lot of time outside the home, in the car or in public places, such as supermarkets, department stores, day care centers, and playgrounds. By using protective devices, learning how to avoid high-risk situations, and teaching your children how to react, you can help protect them from injury in the car and from abduction by strangers.

## Car Safety

Car accidents are the leading cause of death in children after the first few months of life. Of all deaths due to injury, two-thirds are related to motor vehicles. In the one- to four-year-old age group, two-thirds of the children who are killed in car accidents are occupants of a car, and one-third are pedestrians struck by a car. It has been estimated that eighty-five percent of those deaths and sixty-five percent of those injuries could have been prevented by the use of car seats and seat belts.

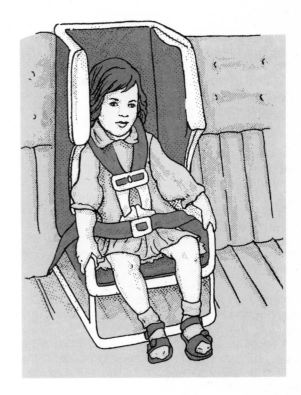

_Car seats and child restraints prevent injury and save lives._

Children can be injured by cars in two major ways. Children playing on the sidewalk may be hit by a car that jumps the curb, or they may be struck if they venture into the street. But, more commonly, a child is hurt when a car in which he or she is a passenger is involved in a collision. When a car stops suddenly, the unrestrained passenger continues to move at the original speed until he hits something that stops him. This is usually the interior of the car, but may be the ground if the passenger has been ejected. Children who are at highest risk of injury in an accident are those who are held in an adult's lap. Not only is the child thrown forward into the dashboard, but he is smashed from behind by the weight of the adult. Even if the passenger is belted in, it is nearly impossible to hold onto a child in a crash. For example, to hold onto a ten-pound infant in a collision at thirty miles per hour requires the same amount of strength as lifting three hundred pounds one foot off the ground!

To prevent an auto injury to your child, you must address the issue of safety from the point of view of each of the ways in which injury occurs. You have to consider both pedestrian safety and auto safety.

To make sure your child isn't struck by a car, teach her to respect the road and to walk defensively. Teach her to play in the yard or on the sidewalk, and to stay away from the street. Try to "keep an eye out" for her. As she gets older, teach her to look both ways before crossing the road. Be sure she knows how to read traffic signals.

To keep your child safe in the car, drive carefully and defensively. Follow the rules of the road. Don't allow your children to distract you—concentrate on driving. Avoid having any sharp or heavy objects in the car that could become flying missiles in a sudden stop or crash. But the most important precaution doesn't concern your driving skills, but rather one simple plastic and metal device—a *car seat*.

Nearly all the states and the District of Columbia require child restraints in automobiles. Tennessee was the first to require them, in 1977. Use of car seats in Tennessee increased from eight to twenty-nine percent in the two and one-half years after the law was enacted. The number of children killed decreased from twenty-two in 1979 to ten in 1981. While states regulate their use, the federal government regulates the construction of car seats. Child seats must meet federal standards for crash protection, standards that are based on dynamic, rather than just static, testing. See Chapter 4 for information about shopping for a car seat.

## Abduction

A child is much less likely to be abducted than to be involved in a car accident. Exactly how much less likely, though, is not clear. It is known that 1.8 million children are reported missing each year. However, ninety to ninety-five percent are runaways or the objects of custody disputes. Estimates of the true number of children abducted by strangers vary widely, ranging from four thousand to fifty thousand a year. No matter what the number, however, the thought of a child being kidnapped frightens many parents. In response, the media have recently paid a great deal of attention to the problem. It is hoped that this attention will produce a heightened awareness in the public—and contribute to prevention of child abduction.

Small children are at particular risk of being victimized. They are taught to respect adults, to be polite, not to question older people, and certainly not to yell or fight. In addition, they are easily swayed by offers of food or treats. Their small size also makes it easy for a stranger to physically abduct them.

Child abductors are often people with serious psychological problems—people who sexually abuse children, or those who have lost a child or are unable to have children of their own, racketeers who sell babies, or even murderers.

When a child is reported missing, law enforcement agencies become involved. Local police play a major role initially. However, because older children often turn out to be runaways, the police tend to wait twenty-four to forty-eight hours before actively pursuing a case. By then, it may be too late. The kidnapper may already have injured the child or may have crossed state lines, making pursuit more difficult. Therefore, the FBI often becomes involved. As of 1982, cases of missing children can be logged into the FBI's National Crime Information Center computer.

Parents' organizations are also taking a vigorous role, not only in helping to locate missing children but also in preventing abductions. The oldest group is Child Find, established in 1980. This group publishes an annual directory of missing children. Other groups provide information and educational materials to parents and lobby for stiffer penalties for offenders.

The individual family still has the major responsibility for preventing child abduction. There are a number of precautions you can take. For example, never leave an infant alone in a car or shopping cart, even for a second. If your child is in day care, be sure the center has a strict policy regarding pick-up. Starting at age three, you can begin to discuss the problem directly with your child. Approach the subject simply and directly. Talk about what to do, but not about the consequences of kidnapping, to avoid scaring your child needlessly. Broach the subject gradually, as different situations arise.

It is important to teach your child exactly who is to be considered a stranger. While Aunt Mary and your next-door neighbor are not, the postman and the kindly old lady in the market are, no matter how friendly they seem. When your child understands this, teach her to say "no" to strangers. She should never accept anything from someone she doesn't know. She should ignore people who ask directions or beckon her closer. If they persist, she should run or yell, and even fight if the person attempts to touch her.

Teach your child his name, complete address (including city and state) and phone number (including area code). Don't buy items, such as T-shirts, with your child's name on them. A stranger could utilize that knowledge to approach your child in a nonthreatening way. Establish a "code word" for emergency use in case your child needs to be picked up by someone else. There are read-aloud books available to help teach your child these lessons.

You may want to keep a file with your child's fingerprints, dental records, and current photographs. The value of fingerprinting, however, is controversial. Though it helps you feel that you are doing something to protect your children, it will not prevent their disappearance. It will only help identify a small child who doesn't know his or her name, or one who has recently been murdered. Some people consider fingerprinting, especially when schools or police are given copies, a violation of a child's constitutional rights to privacy and to freedom from self-incrimination. Others feel it alarms children unnecessarily. Whether to fingerprint your child must be your individual decision.

There are many precautions, then, that you can take to protect your child when away from home, from car seats to careful driving, from fingerprinting to teaching your child to say "no." While you don't want to become excessively wary, you do need to be concerned—for your child's sake.

## Safety and Health Considerations at Playgrounds and Pools

Playgrounds and pools are places for recreation and relaxation. But the laughter can easily turn to tears and tragedy. A two-year-old follows his older brother to the top of a ten-foot-high slide, slips while trying to sit on the top, and falls to the ground, breaking his leg. A one-year-old topples over the edge of the wading pool—luckily, an observant lifeguard rescues her. Knowing what the hazards are at playgrounds and pools and teaching your children how to play and swim appropriately can ensure a safe outing.

### Playgrounds

Playground equipment is ranked sixth on a list of one hundred hazardous consumer products

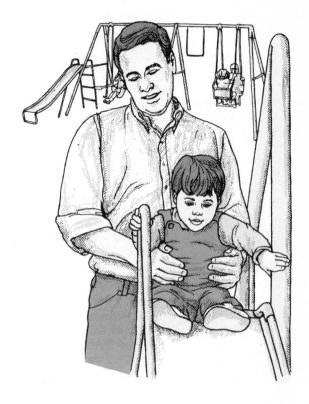

*Parental supervision makes for safe and happy times on the playground.*

published by the Consumer Product Safety Commission. Each year, 155,000 children are injured on playgrounds. On public playgrounds, sixteen percent of those injured are under five years old; on home playgrounds, twenty-nine percent are under five.

Younger children are likely to be injured on the playground because of their stage of development. They are compelled to investigate. They won't be satisfied at the bottom of the slide—they need to see the top, too. But physically, they are not coordinated enough to do what they want. In addition, they can't project the consequences of their actions; they never anticipate falling off.

Slides, in fact, are one of the most hazardous pieces of playground equipment. Other pieces of equipment to watch out for include swings, climbing structures (such as "monkey bars"), and see-saws.

Most children are injured by falling. Seventy-five percent of playground injuries are from falls to the ground or onto other equipment. Fifty percent of these result in head and neck injuries. The most serious injuries occur when children fall onto concrete or asphalt rather than onto a more yielding surface, such as sand. Falls can also result in fractures and lacerations.

Children can be injured in other ways as well. They may be hit by moving equipment or cut by rough or sharp edges, or they may become stuck in the equipment.

The Consumer Product Safety Commission has established voluntary product safety standards for home and public playgrounds. These include equipment specifications and suggestions for everything from the type of base surface to use to design and arrangement of the play area. The standards also stress that safe playgrounds require adequate supervision and maintenance, as well as good design.

It is essential to teach your children how to behave at the playground and to supervise their activities. Teach your children to hold onto all equipment with *both* hands. Teach them to stop before getting off any moving equipment. Teach them to *sit* on the swings and slides, not stand, lie, or hang upside-down. Only one person should be allowed to use playground equipment at a time. Be sure they don't push or shove, and that they walk well away from areas where other children are swinging or sliding. Be sure the equipment your child plays on matches her ability. A ten-year-old can easily climb a jungle gym, for example, but a two-year-old shouldn't follow suit. Teach your children to use equipment as the manufacturer intended. For instance, children should swing on the swings, not twist around.

There is a growing public awareness of environmental hazards. Although little research has been done on the subject, playgrounds may pose subtle dangers. Some parks have been built on previously contaminated landfills. Others, especially those near freeways, may have high lead levels from automobile fumes. Some playgrounds surrounded by open land are sprayed with pesticides. Other playgrounds have wooden equipment that has been treated with wood preservatives or painted with lead-base paint. Better planning by manufacturers and playground owners and greater parental awareness could reduce the risks posed by such toxic chemicals.

## Pools

When most people think of pool-related injuries, they think of drowning and water aspiration. Drowning is the second most common cause of accidental deaths in children, and the third most common in children aged one to four. Two-thirds of the victims are nonswimmers.

Diving injuries also occur and can be very serious. However, older children and adolescents account for most of these. In younger children, falls and cuts are common—children slip on wet surfaces.

Toddlers are at particularly high risk for drowning. Their size makes even a small amount of water hazardous. In addition, they are often unsteady and fall easily, and they seldom know how to swim.

The key, then, to preventing drowning is to teach your children how to swim. Toddler swimming lessons have been controversial, but they can be worthwhile—especially if the disadvantages to them are understood. Children who have had some form of swimming lessons are only one-half as likely to need some type of assistance in the pool as children with no training. Also, toddlers who start swimming earlier are more likely to become competent swimmers as adults.

The biggest disadvantage to toddler swimming lessons is that, afterward, parents believe the child is water-safe and don't watch her as carefully as they might if there had been no lessons. Although your child may be more comfortable in the water after taking lessons, she really can't swim well, nor can she be expected to know how to react to emergencies.

Infant swimming lessons have other drawbacks. Prolonged lessons have been associated with water intoxication. Therefore, the YMCA recommends prohibiting forced submersion and limiting in-water time to thirty minutes. In addition, when children are still in diapers, it becomes difficult to maintain the effectiveness of the pool's chlorination. There have been reports of epidemics of diarrheal diseases from infant swimming classes.

Besides swimming lessons, there are other precautions that may help prevent pool accidents. Fences and self-locking gates around public and private pools may prevent a toddler from toppling in while unattended. Adequate supervision, from both parents and lifeguards, is a necessity. Children should be taught to follow rules in the pool area, such as no running and no diving in shallow water. Finally, use life jackets on young children who don't know how to swim, but don't become complacent—life jackets, too, can fail.

Similarly, bear in mind that inner tubes, air mattresses, and other flotation devices are for fun *only,* and must not be trusted in deep water, or if your child is out of your sight. Toys break, inflatables deflate. Don't place your child in unnecessary peril by trusting such devices.

By their very nature, playgrounds and pools can be hazardous places unless a certain amount of caution is exercised. You can teach your children how to be careful, and keep playgrounds and pools safe recreational places.

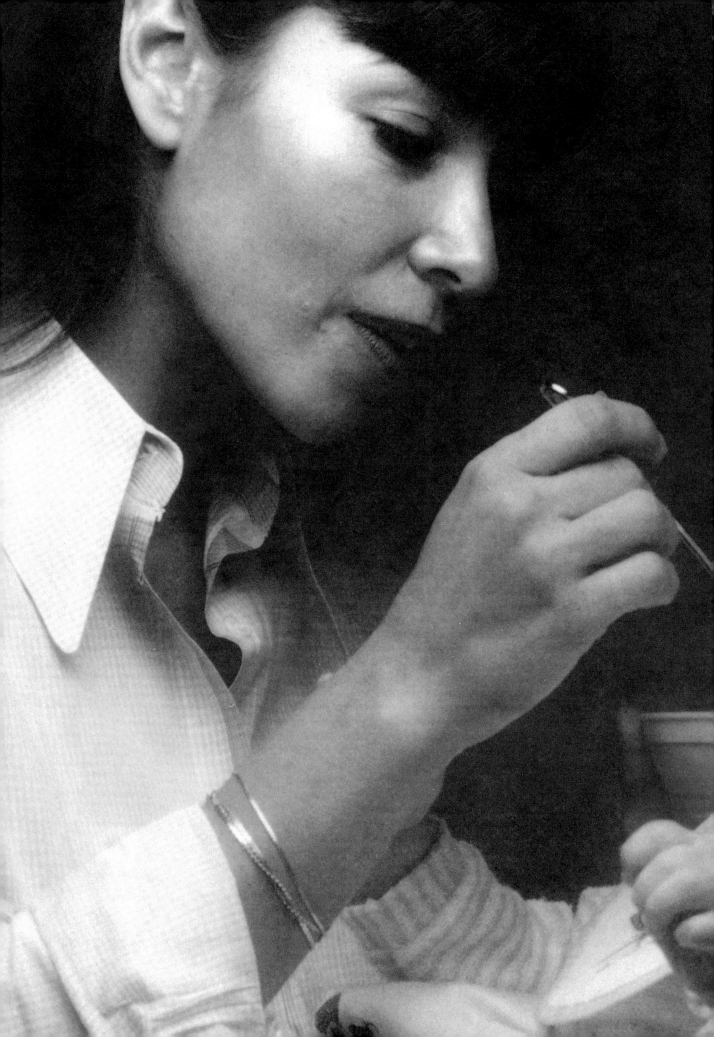

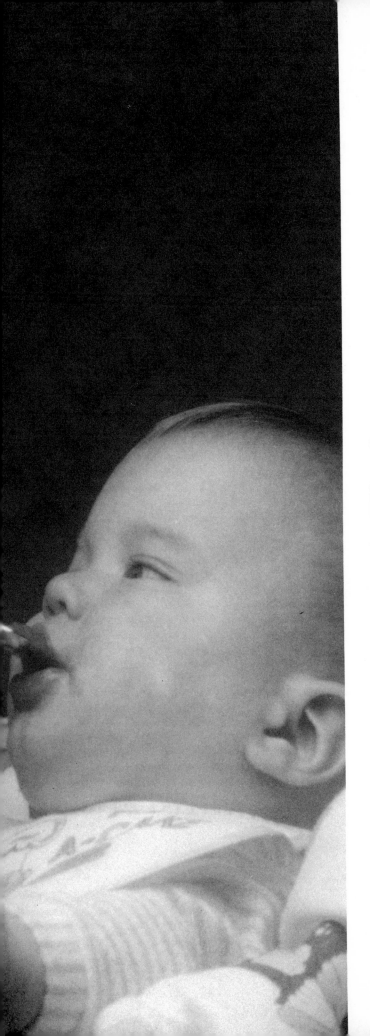

# Chapter 9: Diet for Mother and Baby

## Mother's Diet During the Postpartum Period

You will probably have some very specific concerns and questions about nutrition in the weeks and months after your baby's birth. You, like most mothers, may be concerned about losing the weight you gained during pregnancy. You may also wonder whether a dietary change can help eliminate the fatigue you feel. If you have become anemic, you might want to know how to restore your iron reserves. If you have had a cesarean delivery, you should know what your special nutritional needs are. If you are breastfeeding, you are sure to have many questions about what to eat and what to avoid.

279

## Some General Guidelines for Postpartum Nutrition

Continue eating a good-quality diet just as you did during pregnancy. If you are not breast-feeding, your nutrient and calorie needs will be the same as they were before you became pregnant. If you are breast-feeding, or if you are anemic or recovering from a cesarean delivery, special nutritional management is most certainly in order.

Take a creative approach to nutrition, choosing foods that require little or no preparation. Fresh fruit, raw vegetables, melted cheese on toast, cottage cheese for breakfast, and yogurt with sunflower seeds or granola are quick and nutritious. Broiled meats and fish are faster to prepare than casseroles and can be prepared whenever you find time to eat.

Let friends and family help you by providing nutritious meals during the early months after childbirth. Meals that can be frozen are especially helpful since you can pull them out of the freezer for use on those occasional difficult days.

Nurture yourself by taking time to sit and eat your meals. Eating on the run or standing to eat makes you feel you have not had a meal; this habit contributes to fatigue. Place your baby in a swing or in an infant seat so your hands are free. If your baby needs to be close to you, an infant backpack or sling is helpful. Or you may wait to eat until your baby's quiet time or when she is asleep.

Constipation is a common and unpleasant postpartum complaint. You can relieve constipation by:

- Getting some form of daily exercise, such as walking.

- Making sure you have adequate dietary fiber. Bran muffins, high-fiber cereals, and lots of fruits and vegetables will help.

- Drinking prune juice on an empty stomach followed by several cups of hot water, tea, or other hot beverage. (This works wonders for many mothers.)

- Drinking to quench your thirst, which ensures that you are getting the fluids you need. Two to three quarts of fluids a day is generally recommended.

### Weight Loss After Pregnancy

The pattern of weight loss after pregnancy varies with each mother. Many factors affect your return to your ideal weight. If you were overweight before pregnancy, reaching your ideal weight may take some effort. You may find you are so tired that you do not eat. Your weight loss then may be more rapid than is good for you. If you are breast-feeding, the calories you use to manufacture milk may help you to lose weight, though this is not true for every breast-feeding mother.

As you may have guessed, the best approach to weight loss after childbirth is to exercise regularly, even if only dancing with your baby to music or taking your baby out for walks and fresh air.

You will want to avoid foods with little nutritional value and eat a good-quality diet. Severe dieting is not good for you and not good for your baby if you are nursing. Many communities have special programs to help people lose weight. Choose one that will help you plan your daily diet in a reasonable way. Avoid the "lose-it-quick" methods and diets that rely on powders and pills instead of food for nourishment.

### Dealing With Fatigue

Most new mothers find themselves feeling overwhelmingly tired often or at least occasionally. Getting adequate rest is important for your recovery from birth, for making milk, and for enjoying your baby.

Fatigue also has a negative impact on appetite. With diminished appetite, you eat less, lose weight, and become more fatigued. Severe loss of appetite accompanied by mood swings, uncontrolled crying, and insomnia may be symptoms of postpartum depression.

How do you get rest? Taking time to rest every time your baby rests or sleeps, instead of using that time to clean house or wash clothes, will help. During your rest times, take the phone off the hook so you will not be disturbed. Let your family and friends help you by cleaning house and doing laundry and other household chores. Your rest is important.

There are no particular foods that relieve fatigue. A good-quality diet helps you to feel well, but is not a substitute for rest and sleep. Avoiding caffeine may make it easier for you to fall asleep.

## Restoring Your Iron Reserves

You may find you are anemic after childbirth. Anemia is characterized by a low hematocrit and a low hemoglobin level. (The hematocrit is the percentage of red blood cells in your blood. Hemoglobin is the oxygen-carrying component in those red blood cells.) Anemia may result from having been anemic during pregnancy, from blood loss during vaginal or cesarean birth, or from giving birth to more than one baby.

Your hematocrit and hemoglobin level will be evaluated by your doctor during the postpartum period. If these laboratory tests confirm that you are anemic, treatment will begin immediately. If blood loss was severe during childbirth, you may have had a transfusion. Otherwise, treatment is aimed at restoring iron levels through dietary management and supplements.

Remember to take iron supplements with a food rich in vitamin C, such as orange juice. Do not use antacids, because they diminish the amount of iron you absorb. The very best food sources of iron include organ meats (such as liver), red meats, and egg yolks. Other good sources are whole grains, nuts, legumes, dried fruits, prunes, and prune juice.

## Recovering from a Cesarean Delivery

Having a cesarean section temporarily upsets the passage of food through the digestive tract, resulting in gas production and constipation. Both of these early discomforts can be treated by walking, which increases bowel activity and aids you in passing gas. Be sure to eat, too. There is a temptation not to eat when you feel so bloated, but food will help restore normal bowel action, thereby relieving constipation and gas.

If you are anemic after delivery, following the suggestions given above will help. Treating the anemia will speed your recovery from surgery.

Nutritional management after surgery includes increasing the vitamin C and protein in your diet. Vitamin C contributes to wound healing, and protein helps your body to repair itself.

## Baby's Diet

The decision to breast-feed or bottle-feed your baby isn't an easy one. There are many factors you must consider. Since you are going to be the one taking care of your baby, you must feel comfortable with the decision. Being pressured into one or the other feeding method only leads to discontent.

Perhaps the most important thing to remember is that, on the whole, babies do well whichever way you decide to feed them.

## Bottle-feeding

Mothers have fed their babies formulas for years. In the past, evaporated milk was the main component of formula. Doctors would recommend various additions to it in an attempt to make the formula more complete.

Large companies now manufacture many different types of formula. They are continually improving their products, trying to make them closer to breast milk. There are also a number of special formulas available for babies with certain problems.

The formulas most babies drink use nonfat cow's milk as their base and source of protein. Many different sources of fat are used; soy, coconut, and corn are the most common. Various vitamins, minerals, and trace elements are also added. There is, unfortunately, no way to duplicate the antibodies found in breast milk.

Some formulas use soy protein in place of nonfat cow's milk as the main source of protein. These formulas are for babies with a milk allergy or intolerance.

Babies with digestive problems or acute, severe diarrhea often need formulas that are very easy to digest and absorb. These formulas use casein as their protein source. They are usually used for only a few days, until the baby can get over his diarrhea.

## Selecting a Formula

All the milk-based formulas currently available are similar in composition and nutrient value. There are small differences between them, but they are more similar than different. Despite this, some babies seem to do better on one milk-based formula than on another. If your baby has gas, vomiting, or bowel problems with one formula, switching to another may help.

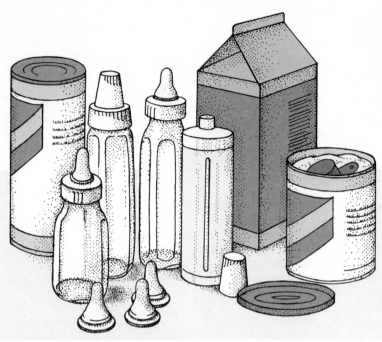

*Successful bottle-feeding requires a variety of supplies and equipment.*

Most formulas are available either with or without supplemental iron. This element is necessary to prevent anemia. Most babies have no problems with the iron-supplemented formulas, and many doctors recommend them. The most common problem from the added iron is constipation. If your baby is constipated, you might temporarily try giving him formula without the extra iron.

Most babies do well on any milk-based formula. Many hospitals give out samples of formula when you leave the hospital. Just because your baby was started on one formula, doesn't mean that he needs to continue on that brand.

### Ready-to-feed, Concentrate, or Powder?

Formulas come in three forms—ready-to-feed, concentrate, and powder. All three forms contain the same protein, fats, and other nutrients. Which you select is a matter of price and convenience. The most convenient, but most expensive, is the ready-to-feed in individual bottles or quart cans. The powder and concentrate are less expensive, but more of a hassle to use.

### Bottles, Nipples, and More

Using formula means you need bottles, nipples, and other paraphernalia. There's really little difference between plastic and glass bottles except that glass bottles are more breakable. Which size you select is also a matter of convenience. Some parents find special bottle/bottle liner systems handy.

Nipples come in many different sizes and shapes. Some are promoted as being "more like mother" because of their shape. What's really important is not what the nipple looks like in the package, but how it works when your baby is sucking on it. If you find a nipple that meets your baby's needs, stick with it.

You may wonder if it's necessary to sterilize your baby's bottles and nipples. If your water supply is safe and clean, there's no need to sterilize or boil bottles and nipples. Clean them with hot, soapy water and then rinse and thoroughly dry them. Some mothers put the bottles in the dishwasher.

### Mixing and Storing Formula

With the concentrated and powdered formulas, water must be added before use. Except when told otherwise by your doctor, never add more water than the instructions say. Overdiluting formula on a regular basis leads to malnutrition.

If your water supply is clean and safe, there's no need to boil the water before adding it to the formula. As a general rule of thumb, if you can drink the water without problems, so can your baby. If you have concerns regarding water quality, check with your local water or health department, or discuss your concerns with your baby's doctor.

If you mix one bottle of formula at a time, you can just add cold tap water to the powder, mix it well, and feed your baby. In areas with fluoride in the water, you won't need to give your baby supplemental fluoride. Avoid using hot tap water—it has a greater tendency to pick up lead from plumbing.

Mixed or open formula can be safely kept refrigerated for twenty-four hours. If you are traveling, the most convenient form is powdered. You simply add water, and you're ready to feed your baby. You should be extremely cautious, however, if there is any question as to water quality—for example, on camping trips or in foreign countries.

## Feeding Your Baby

There's no need to warm up cool bottles of formula. Most babies will take the formula straight from the refrigerator. It's a lot quicker and easier than trying to warm up a bottle of formula when your baby is screaming.

Some parents heat up their baby's formula in a microwave oven. There are potential dangers to this method. If heated in a baby bottle, the formula may cause the bottle to break or leak. Since foods heated in a microwave continue to get hotter for a short while after they are taken out of the oven, the break or crack may not appear until after the bottle has been removed. Another problem is that the formula may become overheated after removal from the microwave; test the formula immediately before feeding to be sure you won't burn your baby.

When feeding your baby, always hold the bottle—never prop it. Your baby shouldn't lie down and feed. He should always be semi-upright or sitting up. Bottle propping causes four problems—increased ear infections, increased cavities, feeding longer than necessary, and decreased emotional and physical satisfaction from being held.

The nipple hole should be large enough that the formula drips out at a steady pace of two drops per second. A flow that's too slow may increase the amount of air your baby swallows. If the flow is too fast, he may choke.

## Breast-feeding

More and more mothers are deciding to breast-feed their new babies. In deciding if you will breast-feed, you will consider many facts; but perhaps the most important one is that breast-feeding gives your baby the best nutrition possible. The more we learn about breast milk and its composition, the more we realize it is the perfect food for babies. Besides the nutritional benefits, a special closeness often develops between breast-feeding mothers and their babies.

### Nutritional Benefits

One of the most convincing arguments for breast-feeding is that human breast milk was designed for human babies, just as cow's milk was designed for calves. Commercially made formulas are attempts at duplicating human breast milk. Formulas are getting closer to breast milk in composition and in the proportion of various fats, proteins, carbohydrates, salts, minerals, and other constituents, but commercial formulas will never be able to duplicate it exactly.

As we learn about the nutrients in breast milk, it becomes more obvious that breast milk provides just about everything a baby needs for good growth and development. All the nutrients are in the perfect balance for optimal absorption and utilization. Earlier research suggested that breast milk is nutritionally inadequate for infants; it now appears that what was inadequate in that research was the study techniques and the information on which it was based. For example, the amount of iron in breast milk was once thought to be inadequate for growing infants. Doctors were concerned about breast-fed babies becoming anemic (not having enough iron in the blood). Further studies revealed that the iron in breast milk is so well absorbed by infants that the small amount present is sufficient to prevent anemia.

Perhaps the only important substance lacking in breast milk is fluoride. No matter how much fluoride a nursing mother takes in, little or none gets into her breast milk. Many doctors feel this is the only type of supplemental nutrient a breast-fed baby needs.

### Immunologic Benefits

Every time you have an illness or receive an immunization, your body develops immunity against

# DIET FOR MOTHER AND BABY

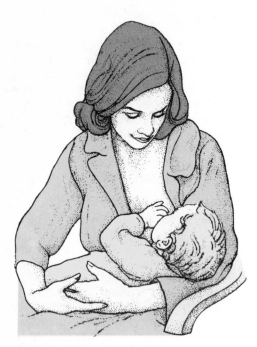

*Breast-feeding offers many benefits to both baby and mother.*

that illness. This means that some special cells become sensitized to a particular type of virus or bacterium. The next time that particular organism invades your body, you are prepared to fight it off. If the immunity is strong enough, you may never come down with that illness again. That's the principle behind immunizations for such diseases as mumps, measles, and pertussis (whooping cough). A vaccine contains inactivated bacteria or virus. Your body is fooled into thinking an infection is present. It develops an immunity against the inactivated virus or bacteria, which also works against the active form.

When you breast-feed your new baby, much of the immunity you have developed is passed on to him through the antibodies present in your breast milk. Many studies have shown that breast-fed babies have fewer illnesses, milder illnesses, and fewer hospitalizations. This increased healthiness is thought to be due to the protection against illness that is passed through the breast milk.

Breast-feeding is no guarantee that your infant will never get sick, but it surely lowers the chances. Many mothers note that once they stop breast-feeding, their infants seem to come down with more colds, runny noses, and so on. This may be due to loss of the protection that the baby received from breast milk.

## Health Benefits for You

Some of the weight you put on during your pregnancy was a special type of high-energy fat called brown fat. With breast-feeding, this extra fat tends to disappear on its own. During the first few months it will almost "melt" away.

## Closeness

Many mothers feel there is a certain closeness they have with babies they breast-feed. It comes from more than just holding and feeding the baby. Many of these women have older children whom they bottle-fed. Although they held and fed them just as much, that special feeling wasn't there. It's the fact of really being the source of nutrition for their growing infants that seems to be important. Unfortunately, the father may feel left out when the mother breast-feeds because he doesn't have an opportunity to feed their new baby. This problem can be offset in a number of ways. One is for the father to occasionally bottle-feed the baby. Another is for him to hold the baby at other times.

## Economic Factors and Convenience

Breast-feeding is much less expensive than bottle-feeding—fewer bottles to sterilize, no formula to prepare, no midnight trips to the kitchen to warm up the baby's meal. You *will* need a breast pump and other equipment; see Chapter 4 for information about breast-feeding supplies.

## Preparation Before Your Baby Is Born

The most important thing you can do to prepare for breast-feeding is to learn all you can about it. There are many good books that discuss breast-feeding exclusively. They range from "how-to" manuals to those that discuss the benefits and the more technical aspects of breast-feeding.

You should discuss your decision to breast-feed with those who are important to you. It is much more difficult to succeed if your husband, parents, or children don't understand why you want to breast-feed your new baby. A young child may be concerned that his new brother or sister is actually hurting you. Your other children may become jealous of all the attention you are giving the new baby. Preparing them for what's to come will make it easier.

Some men become jealous of a new baby, and breast-feeding may make matters worse. Discussing your decision ahead of time is one way to lessen these feelings. Making the father a participant in routine baby care is important.

## Learning the Techniques of Breast-feeding

There are still many misconceptions about breast-feeding. Many women find it frustrating if they don't breast-feed easily and instinctively—they don't realize that they need to *learn* the best way to breast-feed. Years ago, women would learn breast-feeding techniques from their mothers, older sisters, and other women who were breast-feeding. This isn't as likely to happen today. Chances are reasonably good that your mother did not breast-feed you, so she can't really help you with your own breast-feeding.

Classes in breast-feeding techniques are available. Organizations such as the La Leche League offer support and encouragement for women having problems with breast-feeding. If you should experience difficulty, remember that the treatment for most breast-feeding problems is to continue breast-feeding. Rarely does stopping help the problem.

## Getting Started

Most women are now offered the opportunity to breast-feed their newborns shortly after giving birth. Unless you are so exhausted from the delivery that you can't stay awake, you should try nursing your new baby as soon as possible. Often this is done on the delivery table. Don't be discouraged if your baby isn't interested—remember that he's been through a tough and tiring process, too. He may be too worn out to be interested in feeding. Don't take this as a rejection. Some women's breasts don't seem to have milk in them right after the delivery; don't be discouraged—your milk will come in. Feel free to ask questions of your doctor or obstetrical nurse about breast-feeding. Very few new mothers *cannot* breast-feed. Most who feel they have to discontinue just give up too soon. As mentioned earlier, the best treatment for most breast-feeding problems (for example, blocked ducts or insufficient milk supply) is to continue to breast-feed.

When you start, your nipples may be a little sore. This is natural; they aren't accustomed to this type of work and need some time to "toughen up."

## Breast-feeding and Your Diet

You need about five hundred calories a day more than your pre-pregnancy intake if you are breast-feeding. These additional calories, plus the calories available from the three to seven pounds you stored in pregnancy for lactation, supply enough calories to make milk.

Once you reach three to seven pounds above your pre-pregnancy weight (including two to four pounds for the weight of your lactating breasts), let your weight be a guide to the number of calories you consume each day. Your activity level and the amount of milk you are producing for your baby will affect your weight.

In addition to extra calories, your breast-feeding diet should include extra protein for milk production, more calcium-rich foods, more vitamins, and more fluids than your normal diet. Here are some simple guidelines:

- Continue to take your prenatal vitamins (unless your doctor tells you otherwise).

- Drink more milk than when you were pregnant (drink about five glasses a day). If you have a milk-intolerance problem, calcium supplements may be necessary. Let your doctor advise you about this.

- Eat a varied, balanced, good-quality diet.

- Pay special attention to fluids, making sure you drink enough to quench your thirst.

- Avoid junk foods and "empty" calories.

## Foods and Drugs to Avoid

Every breast-feeding mother wonders if something she ate caused fussiness, gas, diarrhea, a rash, or nasal stuffiness in her baby. While almost all foods can be eaten without problem, some foods can cause difficulty. Cow's milk in the mother's diet may cause colicky symptoms in some babies. If this is a problem for your baby, he will draw his legs up toward his body and scream with gas pains after feeding. You can eliminate milk from your diet for four to seven days to see if the symptoms of colic disappear. As your baby grows older, re-introduce milk into your diet, since the reaction to milk is often outgrown. If you eliminate dairy products from your diet, you will need to talk with your doctor about a calcium supplement.

# DIET FOR MOTHER AND BABY

Other foods that may cause problems for breast-fed babies include those that have food additives and dyes, certain gas-producing foods (such as broccoli, cabbage, and beans), eggs, nuts, tomatoes, shellfish, chocolate, corn, strawberries, citrus fruits, onion, garlic, and some spices. To decide if a particular food upsets your baby, eliminate that single food from your diet and see if the symptoms disappear.

Occasionally, consuming food in enormous amounts will cause problems for a breast-fed baby. A half gallon of apple juice or orange juice, very large amounts of fruit, a jar of peanuts, or any other food consumed in unusually large quantities may cause your baby to have diarrhea or gas.

In the past, breast-feeding mothers were encouraged to drink beer to aid milk production. We now know that beer will not increase milk production. We also know that beer and other alcoholic beverages readily enter the breast milk in about the same concentration as your blood alcohol level. Since no safe level of alcohol has been established for the breast-fed baby, it is probably wise to strictly limit your alcohol intake or not drink at all. In addition, alcohol can inhibit letdown (the release of milk from the milk-producing sacs within the breasts to the milk ducts), so your baby will not get the milk he needs.

Cigarette smoking and breast-feeding are not compatible. Heavy cigarette smoking may reduce milk production; increase the incidence of nausea, colicky symptoms, and diarrhea in the baby; and decrease the vitamin C content of the milk. Smoking near the baby increases his risk of pneumonia and bronchitis. As in pregnancy, the best advice is to quit if you can, or at least cut down. Avoid smoking in your home.

Caffeine passes into breast milk and may cause your baby to have an upset stomach and be irritable. If you suspect caffeine is affecting your baby, try eliminating coffee, tea, cola drinks, chocolate, and other caffeine-containing foods from your diet to see if the symptoms disappear.

Vitamin B$_6$ has received some attention lately. In large amounts (more than is contained in your prenatal vitamin tablet) it may inhibit milk production.

Almost every drug or medication makes its way into breast milk. Some medications appear to have no harmful effects on your baby, while others are most certainly not safe. Talk with your pharmacist or pediatrician before taking any prescribed or over-the-counter medications—be sure the medications you take pose no problems for your baby. If you need to take *any* drugs, particularly on a regular basis, discuss it with your doctor. You may have to stop breast-feeding until all the drug has passed out of your system.

## Allergies

It is extremely rare for a baby to be allergic to his mother's breast milk. If there are allergies on either side of the family, particularly to milk or milk products, your baby is more likely to have problems with formula than with your breast milk.

## Diapers and Bowel Movements

Many parents of breast-fed babies notice that their babies' bowel movements are different from those of bottle-fed babies. The bowel movements are soft and yellowish. Changing the soiled diapers of a breast-fed baby may not be as unpleasant as dealing with the diapers of a bottle-fed infant. Because breast milk is so well absorbed, breast-fed infants are rarely constipated. All of this changes, of course, once a baby starts on formula or solid food.

## When Should You Not Breast-feed?

There are very few instances when breast-feeding should be discontinued or avoided. If, for example, you must take a drug that crosses into the breast milk and has the potential for harming your baby, you will probably elect not to breast-feed. In addition, there are certain diseases and infections (although few in number) that may force you to avoid breast-feeding your baby.

Many doctors use the guideline that if you are too sick to bottle-feed your baby, you should not breast-feed.

## Breast-feeding and Working

Some women wonder if they can continue to breast-feed their baby once they return to work. Most women in this situation find that they can, with a little planning. It's important for you to remember that breast-feeding is not an all-or-nothing proposition.

The human breast makes milk on a "supply and demand" basis. The more milk is taken out, the more milk is made. And human breast milk production is very adaptable. Many women have no problems with breast-feeding in the morning before work, when they pick up their baby in the afternoon, during the evening, and, again, at night.

The missed feedings during the day can be taken care of. Properly frozen breast milk can be stored for up to two weeks. You also may be able to pump your breasts at work and refrigerate the milk in a clean bottle. This pumped breast milk can be fed to your baby the next day by your babysitter so that your child's diet consists solely of breast milk.

If you are going to successfully combine work and breast-feeding, you must be flexible. What works for one woman may not work best for you. Experiment with your schedule and the times you feed your baby.

### How Long Should You Breast-feed?

Breast milk alone supplies all the nutrition your baby needs for at least his first six months of life. Many experts now believe that a baby needs nothing but breast milk for his entire first year of life.

If you decide to feed your baby solids, wait until he's at least six months old. Even at that age, he gets most of his nutrients from the breast milk, not solids. A good guideline to follow is that your baby should be old enough, and sufficiently coordinated, to let you know when he's full. If he can't yet do this, he isn't old enough to start eating solid foods. Also, he should be offered the breast or formula *before* you give him any solids until he's at least one year old.

### Stopping Breast-feeding

How long to breast-feed is an individual decision. Most women stop within the first year. Remember, even if you breast-feed for only a few months, you have given your baby that much of a headstart.

Sometimes a baby will decide when it's time to stop. He may lose interest in the breast or prefer solids and a cup to breast milk. Some women breast-feed for two or more years.

### Demand Versus Scheduled Feedings

Arguments have been going back and forth as to which method, demand or scheduled feedings, is best. If your schedule is flexible and you are willing to feed your baby frequently, a demand-feeding program may be best. You feed the baby whenever he seems hungry. A potential problem with the demand-feeding method is that your baby may get used to taking only small amounts of formula or milk frequently and you will end up spending a lot of time feeding him. Using a regular schedule may be easier on you. You know when it's time to feed your child.

It's important not to overfeed your baby. Once he loses interest in the bottle or breast, stop. Don't try to coax him into finishing the bottle. An infant generally doesn't need more than one quart of formula a day.

### A Word About Burping

Babies generally swallow some air as they are feeding, although breast-fed babies tend to swallow less air than bottle-fed babies. To minimize the amount swallowed by a bottle-fed baby, try to always keep the nipple full of formula as you feed. Regardless of the method of feeding, an air bubble will probably accumulate and make your baby feel uncomfortable. To prevent that distress,

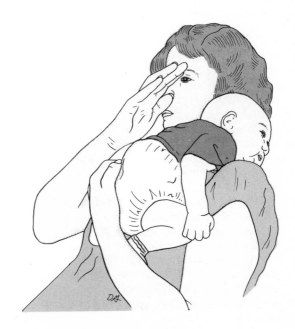

*The over-the-shoulder burping method.*

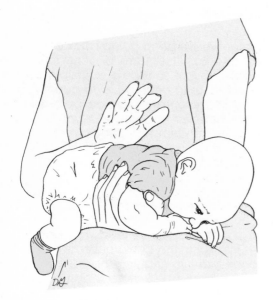

*The across-the-lap burping position.*

you should burp him at the conclusion of each feeding; you may also want to burp him at the midpoint of the feeding, to prevent the buildup of too large a bubble.

There are a number of commonly used positions for burping, and no one of them is the "right" one. You will eventually find the one that is most effective for your baby, although on some occasions you may have to run through the whole repertoire of burping positions until you get results. These positions generally have in common putting some slight pressure on the baby's abdomen—by placing him against your shoulder so that he is facing backward; by sitting him up on your lap, resting his midsection on your forearm; or by laying him face down across your lap—and then gently rubbing or patting the middle of his back. Remember to protect the area beneath his mouth with a cloth because he is quite likely to bring up some milk with the gas bubble; this is usually only a small amount and does not indicate a feeding problem.

Some babies don't accumulate a large bubble or aren't made uncomfortable by one, so if your baby doesn't burp after several minutes of concerted effort, there is no point in exhausting both of you in a marathon burping session. Simply put him face down in his crib as you would if he had burped; that prone position often brings up the bubble by itself. Of course, you want to spare your baby any discomfort that might result from an air bubble, but if your burping efforts aren't success-

ful, the worst that may happen is that your baby will noisily let you know when the bubble is making him uncomfortable, at which point you can simply pick him up and renew your burping efforts.

## A Word to Fathers About Your Role in Feeding

Research has shown that fathers can influence the diets of their families in some very important ways. In one study, eighty-nine percent of the mothers served infrequently or eliminated from the family diet entirely those foods that their husbands disliked. In another study, eighty-one percent of the mothers surveyed planned meals based on the food preferences and dislikes of their husbands. As a result of such studies, nutritionists now urge fathers to recognize the important effect their food tastes have on the nutritional well-being of their families.

Your food preferences and dietary habits are the first important way you are involved in feeding. A nutritious, age-appropriate diet is the very best for your baby. Your role in achieving this is essential.

During pregnancy, you and the baby's mother probably discussed how you wanted to feed your baby—by breast or bottle. If breast-feeding was your choice, your unswerving support during the time your baby is breast-fed is crucial. If bottle-feeding was your choice, being knowledgeable about formula preparation and healthy feeding practices is necessary and valuable. Perhaps your choice was to breast-feed first and bottle-feed later, or to combine the two feeding methods. In any case, your support and involvement with feeding your baby will be helpful to your baby and pleasurable for you.

If your baby is breast-fed, you obviously cannot directly provide milk for your baby, although you can give him bottles of expressed milk if there are times when it is inconvenient or impossible for your wife to breast-feed. There are other important ways you can be helpful during feedings. You can bring your baby to his mother for night feedings and then tuck him back in bed later. You can burp the baby after feedings and take the opportunity to enjoy the quiet but alert time he has after feeding.

Many breast-feeding mothers experience sore nipples, fatigue, and doubts about milk supply.

Your encouragement and nurturing help are important. In fact, one study has shown a relationship between the father's support of breast-feeding and its success or failure.

Another important way you can help is to teach other family members about breast-feeding, so they will understand and support this method of feeding. In the past, less was known about the benefits of breast-feeding than is known today, and feeding practices were different.

If your baby is bottle-fed, you can help by actively sharing the feedings with his mother. Make it your responsibility to mix formula in the proper way and to ensure that the feeding equipment is clean and functioning well.

Always hold your baby when you feed him. He will begin to trust that you love him and are able to satisfy his needs. To provide for normal eye muscle development, hold him sometimes in your right arm and sometimes in your left. Hold him so that his head is slightly elevated. Feeding in a flat position is associated with an increased incidence of middle ear infections.

Discontinue feeding your baby when he indicates that he is through. Burp him during and after feedings. The frequency of burping depends on how much air he seems to swallow.

Whether your baby is breast- or bottle-fed, you can help by keeping feeding times calm. Run interference with the doorbell and the telephone. Anything you do to reduce tension is beneficial.

When your baby is ready for table foods, you can be involved in many ways. You can help by making mealtimes pleasant and happy. Tension during feedings diminishes appetite. Make an effort to indicate pleasure with the variety of foods you offer your baby even if the food does not appeal to you. As tempting as it might be, avoid using food as a reward for good behavior or a special accomplishment.

Never offer your baby junk food or alcohol. Neither is part of a nutritious diet, and each replaces the foods your baby does need for growth and health. In addition, even small amounts of alcohol can be toxic to a young child.

Your involvement with your child's mealtimes is important. You can have a significant effect on your baby's health, and your relationship will benefit from the time you spend together.

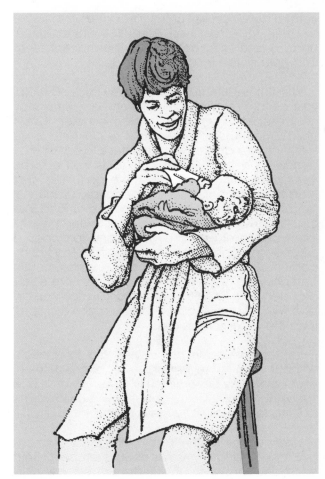

*A new father can bottle-feed even a breast-fed baby.*

## Oral Health

When your baby begins to smile, you will probably see an endearing toothless grin. However, within a few months, you will notice a glimmer of something white or you will hear a clunk when the feeding spoon touches the first tooth. (See Chapter 10 for information about tooth formation and eruption.) By taking a few steps early in your baby's life, you can establish a pattern to help ensure that your baby will continue to have a healthy smile throughout her life.

Many parents overlook the importance of their child's teeth, especially their "baby" teeth (also called primary, or deciduous, teeth). Some parents do not realize that teeth serve functions other than biting and chewing and that prevention is the best method of caring for teeth.

Your baby's teeth (1) help to provide nutrition, (2) help to make speech possible, (3) aid in the normal development of the jaw bones and facial muscles, (4) add to an attractive appearance, and (5) reserve space for the permanent teeth and help guide them into position.

Without healthy, reasonably well-aligned teeth, your child may have difficulty chewing and may not be able to eat a well-balanced diet. If your child's mouth is sore because of cavities, loose teeth, or sore gums, she may refuse to eat or may accept only those foods or liquids that can be consumed without causing more pain. This may lead to additional problems because a variety of foods is needed for a balanced diet and because chewing foods of different textures stimulates and exercises the gums and provides a cleansing action for the teeth. The first stage of digestion of some foods takes place in the mouth, and chewing helps break up foods to more easily digested sizes. If your child swallows too rapidly and without chewing food properly, she may prolong the digestion process.

Your baby's teeth are a vital aid to speech. Without healthy, reasonably well-aligned teeth, your baby may have difficulty forming words and speaking clearly. (Think about how a child who is starting to lose primary teeth speaks.)

Like muscles in other parts of the body, your baby's face and jaw muscles need exercise to help them develop; without well-developed jaw muscles, your baby's jawbones may not develop properly. Sucking provides exercise for your baby's jaw, cheek, and tongue muscles. When your baby is old enough for solid foods, chewing also provides exercise for these muscles. This exercise is necessary for these structures to develop enough for your baby's teeth to come in properly.

Your baby's appearance is as important to you now as it will be to him later. Not everyone naturally has sparkling white teeth and a beautiful smile. Your baby may have inherited tendencies (for example, a tendency toward having large teeth in a small jaw) that will affect the appearance of his teeth. Occurrences during fetal life, like a mother's having a fever or taking certain medications, may also affect early tooth development. But you can help your child learn good oral hygiene habits early, which will help add to as attractive an appearance as possible.

Your child's primary teeth must last five or ten years or longer. As a permanent tooth reaches the stage of development at which it is ready to erupt (emerge through the gum), the roots of the primary tooth it will replace begin to resorb (break down and dissolve). Gradually, the permanent tooth pushes the primary tooth out and takes the place the primary tooth has been reserving for it. If a primary tooth is lost too soon, the permanent tooth will have no guide to follow. Also, the teeth next to a missing tooth may drift into the space left by the missing tooth. Because these teeth are occupying the space meant for another tooth, as their permanent replacements come in, they too will appear in the wrong position. The dentist may provide your child with a space maintainer if a primary tooth is lost too soon. But it is preferable to take preventive measures early so your child can keep all of his primary teeth until they are ready to be shed.

## Fluoride

Fluoride combines with the enamel of the teeth and makes the teeth more resistant to decay. An estimated two of every three potential cavities can be prevented by the use of fluoride. Fluoride can be provided in drops to be swallowed, in a gel to be applied to the teeth, in a chewable form, in fluoride-vitamin combinations, and in toothpaste. The most common source is the community water supply.

Because the enamel of some teeth is forming during fetal life, it is important for the future health of your baby's teeth to obtain an adequate supply of fluoride. If you drink fluoridated water, you will be receiving ample fluoride. However, if you have a private water supply that is not fluoridated (such as your own well) or drink bottled water, check with your dentist about the best source of fluoride for you.

If your baby is breast-fed or fed a premixed formula, he probably will not be receiving enough fluoride and may need a fluoride supplement. Your doctor or dentist can tell you the best supplement to use.

You should also be aware that excess fluoride can cause permanent discoloration of the teeth. Therefore, if your drinking water is fluoridated, it is recommended that you not use additional fluoride supplements.

## Care of Your Baby's Teeth

You should begin checking your baby's mouth on a periodic basis even before the first tooth erupts (see Chapter 10 for more information on tooth formation and eruption). This will give you an idea of the normal appearance of your baby's mouth. Teething may be preceded by whining, crying, or drooling more than usual. Other common signs of teething are changes in feeding habits, trouble in sleeping, and increased irritability. If your baby's gums are red and swollen or if you can feel or see the tip of a tooth, teething probably is causing these changes in your baby's behavior. However, if your baby also has a fever or a rash or is vomiting, something else may be wrong.

Your baby will have a strong urge to chew at this time and should be given a teething ring or dry toast to chew on. Babies will vary in their need for other help at this time. Check with your baby's doctor or your dentist before using any of the commercial preparations to ease teething discomfort. To help soothe your baby's gums, wipe a dampened gauze pad over them two or three times a day.

After your baby's teeth begin to appear, clean them daily with a dampened gauze pad or clean washcloth until your baby is big enough to begin using a toothbrush. When your baby is one and a half to two years old, purchase a child-sized toothbrush. At least once a day—preferably before bedtime—you should brush your child's teeth. Several other times during the day—preferably after meals—let your child "brush" her own teeth; this will consist mainly of chewing on the toothbrush. At this age, make no attempt to try to teach your child toothbrushing techniques. It is more important to establish a pattern of dental care, and even chewing on a toothbrush helps clean the teeth.

Never give your baby a bottle of milk, juice, or a sweetened beverage when you put her to bed, and never put honey, syrup, or another sweetening agent on your baby's pacifier. These practices may help comfort your baby, but they can cause severe destruction of your baby's teeth. Nursing decay syndrome, or nursing bottle caries (dental cavities), can result from such practices. When your baby is awake and sucking on a bottle, the liquid is rapidly diluted with saliva and swallowed. However, if your baby falls asleep while nursing and swallows less often, the bacteria normally present in her mouth have time to turn the sugars in these liquids into acids that attack the tooth enamel. Sweetening agents on a pacifier also permit the sugars to remain in the mouth too long. The teeth most severely damaged are the upper

incisors, and it has been necessary to remove teeth destroyed by this type of decay in children as young as eighteen months old.

Other practices that are just as destructive are putting sugar in a piece of cloth and using this as a pacifier or using a piece of bread as a pacifier. The starches in the bread are quickly converted to sugars in the mouth, which can then serve as a food source for decay-causing bacteria.

Dental decay is among the most common diseases affecting children, and it is the most preventable. Eating a well-balanced diet low in sugars, drinking fluoridated water or using fluoride supplements, toothbrushing after meals, and visiting the dentist at recommended intervals can help prevent most caries or catch decay at an early stage. Caries in the primary teeth must be taken care of to relieve your child's pain and to help maintain the teeth until they are ready to be replaced by the permanent teeth.

Inflamed, bleeding gums are not normal but are a sign of dental problems. Even a young child can have gum disease, which needs the attention of a dentist. Dental decay in primary teeth or gum disease that is not taken care of can lead to infection or other problems that may affect the permanent teeth.

Young children exploring their world by crawling, toddling, and attempting to stand alone may fall or bump into things and injure their teeth and mouths. Any mouth injury that results in excessive bleeding or a chipped, loose, or displaced tooth needs to be evaluated by a dentist. If a tooth is knocked out, put the tooth in a cup of water and take it and your child to the dentist as soon as possible.

Thumb sucking is a natural and satisfying behavior for babies and young children. Most children outgrow this activity by four or five years of age. It should not be a cause for concern in young children.

## Visiting the Dentist

You should begin taking your child to the dentist no later than by the age of three years. The American Academy of Pediatric Dentistry recommends a visit by one year of age.

Usually all the primary teeth have erupted between two and three years of age. Most children

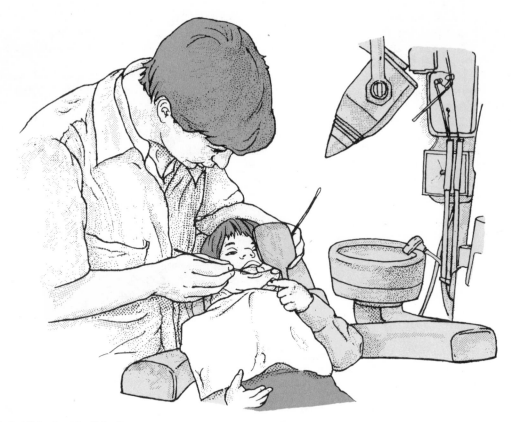

*Your child's first visit to the dentist will occur between the ages of one and three.*

three years old or younger have no or few dental problems, and the first visit to the dentist can consist primarily of an examination and probably a cleaning.

Your dentist is often the best resource for finding a dentist for your child. When your baby is about one year old, talk to your dentist about him. If you live in a small town or a rural area, your dentist probably will be your child's dentist also. However, many dentists, especially those in cities and large suburban areas, prefer not to see child patients. Instead, they will refer you to a pediatric dentist, or pedodontist, a dentist who has specialized in taking care of children. If you have no dentist or are new to an area, check with the local dental society about which dentists in the area treat children.

Most children fear strangers, and the dentist initially will be a stranger to your child. You can help your child to realize that the dentist is another friend by the attitude with which you approach the first and successive dental visits. If you are relaxed and matter-of-fact about going to the dentist, your child also will be. However, if you begin to show signs of fear and tension (such as clutching your child's hand tightly), these fears will be transferred to your child. Avoid situations in which your child hears you or someone else talking about painful details of dental procedures. Such procedures will not be necessary for your child for many years, if ever; hearing about them can result in unnecessary fears and apprehension. Also, never threaten your child with a visit to the dentist or any other health care professional. Be honest with your child if he asks about procedures or pain. Some procedures may be uncomfortable and your child needs to know this, but *only* if he asks ahead of time. If you are unsure of an answer, tell your child that he can ask the dentist about it. Remember also that even painful procedures can be made painless with anesthesia; your child can be told this if he is concerned about pain.

## Diet Progression, Portions, and Scheduling

Infant feeding has changed enormously since the turn of this century. From 1900 to about 1920, most babies were fed only breast milk or occasionally modified cow's milk formula for the first year of life. The first supplements were cod liver oil to prevent rickets and orange juice to prevent scurvy.

During the next thirty years, solids were offered earlier, to supply the iron and vitamins thought to be missing from milk and to accustom the infant to a more varied diet. During that time, mothers were eager to have their babies gain weight rapidly, since a fat baby was considered desirable.

By the late 1930's, the approach to infant feeding was rigid and pat. Formula was more readily available, and it was becoming more "modern" to bottle-feed on an inflexible four-hour schedule. By the late 1940's, more than one-half of babies in this country were bottle-fed. By 1970, more than three-fourths of babies were bottle-fed.

During the 1970's, primarily because breast-feeding was beginning to be considered more "natural," things began to change. By 1975, thirty-five percent of babies were breast-fed. Today, about sixty percent of mothers in this country choose to breast-feed their babies.

Recommendations for infant feeding have changed, too. In 1980, the American Academy of Pediatrics' Committee on Nutrition revised its 1950's recommendations. In 1985, they published *The Pediatric Nutrition Handbook*. These more cur-
continued on page 295

# GUIDE TO INFANT FEEDING

This guide provides information about the physiological and social development of infants during the first year, as they relate to feeding. The recommended diet for each period is provided, along with reminders of what to avoid. Suggested amounts of food are listed, too. Keep in mind that the size of your baby, his growth, and his activity level all affect the amounts he needs. Your baby's doctor can help you decide just the right amount to feed your baby.

| AGE | RECOMMENDED DIET | AMOUNT TO FEED DAILY | PHYSIOLOGICAL AND SOCIAL DEVELOPMENT |
|---|---|---|---|
| **Month 1** | Breast milk (on demand or schedule)<br><br>Vitamin K by mouth or injection at birth<br><br>Possibly vitamin D and fluoride<br><br>*or*<br>Iron-fortified commercial formula (on demand or schedule). No vitamins.<br><br>Possibly fluoride if reconstituting with water containing less than 0.3 part per million<br><br>Avoid: Cow's milk, goat's milk, and milk substitutes for the whole first year. No honey for first year. No solids needed until 4–6 months old. | 14–30 ounces | Limited ability to digest complex proteins, starches, and fats other than those found in breast milk or commercial formula.<br><br>Able to suck and swallow rhythmically.<br><br>Tongue protrudes, so unable to take solids.<br><br>Gastric acid and pepsin (to digest protein) reach adult levels during second month. |

_ continued _

## GUIDE TO INFANT FEEDING continued

| AGE | RECOMMENDED DIET | AMOUNT TO FEED DAILY | PHYSIOLOGICAL AND SOCIAL DEVELOPMENT |
|---|---|---|---|
| Month 2 | Same as above | 22–40 ounces | May be able to take more at each feeding.<br><br>May have longer periods of sleep and wakefulness. |
| Month 3 | Same as above | 24–40 ounces | Has better head control. Recognizes breast or bottle as the source of food. Usually quiets in the nursing position.<br><br>Amylase (to digest starch) increases after month 2. |
| Months 4 through 6 | Same as above<br><br>Some infants begin to show a readiness for solids by sitting forward, indicating fullness, and being able to take food from a spoon.<br><br>By six months, may need supplemental iron. Use one-grain cereals (rice first, 3–5 tbsp. in two feedings).<br><br>Introduce only one new food each week to recognize allergy. | 4 months: 25–42 ounces<br><br>5 months: 27–44 ounces<br><br>6 months: 30–46 ounces | Extrudes foods from mouth less (after 4 months).<br><br>Able to swallow solids at 4–5 months.<br><br>Able to lean forward and open mouth to indicate hunger.<br><br>Able to lean back and turn away when full.<br><br>First teeth may erupt. |
| Month 7 | Breast milk or formula<br><br>Cereal, in two feedings<br><br>Fruits, vegetables, and meat. Offer soft, chewable foods (homemade or commercial baby food or food processed in small grinder). Order of introduction is not important. Add only one new food each week.<br><br>Avoid: Chocolate, oranges, nuts, and tomatoes (for whole first year). | 30–32 ounces<br><br>3–4 tbsp. | Able to sit in a chair and hold own bottle.<br><br>May gag on solids.<br><br>May do well with finger foods, such as banana, steamed vegetable bits, and toast strips. |

| AGE | RECOMMENDED DIET | AMOUNT TO FEED DAILY | PHYSIOLOGICAL AND SOCIAL DEVELOPMENT |
|---|---|---|---|
| **Month 8** | Breast milk or formula | 29–32 ounces | Able to reach for cup and spoon. Able to lift cup. |
| | Cereal | 4–8 tbsp. | |
| | Fruits, vegetables, meat, and bread | 16–38 tbsp. | Expresses fullness by turning away, playing, or activity. Pushes away food he does not want. Begins to have a "regular" pattern of eating. |
| **Month 9** | Breast milk or formula | 26–32 ounces | Pancreatic amylase (to digest starches) reaches adult level. |
| | Cereal | 4–10 tbsp. | |
| | Fruits, vegetables, meats, breads, and assorted finger foods | 18–38 tbsp. | Able to bite off appropriate amount to eat, chew easily, drink from a bottle alone, and pick up food using pincer grasp. |
| **Month 10** | Breast milk or formula | 24–32 ounces | May poke at and play with food. Likes to feed self and is able to use cup. Will turn away when full. |
| | Cereal | 4–12 tbsp. | |
| | Fruits, vegetables, meats, breads, and assorted finger foods | 18–38 tbsp. or as desired | |
| **Month 11** | Breast milk or formula | 24–32 ounces | Able to drink 4–5 swallows at a time from a cup. |
| | Solids, including cereal (as in month 10). May add cheese, cottage cheese, and yogurt unless there is a cow's milk allergy. | 22–50 tbsp. or as desired | Mealtimes may be messy. Likes to squish food in fingers. Able to hold own cup and spoon. |
| **Month 12** | Breast milk or formula | 24–32 ounces | May begin to deliberately spit. |
| | Solids (as in month 11) | 22–50 tbsp. or as desired | Wants to feed self most of meal. May be proficient with spoon and cup. |

continued from page 293
rent guidelines reflect an understanding of the infant's nutritional needs and the maturation of his organ systems, specifically, his digestive capabilities; the nutrients he requires for his rapidly developing and growing brain and central nervous system; and his kidneys' ability to excrete the by-products. The guidelines also recognize the effects of the type of milk an infant receives, the foods he receives, and how much he is fed, on his social and physical development, size, and activity level.

# DIET FOR MOTHER AND BABY

In its guidelines, the committee defines three feeding periods in the *first year of life*. The first period, the *nursing period,* encompasses the time during which your baby is capable only of sucking and swallowing liquids. The second period, the *transitional period,* begins when your baby first gets solid foods and lasts until he is able to take most of his food from the family table with only some modification. The third period, the *modified adult period,* occurs when your baby receives most of his food from your table.

## The Nursing Period

From birth to about four to six months of age, your baby is able only to suck and swallow liquids. His ability to take food from a spoon begins about the fourth or fifth month. During these early months and for the whole first year of life, the very best food for your baby is breast milk. Breast milk provides just the right blend of proteins, fats, carbohydrates, minerals, and calories. It also contains enzymes to aid digestion and minerals, such as calcium and iron, in a form in which they can be almost completely absorbed by your baby. Breast milk contains antibodies, which help protect your baby from infection and disease. If your baby is exclusively breast-fed, the incidence of allergy is greatly reduced.

If breast milk is your baby's only food, certain vitamin supplements may be recommended. Your baby will probably be given vitamin K at birth, by injection or orally, to protect him from hemorrhage. Vitamin K is necessary to help blood clot. If your baby has limited exposure to the sun, he may be given a vitamin D supplement. Your baby's doctor can discuss this with you.

Fluoride supplementation is a controversial issue. Experts disagree about whether it is necessary or advisable. You should speak to your baby's doctor and perhaps to your baby's dentist about this.

Iron supplementation is not usually necessary for a full-term, healthy, breast-fed infant. The iron stores your baby accumulated in the last months of pregnancy in addition to the iron obtained from breast milk should be sufficient until he begins to get iron in his diet in the second six months of life.

If you do not breast-feed, a commercial formula is recommended for the whole first year. If you bottle-feed, your baby needs no supplements at all. All the vitamins and minerals he requires are present in the formula. Fluoride supplements may be suggested if the formula is reconstituted with water containing less than 0.3 part per million of fluoride.

During the nursing period, babies are generally fed milk on demand. Breast-fed infants will probably feed more frequently since breast milk passes readily through the digestive tract. You can expect to feed your breast-fed newborn eight to eighteen times a day. As he grows older, the number of feedings may decrease as he becomes capable of taking more milk with each feeding.

Bottle-fed infants often feed less frequently than breast-fed infants because formula is not as readily digested and tends to leave the stomach less quickly. Whether you feed your infant on demand or on a schedule, be sensitive to when he is finished feeding. Even though it is tempting to have him finish the bottle of formula you have prepared, do not force him—be careful not to overfeed him. (See the chart in this chapter for suggested amounts of milk.)

Some foods should be avoided during this period. They include whole cow's milk, skim milk, 2% milk, and homemade soy milk. All are high in protein and mineral content. The metabolic by-products of these would stress your baby's kidneys, causing your baby to become dehydrated. Skim milk lacks the essential fatty acids necessary for the development of the central nervous system and the vascular system, and it does not provide enough calories for growth. Goat's milk is dangerously low in folic acid, and if it is unpasteurized, it may be contaminated with disease-causing bacteria. Homemade soy milk contains no vitamin K and inadequate calcium (placing an infant at risk for rickets).

Solid foods are inappropriate before four to six months of age since your baby cannot digest and use the starches contained in such foods as baby cereal. Starting your baby on solids too early may cause diarrhea, impair growth, increase the likelihood of obesity, and increase the incidence of allergy.

Honey is another food that should not be given to your infant—in either raw or cooked form—during the first year of life. Honey may contain spores of the bacteria that cause botulism.

## The Transitional Period

The transitional period begins sometime between the fourth and sixth months. By then your baby can show a readiness for solids by being able to indicate when he is hungry and full, to swallow food from a spoon without extruding it from his mouth, and to digest more complex starches, proteins, and fats. You will know he is ready for solids when he shows an interest in what you are eating.

Milk (breast milk or an iron-fortified formula) is still the most important food in his diet. Since he is beginning to deplete his iron stores, an iron-fortified cereal is often the first solid food offered. The cereal can be mixed with breast milk, water, or formula. Start with just a teaspoonful in a very liquid form. During the next months, you might build up to three level tablespoons of cereal a day to supply the seven milligrams of iron your baby needs. Use one-grain cereals at first, such as rice, oats, or barley. Later, you can introduce multigrain cereals.

After cereal, the order of introduction of new foods is not important. However, breast-fed infants might be offered a high-protein food, such as chicken or lamb, because breast milk is somewhat lower in protein than formula. Some parents like to offer vegetables first, hoping to accustom their babies to foods less sweet than fruit. Once you begin to give your baby solids, offer him water too because his kidneys must work harder to excrete the by-products of these new foods.

Introduce only one new food a week so you will be able to identify which food, if any, causes a problem for your baby. You might suspect a food allergy if your baby has diarrhea, vomiting, abdominal pain, eczema, or a chronic runny nose. The most common offending foods include wheat, soy milk, cow's milk, eggs, orange juice, tomatoes, peanut butter (and other nut products), chocolate, fish, and beef. If your family has a history of allergy, be sure to tell your baby's doctor and get some special guidance for feeding your baby.

Foods to avoid in the second six months of life include honey, milks other than breast milk and formula, and allergenic foods, such as tomatoes, orange juice, nuts, and chocolate. Avoid adding salt to your baby's food; he does not need it. Avoid giving him large pieces of meat, hard candy, nuts, and popcorn, which may choke him. Also avoid nitrate-containing foods, such as spinach and turnip or collard greens. These foods have been associated with methemoglobinemia, a very serious condition that interferes with the oxygen-carrying ability of the blood. The American Academy of Pediatrics also recommends not giving your baby juice in a bottle since this predisposes to tooth decay.

For suggestions about how much food to feed your baby and how often during the transitional period, refer to the "Guide to Infant Feeding" chart in this chapter.

## The Modified Adult Period

This period begins about the eighth month of life, when your baby is able to eat chunkier foods and a more varied diet. You will find that he will finally be on a more predictable feeding schedule. Most of his food can come from the family table, although you will have to cut it in smaller pieces and perhaps grind his meat.

For suggestions about how much food to feed your baby and how often during the modified adult period, refer to the "Guide to Infant Feeding" chart.

## The Toddler Period

The rapid rate of growth in the first year of life slows during the second year. Correspondingly, your baby's appetite diminishes as well. She may express some very strong food preferences and refuse to eat foods that she seemed to enjoy as an infant. She may show lack of interest in eating and may dawdle for what seems like hours over her meal. She wants to feed herself but may be very messy with cup, spoon, and fingers. If a food is too difficult to chew, she will take it out of her mouth and not eat it. Cutting her food into easy-to-eat pieces will help.

Since individual children vary so much in their growth, activity level, and interest in food, the amount of food to feed and how frequently to feed vary too. In general, your toddler needs about nine hundred to eighteen hundred calories a day in her second year. The calories should be from a high-quality, varied diet. Milk intake should be monitored by your baby's doctor. Some toddlers do not get enough milk, while others get too many of their daily calories from milk.

Offering your child a balanced, varied diet, including some high-quality protein foods, and avoiding "junk" food is the best approach to feeding. Never force-feed your toddler. Even when it seems she is not eating at all, force-feeding is not the answer; this approach may lead to the development of some unnecessary feeding problems. Let her natural appetite be your guide. If she is offered only good food, then when she does eat, she will eat well.

Each new stage of development offers new feeding challenges to parents. Remember that by offering your baby very nutritious foods, prepared and portioned in a way that is appropriate for her age, you are doing the very best you can to help her be healthy.

## Making Your Own Baby Food

The first foods you offer your baby should be smooth in texture and thin in consistency. Initially, solid foods should, therefore, be offered to her in a very liquid form—that is, pureed. At about seven to eight months, your baby is able to manage soft chunks of food with some substance (such as bits of cheese, flakes of fish, peas, and Cheerios), which she can get from the family table. As a result, pureeing your baby's food is a temporary task.

What is the difference between commercial and homemade baby food? The difference really depends on the quality of the foods used to make the baby food, the care given to preserve the vitamin and mineral content, and the amount of salt, sugar, preservatives, and spices that have been added to the food. In general, homemade baby food is often denser in calories. That is, it often is thicker and has less water. Commercial baby food is required by law to list the ingredients contained in each jar. You will notice that in response to parents' wishes, commercial baby food now rarely contains added salt, sugar, spices, or preservatives.

Homemade baby food may have a higher vitamin and mineral content than commercial baby food if it is made from the very freshest foods and if it is served soon after preparation. A long shelf life and exposure to light may reduce the vitamin content of commercial baby food.

In the preparation of commercial baby food, care is taken to be certain the food is free of bacteria and other organisms that could make your baby sick. Homemade baby food is safe, too, if a high standard of cleanliness is used in its preparation.

If you decide to make your own baby food, the following method may be helpful.

## Preparing Your Own Baby Food With a Blender or Food Processor

1. Use the freshest and best food available. Avoid canned foods, which are high in salt and additives. Avoid using foods that have added sugar, spices, preservatives, or fat, and don't add these ingredients yourself.

2. Wash your hands carefully before handling the food or equipment.

3. Make sure all the cooking utensils, the cutting board, and the blender or food processor are very clean. You can do this by scrubbing all equipment with hot, soapy water and rinsing it well.

4. Prepare the food for cooking by washing fruits and vegetables well and removing skins, pits, and seeds. Remove the fat, skin, and bones from meats.

5. Cook the food by steaming or by boiling in a very small amount of water in a covered pot. Cook until tender.

6. Add a cupful of the cooked food to the blender or processor and puree with just enough of the cooking liquid to allow the blades to spin. Add more cooking liquid or water if necessary.

7. Some foods do not need to be cooked. Fresh peaches, pears, and bananas are examples. These may be processed by cutting the peeled fruits into chunks and then pureeing.

8. The pureed food may be served right away. The remainder should be stored carefully for later use.

9. To store the pureed food, place serving-size portions in an ice cube tray, a paper cupcake liner, or a glass dish or on a piece of plastic wrap and freeze. Two tablespoons is an arbitrary serving size. Make the servings larger or smaller, depending on what your baby eats.

10. To serve stored food, reheat the individual portions. Microwave ovens can be dangerous since they may create hot spots in the cooked food, which can burn your baby's mouth. Be sure to cool the food to a safe temperature before feeding.

Once your baby no longer requires pureed food, a baby food grinder is a convenient way to make baby food right at the table. The grinder should be very clean, and the food used in the grinder should be fresh, unsalted, and without spices, fat, or skins. Place the right portion in the grinder, adding water or cooking water as needed to get the right consistency. You will discover that as your baby grows older, she prefers foods from your table since she wants to eat the same foods she sees you eating.

## Self-feeding

Your baby may be ready to help feed herself when she sits with stability in her high chair, can put objects into her mouth, has begun some chewing motions, and perhaps holds breast or bottle in her hands while feeding. Both she and you benefit from her attempts to feed independently. Though the process may be much slower and is definitely messier than your feeding her, the advantages of letting her try are many. She feels good making her fingers, body, and mouth cooperate as she attempts to satisfy her hunger. Feeding herself stimulates all her senses and provides a wonderful learning experience. She will taste and smell the food. She will feel the texture and temperature on her fingers as she reaches, chews, and swallows her food. She will love the click the spoon makes on her dish or her new teeth. And she will enjoy the bright colors of her squash and peas.

### The Transitional Period

At six months, your baby can put objects into her mouth. She explores her world through her mouth, which makes this time perfect to begin some finger foods. She can also sit with little support. By seven months, she may have some teeth and may begin to make chewing motions with her mouth. She can hold a small bottle by herself and may even begin to take liquids from a cup with your help.

While she cannot be expected to feed herself all her foods at this stage, she can participate by

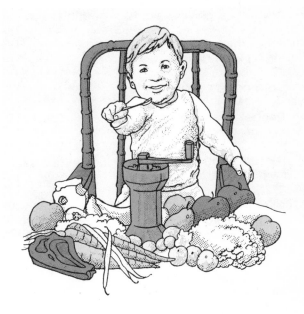

*Self-feeding is a major step forward for your baby.*

feeding herself some foods while you prepare the rest of her meal. She can also have finger foods for snacks.

Appropriate finger foods during this period include those that dissolve easily in the mouth, such as the following:

- Small pieces of toast

- Small pieces of cooked vegetables, such as peas, squash, soft green beans, or broccoli

- Small pieces of very soft meat, such as fish without bones, chicken, or hamburger

- Small pieces of scrambled egg (unless there is a history of allergy)

- Small pieces of ripe peaches, bananas, or pears

- Small pieces of soft cheese, such as Monterey Jack or Colby (unless there is a milk allergy)

- Cheerios or puffed rice

Foods you should avoid include those that may cause choking. Do *not* offer the following during the first year:

- Any dried fruits, such as apricots, raisins, dates, pineapple, or coconut

- Any nuts, such as walnuts or peanuts

- Popcorn, potato chips, corn chips, or crackers that do not dissolve well

- Hard candy of any kind

- Uncooked vegetables, such as carrots or celery

- Hot dogs and other foods that might be of "windpipe size"

Bath time is an excellent time to teach your baby to drink from a cup. She will enjoy the challenge, and you will not need to contend with a mess on the floor or her clothes. Use a plastic shot glass or plastic nipple cover as the first cup; the smaller diameter of the opening makes it easier for her to manage with her small mouth. You can offer her water, breast milk, formula, or juice from a cup.

If you are bottle-feeding, your baby may enjoy helping you hold her bottle. Let her participate by pulling the nipple in and out of her mouth and adjusting the angle of the bottle. Avoid putting her to bed with her bottle, though; as she falls asleep, less saliva bathes her teeth, and she swallows less often. Some milk may "pool" in her mouth and support the growth of bacteria, which leads to tooth decay.

## Modified Adult Period

By the time your baby is eight months old, she can sit without support and reach for a cup and spoon. She may be able to lift a cup by herself. When she is full, she lets you know by turning away from her food or playing with it.

Since she cannot feed herself well yet from a spoon, you can help her by teaching her how to grasp it in her hand and move her hand toward her dish. A good way to begin is to let her hold a spoon while you feed her with another spoon. Every several bites, help her load her spoon and bring it to her mouth. Use foods that "stick" well to the spoon, such as cereal, mashed potatoes, thick mashed banana, or macaroni and cheese. Lots of praise and acceptance of spills will encourage her to learn.

Use a small cup at mealtimes with a small amount of milk or water (to save you work if the contents are spilled). She will probably need help

at first just learning to hold on to the cup without spilling and, of course, she needs your approval.

By nine months, she can chew easily and can bite off a chunk of food from a larger piece. Her pincer grasp (ability to pick up objects with thumb and forefinger) is well developed. Foods that are appropriate at this age include strips of soft cheese or toast, fish sticks without bones (cut into small pieces), strips of bread with cheese melted on top, peeled cucumber cut into small pieces, cooked green beans and broccoli spears, wedges of fresh pears or peaches, or slices of banana. She will do well with peas and blueberries, too. She still needs lots of opportunities to use a spoon and cup.

By ten months, your baby may do well with a cup and may enjoy feeding herself much of her meal. By eleven months, she is able to drink several swallows from her cup at a time. She enjoys squishing foods in her fingers, appreciating the feel and texture. By twelve months, she may be quite proficient with her utensils and may prefer to feed herself most of her meal. At this age she may also enjoy the new skill of deliberately spitting.

These last few months of the baby's first year offer parents special challenges in feeding. Creativity in planning nutritious meals your baby can feed herself helps your baby to become independent at the table. Make it easy on yourself by giving your baby no more food than she can quickly and easily eat or drink. She can always have more put on her plate or in her cup if she finishes. Putting small amounts of food and beverage within reach of your baby helps reduce some of the messiness of this stage. Tipping over bowls and cups and watching your reaction are great fun, and spitting is sure to grab your attention. Remember that sometimes ignoring a behavior you do not like ends the behavior more quickly than expressing surprise or displeasure.

## The Toddler Period

Your toddler can manage cup and spoon with ease. She can chew well and take foods that are too difficult to chew out of her mouth with her fingers. She is a messy eater who may express some strong food preferences. She has a diminished appetite at this stage, corresponding with her slower rate of growth.

Mealtimes will call for creativity and patience on your part. Your toddler needs foods she can easily eat by herself. Since her appetite is not large, take advantage of snack times as well as mealtimes to provide her with nutritious foods. Use her natural hunger as your ally.

Try offering vegetable strips as snacks. To make zucchini, broccoli, and cauliflower more interesting, try a yogurt dip with dill seasoning. Fortify milk shakes with an egg, wheat germ, and fruit. You might also try adding a small amount of grated carrot, apple, or zucchini to pancakes.

Always offer foods that are nutritious. Then you can relax and avoid the food battles that result from forcing foods on a resistant toddler.

## Instilling Good Dietary Habits

Your attitudes about nutrition and how you eat directly affect the development of your child's food attitudes and habits. You are your child's first model of how to eat and what to eat. Take time to consider your use of salt and the amount of sugar you consume. Think about which of your dietary habits you want to pass on to your child. Are there modifications you would make? Right now is a good time to make changes in your diet, if change is necessary, so that your eating habits are in harmony with what you want for your baby.

Informing yourself about what constitutes a good diet for your baby and growing child is a good place to start. You will learn that, in excess, salt is not a healthy thing to add to your baby's diet or your own. You will learn, too, that Americans consume far more sugar than they need, which may contribute in part to obesity and tooth decay. As you grow to understand more about your child's nutritional needs and his normal growth and development, you will be able to see why food battles occur in some families. You also will come to recognize when it is normal for your child to be picky or to dawdle over his meal.

## Salt

The American diet contains, on the average, ten times more sodium (one of the chemicals in salt) than is required for good health. You get sodium naturally in the foods you eat and, as a result, generally do not need to add salt to your diet. High sodium intake has been directly correlated with the development of hypertension (high blood pressure). Hypertension is dangerous because it can lead to heart disease and stroke.

Some people seem to be genetically more at risk for developing hypertension. A family history of high blood pressure should alert you to be prudent with the use of salt in your diet and your baby's.

When should you first be concerned about salt in your baby's diet? Research indicates that overuse of salt should be avoided right from birth. Breast-feeding or choosing a formula that is most like breast milk ensures your baby's getting just the right amount of sodium. Once your baby begins to eat solid foods, feed him foods to which no salt has been added. Processed foods, such as hot dogs, bacon, soup, canned vegetables, canned meats, catsup, pickles, and puddings, as well as salty-tasting foods, are usually high in sodium and should be restricted. Take care not to add salt to the baby food you make at home, even though it may taste bland to you.

Research shows that a baby who has high levels of sodium in his diet from birth and who continues this pattern throughout his life has an increased risk of developing high blood pressure as an adult. Your baby's food tastes are established in infancy; if he grows accustomed to salty foods and enjoys them, it will be more difficult for him to give up salt later. Remember, too, that if your baby sees you salt your food or eat potato chips, he will want to do the same. Reducing salt in your baby's diet means reducing salt in the family diet.

## Sugar

Sugar is not an unhealthful food. You need some sugar in your diet and get a form of sugar every time you eat fresh fruits and vegetables. Refined sugar in limited amounts is all right too, except when it contributes too many of the calories your baby eats each day. A diet too high in sugar is a diet that probably lacks other nutrients.

Sugar comes in many forms. Fruit sugar naturally sweetens the fruit you eat. Corn syrup is used to sweeten soda pop and some fruit juices. Honey is simply another form of sugar—it is no more healthful than granulated sugar. (In fact, because of the threat of botulism, honey should not be given to a child under one year of age.) Molasses, besides sugar, contains other nutrients, including iron. Milk contains a sugar called lactose.

Probably the best way to get the sugar you need is from fruits, vegetables, and other fresh foods. An occasional cookie or piece of pie, cake, or candy is not bad unless it replaces the food you need or diminishes your appetite for nutritious foods.

Babies prefer sweet foods. Your baby's first food is breast milk or formula. If you taste these milks, you will discover that both are very sweet. Since your baby gets all the sugar he needs from his milk and later from the good foods he eats, you should avoid giving him too many cookies or sweet desserts. Eating cookies and sweets before meals quickly raises the blood sugar level, which is likely to ruin your baby's appetite.

Frequent bathing of the teeth in sugar promotes tooth decay. Since sugar is in milk and other foods, the additional sugar found in soda pop, gum, sticky dried fruits, and other sweet snack foods increases the likelihood of tooth decay. Restricting sugar consumption and giving your child low-sugar snacks, such as fresh vegetables, toast strips, and cheese chunks, is advisable.

### Overeating and Obesity

Overeating and overweight often begin during infancy. Obesity results when more calories are consumed than are needed for growth, when the choice of foods is poor, and when the activity level does not require the caloric intake to be as high as it is. Obesity tends to run in families. Children with one obese parent have a forty percent risk of becoming obese, while children with two obese parents have an eighty percent risk of becoming obese.

You can start right after your baby's birth to prevent overfeeding and obesity. If your baby is bottle-fed, let him decide when he is finished with each bottle instead of encouraging him to empty it. Starting solid foods too soon, before four to six months of age, can lead to excessive weight gain. As your child grows older, let him eat to satisfy his natural appetite. Your baby's doctor can tell you if his weight gain is too much for his height.

If overweight or obesity does become a problem, measures may be taken to slow the rate of your baby's weight gain. He should not actually lose weight; rather, he should be helped to get his weight in proportion to his height while still getting the nutrients and calories he needs for growth and development.

You can aid your baby or child by taking the following measures:

- Be sensitive to his cues that he is full. He may pucker his face, pull back from the table or bottle, turn his head away, dawdle, spit out his food, or begin to play with it. These are all signs that he is finished eating.

- Milk is your infant's most important food. Water is generally necessary only as an additional fluid (for example, on very hot days). Juice is *not* a substitute for milk.

- Limit or eliminate high-calorie foods. Fresh fruit makes a tasty substitute for a cookie. Avoid sauces and gravies, which provide a lot of calories and limited nourishment. Broil or steam foods rather than frying them. Limit the use of butter, margarine, and mayonnaise.

- Give your child fresh fruit instead of canned fruit or fruit juice. Fresh fruit has fewer calories.

- Provide your baby with lots of opportunities to exercise. As you play with your baby, give him a chance to move his body as he interacts with you. As he grows older, give him space to run and opportunities to walk. He is more likely to exercise if you are involved with him. See Chapter 10 for useful information about exercise.

- If you prepare your own baby food, make it less caloric by not adding sugar, margarine, or butter. Take all the fat off meat before cooking.

- Remember that babies cry and fuss for reasons other than hunger. If your baby has just been fed, try other methods of soothing him before again offering breast or bottle. Try walking or rocking him. Maybe he just needs to suck. Let him suck on your finger, his finger, or a pacifier. Perhaps he is bored and needs a new position or toy or change of room.

- Offer nonfood rewards for achievement or good behavior. It is tempting to give candy or a cookie for an accomplishment or an ice-cream cone for good behavior on an outing, but the overweight child needs other rewards. Your verbal expressions of pleasure and hugs are wonderful rewards. For special accomplishments, a book, a toy, or a record might be in order. You will probably need to enlist the support of other important adults, such as grandparents and babysitters, in this approach.

A word of caution: Let your baby's doctor decide if your baby is overweight or obese. The doctor can follow your baby's growth on growth charts and will be able to tell you if you need to be concerned. Do not decide your baby is overweight because of the way he looks or because someone tells you he looks fat. Most babies have a cherubic appearance. They do not look like lean mini-adults. Your baby or toddler will have a rounded abdomen. He may appear to have no neck and may have a double chin and dimpled skin. Despite his appearance, he may be just right for his height. Since good nutrition is so important to the development of your child's brain and his general growth in the first two years, restricting calories and nutrition unwisely may have a poor effect on his development. Children do change in appearance over the years, and the baby you thought was so round may become a lean toddler or preschooler.

## Food as a Reward

You probably already know that using food as a reward is not a good idea. In practice, though, it is difficult to avoid. When a parent says, "Eat your broccoli first and then you can have dessert," he is implying that broccoli must be endured so the child can have the "good stuff" as a reward. Offering a cracker or cookie whenever a child fusses rewards fussing. And using food as a bribe for an achievement is not always the best reward.

It is wonderful to celebrate your child's new skills or abilities. Sometimes food is an appropriate and convenient way to celebrate or reward. What happens, though, when food is the usual or the only way of rewarding an accomplishment or behavior? Patterns of reward and celebration are often set in childhood, and you will have to decide if using food as a reward is what you want to teach. Try varying the rewards. A hug, a compliment, an invitation to play a game with you or help you with a task, and time set aside for a story or book are some good alternatives.

When your baby fusses, cookies and food often work to quiet him temporarily. Examine the cause of the fussiness. As your baby grows older, his fussiness may be the result of fatigue, new teeth, overstimulation, or boredom. Try some other cures for fussiness if it does not seem likely he is hungry. The cure is sure to be longer lasting if it is directly aimed at eliminating the cause of fussiness.

Food is punishment if a baby or child is forced to eat it. You can probably remember foods you were forced to eat as a child, and you probably do not like those foods to this day. Force-feeding and then rewarding for eating certain foods is never a good idea. You are setting yourself up for food battles, which have ruined many family mealtimes.

## Picky Eaters and Dawdlers

Babies and toddlers have days when they are more hungry than on other days. During the toddler years, appetite diminishes in relationship to a slowed rate of growth, and strong food preferences are normal. Illness affects appetite, as does teething. And adding new foods and textures to your baby's or toddler's diet may slow him down or cause him to lose interest in his food. You can expect that there will be times when your baby dawdles during his meals or gets very picky about what he will eat.

Here are some tips to help you cope:

- Make sure the portions are not too big. Too much food may appear overwhelming and thus diminish appetite.

- Avoid force-feeding and making food an issue.

- Make sure the food you serve is in a form he can eat easily. (For instance, if your baby has no teeth, his foods need to be soft; your toddler may need to have his meat or noodles cut into small pieces.)

- Be sure there is an adequate interval between meals and snacks.

- Avoid high-sugar foods and between-meal snacks, which may blunt his appetite. This includes juice before meals.

- Serve a variety of foods.

- Serve food in a colorful and creative way. Eye appeal stimulates the appetite.

- Make mealtime pleasant. The atmosphere at the table has an enormous effect on appetite.

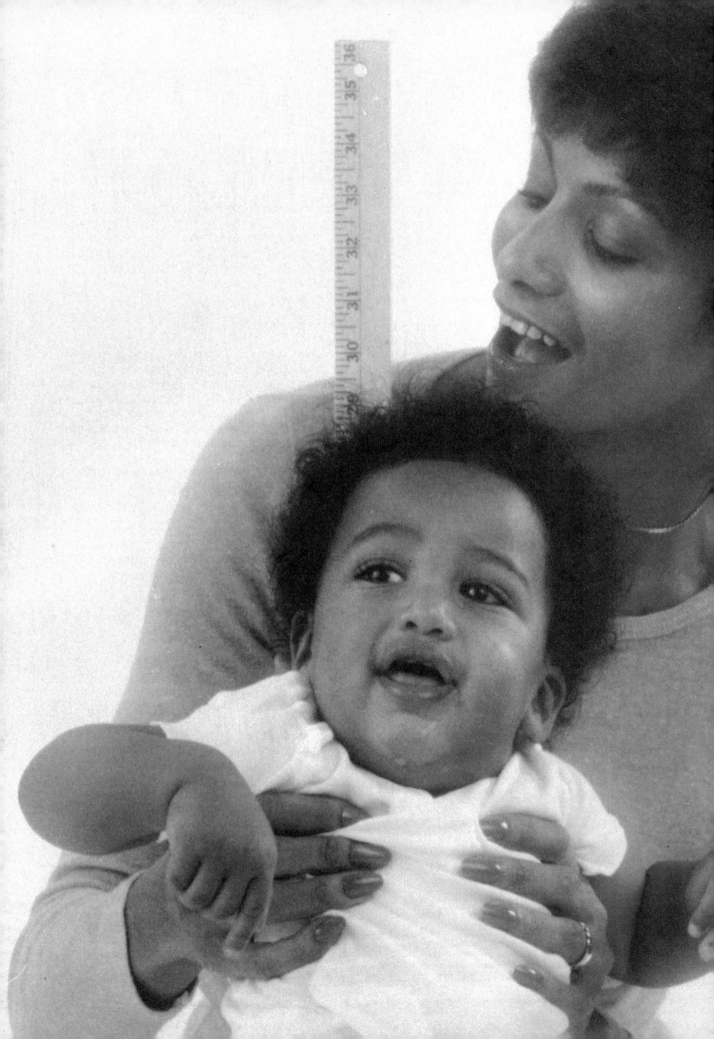

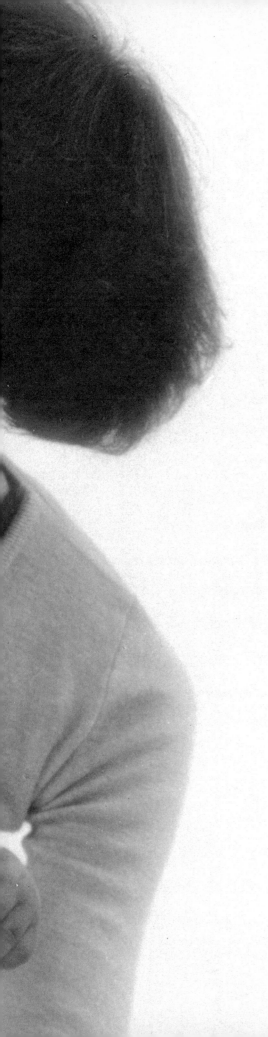

# Chapter 10:
# Physical
# Development
# and Exercise

### Introducing the Newborn

After nine months of anticipation, the two of you may feel that you have had ample time to consider the consequences of your pregnancy, perhaps even time enough to read about babies or to attend a parenting class. But unless you have actually had hands-on experience with a newborn, your baby's appearance may surprise you. Since many movies and television programs cast an older baby for the part of a newborn in tender scenes with parents after the delivery, it is no wonder that many first-time parents expect to give birth to a sturdy, smiling three-month-old baby.

If you feel amazed upon first seeing your newborn, think of the astonishment he must feel. Although all his senses had been intact since the twenty-eighth week of gestation, his perceptions were muted while he was within the confines of the uterus. He was able to hear sounds, such as your muffled voices and his mother's heartbeat. Occasionally he could see soft light filtering into his world. He felt his mother's movements and the gentle pressure of your hands as you caressed the outlines of his body.

Throughout the pregnancy the uterus underwent many changes. As the fetus grew larger, his movements became restricted as the ability of the uterus to stretch reached its limits. With the onset of labor, increasingly stronger contractions began pushing him outward. His head squeezed through the bony pelvic outlet or was pulled by strong hands through a cesarean incision. His soft body followed. Suddenly, his delicate skin was no longer cushioned by warm fluid. The air felt relatively cooler. Unfamiliar hands and fabrics rubbed against him. Brighter lights and louder voices bombarded his senses. Once separated from you, he had to take over all the life-sustaining functions you had controlled for him. He was forced to take his laborious first breath. For him, birth represented a dramatic change.

Once in your arms, he began to feel better. With his head snuggled against your chest, he heard that familiar heartbeat and felt reassured. Your voice also comforted him. As your adoring face moved close, he scrutinized it.

In the next few days, he began to make the enormous adjustment to his strange new environment. Having survived birth is a testament to the fact that he is not as fragile as he looks.

## Physical Appearance of the Newborn

A newborn looks very different from older babies and children. Her head is relatively large, measuring one fourth of her entire length. Her disproportionately short legs are only one third of her length. Clearly, in humans, brain development takes precedence over development of the rest of the body.

### Head

Aside from being large, her head may look misshapen and even a little bruised. The bones of the skull are separated, rather than fused as they are in adults. This separation allows the bones to slide over each other as the head passes through the narrow birth canal. Also, this mobility is essential to accommodate an infant's rapid brain growth.

If you caress the top of her head, you will feel the "soft spots," or fontanels, in the skull. Here the bones are widely separated, but the brain is covered by a tough membrane and scalp. You won't hurt your baby by *gently* touching these areas. The anterior fontanel, located in the midline on top of the head, usually closes between nine and eighteen months after birth. Behind it is the smaller posterior fontanel, which closes by four months.

### Eyes

Your baby's eyelids may be red and swollen from pressure during the delivery. In most hospitals, antibiotic drops are applied to the newborn's eyes. The drops may cause mild, temporary inflammation.

As your baby studies your face, you may notice that one eye wanders or that the two eyes don't move together smoothly. Unless one eye seems to be almost fixed in position (cross-eyed or walleyed), this wandering is normal and will be corrected as the baby gains strength and coordination in the muscles that move the eyes.

### Ears

The cartilage in the outer ear is very flexible in the newborn. If an ear looks folded, don't worry—it will probably straighten out. If the problem continues, talk to your doctor.

### Nose

At birth, the nose and mouth are often filled with mucus. After the delivery, suctioning by hospital staff with a rubber syringe clears the airways and helps your baby to breathe. Her own sneezing helps clear her nasal passages and is not necessarily the sign of a cold.

### Mouth

An occasional baby already has one or more teeth at birth, which usually fall out. Your doctor may want to extract these teeth so that your baby doesn't later choke on them. If your baby did a lot of sucking in the womb, blisters may be present on the upper lip, as well as on the fingers, hands, or forearm.

### Skin

Your baby's skin is wonderfully soft. It may not, however, appear as flawless as the complexion of an older infant. The newborn's skin often has a ruddier hue. For the first few days, the hands and feet may appear to be tinged with blue. Soon, the baby's circulation will improve and the skin color will be more uniform.

Over half of newborns have some degree of jaundice in the first week of life. In most cases, this condition is due to the immaturity of the liver and is not a threat to the baby. The liver is the organ that helps to clear *bilirubin,* a waste product of broken-down red blood cells. Since the liver is not completely mature at birth, babies are often not able to excrete bilirubin as well as adults. It is the deposition of bilirubin in the skin and the whites of the eyes that gives them a yellowish tinge.

Jaundice first appears on the face and spreads downward as the bilirubin level increases. Normal newborn, or "physiologic," jaundice usually is first visible between the second and fifth days of life, peaks between the fifth and seventh days, and clears within one to two weeks. In some breast-fed babies jaundice may last a bit longer.

Unless your doctor determines that the bilirubin level is too high, you can probably manage your baby's jaundice at home. The mainstay of home treatment is frequent feedings at breast or bottle. Bilirubin is eliminated in the urine and feces; the elimination can be accelerated by increasing fluid intake. Bilirubin is broken down in the skin, and light stimulates the action. The wavelength of light that hastens bilirubin breakdown in the skin passes through glass and plastic. Because this is so, placing the baby near a sunny window (for short periods of time) is beneficial.

Your doctor may follow your baby's progress by checking the bilirubin level with a simple blood test. If the level rises excessively, the baby will require hospitalization for phototherapy treatment (exposure to light at a wavelength similar to that of ultraviolet light) and to determine whether the jaundice is due to something more serious than immature liver function.

In most babies, the jaundice resolves spontaneously. If your baby has jaundice, your doctor will tell you what to do to speed its disappearance.

Birthmarks are a fairly common skin condition of the newborn. Babies of darker-skinned parents may have "mongolian spots," due to a bluish pigmentation under the skin over the lower part of the back and the buttocks. "Stork bites" (also called "angel kisses") are red, flat birthmarks usually located on the bridge of the nose, the upper eyelids, or the back of the neck. They usually disappear by the second birthday, but may reappear with crying. Sometimes the spots on the nape of the neck persist into adulthood.

Rashes often develop within the first few days of life. Although parents tend to worry about these skin blemishes, most of them are harmless and go away on their own. *Milia* are small white "pimples" on the face, caused by maternal hormones. They go away in several days without treatment. *Erythema toxicum*—a rash of red bumps with yellow centers and a generally "flea-bitten" appearance—occurs in half of all newborns. It is harmless and disappears on its own in a week or so.

The skin of most babies peels a little after birth. Peeling is most noticeable on the palms and soles. It is more marked in babies born after more than forty weeks of pregnancy. You might also notice a flaky condition known as "cradle cap" on the scalp. This flaking goes away by itself. Daily washing with soap and water is helpful.

### Chest
Your baby breathes at a faster rate than you. The normal newborn breathes between thirty and fifty times a minute. The rate is often irregular. If you watch closely, you may see a faint motion of the heart beating against the left chest wall. The pulse in new babies is also fast—130 to 160 beats per minute.

You may also notice that your baby's breasts are enlarged. This enlargement, caused by exposure to high estrogen levels while in the uterus, is temporary.

### Genitals
Exposure to maternal hormones may also cause swelling in the baby's genitals, especially the labia in girls. In the first few weeks, girls may have a white, blood-tinged, mucous discharge from the vagina due to withdrawal from those hormones.

In boys, the foreskin that covers the penis is not easily retractable. Don't try to force it back, as this may hurt your baby.

### Abdomen
After the umbilical cord has been cut, a stump remains. If it is kept clean and dry, it will fall off

within ten days. Many hospitals recommend that you gently clean the base of the stump with a cotton ball and rubbing alcohol.

Your baby's first bowel movements will be sticky and greenish-black. This tar-like substance is called *meconium.* After your baby has been drinking milk for a few days, her bowel movements will appear yellow to brown.

### Arms and Legs

Your baby can move all four extremities quite well. He prefers to keep them flexed and close to his body. Their exact position may resemble his posture during the last few weeks in the uterus. The legs often flop open at the hips, giving him a frog-legged look.

Extending his arms and legs makes him feel insecure. When he is fretful, you may be able to make him more comfortable by wrapping him snugly in a blanket and holding him close to you.

### Hair

The amount of hair on the head is variable. Any amount is normal. Most of this hair will fall out and be replaced. The color and texture of the new hair may be quite different from those of the hair he was born with.

Inside the womb, the baby's body was covered with fine, downy hair called *lanugo.* Unless your baby was premature, most of this body hair will have disappeared, except for some fuzz on the back. Even this residual lanugo will be gone in a few weeks.

## The Newborn as a Reflexive Being

After making the dramatic transition to life outside the womb, your baby is faced with the task of learning to survive in his completely new environment. Fortunately, nature has provided him with many reflexes to maximize his success until he is able to do certain things voluntarily. Your own instinctual responses will guide you in meeting your baby's needs.

Just as a mother's breasts are programmed to provide milk to nourish her newborn, a baby automatically knows how to respond to attempts to feed him. When you stimulate his cheek, mouth, or lips with the nipple of a breast or a bottle, his head will turn toward it, his mouth will open, and his

tongue will move forward. This movement of his head and mouth is called the *rooting reflex* and helps him find a source of nourishment. As soon as the inside of his sensitive mouth is stimulated, he will automatically suck and swallow in a coordinated fashion.

A similar reaction, the *hand-to-mouth reflex,* occurs if you stroke your baby's cheek or the palm of his hand. His mouth will "root" and his arm will flex. After his hand and mouth find each other, he may suck his fist energetically for several minutes. This reflex helps babies suck and swallow any mucus that might have been clogging their upper airways (nose and mouth) after birth.

If you slowly pull your baby to a sitting position from his back, he will make a gallant attempt to keep his head upright. This response is called the *righting reflex.* Because his head is heavy and his muscles are not yet strong enough to hold it steady, his head will wobble back and forth. You will quickly learn to support his head when you pick him up.

For the first few weeks, your baby will lie with one cheek down when on his back. As his head turns to one side, the arm on the same side straightens and the opposite arm bends. This posture resembles a "fencing position" and is called the *tonic neck reflex.* Lying in this position gives your baby an opportunity to discover his own hand in the weeks to come. Because it is difficult to turn over on an outstretched arm, this reflex will have to fade before your baby can roll over.

A newborn baby has a very strong *grasping reflex.* If you place your finger in his palm, his fingers will curl tightly around it. The automatic grasp reflex fades over the first two to three months to enable your baby to grasp objects voluntarily. Gentle pressure against the sole of his foot causes his toes to curl downward. Stroking the side of his soles will cause his toes to spread and the big toe to extend upward. This *Babinski reflex* is the opposite of the normal adult response, in which the big toe turns downward.

Holding your baby upright and pressing the sole of one foot at a time to a firm surface will elicit the *stepping reflex.* He will alternately bend each leg as though walking. This remarkable reflex fades rapidly but reappears months later, as your baby prepares himself for voluntary walking.

Stroking one leg causes the other to bend, cross the first leg, and push away the offending object. He moves as though to escape from a harmful stimulus.

When placed on his belly, your baby will lift his head and turn it from side to side. He may even attempt to crawl. His responses make it virtually impossible for him to smother when he is lying on his stomach on a firm, flat surface. (For this reason, you need not worry that your baby will have trouble breathing while prone. You should, however, keep excess bedclothes, toys, and stuffed animals out of the way.)

The most dramatic reflex is the *Moro,* or *startle, response.* A loud noise or rough handling will cause your baby to throw back his arms and legs, extend his neck, and cry out. Then he will bring his arms together in an embrace and flex his legs. Unfortunately, your baby's response disturbs him further. His own furious crying only serves to startle him again. You can help break this cycle by calmly bringing his flailing extremities close to his body; applying steady, gentle pressure with your hand against his chest and abdomen; or simply holding him securely against your own body. By three months of age, this reflex will disappear.

## The Newborn as a Responsive Being

Your baby is not simply a bundle of reflexes. Each baby is unique. From day one, your baby asserts her individuality and makes known her temperament. You will soon discern her particular style in responding to the environment.

Within a few weeks, you will see her express her pleasure with coos and fleeting smiles and communicate her hunger, pain, or fear by varying cries of distress. You will learn to read each other. If you are responsive to her needs, she will learn to trust you. Your fostering of a sense of security will encourage her to continue to reach out to you. This circle of positive interaction will be gratifying to you all.

Many parents worry about "spoiling" their baby. Everyone would agree that a child who is rude and selfish is unpleasant. Your infant, however, does not yet have the intellectual maturity to be manipulative. At birth, she doesn't know about people; she doesn't recognize that she is a being separate from you. She is merely aware of her needs and expresses them as best as she can.

Don't worry about picking up your newborn when she cries. From her perspective, she was car-

ried about for nine months. Gathering her into your arms to comfort her only makes sense. It is probably safe to say that you can't hold your baby too much during the first three months.

As your baby gets older, responding to her includes replying to her babbling sounds. Your verbal responsiveness promotes her listening skills and language recognition. Many specialists in infant development feel that holding and talking to your baby are the most important contributions you can make to her future development.

## The Special Senses of the Newborn

Your new baby is constantly receiving and responding to stimuli in his environment. By his seventh month in the womb, all of his senses were developed. As a newborn, he can already see, hear, feel, taste, and smell. Some of these senses need time to fully mature. Yet, from birth, he is ready to learn about his new world and everything in it.

Failure to stimulate his senses can have disastrous effects on his future growth and development. Happily, you, as loving parents, will know how to provide just the right kind of sensory input for your baby.

### Touch

One of the most important means you have for communicating with your baby is touch. Babies enjoy gentle handling and rhythmic motion. While inside the womb, your baby became accustomed to being rocked by your movements. After birth, that same swaying motion comforts him. A fretful infant will often become quiet if you gather him close to your body and gently rock him.

Even the most mundane activities—feeding and bathing him, changing his clothes and diapers, holding him, walking with him in your arms—stimulate your baby's sense of touch and movement.

### Smell and Taste

At birth, babies demonstrate that they discriminate odors by turning away from unpleasant smells. Your baby will quickly learn to recognize familiar smells, especially your scent.

Although his taste buds aren't completely mature at birth, your baby can tell sweet from sour and much prefers the former. It is no coincidence that breast milk is very sweet.

## Hearing

During the last trimester of pregnancy, a baby listens to his mother's muffled voice as well as to the sounds of her heartbeat, breathing, and digestion. When your baby's head is pressed against your chest, he no doubt finds those familiar sounds comforting. You may notice that he selectively listens to higher-pitched voices. Even men unconsciously raise the pitch of their voices when speaking to babies. As your baby gains more control over his head movements, it will become clear that he not only can hear, but can accurately determine the location of a sound source.

Loud, sharp noises often upset babies. Soft, rhythmic sounds are calming. Music boxes, toys that make pleasant sounds, and soft music will stimulate your baby's sense of hearing. He will enjoy listening to you sing and talk to him. Soon the monologue will turn into a delightful dialogue as he starts replying with his own babbling sounds.

## Vision

Upon emergence from their dim intra-uterine environment, babies exhibit a protective reflex of tightly shutting their eyes against bright light. This response is called the *blinking reflex.*

Once you and your baby have settled into an environment more subdued than the delivery room, you will notice your baby scanning your face with wide-eyed interest. Although his visual system is immature, a newborn sees quite well at a distance of eight inches from the bridge of his nose. Parents instinctively bring their faces that close to inspect the new member of the family.

Like an old-fashioned camera, your newborn infant has "fixed" focus, that is, he is not able to adjust his eyes to clearly see images closer than eight inches or farther away than ten inches. He will quickly learn to accommodate (to focus the eyes with changing object distance). By six weeks of age, he will be able to focus at a distance of approximately twelve inches. The ability to accommodate matures by four months. In fact, at this age, infants not only see distant objects well, but can focus on images that are very close better than an adult can.

The muscles that move the eyes to help them both focus on an object to produce a single im-

age are immature at birth. You may notice that one eye or the other occasionally wanders. As long as that eye is not always deviated in the same direction, this wandering is normal. Visual coordination is much improved within a few weeks. By the age of six weeks, he will be able to smoothly move both eyes in concert as he follows a moving object. By eight weeks, your baby will be able to converge both eyes perfectly when viewing a stationary object.

The ability of both eyes to focus on the same image is essential to the development of depth perception, the capacity to distinguish near from far. Infants less than two months of age are probably not able to perceive depth. Your baby will be able to discern relative distances by four to six months. His ability to estimate distances matures after he has the experience of reaching and crawling. Until your baby has had experience with propelling himself around his environment, he probably will not have any fear of heights. If you leave him on a raised surface, for instance, he will blithely scoot over the edge.

Color vision is probably immature at birth. Color discrimination is learned early, starting with yellow and ending with blue. By four months, babies can see all colors well and often prefer red.

### What Your Baby Will Enjoy Looking At

At birth, babies prefer high contrast. Black and white designs provide the most contrast. At first, babies prefer geometric patterns with stripes and angles. Soon they shift their preference to circular patterns, such as a bull's-eye.

Within three weeks, the most exciting image in his visual field is the human face. Because your hairline and your eyes offer the most contrast, he will at first concentrate his gaze between your nose and your forehead. Between four and eight weeks, your baby may break into his first social smile while studying your face. At three months, he will be able to distinguish your face from a stranger's. By rewarding you with a special smile, he lets you know that he recognizes you. By four months, his vision has matured. Like you, he enjoys looking at things that are colorful, novel, and in motion.

How do you know when your baby finds something visually interesting? An alert, calm baby will respond to a pleasing object in his visual field by brightening his face and moving his arms and legs rhythmically. An active baby will stop moving and carefully scan the object with his eyes. He will signal to you when an object doesn't interest him or when he has had enough stimulation by turning away and withdrawing.

Avoid bombarding your baby with visual input during the first two months of his life. During this time, while he is getting settled, all stimuli should be low-key. In these first weeks, he is becoming familiar with his hands and should not be exposed to a lot of jazzy visual stimuli that will distract him from that familiarization process. Later, when he has begun to master basic visual skills and has gained control over his head and hand movements, he will be ready to explore his visual environment. As always, take your cues from him.

---

## Things That Stimulate Visual Development

- Black and white geometric patterns

- Your face

- Toys with faces

- Out-of-reach mobiles (remove them when the baby can sit, to avoid entanglement)

- Mirrors (choose stainless-steel mirrors he can't break)

- Being carried about with you

- Being placed in an infant seat (always fasten the lap belt and never leave him unattended)

---

## Patterns of Growth

A baby's growth and development begin inside the womb. In fact, her most rapid rate of growth will occur during the first four months of the pregnancy. After birth, she will continue to grow rapidly. Each baby's pattern of growing and developing is unique, influenced by gestational age at birth, birth size, body type, general state of health, quality of diet and exercise, and the sizes and growth patterns of the parents.

### Birth Size

After spending approximately forty weeks inside the womb, the average newborn weighs seven and a half pounds. Most babies weigh between five and a half and ten pounds. The average length of a newborn is twenty inches (fifty centimeters), with a range of eighteen to twenty-two inches. The average head circumference (the distance around the head) is fourteen inches (thirty-five centimeters).

At each visit, your doctor will chart your child's growth. The best indicators of growth are weight, height, and head circumference. Plotting these growth measurements is a simple and extremely useful way of monitoring your child's state of health.

### Rate of Growth

During the first few days after birth, you can expect your baby to lose six to ten percent of her birth weight. Most of the weight lost is in the form of extra body water. If you are a mother who plans to breast-feed, your milk will be "coming in" during this time. The first milk, or *colostrum*, albeit scanty, is high in protein and will sustain the baby as your milk supply increases.

After three to four days, the baby will begin to regain weight and should attain or surpass her birth weight by ten to fourteen days. For the next three months, your infant will grow at the astonishing rate of approximately an ounce a day. Between three and six months, her weight gain will decline to four to five ounces a week. Between six and twelve months, the weight gain slows to two to three ounces a week. After the first year, the growth rate further tapers. During the second year of life, appetite sometimes diminishes as physical activity increases, resulting in temporary plateaus in growth.

If you have an average-size baby, you can expect her to double her birth weight by five months, triple it by one year, and quadruple it by two years. The average gain in length or height is ten to twelve inches in the first year and five inches in the second year. Keep in mind that these predictions are estimates for the average-size baby. If your baby was smaller at birth, she may grow faster; if she was larger, she will probably grow at a slower rate.

The growth curve isn't always smooth. Babies often grow in spurts. If your baby is ill or preoccupied with acquiring a new physical skill, her growth rate may temporarily decline (she may be burning more calories, and may be less interested in eating). Also bear in mind that bigger is not necessarily better. Obesity at any age should be avoided.

## Tooth Formation and Eruption

Tooth buds for your baby's first teeth begin to form at about six weeks of fetal life. Between the fourth and fifth months of fetal life, some tooth buds become evident. By about the seventh month of fetal life, the tooth buds for all of your baby's primary (deciduous) teeth are formed. At birth, the crowns—the portions of the teeth visible above the gums—of your baby's front teeth are already formed and contain most of their enamel covering. The crowns for some of the other primary teeth are partially formed, and the tooth buds for some of the permanent molars are forming. By the time your child is three years old, the crowns of some permanent teeth will be fairly well formed, and the tooth buds for the last molars will have formed.

As early as three months of age, your baby may begin teething. Teething is marked by drooling, fretting, and chewing on things in an attempt to reduce the discomfort of sore, swollen gums. Some babies will exhibit these symptoms for up to four months before the first tooth finally erupts. If your baby seems uncomfortable, you can help reduce the pain and swelling in her gums by giving her firm, smooth, cool, unbreakable objects to chew. Massaging the inflamed gums with a clean fingertip may also be helpful. Medications to numb painful gums are also available.

Don't be alarmed if your baby seems less interested in the breast or the bottle while teething; sucking increases the blood flow and hence the swelling and pain of the gums. If she's old enough, you might try offering her fluids from a cup.

Your baby's first tooth should appear when she is four to eight months old. It is not unusual for a child to be ten or more months old before the first tooth appears, though, and occasionally a baby is born with one or more teeth already erupted. Although most babies will have cut six to eight teeth by their first birthday, some normal babies will have just two teeth or fewer. If your baby is approaching the age of one year and no teeth are evident (you may see the outlines of teeth before they erupt), you should talk to your baby's doctor about having a dental evaluation.

Even though all of your baby's teeth may have erupted by one and a half or two years of age,

### Eruption of the Primary Teeth*

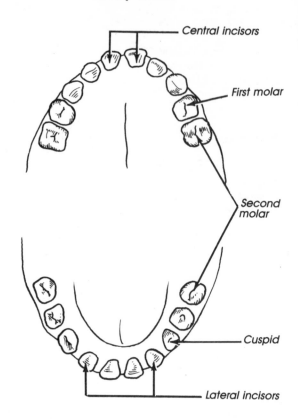

| Tooth | Upper Jaw† | Lower Jaw† |
|---|---|---|
| Central incisor | 8–12 months | 6–10 months |
| Lateral incisor | 9–13 months | 10–16 months |
| Cuspid | 16–22 months | 17–23 months |
| First molar | 13–19 months | 14–18 months |
| Second molar | 25–33 months | 23–31 months |

*Compiled from information furnished by the American Academy of Pediatric Dentistry.
†These eruption times are average and can normally vary by two months.

you will have to exercise care in the foods you give her. A child's chewing ability usually is not fully developed until about the age of four years. Children younger than this should not be given such foods as popcorn, nuts (especially peanuts), raw vegetables such as carrots, whole grapes, hot dogs, and round candies. If these and similar food items are not properly chewed, they may lodge in a small child's windpipe and cut off the air supply.

Because a baby's teeth begin to form so early in fetal life, what the mother ate, or did not eat, during pregnancy can have an effect on the development of the baby's teeth. However, the nutritional needs of the teeth and their supporting bones and muscles are easily met by a well-balanced diet; an ample supply of calcium is essential. After birth, the diet recommended by your baby's doctor will contain the proper nutrients for your baby's healthy growth and development, including healthy tooth formation. (For more information on tooth care, see Chapter 9.)

## Development of Physical Skills

While your baby is busy growing taller, gaining weight, and cutting teeth, he will also be learning how to interact physically with his environment. That is not to say that your baby's physical development does not begin until after birth. No doubt you were well aware of your infant's intra-uterine acrobatics.

During the first three months of your baby's life, however, reflexes govern much of his behavior. As these newborn reflexes fade, they are replaced by more purposeful movements. As he gains strength and coordination in his muscles, your baby is able to explore and manipulate things in his environment. Each day, he moves more competently.

Physical development is divided into two categories: *fine motor* and *gross motor*. Fine motor skills require precise coordination of the small muscles. Acquisition of hand-eye coordination is the focus of fine motor development. Gross motor skills are governed by larger, stronger, less exacting muscles. These skills include holding up the head, sitting, crawling, and walking.

Acquisition of developmental skills occurs in an orderly, predictable sequence. The precise timing of the mastery of any one skill, though, is subject to much normal variation—something to keep in mind when you are tempted to label your baby as "early" or "late" in development.

Each baby approaches the world with his own unique style. Resist comparing your child with your friends' children. When you hear that another child is walking at nine months, don't despair because your child is still perfecting his crawl. Instead, focus on his special talents. For instance, your baby may be much better than another at picking up and examining small objects. No matter when it occurs, celebrate your child's every accomplishment with him.

Physical development follows three general patterns:

1. *Muscular development progresses from head to toe.* In other words, your baby will learn to lift and hold up his head before his torso is strong enough to maintain a sitting posture.

2. *The strength and coordination of the limbs begins close to the body and moves outward.* Your baby will coordinate his arm movements at the shoulder, then the elbows, then the wrists. Skillful manipulation of the fingers comes last.

3. *Motor responses are general at first. Later, they become more specific.* For example, if you hold a red ball before your baby when he is three months old, he may smile, wave his arms and legs, and finally make an attempt to swipe at the ball with one or both arms. A few months later, he may still smile at the ball, but will quickly, smoothly, and deliberately grasp it with one hand.

### Gross Motor Development: Controlling the Big Muscles

*Head Control*

The first motor hurdle your infant must clear is to gain control over his relatively large head. If you imagine trying to lift your head while balancing a huge, unabridged dictionary on top of it, you will have some idea of the challenge facing your baby. He will spend the first three to four months learning to control his head movements.

Gradually, his neck muscles will strengthen and his head will become less wobbly. In the meantime, you will need to support his head when you pick him up. By three months he will be able to control his head when gently pulled up to sit, though his head will still bob a little if you hold him in a sitting position. By four to six months, his head doesn't fall backward as you sit him up; and once sitting, he can hold his head steady.

Despite the head's relatively large size, your healthy newborn can raise his head long enough to move it from side to side when lying on his stomach. Hence, he can avoid suffocation. Over the next three months, he will develop enough strength to lift his head ninety degrees away from a flat surface. Between two and four months, if his arms are extended in front of his chest, he can raise his head and chest above a surface.

*Sitting*

As your baby gains strength progressively down his torso to his hips, he will be able to sit. Around four months of age, he will be able to sit with support for ten to fifteen minutes. At this point, he will enjoy sitting with his back supported by an infant seat, pillows, or friendly hands. Stroller rides become much more fun because he is able to sit up and observe the world. He might even enjoy brief outings in a baby backpack. During meals, he can sit in a high chair with a pillow or blanket supporting the lower part of his back.

Between five and seven and a half months, if you set him down with his legs spread apart, he will be able to sit alone. You may still want to place pillows or blanket rolls around him to pad his fall should he topple over. For a while, he will still need to lean forward on his hands to maintain his sitting posture. But soon he'll be able to balance, freeing his hands to finger interesting objects. By nine months, he will be able to push himself into a sitting position. His increasing independence will give him hours of delight as he sits and plays with his toys.

*Rolling Over*

Rolling represents your baby's first whole-body maneuver and his first means of locomotion. As the tonic neck reflex fades, his arm no longer automatically extends as he turns his head. When he has enough control over his head, torso, and legs, he can tuck his arm under himself and roll. His weighty head initiates the rotation.

At about three months, babies start to turn by rolling to their sides. Between four and six months, your baby will probably first roll from his stomach to his back. A month or so later, he will master rolling in both directions. Never leave a baby of any age unattended on a raised surface, as even young infants can accidentally flip themselves over.

*Crawling*

During the same time that your baby is learning to sit, he may also start to crawl. The onset of crawling is extremely variable. Some babies prefer to bounce along on their buttocks from a sitting position. A few babies seem to decide that they would rather omit crawling and proceed directly to walking.

If crawling is to occur, first attempts can begin as early as five months of age. If yours is a very active baby, he may then travel by half rolling and half pushing himself in the desired direction. He may start to crawl at seven months.

The average baby begins by creeping in the sixth or seventh month. Because a baby's arms are stronger and better coordinated than his legs, he may drag himself around by pushing with his arms, dragging his legs behind. His first progress may be in a backward direction. Later, he will begin to dig in with his toes and knees. By eight months, he will probably be scooting about on hands and knees in the traditional crawl position.

Once crawling begins, your child will be jubilantly exploring all the things in the house he had to passively view from a distance for so long. He will be able to entertain himself for longer periods. The trade-off is that you will need to be especially vigilant about his activities. You must "baby proof" your house (check for safety hazards) before your baby can navigate on his own. He may be as curious about the electrical outlets in your house as he is about his toys. See Chapters 4 and 8 for important information about baby safety.

*Standing*

Between three and six months, your baby will bear some weight on his legs when you stand him up. At first, he will stiffly lock his legs. A few weeks later, he will bounce by bending and straightening his legs. Check to see that he can stand with his feet flat; "toe walking" may be a sign that he is bearing his weight on his legs too early.

Your baby may begin pulling himself to a standing position as early as six months or as late as ten months. Most babies pull to a stand between the eighth and ninth months. You can help your baby by providing him with stable objects that won't topple over with his weight. Surrounding him with pillows will cushion him if he falls; but keep an eye out to make sure he doesn't suffocate.

At first, he will be delighted with his upright posture. Happy gurgles may turn to wails of despair, though, when he discovers he doesn't know how to sit back down. You can help him learn to sit by sliding his hands down the supporting object to lower his buttocks to the floor.

During the eleventh month, your child will probably be able to stand well alone. About this same time, he may get himself to a stand by bending his knees and pushing off from a squatting position.

*Cruising and Walking*

After he can pull himself up to a stand by holding onto a piece of furniture, he will start to

## Motor Development "Milestones"

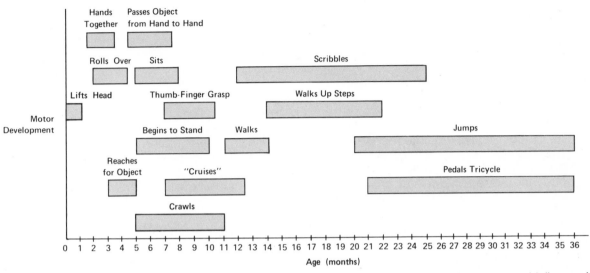

*Keep in mind that babies vary greatly in their physical development. The indicated age ranges are guidelines, not absolute requirements.*

"cruise." Cruising consists of taking steps while holding onto the furniture for support. At first, he will probably face the furniture and shuffle sideways. As he gains confidence in his balance, he will slide one hand as he walks in a forward direction. Cruising usually begins in the ninth month, but can begin as early as seven and a half months and as late as twelve and a half months.

When your child bravely lets go of the furniture and takes his first solo steps, walking has begun. This milestone of development is as exciting for you as it is for your child. Walking with or without assistance usually occurs by a baby's first birthday, and most babies walk well by fourteen months of age.

Your baby will quickly grow more nimble and confident. By eighteen months, he will be able to walk backward. Between fourteen and twenty-one months, he will learn to walk up stairs, though it may be a couple of months longer until he can confidently walk *down* the stairs. At eighteen months he will be able to run stiffly. In just a few months more, he will not look so precarious as he runs toward you.

### Fine Motor Control: Coordinating Hand and Eye

As your newborn looks about her world, her own fisted hand randomly passes through her field of vision. This strange object may interest her, but she has no idea of what it is or how it got there. By compelling her arm to extend in front of her face when she turns her head to the side, the tonic neck reflex creates plenty of opportunities for her to study her hand. During the first six weeks, she devotes more and more time to regarding her own fisted hand.

As the grasp reflex fades, she is increasingly able to unclench her fist. Similarly, her body unwinds from its flexed position. As the tonic neck reflex disappears, she spends more time looking up rather than looking to the side when she lies on her back. Hand-to-mouth activity, which began as a reflex at birth, becomes a more deliberate, conscious act. She moves her hands over her chest where she can look at them, explore them with her mouth, and finger one with the other.

Until three months of age, she will look at things without touching them and finger objects absently without looking at them. Then, the two systems for examining the world fuse. She feels something and turns her head to see what it is. She sees something interesting and reaches out to learn more about it by touch.

Her first attempts at hand contact consist of broad swipes. Her entire arm sweeps in a grand gesture as she bats at, and occasionally contacts, an object. The coordination of her arms begins closest to her body—at the shoulder. At six to fourteen weeks, sturdy objects suspended within an arm's length of your baby make good toys.

After this swiping period, you may notice that your baby begins to make slow, labored attempts to reach out and touch an object with one or both hands. If you watch carefully, you might see her glance back and forth between the object and her hand as she calculates the remaining distance. Having not yet mastered the correct sequence for grasping, she may close her fist before she reaches the object. During this time (between fourteen and twenty-three weeks), try to be patient when you hand her a toy. Give her plenty of time as she laboriously tries to reach out and grasp it. Practicing this sort of hand-eye coordination is important for her development.

Between four and six and a half months, she will have mastered the ability to smoothly lift her hand and accurately grasp an object. This is the time to introduce toys that make things happen—toys that help her to learn cause and effect (such as squeaky ducks or spinning bathtub toys).

During her sixth through eighth months, your baby will avidly explore everything in sight with her eyes, hands, and mouth. She will use both hands simultaneously to explore objects; while holding an object in each hand, for instance, she may delight in banging the two together. Given a small block, she will be able to transfer it from one hand to the other.

At six months, most babies can deliberately, but perhaps awkwardly, let go of an object. By ten months, your baby will be quite adept at uncurling her fingers at will to release an object. Over and over, she will grasp something and drop it for the sheer pleasure of watching it fall. For a while, she will rely upon you to retrieve these objects.

Between eight and fourteen months, your baby may spend long periods of time examining small objects. She will learn to prod an object with a single index finger. Rather than raking at things with her whole hand, she will begin to oppose her thumb and index finger in a "pincer grasp" to pick up a small object. At first, your baby may need to steady the side of her hand against a firm surface as she learns the pincer grasp. By her first birthday, your child will be an expert at plucking the smallest crumbs from the kitchen floor.

Your doctor will be keeping track of when your baby masters these motor skills.

## Growing Up With Exercise

There are many habits we want to impart to our children—brushing their teeth, picking up after themselves, having good personal hygiene—but none will have as much total impact as good fitness habits.

Start by simply putting your new little person on a blanket to watch you exercise. Let your baby see you doing exercises, enjoying them, and looking and feeling great. Children of exercising parents grow up accepting the exercise habit as both natural and necessary, which is the first step on the road to an active and healthy lifestyle.

## One to Twelve Months

Proud parents always seem to have an endless supply of photos of and stories about their cherished little one. Wouldn't they love to tell others that their child talked sooner than any of the other babies on the block? And when that baby reached toddler age, wouldn't they love to point out how she ran, jumped, and tumbled with surprising strength and balance?

Why is it that some children seem to develop at a faster rate than their peers? These children may have only one special advantage over others—parents who actively care about their growth, both physical and intellectual. Sadly, though, many parents who are very concerned about mental development give little thought to exercising their babies.

Babies who have reached the age of one month or who have recovered their full birth weight need movement. At this stage of life, babies need their parents' encouragement to move. As the baby gets older, movement and exercise will help him to learn to maintain balance, develop strength, and use new muscles.

### The Need for Exercise

There are three basic reasons why babies should be active: their learning habits, both motor and verbal, benefit; they establish a habit of activity that will carry over into adulthood; and they experience the pure joy of movement.

Researchers have shown that babies exercised vigorously from the age of one month seem to out-learn their unexercised counterparts. And these researchers are talking about intellectual development as well as physical, for the former seems to depend not only on early mental stimulation but also on early physical stimulation.

This exciting discovery was the result of a controlled study conducted in Czechoslovakia by Dr. Jaroslav Koch, a psychologist at the Institute for the Care of Mother and Child in Prague. The investigation concerned three groups of infant boys; two of the groups performed exercises prescribed by Dr. Koch, and the third did not exercise.

The first group consisted of ten boys born at the Institute and kept there for six months. The Institute staff exercised the babies according to Dr. Koch's wishes.

The second group of twenty boys was raised and exercised at home, but the boys' mothers came to the hospital every two weeks for instruction from Professor Koch.

The ten boys in the third group had no contact with the physician other than regular checkups every three months.

The exercise program began when the children were one month old. The hour-long exercise periods, with the children nude to provide complete freedom of movement, included rhythmic exercises using large body muscles. For example, the infants were encouraged to roll over. Other activities worked their arms, legs, and the upper part of their bodies. In addition, the program (which lasted about a year) included such precision work as grabbing onto an overhead rubber ring and fitting pegs into holes.

At the end of the study, all three groups were tested at the Institute for Mental Development and Physical Progress. The tests indicated that the motor-stimulated babies, both those exercised at the hospital and those exercised at home, developed faster than the unexercised control group in several ways. For one, they learned to talk sooner. The average year-old child has an active vocabulary of about five words, but the exercised groups displayed vocabularies of ten to twenty words at the same age. Dr. Koch also found that the babies trained in motor activity and problem-solving seemed to understand a great deal of everyday conversation, something most one-year-olds are seldom capable of doing. The exercised children's movement patterns, strength, and coordination also were superior to those of the control group.

Many educators argue that any child learns quickly if he is exposed to reading, conversation, music, and other cultural phenomena. But Dr. Koch maintains that the early stages of growth are highly dependent on physical activity. Some pediatricians have questioned the validity of Dr. Koch's testing procedures and conclusions, but most endorse the value of exercise per se, for young and old alike.

Earlier societies, either by accident or design, seemed to know that a child's mental development could be fostered through physical development. Ancient cultures considered physical activity indispensable for survival. The Greeks stressed that the body had to be cultivated along with the mind, and it did not matter whether the Greek was a Spartan interested in military proficiency or an Athenian interested in culture.

## What You Can Do

The first step toward promoting physical activity in your child is to be active yourself! A child's attitude toward exercise is definitely shaped by that of the parents. Active children generally have active parents who encourage their children to exercise. Conversely, inactive youngsters frequently have sedentary parents who do not promote physical activity.

Dr. Koch's study seems to indicate that the active child learns more. Movement, manipulation of various objects, and a variety of body positions stimulate the child's brain and nervous system and enhance his learning experience. On the other hand, the parent who confines a child to a crib or playpen all day does the offspring a grave injustice. A child needs activity and explorative movement—not restraint!

Try not to put your child in a playpen or crib unless it is nap time. When he is awake, give him every possible opportunity to crawl around on the floor and explore. If the child must be in a crib or playpen, supply objects—rings that go on a spool, blocks, nesting boxes, toys with dials—that stimulate manipulatory skills.

You can start exercising your child when he is about one month old or has regained his birth weight. While any time is appropriate for an exercise session, bath time or the evening is probably the best. The session can be long or short depending on your child's response. The session should be consistent in length and held at the same time every day. The idea is to fit exercise into the daily routine of both parent and child.

If the exercises are conducted in the same place every day, the child will become familiar with the feel of the floor, the bed, or the towel. Consequently, when placed in that position she will show readiness by kicking, cooing, twisting, and smiling.

While exercising, the child should be dressed in loose-fitting diapers, a little swimsuit, or—if you and the baby don't mind—a "bare bottom." The room temperature should be comfortable.

If you turn on some music, you will give the child a chance to make a pleasurable association between sound and exercise.

Most important of all, make sure that you exercise with the child!

As the infant grows older, the whole family should join in the fun. It has been said that our overurbanized, mechanized society is driving each member of the family his or her separate way. His job may cause a father to travel extensively; children may be in a nursery school or a day care center, particularly if a mother is employed; the mother who is not employed frequently devotes time to community or social activities. Consequently, the family has less time together to communicate, less time to touch, less time to share.

All too often, individual family members are involved in exercise programs that reduce their "together time" even more. Dad goes off to play golf, while Mom goes to a health club. These efforts toward fitness are often inadequate, and the absence of family members makes the family suffer. An opportunity for real family togetherness is wasted.

Learning together, touching, talking, and sharing improve human relations. Creating a family gymnastics program and enjoying it on a regular

basis is a terrific way to enjoy time together as well as to keep in shape. After all, you owe it to your toddler, who, having enjoyed the "diaper fitness" program, expects to learn new skills.

Set time aside in the evening for free play. Turn off the television early enough to allow thirty minutes of gymnastics, tumbling-type activities, or family wrestling.

## Suggested Exercises: One- to Four-Month-Old

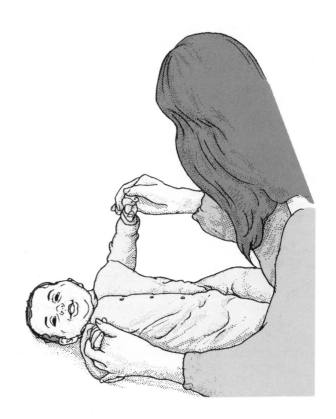

### Grip

Lay baby on his back on the floor. Wrap your baby's hand around your forefinger; hold in place with your thumb and third finger. Stretch out baby's arm by gently drawing his hand toward you. Do not pull baby up off the floor. Return to the starting position. Repeat five times with each arm.

## Suggested Exercises: Five- to Six-Month-Old

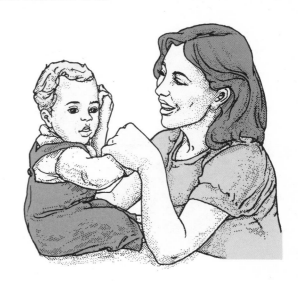

### Chest Cross

This time, hold both the baby's hands in the Grip position. Spread baby's arms out to the sides, bring them in across his chest, and spread them out again. Do this exercise slowly and gently, repeating the movement five times. As an alternate, you can raise baby's arms upward and downward.

### Pull-Up

Grasp your baby's forearms. Keeping his back straight, pull baby up slowly to a sitting position. Then slowly and softly return baby to the floor. Repeat four times.

## Suggested Exercise: Three- to Four-Month-Old

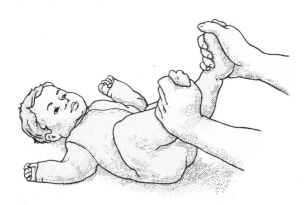

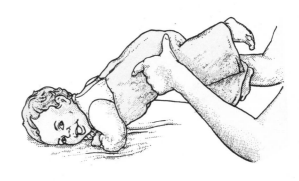

### Bicycle

With baby lying on his back, hold his feet or lower legs and gently push one leg up toward his chest while extending the other. Alternately push and extend each leg three times. Stop and then repeat a second time. After you finish, let baby kick freely.

### Elbow Stand

Lay the child on his stomach, and place his elbows directly underneath his shoulders. Grasp and lift baby's hips and trunk to form a forty-five-degree angle with the floor. Let the child rest on his forearms. Try to lift the legs up a little higher, but make sure the baby doesn't bang his nose.

# PHYSICAL DEVELOPMENT AND EXERCISE

## Suggested Exercises: Seven- to Eight-Month-Old

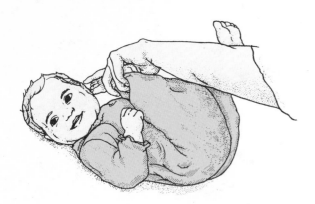

### Toe to Ear

Lay the baby on his back. Slowly bring his right big toe toward his left ear (do not force it), and then guide it back to the starting position. Then bring the left toe toward the right ear. Keep the leg straight as you move it. Repeat five times with each foot.

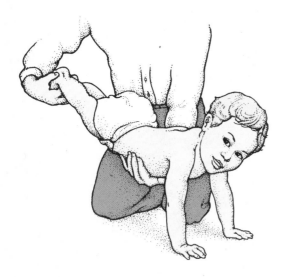

### Wheelbarrow

With baby lying on his stomach, place your hand under his belly and pelvis, and lift the lower part of his body. The child should support his own upper body weight using arms and hands. Notice that baby will hold his head up and look forward. Hold for a slow count of three (count 1001, 1002, 1003).

## Suggested Exercises: Nine- to Eleven-Month-Old

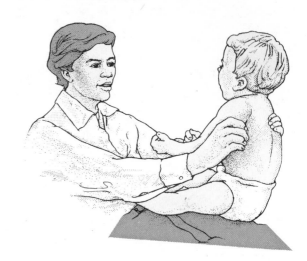

### Mountain Climbing

Sit on the floor, with legs extended and knees slightly bent. Hold baby on your lap facing you and grasp him around the rib cage. Lean back slightly, and let baby walk up the front of your body. This is a good exercise for young legs.

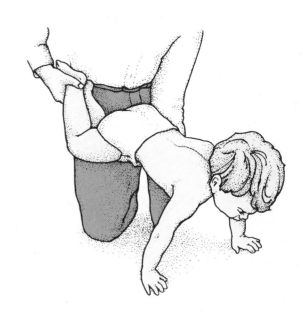

### Hand Walk

This exercise is identical to the Wheelbarrow, except baby walks forward on his hands. Again, support baby's pelvis and trunk with your hand.

## Twelve- to Twenty-two Months

Babyhood is gone. From now on, when your child is awake, she will be on the go. More and more, she exhibits her own personality, strengths, and abilities. Development of language, social, intellectual, and motor skills accelerates.

What does this have to do with exercise? Your child is constantly learning. By exercising your toddler every day, you are helping her learn to control her body; becoming stronger and more coordinated means fewer bumps, bruises, and spills in her exploration efforts. Understanding her growth and development stage will help you tailor a program according to your child's individual personality and temperament.

Trunk exercises for abdominal muscles are often overlooked. Abdominal and lower back muscles control and support the body. Strengthen the trunk muscles first, then the arms and legs. As abdominal strength increases, other movements change and become smoother.

Your child's attention span is short. Take this into account when exercising together. Change exercises every twenty to thirty seconds. This will increase coordination and concentration while decreasing the chance of injury or muscle soreness from overuse. We've provided a large variety of exercises, so you can change from one to another frequently and avoid boredom.

In this age group, your child will sometimes follow directions. After she is familiar with the exercise routine, she may initiate the exercises herself when you sit down together. However, the easiest and most fun way for both of you is for you to do it with her.

In general, thirty to forty-five minutes is a good period of time for your child's exercise program, but on some days, even ten minutes will be too long. We all have days when we need to rest, digest new information, and have a time-out from new experiences. Grown-ups call such periods a "vacation" or a "holiday." Toddlers use a few hours or a day here or there. Give your child this time to consolidate and solidify her learning.

Toddlers respond to music. Be sure to add various kinds to your routine. Music helps develop a natural rhythm and coordination that will last long after the music fades.

## Lay-Back

*Benefit:*
* Strengthens abdominal and arm muscles

1. Sit with your toddler lying between your bent legs, as shown. Hold hands, supporting her forearms with your fingers.

2. Slowly pull her to a sitting position (let her use her arms and abdominal muscles as much as possible).

3. Slowly lower your toddler back to the floor. *Caution:* Be sure her head is in line with her spine and not hanging backward. Repeat five times.

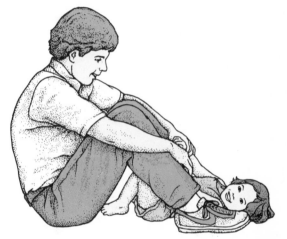

**Step 1**

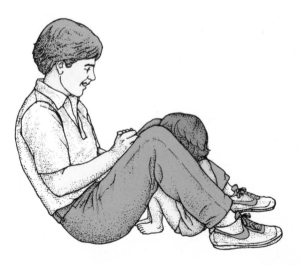

**Step 2**

# PHYSICAL DEVELOPMENT AND EXERCISE

## Touch and Hug

*Benefits:*
- Strengthens legs, shoulders, upper back, and arms
- Increases flexibility
- Provides body contact and closeness

1. Position your toddler as shown, letting her lean against you. Holding her right ankle and left hand, slowly bring the foot and hand together. (Do not force the limbs together.)

2. Stretch out the right leg and the left arm (high overhead). Repeat three to five times.

3. Change arm and leg. Repeat three to five times.

4. Holding your child's wrists and hands, cross her arms over her chest. Hug!

5. Slowly, stretch both of your child's arms above her head. Repeat from previous step three to five times.

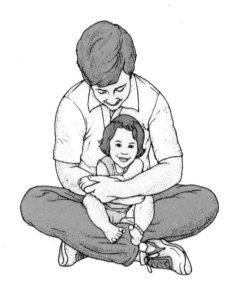

Step 4

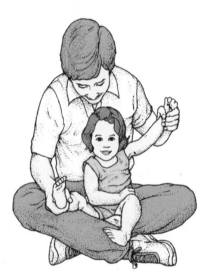

Step 1

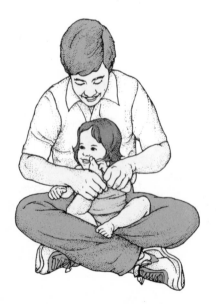

Step 1

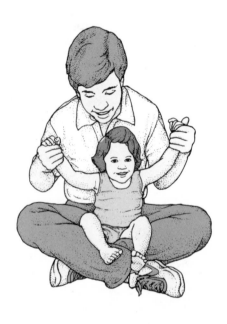

Step 5

## Let's Squat!

*Benefit:*
* Strengthens entire leg, especially quadriceps muscles (fronts of thighs) and knees

1. Stand next to each other. Feet should be shoulder-width apart, with toes pointing forward. Place hands on hips.

2. Bend the knees, lowering hips and buttocks toward floor. Buttocks should be pushed back (out) as you squat. Do not try to squat straight down or drop buttocks lower than backs of knees. You can place hands on the floor in front of you for stability, if needed.

3. Push up and repeat eight times.

## Hip Lift

*Benefits:*
* Strengthens back muscles
* Increases flexibility

1. Lay your toddler on her back, with her knees bent and her feet flat on the floor. Slip your hands around her waist, at the same time supporting her back.

2. Help your toddler lift the trunk of her body two to four inches off the floor; encourage her to use her leg and buttock muscles. Hold for two to three seconds.

3. Lower your toddler slowly back to the floor, keeping her knees bent.

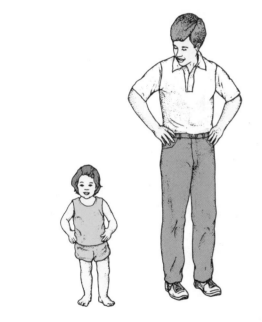

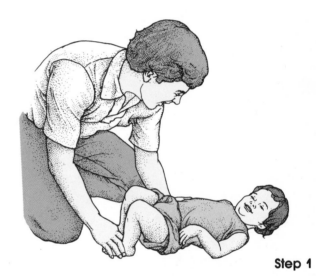

**Step 1**

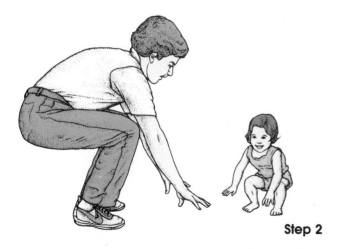

**Step 2**

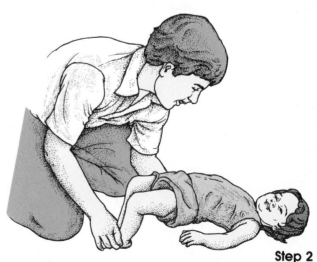

**Step 1**

**Step 2**

# PHYSICAL DEVELOPMENT AND EXERCISE

## Curl-Down

*Benefit:*
• Strengthens abdominal muscles

1. Sit facing your toddler, with your legs crossed (or with knees bent and feet flat on floor). Have your toddler sit with her knees bent and feet flat. Arms may be crossed (as shown) or held out straight toward you. Hold your toddler's ankles (not feet) so knees remain bent and feet flat.

2. Have her tuck her chin to her chest and round her back, as she slowly curls down to the floor to a count of four.

3. Return to the starting position by pulling your toddler up or having her push herself up. Repeat sequence five to eight times.

*Caution: Never let your child perform this exercise with a straight back; it could strain the lower back, causing pain or injury. Be sure your toddler breathes normally during the downward move. If you find she is holding her breath, remind her to breathe—she should count, sing, or talk. Also, she should try to curl back without leaning to one side or the other.*

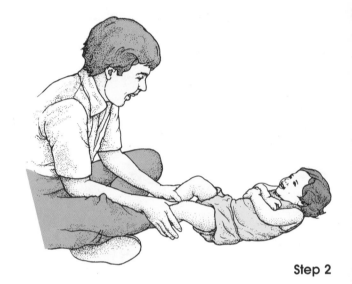

Step 2

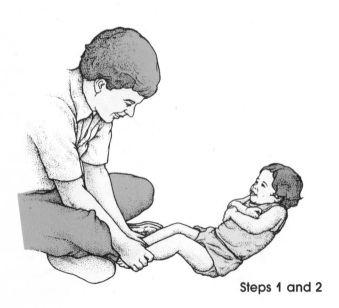

Steps 1 and 2

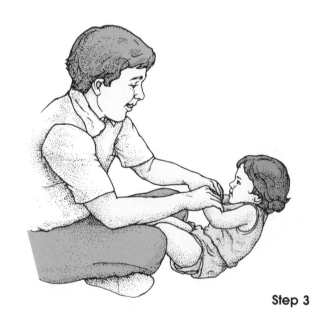

Step 3

## Head-to-Toes

*Benefits:*
- Increases lower back flexibility
- Strengthens abdominal muscles

1. Sit side by side or facing each other. Each of you place the soles of your feet together, well away from your body, and relax your legs.

2. Round your back and slowly curl your body toward your feet.

3. Curl back up (head will be the last thing to come up) to starting position. Repeat ten times (or more, if your toddler is agreeable).

## Train Tracks

*Benefits:*
- Greatly improves overall coordination
- Strengthens leg, abdominal, and lower back muscles
- Improves eye-foot/leg coordination

1. Place two two-by-fours on the floor, about one foot apart and parallel to each other. Your toddler should stand at one end, with one foot on each board.

2. Hold your toddler's hand as she walks the length of the boards. Repeat four times.

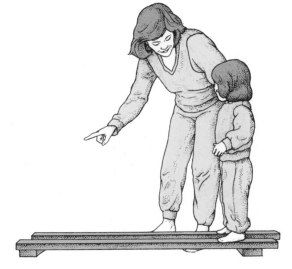

Step 1

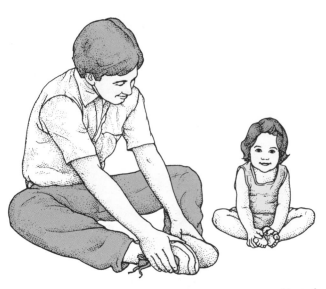

Step 1

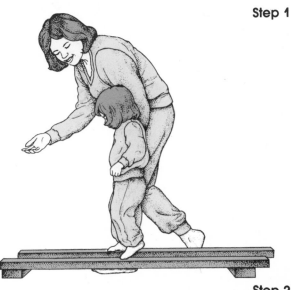

Step 2

Step 2

# PHYSICAL DEVELOPMENT AND EXERCISE

## Board Walk

*Benefits:*
* Improves balance
* Increases eye-foot coordination

1.   Use a two-by-four, slightly raised from or flat on the floor, for this exercise. Place your child at one end with both feet on the board, one in front of the other.

2.   Stand beside your child. Hold one hand while you place your other hand under her other arm.

3.   Encourage your child to walk from one end of the board to the other. Repeat the sequence four times, twice in each direction.

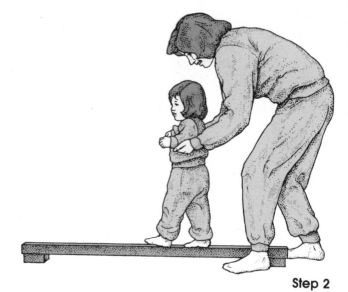

**Step 2**

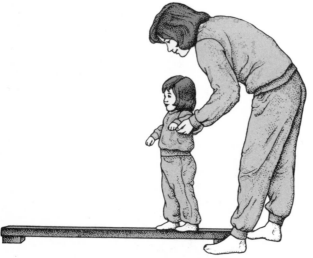

**Step 1**

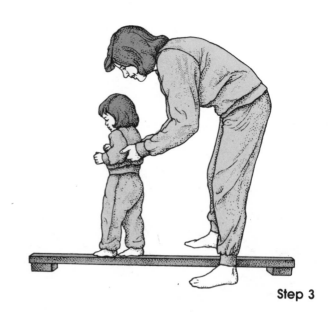

**Step 3**

### Ball Toss

*Benefits:*
- Improves concentration
- Increases eye-hand coordination

1. Sit close to your toddler, so that you are facing each other. Hold a large, bright, lightweight beach ball in front of you. Roll the ball to your child. Have your toddler roll or throw the ball back to you. Repeat eight to ten times, or as long as interest lasts.

2. This time, your toddler sits and you stand. Throw the ball to your child. Have her return it to you any way she can. Repeat eight to ten times.

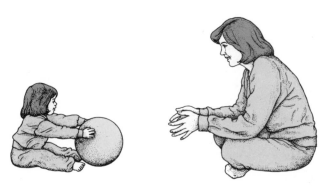

**Step 1**

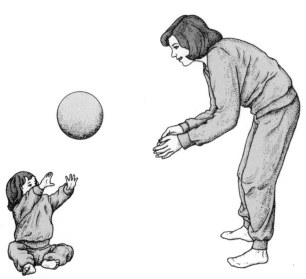

**Step 2**

### Twenty-Three Months to Three Years

A child this age will keep you busier than ever. He can hold a thought and he enjoys solving problems—like how to get on top of that counter or out the front door faster than you! He is physically strong, has a good memory, and is a constant surprise. Climbing and running are his choice activities. Even a parent in good physical condition will be awed by his seemingly inexhaustible energy level.

Exercise will refine his skills and help him learn to master his body. Cardiovascular (aerobic) exercises for his heart and lungs should be encouraged and fostered during play, like running, chasing, and kicking balls to a partner. Try for twelve minutes of nonstop action to develop his stamina and endurance (aerobic fitness).

Adding some new equipment to the routine will increase interest and variety. Mastering new tricks is a challenge; repeating old ones is reassuring. Children love new experiences as well as repetition.

At this age, children sometimes develop fears. Don't force a new experience. Hug and hold your child. Reassure him to help him feel safe. Fear will pass.

Choose a time when your child is naturally active for your exercise time. Although no special clothing is needed, children love to dress up for the occasion. A warm-up suit or leotard may increase the fun.

Don't forget music! When possible, let your child decide what music to use, and offer him a wide variety.

If you wish, you can use your favorite exercises from the previous section in addition to those that follow.

# PHYSICAL DEVELOPMENT AND EXERCISE

## Squat Bend

*Benefit:*
* Strengthens entire leg, especially quadriceps muscles (fronts of thighs) and knees

1. Stand next to or facing each other. Feet should be shoulder-width apart, with toes pointing forward. Place hands on hips.

2. Bend the knees, pushing buttocks out and back. Lean upper body slightly forward so abdomen is over tops of thighs. At all times, keep heels flat on the floor, with weight distributed evenly on soles. Do *not* (1) try to squat straight down, (2) turn toes out, or (3) drop buttocks lower than backs of knees.

3. Concentrating on your leg muscles, push up to the starting position. Keep knees "soft" as you reach the starting position. Do not snap them into a locked position by pushing kneecaps backward.

4. Repeat four to eight times.

## Jack-in-the-Box

*Benefit:*
* Strengthens quadriceps muscles (fronts of thighs)

1. Stand next to each other and squat (as in Squat Bends), placing your hands on the floor in front of you.

2. Push up quickly (using legs), popping up as high as you can. Straighten body as much as you can. Bend knees as you land, returning to squatting position. Repeat four to eight times.

*Caution: Do this one on a hardwood floor, a carpet, an exercise mat, or grass. Do not perform on a linoleum or concrete floor with no "give."*

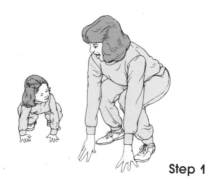

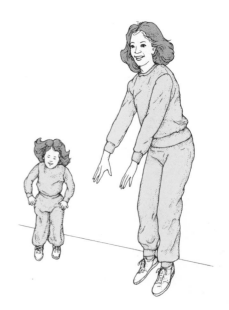

**Step 1**

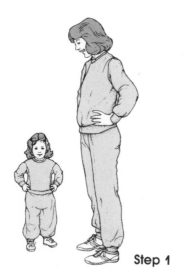

**Step 1**

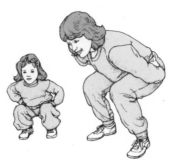

**Step 2**

**Step 2**

## Toe Touch

*Benefits:*
- Strengthens abdominal muscles
- Increases leg and lower back flexibility

1. Sit close to each other, with legs in front of you. Hold one foot with both hands.

2. Bring toe to your nose (not vice versa). Lower leg to starting position. Repeat five to ten times.

3. Change feet and repeat sequence.

## Rowing

*Benefits:*
- Strengthens arms, back, chest, and abdominal muscles
- Increases hamstring (back of the thigh) flexibility

*As you do this exercise, try singing "Row, Row, Row Your Boat"—it's great fun!*

1. Sit facing your child, as shown, with your child's feet touching the insides of your knees. Hold a dowel or stick between the two of you, with your hands snugly but gently over hers.

2. Slowly lean slightly backward, pulling your toddler toward you.

3. Reverse the action as your toddler leans backward. Legs should be as straight as possible, but keep knees slightly bent, not locked. If your hamstrings are tight, making it uncomfortable to sit with straight legs, bend your knees as needed. Repeat sequence ten to sixteen times.

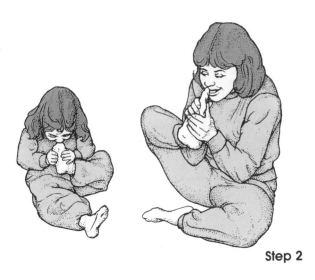

**Step 2**

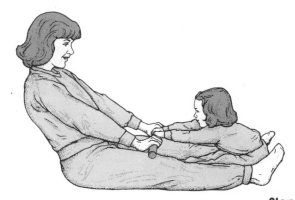

**Step 2**

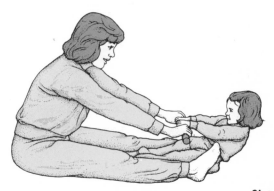

**Step 3**

# PHYSICAL DEVELOPMENT AND EXERCISE

## The Hill Walk

*Benefits:*
- Offers a safe challenge
- Improves balance and coordination
- Increases body/spatial awareness

*Use a homemade ramp, one purchased at a teacher's supply store, or a four- to five-foot-long, one-foot-wide platform (or board) with one end securely propped one foot off the floor.*

1. Holding your child's hand, have her walk from the low to the high end. (Telling her which foot she is on as she walks will help her learn right and left.) At the high end, while still holding her hands, have her jump off—she'll need no encouragement! Tell her to land on both feet and keep her knees bent. (If your child is very small and a distance of one foot is too high to jump, or if she seems reluctant, you can either lower the board or have your child sit down at the upper end, then jump off.) Repeat four to six times.

2. Reverse the walk, going from the high end to the low end.

3. As your child feels more comfortable with these moves, have her walk forward up the ramp and backward down the ramp. Then let her walk down and then up the ramp backwards.

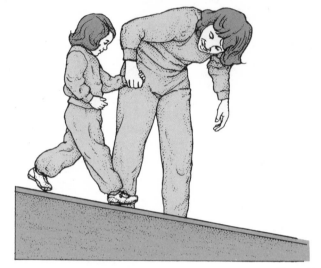

**Step 2**

## Hug Yourself

*Benefits:*
- Improves flexibility in arms, upper back, and shoulders
- Improves coordination

1. Sitting or standing, bring arms snugly around chest. Relax shoulders. Hold for a slow count of eight to ten.

2. Reverse arms and repeat.

3. To increase stretch, "walk" fingers slowly toward back. Hold.

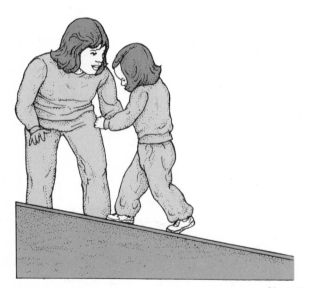

**Step 1**

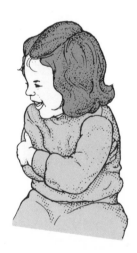

### Balance Beam Walk

*Benefits:*
- Improves balance, poise, coordination, and confidence
- Enhances self-esteem and body awareness

*If you have been working with your child on a two-by-four on the floor, you can introduce her to something higher. Use a four-inch-wide board on a sawhorse (clamped or nailed securely) or a balance beam. Stay close. She may exhibit some fear in the beginning.*

1. Place your child at one end of the beam. Standing beside her, hold her left hand in your left hand, with your right arm around her back and holding her right arm. Have your child take a step forward, while telling her which foot she is using.

2. Continue walking your child to the end of the beam. Repeat the sequence at least twice (more if your child is willing).

*After your child gets comfortable walking on the beam, try this:*

3. Place your toddler on one end of the beam, facing you. Hold both of her hands.

4. Have her walk backward, slowly, to the end of the beam. Tell her which foot she's using. Repeat this sequence at least twice.

*Note: Remember to securely hold your child at all times; floor padding beneath the balance beam is also a good idea. Teach your child never to climb on this piece of equipment unless you are present.*

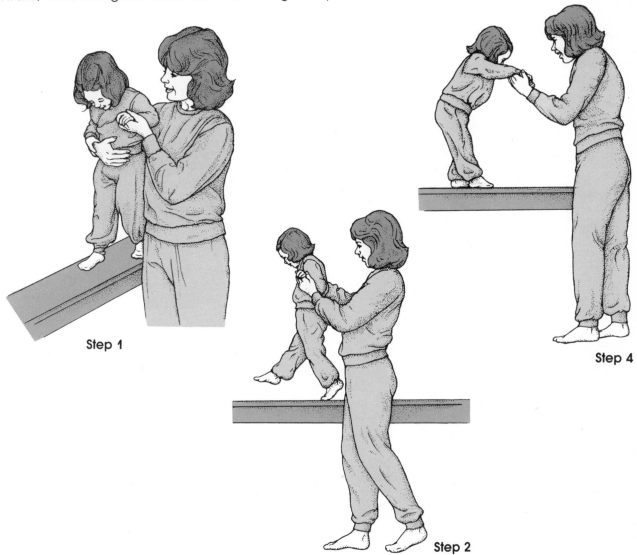

Step 1

Step 2

Step 4

# PHYSICAL DEVELOPMENT AND EXERCISE

## Basic Push-Up

*Benefit:*
* Strengthens arms, shoulders, back, and chest muscles

*This is a modified version of the all-time best upper body exercise. It doesn't have to be super-hard to be effective. This version will give both of you results.*

1. Kneel, facing each other or side by side, with hands and chin resting on floor. Keep hips and buttocks in the air, as shown. Keep your abdomen tight, and don't let your back sag.

2. Lift your upper body by straightening your arms. Back should be flat and parallel to the floor. Repeat six to eight times, working up to twenty.

*Caution: Keep neck in line with spine. If you curl or flex your neck up, to look at each other, you may experience discomfort or pain in the neck. It's best to look down at the floor.*

## The Angry Cat

*Benefits:*
* Strengthens abdominal muscles
* Stretches lower back muscles, increasing flexibility

*For fun or while telling a story, make cat noises while doing this exercise.*

1. Begin on hands and knees, side by side, facing the floor. Keep your back flat; don't let it sag.

2. Slowly, pull in your abdomen by tightening your abdominal muscles and round your back. (All the action should come from the abdominal muscles; do not push with your arms.) Breathe normally. Hold for a slow count of eight to ten. Return slowly (no sharp, jerky movements) to starting position.

3. Repeat four to eight times.

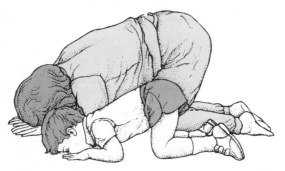

Step 1

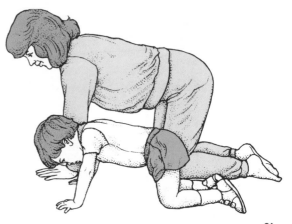

Step 1

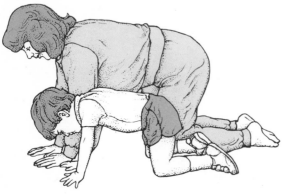

Step 2

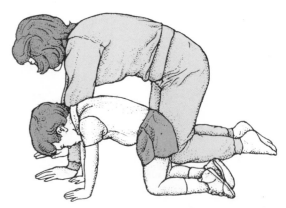

Step 2

### Jump in the Hoop

*Benefit:*
- Enhances coordination, concentration, and balance

*Sometimes young children have difficulty getting both feet off the ground at the same time. Be patient and offer help if your child has difficulty.*

*Caution: Do this exercise on a padded carpet, grass, or a wooden floor. Do not jump on concrete or linoleum floors. Both knees should be bent before jumping. As your child lands, tell him to bend his knees.*

1. Have your child stand outside a hoop placed on the floor. Remember, knees should be slightly bent.

2. Have your child push off the floor, landing inside the hoop. He should land on the front part of the foot and immediately press his heel down and bend the knees. (Cheer and clap for encouragement.)

3. Have him bend his knees and get ready to jump.

4. Have him push off the ground, landing outside the hoop. Repeat sequence four to eight times.

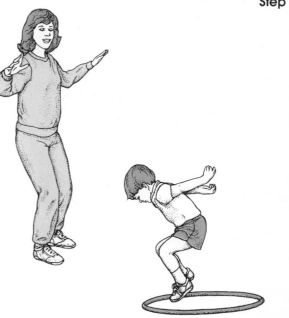

**Step 2**

**Step 4**

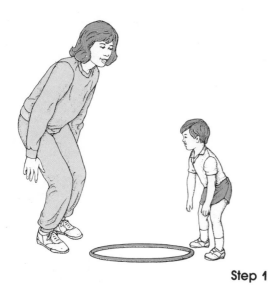

**Step 1**

The three-year-old is a true delight. Tears and temper tantrums are gone. She has even developed some patience. Her vocabulary has grown, and she is able to cooperate more and more each day.

Use these exercises and make up stories to go with the moves. The same can be done with any equipment or combination of pieces of equipment. Now is the time to be creative and imaginative. Equipment might include Frisbees, hoops, ladders, a slant board, one or more two-by-fours with supports, balls, balloons, and wooden dowels or sticks. Use your imagination!

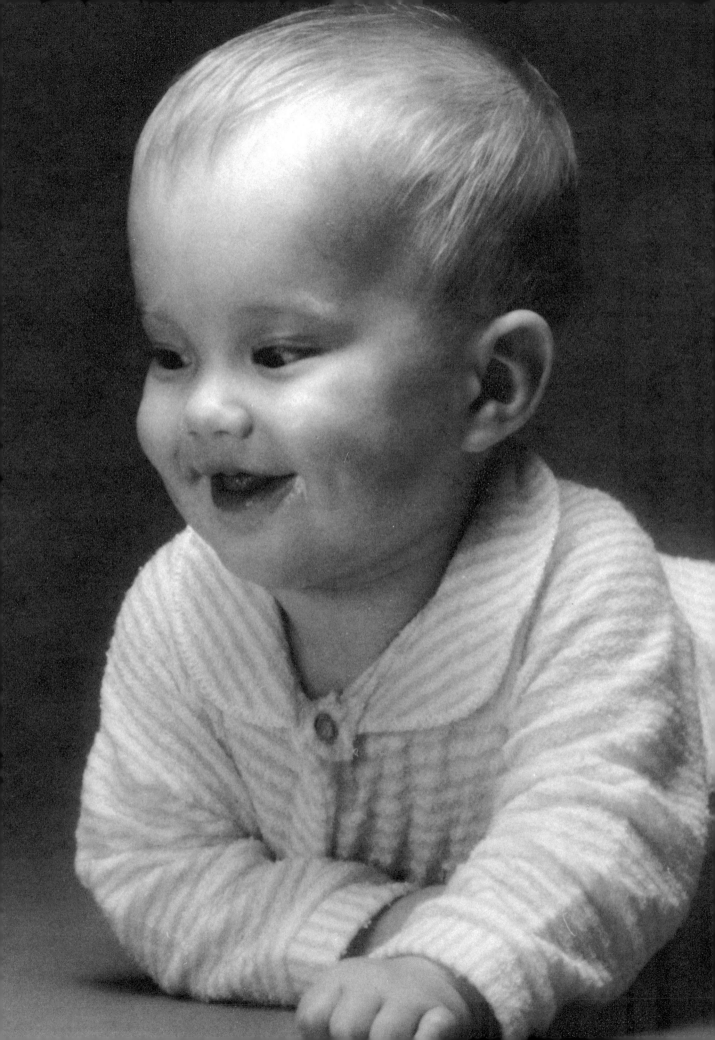

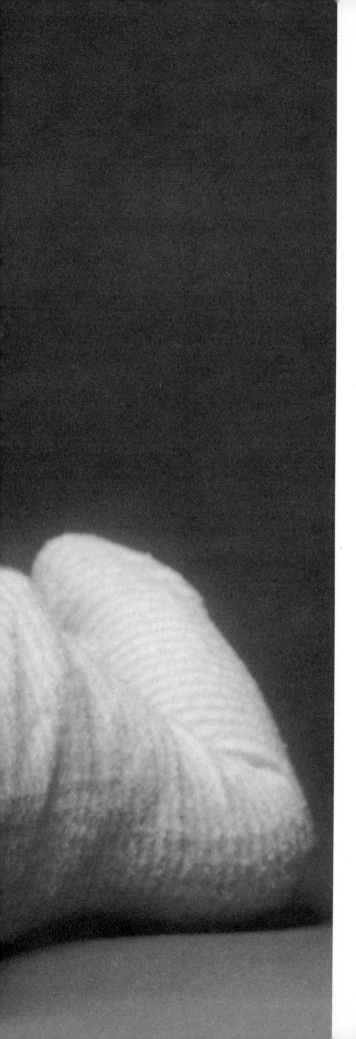

# Chapter 11:
# Learning
# and Cognitive
# Development

## Your Baby's Cognitive Development

In passing suddenly from the watery, dark environment of the womb to an existence outside the mother's body, the newborn is cut off from his former dependence on his mother's blood supply. The baby must begin to use his own lungs to breathe air and his own stomach to digest food. An infant spends his first days recovering from his mother's labor. Mechanisms for breathing, digestion, circulation, elimination, body temperature regulation, and hormonal secretion must be stabilized to begin this new and independent life. As this reorganization is taking place, infants are at the mercy of their reflexes, startling easily in response to sudden changes and flinging their arms out in panic if they feel themselves falling. Thus begins an increasingly independent existence for the baby, a process we call "development." *Cognitive* development is associated with knowing, with acquiring knowledge in the broadest sense, including memory, perception, and judgment as well as the accumulation of facts.

In the seventeenth century, English philosopher John Locke described the infant mind as a *tabula rasa,* or blank tablet, waiting to be written upon. Two hundred years later, William James said that the infant is so heavily "assailed by eyes, ears, nose, skin and entrails at once" that surroundings are seen as "one great blooming, buzzing confusion." As recently as 1964, the author of a medical textbook said not only that the average newborn was unable to fix his eyes or respond to sound, but also that "consciousness, as we think of it, probably does not exist in the infant."

Now we know better. In the past five years, the number of studies of infant cognition has tripled. There are many disagreements about various findings, but researchers definitely agree that the newborn comes into the world, not as a passive "receiver," but as a participant, ready and eager to interact with the environment. For example, although by adult standards the newborn has extremely poor vision, he can still discriminate between light and dark and focus on objects from eight to twelve inches away. Babies' intellects are working, and working very well, long before they can talk. They perceive a great deal, and they have decided preferences as well. From the beginning, you will see that your baby prefers to sleep in one position or another. By eight weeks, your baby will be able to differentiate between shapes, liking faces more than inanimate objects, and will see colors, reacting especially strongly to the bright primary colors red and blue. Your baby will be able to distinguish the sweet taste of sugarwater and will prefer the smell of bananas to that of shrimp. Infants prefer the sound of women's voices, and within a few weeks, your baby will recognize and respond to his mother's voice. In short, the senses participate in the developmental process from the moment of birth. As a Yale University psychology professor who has studied infants for more than thirty years has said about the newborn's zestful approach to life, "He's eating up the world!"

## Genetics vs. Environment

Infants vary tremendously in their capabilities, just as adults do. Some of this variation can be traced to inherited differences. Recently, in fact, geneticists have postulated that, in addition to controlling skin, eye, and hair coloring, genes may control behavior under certain environmental conditions. No matter what a baby's genetic inheritance, though, her environment must supply warmth and nourishment, both emotional and physical, if the baby is to reach her full developmental potential.

There is a great deal of conflict over the degree to which intelligence is inherited. It does seem clear that intelligence is not fixed at a rigid level at birth and that many environmental factors can affect the level of a child's intelligence throughout her development. Some cognitive psychologists today believe that while perhaps the outer limits of intelligence are fixed at birth, a child's environment can make a difference of as much as forty points in her IQ (intelligence quotient, the number indicating the level of a person's intelligence as shown by special tests). This is a staggering figure when one considers that it is the same as the range between the value for borderline mental retardation (eighty IQ points) and the value for the average college graduate (120 IQ points). Other psychologists who have conducted classic studies of identical twins separated at birth have been more conservative, saying that environment can cause a difference of as much as twenty IQ points.

Theories about the genetic inferiority or superiority of certain ethnic or racial groups cannot be proved. The differences among the environments of home, nation, tribe, and culture make genetic comparisons of entire races or ethnic groups scientifically unverifiable. Given the tremendous differences in the family of man, the best we can do is speak of "developmental potential" when trying to gauge intelligence in a young child.

## "Normal" Development

Remember that everything you read or hear about what is "normal" development for a child at a certain age refers to what is expected of the "average" child. Your baby may be ahead of others the same age in some ways, behind in others. We will discuss reasonable expectations you should have and the folly of comparing your child with others later in this chapter. Whatever his individual differences from the norm, you can expect your baby to develop at an incredible rate during the first year of life, in a head-to-toe direction. That is, he will gain control over his eyes, neck, and hands before learning to use his legs for walking. In the beginning, your infant is very much mouth-oriented; the sensations of sucking and mouthing give the most pleasure. Soon, the ability to use the hands develops. At about five months, your baby will be able to grasp toys, and his learning will be related to the ability to manipulate. By about ten months of age, your baby will smile at you and other familiar people and will display anxiety when strangers are present. At about the same time, the baby will probably become expert at crawling—and at getting into things. At about one year, he will begin to walk alone, a true milestone in his development.

In the second and third years, toddlers become increasingly independent and curious, a combination that makes them dangerous to themselves and everything about them. You will have become aware of the necessity for careful childproofing of your home by the time your baby can crawl, but the hazards increase dramatically as your child becomes more agile and more investigative. During the second year, your child's rapid increase in the ability to communicate through language will represent a big breakthrough. "No" will become a favorite word, and temper tantrums may be frequent as she encounters frustration over boundaries you must set. Typical toddlers are torn between the drive toward growth and maturity on one hand and dependency and regression on the other.

As your child grows and changes, you will probably notice that her development seems not to occur steadily, in an even line, but rather in spurts or "giant steps." It is normal for children to have critical periods, times when internal and environmental factors come together and they learn a great deal or become proficient at some physical skill. Then they hit plateaus, so to speak, when their minds and bodies catch up with each other. It is said that if these critical periods are somehow bypassed, they are difficult to make up later in a child's development.

## How You Can Promote Your Child's Optimal Development

Children who are loved for what they are, not for what they will become, develop a sense of security and belonging. Parents who promote a feeling of basic trust allow their children to develop deeper human relationships in later life, and they thereby contribute in a positive way to the formation of their children's personalities. By building on feelings of trust, honesty, integrity, and reliability, parents can do a great deal to promote optimal development.

Ideally, your role in promoting your child's development starts at the moment he is born, with the close body contact that begins the bonding process. When that initial physical closeness with the mother is not possible for one reason or another, bonding can be accomplished later through loving and touching. The first three years of a child's life are extremely important developmentally, and the greatest gifts you can give your child during that period are your time and your enthusiasm for his developing skills. Your child will be learning during every waking moment, and your best function is not so much to teach as to provide a stimulating environment and an emotionally supportive atmosphere. Follow your child's lead; don't push and don't try to rush him. For play to be rewarding and creative, your child needs appropriate toys, but he also needs warm and nurturing attention and guidance. If the daily care of your child will be entrusted to someone else, choose that individual carefully. Children must be with people who love and value them if they are to learn to love and value themselves and others.

Even infants need privacy, time to themselves. The environment in which your baby learns and develops should be a protective one, safe and secure. She needs a quiet, peaceful place to sleep, and when awake should not be constantly at the center of an overly active household. Visual and auditory stimuli should be toned down to provide a calm atmosphere in which your baby will develop her perceptions of the outside world.

Toddlers also need periods of peace and quiet away from people and activities. They need time to "recharge their batteries," to rest, and to organize their inner lives. Children who are overstimulated, spend their days in crowded quarters, and are never alone except during sleep tend to be excitable, dependent upon others for their entertainment, and unaware of their own abilities.

Another essential in your child's development is your guidance—the setting of limits, the enforcing of boundaries. A child needs parents who will set limits that are appropriate to his age level at each step of development. Self-control and inner discipline develop only after limits are firmly set. Overall consistency is important because it builds up feelings of security in the child.

The basic idea is to try to achieve for your child balances between routine and variety, sameness and contrast, protection and freedom. Trust your own instincts, advises prominent pediatrician T. Berry Brazelton. Children are remarkably adaptable, and you cannot fail to be successful in promoting your child's optimal development if your aim is to provide a deep and warm personal relationship with your child as well as an appropriate world of toys, experiences, and instruction.

## Recognizing Your Child's Uniqueness

Environmental influences alone cannot explain the variability in a child's development. Your child's temperament will play a significant and active role through interaction with your own parental style. Unfortunately, mismatches sometimes occur between the temperaments of parents and their children. However deep their love and respect for each other, these parents and children simply have trouble getting along, sometimes all their lives. It is important that parents come to understand the differences between themselves and their children, what makes their children "tick," and how they can best help and guide them. In especially difficult cases, a specific management program instituted by a therapist can help improve the "fit" between a parent and a child.

The term "temperament" means the unique behavioral style of each individual. Many psychologists and others have described what they feel are the most easily identifiable characteristics of various types of temperaments and personalities. A favorite system of classification of those who have worked with pediatrician Arnold Gesell is called constitutional psychology, developed by William Sheldon. This system proposes that we can predict how any child will behave from an observation of his or her body build. No individual is of one type exclusively; we are all combinations, but in most people one or another is dominant.

The body of the *endomorph* is round and soft. The arms and legs are comparatively short, with the upper part of the arm longer than the lower. The hands and feet are small and plump, and the fingers are short and tapering. The endomorphic individual is gregarious and loves to eat. The child who is an endomorph is easygoing and easy to get along with.

The body of the *mesomorph* is hard and square. The extremities are large, with the upper portions of the arms and legs equal in length to the lower parts. The hands and wrists are large, the fingers squarish. The mesomorph likes athletic activity and competitive action, is loud and active, and may be given to noisy temper tantrums.

The body of the *ectomorph* is linear, fragile, and delicate. The arms and legs are long in comparison with the body. The hands and feet are slender and delicate, and the fingertips are tapered. The ectomorph likes to be alone and is most interested in watching, listening, and thinking about things. He may have allergies to foods, and may have a hard time sleeping through the night.

Three other categories of temperament are familiar to parents and perhaps more often referred to. The "easy child" is characterized by biologic regularity (of the bowels, bladder, and feeding cycles) and adaptability. The "difficult child," at the other end of the spectrum, displays biologic irregularity, withdraws from new situations, has negative moods, and adapts slowly. The "slow-to-warm-up child" is somewhere in the middle, combining some of both kinds of traits.

## The Experts on Cognition

Rearing a child is not like producing a piece of craft work. There is no single set of instructions that, if faithfully followed, will assure you of perfect results. Too much human variation and experience not embodied in any particular theory must go into parenting, making it impossible as well as unwise to try to follow just one method of child-rearing. This does not mean that parents should not be interested in the findings of child-development researchers. The better informed they are, the better able they will be to choose from among the many attitudes and viewpoints of the experts those they believe will work for them and be compatible with their temperaments and lifestyles.

A single book such as this cannot possibly cover all the work that has been done on cognition. Following is a "sampler" that attempts to put into perspective the basic premises of four of the major theorists: Piaget, Gesell, Erikson, and Spock. All believe that there are stages or periods of development, but each emphasizes a different approach to the study of a child's thinking and learning patterns.

*Jean Piaget* was a Swiss psychologist who may be called an interactionist. That is, his theory is that intellectual development results from an active, dynamic interplay between a child and her environment. *Arnold Gesell*, an American pediatrician who did his research at the Yale Child Study Center, may be called a maturationist. His theory is that heredity promotes unfolding of development in a preordained sequence—on a timetable, so to speak, with few individual differences. Both men have contributed a tremendous amount of knowledge about the growing infant and child. Although they stand at opposite poles, both have recorded facts useful to parents and professionals alike in making meaningful observations of child behavior. Piaget's contributions to learning theory have helped shape many educational programs in our schools, while Gesell's schedules of behavior development are still used as clinical and diagnostic tools by pediatric developmentalists.

*Erik Erikson,* a psychoanalyst of children at the Institute of Child Welfare in California, and *Benjamin Spock,* the dean of American pediatricians, may be discussed together. While Piaget and Gesell emphasize motor and intellectual development, Erikson and Spock are most interested in the emotional development of children. Although they, too, think of development in terms of stages or periods, they differ from Piaget and Gesell in their stress on the importance of individual differences among children.

## Jean Piaget

Piaget describes four theoretical periods, or stages, of child development: sensorimotor, preoperational, concrete operational, and formal operational. Consideration of these periods has spurred a great deal of research, most of which has tended to support Piaget's conclusions about children's cognitive development.

The four stages are very different from one another; each reveals a different way in which an individual reacts to her environment. As an interactionist, Piaget feels that each stage in development occurs as a result of interaction between maturation and environment. He believes also that intelligence or intelligent behavior is the ability to *adapt.* Even nonverbal behavior, to the extent that it is adaptive, is intelligent.

- In the *sensorimotor stage* (birth to two years), infants are transformed from creatures who respond mostly with reflexes to those who can organize sensorimotor activity in response to the environment—to reach for a toy, for example, or to pull back from a frightening stranger. Babies gradually become more organized, and their activities become less random. Through each encounter with the environment, they progress from a reflex stage to trial-and-error learning and simple problem solving.

- In the *preoperational stage* (two to seven years), children's thinking, by adult standards, is illogical and focused entirely on themselves. They begin to use symbols to represent objects, places, and people. Symbols—images that represent some object or person—are sight, sound, or touch sensations that are evoked internally. In play, children act out their views of the world, using a system of symbols to represent what they see in their environment.

- By the *concrete operational stage* (seven to eleven years), children begin to gain the ability to think logically and to understand concepts that they use in dealing with the immediate environment.

- They have arrived at the *formal operational stage* (twelve years and over) when they start thinking in abstract terms as well as concrete ones. Adolescents, for example, can discuss theoretical issues as well as real ones.

In Piaget's view, then, the development of knowledge is an active process and depends upon interaction between the child and the environment. The child is neither the possessor of a preformed set of mental abilities that gradually unfold nor a passive recipient of stimulation from the environment. From infancy onward, movement increasingly gives way to thought, and learning continues to be an interactive process.

## Arnold Gesell

Like Piaget, Gesell de-emphasizes individual differences among children and stresses the importance of maturation. Unlike the Swiss psychologist, however, Gesell sees maturation following an inherited timetable; abilities and skills emerge in a preordained sequence.

Gesell believes that because the infant and the child are subject to predictable growth forces, the behavior patterns that result are not whimsical or accidental by-products. Those patterns are, in his view, predictable end-products of a total developmental process that works within an orderly sequence. He describes four fields of behavior: *motor, adaptive, language,* and *personal-social.* In his view, the organization of behavior begins well before birth and proceeds from head to foot. In a summary of behavior development, Gesell describes the following landmarks:

- In the first quarter of the first year of life (birth to sixteen weeks), the newborn gains control of muscles and nerves in the face (those that are involved in sight, hearing, taste, sucking, swallowing, and smell).

- In the second quarter (sixteen to twenty-eight weeks), the infant starts to develop command of muscles of the neck and head and moves her arms purposefully. The baby reaches out for things.

- In the third quarter (twenty-eight to forty weeks), the baby gains control of her trunk and her hands—grasping objects, transferring them from hand to hand, and fondling them.

- In the fourth quarter (forty to fifty-two weeks), control extends to the baby's legs and feet, and also to the index fingers and thumbs, to allow plucking of a tiny object. The baby begins to talk.

- In the second year, the toddler walks and runs, speaks some words and phrases clearly, acquires bladder and bowel control, and begins to develop a sense of personal identity and of personal possessions.

- In the third year, the child speaks in clear sentences, using words as tools of thinking. No longer an infant, she tries to manipulate the environment. Tantrums are displayed.

- In the fourth year, the child asks many questions and begins to form concepts and to generalize. She is nearly self-dependent in home routines.

- By the age of five, the child is very mature in motor control over large muscles; she actively skips, hops, and jumps. She talks without any infantile sounds and can tell a long story and a few simple jokes. She feels pride in accomplishment and is quite self-assured in the small world of home.

### Erikson and Spock

While Piaget and Gesell emphasize motor and intellectual development, Erikson and Spock are most interested in the emotional development of children. Although they, too, think of development in terms of stages or periods, Erikson and Spock differ from Piaget and Gesell in their stress on the importance of individual differences among children. The classifications below are Erikson's; Spock's findings are included under the appropriate headings.

- The *period of trust* covers the early months in an infant's life and is so called because babies need to establish confidence in their parents and in their environment. This period of trust provides a solid foundation for further development. Spock calls infants at this stage "physically helpless and emotionally agreeable." Some babies, however, are more difficult to understand and their cries for help are not clear. The parents can't separate the cry of hunger, fatigue, or discomfort from wet diapers from the cry for attention. Problems frequently occur because of parental inexperience or because there are marked differences in temperament between parent and infant.

- The *period of autonomy* is one in which toddlers strive for independence; it represents the development of self-control and self-reliance. Spock speaks of the child at this stage as having a "sense of his own individuality and will power" and as vacillating between dependence and independence. Parents of such a child must learn to accept some loss of control while maintaining necessary limits.

- The *period of initiative* covers the preschool years, during which a child gains considerable freedom. Spock calls what the child does during this period "imitation through admiration." Fears are a common problem, and the child has an active fantasy life. Preschoolers frequently have difficulty separating from their parents, often caused or reinforced by the parents' own problems in separating from their offspring.

- The *period of industry or work completion* is one in which the school-age child learns to win praise by performing and producing results. Spock describes this period as one in which the school-age child is trying to fit into an outside group of friends and to move away from his parents. Parents react to this declaration of independence in several ways, frequently being hurt or disappointed. School-age children still need plenty of parental support despite their surface attempts at self-assurance. Parents should give support in a way that shows respect for the child's feelings and pride.

- *Adolescence* is Erikson's fifth and final stage of development. He describes the teenager's task as one of establishing "identity," finding out who he is and what he wants to make of his life. Teenage experiments with relationships

## Social Development "Milestones"

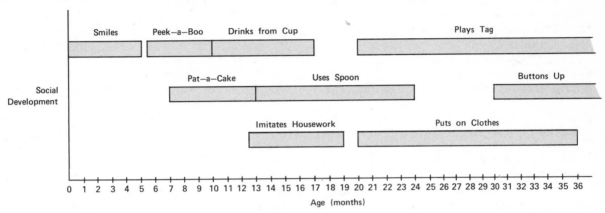

Keep in mind that babies vary greatly in their social development. The indicated age ranges are guidelines, not absolute requirements.

and development of a view of reality through constant testing may be very hard on parents. Spock describes adolescents as being very "peer-oriented." He stresses the need for parents to continue to set appropriate limits, instill worthwhile values, and provide positive role models.

## Your Child's Social Development

Social behavior begins very early in the lives of human beings. Infants respond to people almost from the moment of birth. In fact, if you began the bonding process with close skin contact immediately after your baby was born, you probably felt that she was definitely aware of you, reaching out to you. Newborns are attracted to human faces, and they like the sound of human voices, especially female voices. Soon your new baby's eyes will follow your movements in a room, then her head will turn to watch you. At three or four months, your baby will respond happily to smiling people, then will smile at the sight of any approaching face. The baby will smile—you will smile—her smile will broaden. Thus, social interaction begins; the baby has learned to get a reaction from another person. She will even try to mimic you when you stare, stick your tongue out, or make faces. One day you'll notice that your baby quiets if you speak or sing as you come near the crib. It won't be long until she will make a sound in response to your voice.

At five to eight months old, your baby will probably be learning how to be "cute," how to get your attention by pretending to cough or by doing something that has made you laugh before. She will know the difference between familiar people and strangers and may show fear of strangers. When your baby is somewhere between the ages of eight months and a year, you'll be getting cooperation in the singing games and finger plays with which you've been entertaining her. Soon she will adore having an audience and will delight in performing the "bye-bye" ritual and any others that get attention.

Between the ages of one and three, your child will be ready to branch out socially. Though learning to actually play with other children effectively will take a while, she will want to be around them, if only as an observer. She will learn a great deal from this observation.

### The First Social Set: The Family

The immediate family—mother, father, siblings, and a care-giver, if the baby has some kind of day care—is your baby's first social set, a select and fortunate group. All of you will outdo yourselves to entertain and please the baby, and your greatest thrills will come when he responds and reciprocates. Remember, though, that the key word in all human behavior is *unique*. Your baby is as different from all the other babies in the world as each snowflake is different from all others. Antics that sent your older child or your neighbor's baby into paroxysms of giggles and gurgles may very well make this baby cry and pull back. Take your cue from your child: if he startles easily or seems frightened by your loud noises, funny faces, or sudden actions, ease up.

# LEARNING AND COGNITIVE DEVELOPMENT

At about a year, your child will be extremely sociable. He will love being part of any and every family gathering and will obviously adore everyone. The baby will happily go on your rounds of shopping and errands with you, pay and receive social visits with you, and thoroughly enjoy just being with you around the house. Anything goes, in fact, as long as a family member is close at hand.

Unfortunately, things will change. The push toward independence you've read and heard about will become reality, and at a point somewhere around eighteen months, your baby will appear to have outgrown any need for you. He will barely acknowledge your presence in daily life, except to say *no* a great deal. Walking, running, climbing stairs, exploring, and satisfying curiosity about everything and anything will be all-engrossing. There will be occasional reversions to the old baby ways of love and play, but in general the child at this age is concentrating so hard on self and environment that adults seem to exist for no reason other than to satisfy his desires. The exception to this behavior will be when there's trouble; no one but Mommy or the primary, daily care-giver can handle a cut or bruise or make a stubborn toy work the way it should.

Sociability will return, in time, but by the time it does, your baby's social set will include playmates and others outside the family. You will never again be as all-important to your child as you were for the first year, which is as it should be. Learning to let go is among the most important of parents' lessons.

## Separation Anxiety and Other Fears

Love takes many forms, and your baby may often show her love for you by resisting any separation from you. This is completely natural. Your baby is aware of total dependence on you for survival; if you are absent, fear takes over. Contrary to what many people think, you will not "break" your baby of needing you by forcing frequent or lengthy separations. The truth is that the more secure you can make her feel, by being present and by holding, cuddling, and reassuring, the more confident and unafraid she will be. You will notice that something frightening—perhaps the vacuum cleaner—is no longer so from the safety zone of your arms. Other unreasonable fears come and go suddenly; some common ones are fear of dogs or cats, the ghosts and monsters that come in the night, emergency sirens, thunder, and people in "unusual" garb, such as doormen and nuns

in habits. These frights pass and are forgotten if you support your child through them.

If your baby seems unable to be without you for a single waking moment, realize that this is one of the many phases she will go through and do your best to go along with it. Don't force a stint in the playpen or an exercise period in the middle of the living room floor if your infant seems terrified of being in the center of all that empty space. Don't make an obviously reluctant baby go to someone else, even if it's a relative whose feelings are apt to be hurt by the rejection. Leave the door to the baby's room ajar at bedtime, and reassure her that you're near by letting your voice be heard from wherever you are in the house. Try not to show irritation at what you know to be foolish and unreasonable fears; you will only make your baby feel unloved and less secure than ever. Don't worry about "spoiling" a clinging baby or overprotecting her by avoiding situations you know are frightening. She has a built-in human drive to be mature and to be independent.

Many babies are reluctant to be left with baby-sitters. When Mommy is out of sight, she is *gone,* and children under the age of about two cannot yet reason well enough to know that she will be back. Some parents feel they simply must not leave their children at this point; others insist that they must get out and that both they and their children are better for an occasional separation. If you're in the latter group, someone your child knows will be your best choice for a sitter at first—Grandma or another relative is often ideal. You may wish to have a sitter your baby doesn't know come for a visit or two when you will be home, so the two can get to be friends.

If you must leave a comparative stranger in charge, have the babysitter arrive early enough to get acquainted with your baby while you are still there. Never sneak off, say most parents; use a regular good-bye ritual that includes kissing good-bye and waving. Come home when you've said you will, and set the time as "after your nap," instead of "at three o'clock," for a small child who doesn't live by the clock yet. If you drop your child off at the sitter's house, even if a loving and beloved Grandma is the sitter, be sure to take along the favorite stuffed animal or blanket.

## Siblings as First Friends

Your baby's siblings will be his first friends. With luck, your children will remain good friends for life.

At first, your concern will be to help your older child handle jealousy at being "replaced" by involving her in the care of the baby. As you teach the older child how to play with the baby and how to amuse him, you'll see the baby responding. Admiration for an older child's skills and accomplishments and the pure pleasure of just being allowed to be in her company will be the baby's very obvious emotions. Later, the younger child will probably be jealous of the older because of those very skills and accomplishments, but in the early days there's nothing like having a big brother or big sister to watch and love.

## Grandmas and Grandpas, Aunts and Uncles

The time to start a loving relationship between grandparents and other older relatives and your child is in the beginning. The way to keep such wonderful relationships thriving is to keep the companionship and communication open and frequent. Ideally, Grandma and Grandpa live down the street or around the corner, and the other relatives live not much farther away. Holidays are shared, and the families are often in one another's homes for quick visits or meals. When the kids are a little older, they look upon every home in the family as partly theirs. The child who sees and shares time with elders in this fashion will learn to love and trust them and to look upon them as beings similar to, but different from (and in a special way), her parents.

Unfortunately, not all those in the extended family are always within easy visiting distance, perhaps not even in the same state or region of the country. Some of those whom you want to be closest to your baby may be able to see her only rarely, when either they or you pack up and drive or fly to visit. Between visits, it will be up to you to help your child remember the relatives and to help both the elders and the child feel close to one another. Use the telephone and the mail to keep your relatives informed about your child's development; pictures and tapes will help. Show your child pictures of the relatives, use their names often, and tell stories about your childhood that include them.

A sad fact is that long-distance visits are sometimes exhausting for parents, elders, and children alike, unsatisfactory for all because of unreasonably high expectations and too much "togetherness" in too short a period of time. Routines are upset, and the schedule of activities may be too crowded; there may be neither enough room in the house nor hours in the day for anyone to have the privacy and time alone that everyone from the oldest grandparent to the youngest infant needs.

Handling family visits with grace takes practice, along with consideration and goodwill. Lowering your expectations will help. Don't expect that the elders will find your child perfect and your methods of child care irreproachable. Don't for a minute think your child will not, at some time during the visit, display unattractive habits and perform naughty acts normal for her age, plus some that are far advanced. Don't dream that you can go all the places, see all the people, and do all the things you want to and should. Above all, don't worry about the elders spoiling your child. A little coddling and extra attention and a little relaxation of the rules will make a visit more special and memorable.

## Playmates and Peers

Your baby's social life with his peers will begin just as soon as you see to it that he has opportunities to see other babies. You can put two babies in a playpen or on a blanket on the grass at three months old, and if they are both in happy moods, they'll make a picture both families will always treasure. Cooperative play with other children, the kind most adults consider "real" play, doesn't start until kids are about three, but they all need the companionship of other children long before that. Of course siblings often make wonderful playmates, but it is important for your baby to be around others who are close to him in age and size.

Finding suitable playmates may or may not be easy, depending upon your neighborhood, your own circle of friends, and your personal inclinations and abilities in making new friends. If there's a public park near you, you may find this "fresh air playroom" the ideal place both for your child and yourself to take a break from the home routine. Many lifetime friendships, for both parents and children, have begun in parks. The parents socialize and trade child-care tips as their babies doze in carriages; then later they share supervision duties as their children play on park equipment and learn to get along with others.

Some who have watched their own children or others' closely as their social lives developed have noted that play progresses in quite predictable stages. The first stage is not play at all; ba-

343

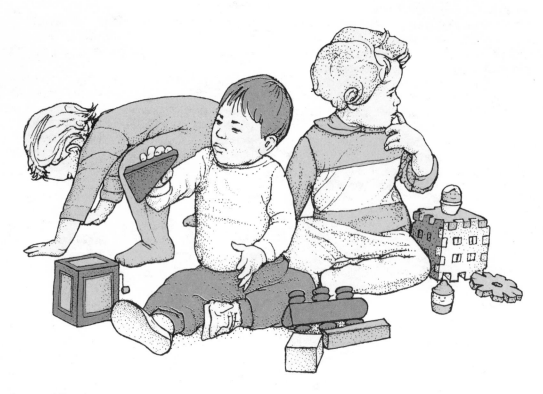

*Parallel play is one of the steps on your baby's road to true social interaction.*

bies under a year old are *watchers*. They examine their toys and everything they get their hands on very closely, and they stare at other people. You'll probably notice that your baby is especially interested in other babies and small children and is well aware that they are different from adults.

Toddlers begin what's called *parallel play*. They play side by side or back to back, paying little or no attention to each other. They like being together, and they may occasionally enjoy watching each other play, but most of all each is interested in what he is doing. When your child is about eighteen months old, you're likely to see some aggressiveness. Toddlers don't really know how to play yet; they don't understand sharing, and they haven't learned that it's not right to hit and shove and bite other people. Use common sense in handling a battle between two toddlers; remember that you are the adult. Of course you can't stand by and see a child get really hurt, but be careful you don't teach your toddler that it's all right to hit others because Mommy will see to it that the others don't hit back. And be aware that if you spank your toddler for being overly aggressive, you'll be teaching him that the way to stop hitting is to hit.

*Associative play,* in which children really play together, follows soon. This is unstructured play; there are no rules, but two children will talk to each other and use some of the same toys. Both attention spans and tempers are short, and egos are all-important, so you can't expect the fun to last more than about a half hour in most cases. You'll hear the word "mine" often. If the eyes of two children happen to light on the same toy at the same time, they'll both reach for it whether or not they really want it. In fact, toddlers of this age really do want everything they see, unselectively. Reason won't solve the problem of contention; these children are not yet old enough to grasp the idea of sharing. You may be able to make use of a timer to set the end of one child's turn and the beginning of the other's, but sometimes you may simply have to put a toy away.

Remember that the quarrels that annoy you because they seem senseless help children develop social skills. If you interfere in any but the most serious, you will be depriving the children of a chance to learn how to get along with others. At this point, children almost always do best with just one other child, and will get along better and be able to play longer with one than with another. It is important now that your child see as many others as possible, so as to be able to select the ones with whom she most enjoys playing.

By about the age of three, your child will have become proficient enough at social relationships to begin *cooperative play,* which involves rules and sharing and turns and fairness—in playing house, the "mother" must act like a mother; it's not fair for one child to knock down a tower of blocks two have put up together; your child will know that she can't use the swing while it's the playmate's turn. If you have older children, it's at about this point that you begin to see the sibling companionship you've been waiting for. While previously the older kids have probably enjoyed playing with the younger one as a sort of living toy, now little brother or little sister has learned enough to make proper responses in play situations and has become much more interesting. Imaginative role playing—"school," "house," "office"—is fun for both the older and the younger kids.

Parents often worry if they see what they think are signs of shyness in their child. Some shyness is simply the result of a developmental phase; the child will soon outgrow it and become outgoing and friendly. You can help your shy toddler or preschooler by encouraging nonthreatening play with just one or two low-key children, not a crowd of boisterous ones. Be aware that some children are simply less gregarious than others, just as some adults are. Don't push too hard.

*Play Groups*
One way to provide your child with a regular source of playmates of the right age is to form a play group with other parents. It's not too early to start a group when the children of three or four congenial parents who live close to each other have reached the age of eighteen months to two years. Some parents choose to meet all together, children and adults, once or twice a week. Others prefer to take turns being in charge of the children. This approach makes the play group more like "school" and gives all the parents some time off. The parent in charge will need to devote total attention to the group to be sure none of the children gets in trouble, so everything must be in readiness before a session starts. Sessions should not last longer than two hours. An elaborate array of toys is not necessary; the ones your own child has will probably be sufficient (see Chapter 4 for information on toys). By the time the children are about two years old, the play group may be expanded. Parents will probably then work in shifts

of two, and you may arrange for meetings to be held in a public place, such as a school or church.

*Birthday Parties*
Your child will learn that his birthday is a very special day when you bring out the cake with its single candle and the whole family cheers and sings. A balloon or two, the lighted cake, the singing of "Happy Birthday," the flash of the camera, and a few presents will probably be enough to overwhelm all but the most sophisticated of babies. Some parents do like to include a few friends and their children in the celebration. This is best handled very simply, perhaps in a park or in the backyard if possible. Ideally, every child will be accompanied by at least one parent. If you have a party at home and you can possibly manage it, provide nap space for exhausted babies.

By the second birthday, your child may have been to a party or two and may have some idea of what to expect. Still, even many three-year-olds are not yet ready for the full-scale party some parents like to put on. By the preschool and kindergarten years, kids can handle theme parties that involve six to a dozen guests and feature clever decorations and full-meal refreshments, games with prizes, craft-making sessions, and even professional entertainers, such as clowns or magicians. Until then, though, keep parties small and short, and plan simple and noncompetitive activities. Balloons, favors to take home, and the traditional ice cream and cake will make as exciting a party as most toddlers are up to. Many excellent books on children's parties are available, and most have ideas that are suitable for toddlers and young preschoolers.

## Parental Expectations

Comparing your child's development with that of the children of your friends and neighbors is futile and unproductive. A common failing of parents is to exaggerate a bit as they try to show their children in the best light, and what you hear is not always the truth. The most glowing (and the most overstated) accounts of babies' accomplishments are likely to come from parents whose children are long past the stages about which they speak. You will hear that one friend's baby slept through the night at two weeks, another's walked at nine months and spoke complete sentences at eighteen months, and still another's was completely toilet trained at a year. If you worry that your child isn't living up to standards set by others, you will upset your own tranquility and find it impossible to enjoy and appreciate your baby. In addition, you'll be setting your child up for a life of low self-esteem and an endless struggle to meet your impossible expectations.

Even the most accurate and realistic of developmental schedules worked out by pediatricians and psychologists after their observations of thousands of children will not tell you exactly what your baby should be doing at any given period. These schedules are helpful if not taken too literally, *but they should be used only as guides,* to give you a general idea of what to expect from your child. Every baby develops at a different rate, and if yours is slow to roll over or build a tower of blocks, it doesn't mean he is less intelligent than your friend's or neighbor's child or than the "average" baby profiled on the development charts.

A child's maturity level may be more likely than his IQ to determine the rate of development. Some children simply mature more slowly than others; they're called "late bloomers," and often their accomplishments ultimately equal or surpass those of others. Some children develop at an average or above-average rate in one area, such as motor skills, and at a below-average rate in another, such as language. You may wish to take the sex of your child into consideration, too. In general, girls mature more quickly than boys. They usually walk earlier, talk sooner, show more early interest in "intellectual" skills, such as printing and drawing, and become toilet trained earlier.

Promise yourself from the beginning that you will respect and love your baby as a unique individual, different from any other, with his or her own beauty and charm. Constantly practice the art of accepting your child as is, without ranking or comparing him with others. Be aware that while the environment you provide is, of course, important, certain facets of a child's potential are genetically controlled. It will not be your fault if you do not rear a genius, nor will it be entirely to your credit if you do.

## Possible Causes for Developmental Problems

Some infants have inborn defects, such as brain damage and incomplete development of the brain, that prevent normal development. Others suffer from conditions or diseases that can be treated once they have been identified. One rare inherited metabolic disease, for which infants are almost always tested before they leave the hospital, is phenylketonuria (PKU). Untreated, the disease leads to mental retardation, but early detection and prompt treatment through diet usually assure development of average intelligence. Another test given newborns is for congenital hypothyroidism, which is also rare and also capable of causing retardation if untreated.

Infants born with some defects may not appear abnormal immediately, but most display marked delays in development that their parents observe or their doctors notice. At each checkup, the pediatrician will observe your child's behavior as a clue to development. She, or an assistant, may also do quick screening tests at certain ages in your child's life. In both the observation and the tests, the pediatrician is looking for possible danger signals.

Other infants, normal at birth, suffer later from incompetent or insufficient nurturing. Environmental problems are often more difficult for a pediatrician to identify than inborn defects, and they can pose serious hazards to a child's development. Some of the clues that alert the physician are these:

- Disturbances of eating or sleeping (either insufficient or excessive). Both the quantity and the quality of parental care influence an infant's own regulation of eating and sleeping.

- Physical symptoms, such as frequent vomiting, diarrhea, and skin rashes.

- Failure to grow normally in height and weight. An infant deprived of loving nurture may fail to grow in spite of adequate food intake. If a lack of nurturing can be ruled out, the pediatrician will investigate suppression of growth factors in the baby's brain.

- Marked delay or deviation in specific areas, such as motor development, verbal ability, intellectual development, and general learning, or in development of relationships to others, a sense of self, or the capacity to play.

Frequently, when the necessary nurturing ingredients are lacking, children develop various medical or psychological problems. For instance, if bonding does not occur between mother and infant, it is not unusual to find "failure to thrive" behavioral problems as well as a disturbed mother-child relationship. This does *not* mean there will automatically be trouble if the *ideal* bonding process does not take place immediately following birth. Recent studies have shown that mothers of cesarean-birth, premature, or adopted babies can successfully bond later.

Likewise, parents who are aware of their own imperfections and lack of knowledge need not worry that their baby's ability to develop will be automatically damaged. Babies have a strong drive toward normal development that helps them resist potentially damaging environmental factors. Clearly, the ability of infants to develop can be damaged in situations of poor care, but none of us is without flaws. We should do the very best we can for our children, but we need not be perfect in order to raise fine human beings.

Parents who are concerned about some aspect of their infant's or child's development or, later, about behavioral problems should turn first to their pediatrician. Sometimes one's inclination is to avoid "bothering" the doctor, and it is true that time is a precious commodity for a pediatrician. Still, if the doctor seems unwilling to discuss what the parents see as a problem, or refuses for some reason to become involved in the parents' worries, it would probably be wise to choose another pediatrician. If more than average time is required for an office visit to discuss behavioral problems, some pediatricians charge more, but you can count extra fees as money well spent if you are able to head off serious problems.

### Special Developmental Evaluations

Occasionally a child whose problems may be as specific as slow speech development or as general as overall slow development needs the attention of a *developmentalist,* a pediatrician whose subspecialty is early childhood development. Parents who suspect a developmental lag in either motor or cognitive development, or see signs that their baby is refusing to be socialized or is withdrawn and depressed, can ask for an evaluation by such a specialist, or their pediatrician may recommend it. The developmentalist, perhaps working with a team of other professionals, such as social workers and psychologists, observes the child performing various functions in a play-like situation to determine the existence and extent of developmental problems. Other specialists may be called in as consultants.

After an assessment, the developmentalist will discuss with the parents his findings and recom-

mendations for treatment. Unfortunately, some parents will learn that their fears of retardation have been confirmed. (See Chapter 8 for discussion of the physical aspects of retardation and disability.) Others will receive the relief of assurance that their child can develop normally, perhaps with special help. Whatever the outcome of the evaluation, parents should strive for a proper balance in their reactions. Hysterical overconcern will help neither their child nor themselves, and trying to insulate themselves against pain and hurt by noninvolvement is just as bad.

## Disabled Children

### Assessing Disability

All children can learn and develop. But children do not learn and develop in the same way or at the same rate. Sometimes parents will notice an overall pattern of slowness in a child's responses to the world around him. Parents may notice that the child's general physical growth and achievement seem to lag far behind those of other children.

Some children don't seem to develop normal sensory responses. Vision-impaired children, for instance, may not focus or follow with their eyes. A hearing-impaired child may not respond to sounds or may fail to speak or make pre-speech sounds, or she may babble later and less frequently than children with normal hearing.

When parents perceive a consistent pattern of delays, they will want their child evaluated by a professional. Part of that assessment will include an effort to determine possible causes of the problem or problems.

The causes cover a wide range of possibilities. Early in the development of the fetus, for example, a spontaneous change in the chromosomes or in individual genes may lead to Down syndrome, a disabling condition that causes affected children to develop and grow more slowly than normal children. Premature birth can sometimes lead to developmental difficulties in a child. Certain infections carried by the mother may affect the fetus in its early stages, and may lead to retardation and other abnormalities. A trauma suffered during birth or shortly before or after birth may adversely affect a child, and can lead to such conditions as cerebral palsy. Certain childhood illnesses, like encephalitis and meningitis, may also leave a child with mental or physical handicaps.

# LEARNING AND COGNITIVE DEVELOPMENT

It is not always possible to determine the cause of a disabling condition; some developmental delays are difficult to diagnose. An IQ (intelligence quotient) score below 69 indicates a child may be mentally retarded (90 to 109 is considered average). But the diagnosis of a handicap should not rest solely on an IQ test score. A child's adaptive behavior—his ability to respond to stimuli, to learn and grow—should also be measured. There are, however, no absolute tests that can tell us how quickly a handicapped child will move through developmental stages, or how much that child will eventually be able to accomplish.

## Stimulating Developmental Potential

From the moment they are born, children begin learning about the world around them. They learn through their movements and through their senses of taste, touch, smell, sight, and hearing. When one or more of these senses are impaired, the child's view of the world is altered, and her ability to learn from it changes. Yet with advances in medicine, technology, and our understanding of how babies grow and learn, we can frequently expect far greater physical and mental development from disabled children than was possible even a decade ago. How *much* development depends upon the extent of the handicap, how soon it is correctly diagnosed, and how quickly the child can be placed in an appropriately stimulating environment. Mentally handicapped children, for instance, need frequent and consistent stimulation because they often have difficulty in focusing their attention and remembering. They may also have perceptual difficulties that make it hard for them to understand what is happening around them and why it is happening.

In many cases, a child's abilities can be improved by stimulating the impaired sense. Children with muscular dystrophy, Down syndrome, and cerebral palsy often can benefit from a physical therapy program that exercises all their muscles. Exercising the legs and feet of children with severe cases of spina bifida prepares them for walking with braces and crutches. Children with hearing impairments can learn to use their residual hearing with the help of high-power hearing aids and auditory training that increases and expands their listening ability. Children with severe visual impairments can sharpen their other senses to help compensate for their lack of sight while they learn about their world. Children with Down syndrome and cerebral palsy may also benefit from vision, speech, and occupational therapies.

Stimulation programs geared for children from birth to age three have demonstrated that even children with severe disabilities can learn, grow, and participate in the world around them. Parents can lead many of the exercises in such programs themselves, but they will almost always benefit from the supervision of a trained therapist. Your local health department, public school, or state department of disabilities may have an appropriate infant stimulation program, or may be able to recommend a trained therapist who could visit your home on a regular basis to help your child and teach you appropriate exercises and play. University teaching hospitals and private agencies that serve handicapped children may also be good sources of information.

Play is an important way of learning for all children. Disabled children who can't move around to explore on their own can still learn about their neighborhoods through trips with the family. Within the home, children can be carried or guided from room to room to touch, feel, see, smell, or hear various objects. Vision-impaired children can use their hands, faces, feet, and other parts of their bodies to explore and learn. Hearing-impaired children need constant language stimulation and, like all children, need to hear explanations for what is happening around them. Pictures in books and magazines are another way of exposing sighted children to places, people, animals, and ways of life outside their immediate experience.

Toys provide another means of understanding our bodies and the world. Disabled children may have trouble playing with conventional toys, but parents can often adapt them to their child's needs or create appropriate play objects. Many communities have toy libraries (known as *Lekoteks*) that serve as resources by providing specially designed or selected toys for handicapped children.

## The Role of Parents

No two handicapped children—even those who have the same type of disability—are alike. Nor are their needs alike. But a handicapped child's primary need is the same as that of all children: the love and support of his parents. Sometimes parents become so absorbed in the need to stimulate their child and to compensate for his handicap that they forget that the most important task is to love him and to take pleasure in him as a human being. When a child sees that his parents enjoy being with him, his sense of self-worth is nourished. That growing sense of self-worth is an important measure of a parent's success with a handicapped child.

If you are the parent of a disabled child, your goals are to foster independence and to help your child develop a sense of self-worth and personal fulfillment. Through therapy and play, you are striving to help your child deal with his handicap while realizing his full potential. How much independence your child achieves will depend, to a great degree, not only on your child's handicap, but on how much you let your child do for himself at each stage.

All children reach plateaus in their development—times when they seem to stop moving forward, or when they may even take a step back. This can be a particularly difficult time for parents of handicapped children, who have to learn to measure the progress of their youngsters in inches rather than yards.

When your child reaches a plateau, it is helpful to look back and focus on how far he has progressed. This may also be a good time to focus on short-term rather than long-term goals—finger-feeding, getting dressed, repeating the first intelligible word or phrase, finally mastering toilet training. When parents focus all their energy on a single, short-term goal, a handicapped child may begin to move forward again. By stopping to observe how a handicapped child copes with such challenges, how he adapts to new and greater demands, parents can help themselves to develop realistic expectations for their child.

Children progress best when their parents function as advocates for them, choosing the most appropriate educational settings, setting reasonable goals, and providing a warm and nurturing environment. Parents should view themselves as partners with professionals in planning the care of their handicapped children.

## Choosing a Special Program

Many disabilities have national associations, like the March of Dimes for genetic disorders, that provide information and recommend programs or resources. Many of those associations have local chapters and parent-support groups. See page 266 for addresses and phone numbers of the March of Dimes and other national organizations.

If you are lucky enough to have a choice of programs, how do you choose the one that will be best for your child? Decisions should be based on how comfortable you are with the professionals in the available programs and with the therapies being presented. Some therapies, such as patterning (manipulation of head and limbs to prompt desired behavior) for brain-damaged and learning-disabled children, are less well known and not as widely available as other therapies. Frequently, educators will differ on the subject of learning sequence; some educators of the deaf, for instance, believe in introducing sign language to children almost immediately, while others believe children should have strictly auditory/oral training before any signs are introduced. Because the opinions and methods of professionals differ, be sure to investigate a number of programs before committing yourself and your child to a particular one. If you consider a private program with private therapists, remember that the cost of a program is not necessarily an indication of its quality or appropriateness.

While factors of cost and convenience will certainly influence your decision, parents should also consider other factors:

- How long will the program be able to serve your child?

- Is it a new program using experimental techniques, or an established program using therapies that are widely accepted?

- How well trained are the therapists who will work with your child?

- Who supervises the therapists' work?

- What does the therapist expect of you?

- Does she seem willing to share her expertise with you?

- Does she want you to understand her methods?

- Does she seem capable of establishing a good rapport with your child?

- If the program is new, will it continue to receive funding, or do sponsors need to raise funds each year?

- How many children are being served, and what is the ratio of staff to students?

- Are children with multiple handicaps combined in classrooms with children who have only one or two clearly defined disabilities?

Perhaps the most important factor in choosing a program is the expectations of the professionals involved. Each child is different and will bring to the program his own determination to succeed. Parents may see strength and recognize progress that professionals miss. If the professionals' expectations are too low, your child may not proceed as quickly as you feel appropriate. And if their expectations are too high, your child may feel frustrated.

## Your Relationship with the Professionals

Most professionals welcome and encourage active parental involvement in decisions affecting the child. However, professionals are human, with human emotions and responses. While it is safe to assume that most professionals who deal with handicapped children have an interest in seeing them well taken care of, professionals may bring to their work certain prejudices and preconceptions that do not serve the interests of all children. You will have your own opinions; express them. You should be able to talk openly with professionals about your concerns and questions. If the therapist is "too busy" for or is resistant to such discussions, or if you find such meetings unproductive and unsatisfying, you should consider finding a new program or therapist. While it is in the interest of the child to have continuity of care over the long run, it is best to change programs if you believe your child is not being adequately served.

## The Handicapped Child and the Educational System

As handicapped children move into the toddler stage, parents may wish to consider preschool or nursery school. Should you send your child to a special school where she will be with other children like herself, and where teachers are trained to deal with your child's handicap? Sometimes no special school exists, or it is very far away, requiring that your child make the lengthy trip to school each day or that she become a resident at the school.

Even when special schools are close, you may wish to consider "mainstreaming" your child—sending her to a regular nursery school class.

Many experts feel that young children with mild to moderate disabilities do better if they can be kept in a normal environment for as long as possible. Young children are usually more accepting of differences than older children and adults are, so a disabled child will not necessarily feel odd or left out in a normal nursery school. Many nursery schools are willing and able to accept children with mild to moderate handicaps. Some are willing to accept children with more severe handicaps.

Certain philosophies of education lend themselves more readily to integrating handicapped children. If you cannot find a school in your area that has had experience with handicapped children, you may wish to approach a Montessori school or other school with a nontraditional approach to nursery school education.

If you are considering mainstreaming in a school that has had little or no experience with your child's handicap, take time to observe and to talk to the director and the teachers who will have your child. Be honest about your child's deficiencies and her needs. Ask about the school's attitudes toward handicaps in general and toward your child's handicap in particular. How do teachers normally handle problems of discipline and teasing? How will they handle questions asked by other children about your child? Do you feel that their expectations are reasonable and consistent with your own for children in general and for your child in particular?

If you decide to mainstream your child, be prepared to serve as a resource person for the school. You may want to talk to the children about how a hearing aid works, about why your child wears braces, or why she looks or talks the way she does. Be prepared for some frustration, especially in the beginning, as parents and other students work to understand your child and how to relate to her. Plan to observe school routine fairly often. If your presence upsets your child's routine, enlist the aid of friends to observe. When you observe, don't focus solely on your child. Parents of handicapped children are frequently—and pleasantly—surprised when they observe how much like other children their child is.

## Your Rights Under the Law

The Education for All Handicapped Children Act (Public Law 94-142) went into effect in 1978. The law requires states to provide a free, appropriate education to all handicapped children regardless of the severity of their disability. Under the law, each child has an individualized education program (IEP) that indicates what kinds of special education and related services the child will receive. Parents have the right to participate in every decision related to the education of their child, and parents have the right to challenge and appeal any decision regarding the identification, evaluation, or placement of their child.

P.L. 94-142 covers handicapped children from ages three to twenty-one, except in states where public education is not provided for children under five and over eighteen. However, you may find many local school districts that provide programs for children under three even when they are not required to by state law. Many of those programs receive federal funding.

While the law has tried to provide for the education of most handicapped children, it has not standardized the *quality* of education, which can vary widely from state to state and from one school district to another. Even within school districts, certain handicaps are better served than others. Further, government budget cutbacks have had particular impact on educational programs, many of which have been truncated or eliminated altogether. Be aware that your best-choice program may not be available in your area. Many school districts provide information on what is available, as well as guidelines for parents that describe their children's educational rights. If your local district cannot readily provide you with information and a copy of applicable laws, contact your state board of education.

# Bright and Gifted Children

It used to be said that if the membrane enveloping the head of a fetus remained intact through a delivery, the baby was born wearing a "caul," and would be lucky, or gifted, or both. Now we know that is only a superstition.

We have also found that it is difficult to determine precocity of mental development in a child by any means at all, and it is particularly difficult to assess in very small children. Educators recognize two kinds of giftedness, intellectual and creative, and programs for gifted children today are labeled "for the gifted and talented." Intellectually gifted individuals are logical thinkers, capable of heavy inner concentration, and they have IQs of 130 or higher. Creatively gifted people are

imaginative, adaptable, and likely to be involved in artistic pursuits; they have IQs of at least 120.

Bright and healthy children from stimulating environments often show signs of falling into one of these classifications. They are typically very inquisitive about the world around them, often creative with words as they learn to talk and with their toys as they play. Some especially love books and teach themselves to read long before they are old enough to go to school. They're eager to learn, and many show early indications of special interest in and talent for music, art, drama, and dancing. The world of fantasy appeals strongly to some, who use their imaginations creatively.

## Assessment for Gifted Children

If you are the parent of a child who may be gifted, you are probably delighted—we all like to think of our children as well above average—and at the same time worried. You may feel as if you are caught in a bind between pushing too hard and providing enough stimulation to challenge your bright child. Formal assessment is the most reliable means of determining whether a child's development puts her into the official "gifted and talented" classification. A child who can read at three or four is considered ready for testing, but parents should be aware that an assessment at this early age will probably not be as accurate as one made later.

Assessment should be performed by an individual or service experienced with young children as well as with appropriate tests and methods of interpretation. It involves the use of certain standardized tests that measure ability levels and skill development, but almost never the use of intelligence tests, because of the instability of IQ at young ages. The results of the assessment give indications of which areas of learning a child may begin to master at an early age and of the child's appropriate reading level. Once the results are known, options such as early entrance to school and enrollment in special programs can be considered. Parents who are interested in having assessments made may be able to work through their pediatricians or through social agencies or gifted programs. One such program is The Johns Hopkins University Center for the Advancement of Academically Talented Youth, 34th and Charles Streets, Baltimore, MD 21218.

Many gifted and talented children do not read before they go to school; early reading is not the only criterion for exceptional mental or creative ability. If you are interested in having an assessment made of your child, and he or she cannot yet read, it is a good idea to accumulate informative evidence by keeping a written record of your observations of your child's advanced behavior. Use examples, and note such things as these:

- Early talking, with adult-like vocabulary, and unusually clever or perceptive questions or observations

- An excellent memory

- Special ability in drawing or other artwork

- Ability to concentrate on an activity for a long period of time

Educators also suggest that you continue to encourage your child's natural inquisitiveness into the whys and hows of things, without pushing or forcing. Offer whatever enriching experiences you can, particularly those that your child enjoys. Take advantage of local opportunities in libraries, children's museums, and such. Try to find another parent or two willing to join you, and share your knowledge and enthusiasm as you take your children on suitable "field trips" together. Look around your neighborhood for opportunities: a construction site, where trucks, machinery, and building materials can be seen; your local fire station, where personnel will probably be willing to arrange a real tour if you call ahead; a bus trip across town, which can be an exciting experience for a child who usually is taken places in a car. Learning experiences are available almost everywhere you go with your child.

Do remember that the most gifted of children are children first, gifted second. However easy it may be to treat your child as you would one much older, she is undoubtedly immature in some ways. While your bright child of three may have the cognitive ability of a child of five, for example, she may also have the bodily coordination or the emotional and social development, or both, of a child of only two and a half. All children, whatever their potentials and capabilities, are in need of the love, attention, and guidance of parents who do not try to make miniature adults of them.

## Early Learning Programs

Should you follow one of the various programs available today that urge parents to help their children's mental development by teaching them to read, do math, and learn foreign languages while they are still babies? Some eye specialists have warned that visual skills needed for working with print do not fully evolve until a child is about six years old, and that such early activity may heighten the possibility of vision problems. Other experts do not see a link between early reading and vision difficulties.

The controversy may never be definitely resolved. Most educators say imaginative play is far more important than academic learning for any preschool-age child. Programs designed to "educate" your child or raise his IQ will probably do no real harm to a child who is only bored and confused by them or to one who seems to enjoy them, but they probably will not do a great deal of good, either. Much research suggests that most children read at age six or seven, when real lessons are started.

Pioneer researcher Arnold Gesell recommended that as much flexibility be used in matters of academic readiness as in those of walking readiness. The conviction that it was actually harmful for children to learn to read before they went to school is outdated now, and there are children who, in effect, teach themselves the skill. This is a heady, delightful boost to a child's ego, an accomplishment as great as were the first independent steps taken. If your child is full of questions about numbers and letters, by all means answer them. Give the child as much information as she wants, but do not waste time for either of you in formal schoolroom lessons.

What you *can* do is help any child—gifted or average—to learn to think and to remember, both skills that he will need. Give your toddler practice in comparing and classifying by sorting laundry, arranging a collection of pretty stones picked up on walks first by size and then by color, and stacking pans in the cupboard. Ask your preschooler to conjecture about things. For example, why is the dog across the street limping? Are the children in the picture happy or sad? Ask the child for his reasons or observations. Is a rejected food too soft, too crisp, too sour, too sweet? Why does it seem as if it will rain today?

Your toddler won't be able to remember what you say will happen a week from Tuesday, but what's coming after naptime will present no problems. Stretch out the time lag, a little at a time. He won't remember a series of instructions, but will be able to handle two commands, such as, "Pick up your book and put it on the shelf." Give three commands next time.

## The Question of Preschool

Another question about early education often bothers parents of toddlers: Is nursery school or preschool necessary, advisable, or even good for very young children? Some parents don't consider it; their children have plenty of time ahead for school, they say. Others feel that the social experience is important for their children and that learning to do such things as form a line, sit still for a period of time, and pay attention to a teacher gives a child a good start in regular school. Working parents often choose the preschool experience for their children instead of babysitters or ordinary day care for a variety of reasons, ranging from convenience and expense to the conviction that the experience is valuable. Some researchers have said that it is not until age three that children have the minimum level of socialization necessary for successful experiences in any kind of school. It is at that age that they begin to relate to other children as helpmates in carrying out such activities as building and destroying, playing, and getting into mischief.

In choosing any nursery school or preschool, it is important first to decide just what it is you want from the facility and what you think will most benefit your child. Is it simply the opportunity for socialization with other children? Preparation for academic education? An atmosphere that concentrates on imaginative and creative activities? Ask yourself, too, if your child will be more apt to thrive in a school where the program is very structured or in one where the children are given some leeway in choosing their activities. Your child's personality will be a major factor in your decision.

Visit any school alone at least once, so you can talk with staff members and observe them closely as they interact with the children. Stay for several hours, so you can see how the program works. If the school is a large one, find out how the children are split up (strictly by age or in groups of all ages) and into what size groups. Determine the teacher-child ratio and question the director or teachers about the school's policies and theories of discipline. Ask what is served for snacks or meals. Watch to see how staff members handle the inevitable conflicts between children. Look carefully at the school's facilities. Is play equipment safe and in good condition and is there enough of it for the number of children enrolled? Are the toys and art supplies adequate and of the kinds your child likes?

When you have found the school you think best, take your child to visit. If you have decided he will definitely be attending, do not ask questions that give an opportunity to say no; make them open-ended, for example, "What area of the big playroom do you think you'll like best?" rather than "Do you want to go there every day?" Be prepared to be put on a waiting list. When your child starts attending, try to keep your home environment very stable. The first weeks are not good ones for you to move, start a new job, or make other big changes in your family life.

## Stimulating Your Child's Mind and Curiosity

In their efforts to supply the best for their children, parents sometimes buy many toys and learning devices proclaimed by their promoters to aid the development of a multitude of skills. But the most creative, colorful, and expensive of these will be helpful to a child only if her basic needs for food, warmth, and nurture are being supplied by a loving adult. The skill development that toys encourage is only a part of the total picture; children must develop as total human beings—body, mind, and spirit. Your child will sense your values by the quantity and quality of time you devote to her and by your attitudes toward imaginative play, reading, and music. Your interaction with your child is more important than *things*.

According to the American Academy of Pediatrics' Committee on the Infant and Preschool Child, parents may be wasting money if they buy educational toys with the specific intention of increasing a child's IQ. Similarly, learning devices do little to advance social behavior. Developing a few deep relationships with people will do more to advance your child's social skills than will any object you can buy.

Granted, toys are important. All play is learning, and your child's toys are her tools. The best way to use toys is to be aware of their limitations—aware that while they may enhance development, they can never substitute for contact with the parent. You yourself are your newborn's first, best, and most amusing learning device—you have an expressive face with changing expressions and moving eyes; you make sounds your baby likes; you have ten fascinating fingers to grasp and hold and pull.

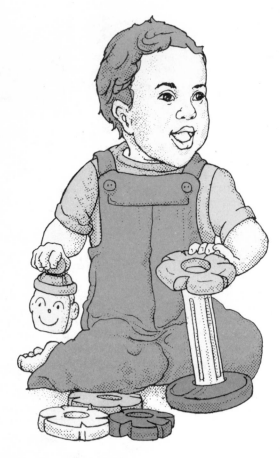

*Well-chosen toys will entertain your baby and stimulate his development.*

Many of the best toys are homemade; others are household articles in general daily use. For example, a child under a year old will love and learn from dozens of perfectly safe things in your kitchen: measuring spoons, nesting plastic bowls or cups, and pans and kettles. When the baby is mobile, store some of these entertaining supplies in a lower cupboard where she can get at them without your help. For several minutes' amusement any time, put a new four-inch rubber ball onto the high-chair tray. Don't throw away any clean, sturdy box, including cylindrical oatmeal boxes and those that hold the store-bought toys and that are often more interesting to your baby than their contents.

A little later, give your toddler a wooden or plastic bowl, plastic measuring cups, kitchen utensils such as your flour sifter and colander, and old magazines to tear up. Water play is endlessly fascinating, and the best bathtub toys are often plastic bowls and cups to measure with and pour

from. You'll find that your child of two or three will often enjoy the real things more than the expensive and often less sturdy "play" ones: a disconnected telephone, a padlock, a magnet, a plastic magnifying glass, a flashlight (securely taped so the child can't unscrew the ends), a plastic lunchbox, and a box full of dress-up hats and shoes and empty handbags from the back of your closet or from thrift shops or garage sales.

## Choosing Toys

Your shopping preferences, your budget, and the amount of time you have to spend will determine where you buy toys—in exclusive toy stores, gift shops, or children's shops; from catalogs that come in the mail; in department stores, supermarkets, drugstores, or discount outlets. One of your first considerations may be price. "You get what you pay for" is true of some things, but it's not necessarily a good guide in buying toys. You may pay a high price for a big name or to follow a fad, when something that costs considerably less would be just as good and would give your child as much satisfaction. Or you may buy something that's well made and worth the price, but that your child will never play with. One way to look at the real value of toys is to consider the amount of pleasure they give in comparison to their cost. For example, it's worthwhile to pay a substantial price for a teddy bear that will be dragged around the house and slept with every night for several years. But the cute jack-in-the-box that breaks after a few minutes of play is a bad buy at any price.

There are other things to consider besides cost. One is fun; your child should *like* the toy you buy. Every child should have access to certain classic kinds of toys: things to build with, things to love and cuddle, things to work with and operate. But a child's preferences, which will start to show up early and continue to grow and change, should also be considered. One baby will like balls better than another; one will like soft dolls best of all; one will turn again and again to the mirror fastened inside the crib. On the basis of those preferences, you may sometimes buy a fad toy that you suspect is overpriced, simply because your child wants it and you like it.

Ask yourself a few questions when you're selecting a toy: Will you have to supervise the use of the one you're considering? If you have to teach your child to use it, are you willing or able to find the time? Is the toy so fragile or so expensive or so noisy that you will curtail your child's use of it? Does the toy suit your family's lifestyle (farm or city, big house or small apartment)? Do you have storage space for the toy? Does the toy promote sex stereotyping?

A very important question is whether the toy is appropriate for your child's age. Manufacturers give suggested ages, but you must use your own judgment, too, and your knowledge of your child's ability to manipulate, maneuver, and solve problems. The age range given is often so wide that you will be tempted to buy a toy too soon. Remember that you want to challenge and intrigue your child, not frustrate and anger her. A toy that requires the skill and experience of a two-year-old will be wasted on your one-year-old and will probably never be used at all.

Above all, toys must be safe. First, be sure that what you buy *is* a toy. Some ornaments and decorations, however colorful and attractive, are not meant to be used as toys and are not manufactured in accordance with standards for toys. Do not assume that every toy you see is safe, however reputable the store that stocks it. Every year the U.S. Consumer Product Safety Commission (CPSC) directs the recall of many kinds of toys that can't take the "normal use and abuse" young children are expected to give them. Watch for notices of these CPSC recall directions in magazines and newspapers, inspect toys carefully before you buy them, and check them often as your child plays with them.

Your child's toys should be nonflammable, nonbreakable (remember that brittle plastic may break as easily as glass), and nontoxic, of course. They should be washable and should have no sharp edges, no splinters or nails sticking out, no traps in which small fingers can get caught, no pins or buttons that can be pulled off. Infant toys should not be small enough to be swallowed, and they should not have detachable parts that could find their way into your baby's windpipe, nose, or ears. No infant toy should have a cord longer than twelve inches that could become wrapped around the baby's neck. If you have older children, it's important to be aware that many of their toys may be dangerous for a baby or smaller child.

To list and evaluate every kind of toy available for babies and toddlers is impossible. We try here to discuss the classic groups of toys that all children enjoy. Many can be homemade, some can be shared by two children close in age, and some can be passed down from one child to another.

However, children often become so attached to some things, such as dolls and books, that they can never let them go. Some of the toys listed here for babies will be the start of collections that will be added to with more sophisticated or complicated items over the years. Books and musical toys will be discussed in the next two sections of this chapter.

*Toys for Babies (Birth to Twelve Months)*
Your baby's very first toys should be those that will awaken and sharpen his senses of sight, hearing, and touch. Bright colors, melodic and appealing sounds, and interesting and varied textures are what you look for. The youngest infants are fascinated by moving objects and are eager to touch, hold, and manipulate. Between three and six months of age, your baby will be able to grasp objects. By six months, he will enjoy putting one thing inside another, banging and hitting objects, exploring them, and opening and closing doors and drawers. Do remember that during the first year, and often for some time after that, babies tend to put *everything* in their mouths.

*Rattles* will probably be your baby's first gifts. They range from sterling silver keepsake models to those made of plastic.

*Stuffed animals* and *soft dolls* are also among a baby's first toys, and they remain favorite gifts for many years. Your baby's first ones should be brightly colored, lightweight, and small enough that he can hold and cuddle them.

*Mobiles*, some of which are musical, are excellent for developing your baby's attention to specific objects and his ability to track things visually. Attach them to the crib or playpen or hang them from the ceiling.

*Mirrors* delight all babies. Safely constructed of unbreakable, polished stainless steel, they come in hand-held models to shake and rattle and in large sizes to attach to the inside of the crib or playpen.

*Balls* of every description are among the best toys for babies. Try to have some of different textures—soft, rough, fluffy, smooth. Some are of cloth, with "grips" for little hands; some are of heavy plastic, weighted, and embedded with chimes or figures.

*Activity boxes* are usually made of plastic and can be mounted on crib or playpen sides or nailed to the wall. They usually include a mirror to look at, wheels and dials to turn, buttons to push, doors to slide open, and objects to slide along built-in tracks. Manufacturers often recommend activity boxes for infants three months and older, but until your baby can sit up well, chances are a box won't be much fun.

*Toys for Toddlers (Twelve to Twenty-four Months)*

By one year of age, your child's large motor skills are developing rapidly, and progress in eye-hand coordination is noticeable. Toddlers are interested in moving objects, and toys to pull and push, especially those that make sounds as they move, are often favorites. Your toddler will also enjoy opening and closing, putting in and taking out, and playing peek-a-boo.

*Blocks* are ideal toys, all-time classics, because they are toys that can be used in more than one way and that can be adapted for use by children of different ages. Blocks for your toddler should be good-sized, with rounded edges and corners. Start with just a few made of cloth, foam or foam-filled vinyl, or molded plastic. As your child gets older, add to the block collection, including all the variations on this classic toy that appeal to you and your child.

*Sorting toys* help your child learn colors and develop manual dexterity. The most popular of these consist of four or more colorful rings in varying sizes that stack on a cone set into a solid or rocking base. The ones in which the rings will fit on the cone only in decreasing order of size are best saved for older toddlers.

*Shape-recognition toys* are suitable for toddlers closer to two than one. They are composed of bright wooden or plastic cubes or other geometric shapes that the child drops through matching holes into a box or other holder. These toys will help your child develop eye-hand coordination, matching skills, and shape recognition. They provide challenging learning activities, but if too many pieces are involved, a child may become frustrated.

*Riding toys* are for children who can walk by themselves. A child should be able to climb on and off without difficulty and should be able to maneuver the toy capably. Look for sturdiness, ease of movement, and secure seating. Your child's first riding toy won't have pedals, and it may come in molded plastic or wood in the shape of a horse or other animal, a wagon, or a car or truck.

*Push/pull toys* will be among your child's favorites when he can walk independently because of their movement and noise-making characteristics. Be sure the handles are covered with large safety balls. Your child can load wagons or trucks with other toys, and some come equipped with block sets. More elaborate push/pull toys for older toddlers are called *action toys*. Favorites are such things as school buses and airplanes outfitted with small wooden passengers that fit into color-coded seats. Younger toddlers will need to be supervised—or you may want to keep small "people" put away until your child is beyond the mouthing stage.

*Pounding toys* are benches with pegs or balls to pound through holes. Some are large enough that your child will be able to sit on them as he develops eye-hand coordination and both gross and fine motor skills. Wooden hammers present safety hazards for a child whose pounding action is still uncoordinated, and they can be dangerous when two or more children are present, so this is not a toy you want to buy too early unless you're willing to supervise its use.

*Dolls* are a good example of toys that have moved out of the era of sex stereotyping as the needs of boys, as well as girls, to cuddle and love have been recognized. Boy and girl *dressing dolls* are outfitted in special clothes that offer practice in the skills of zipping, buttoning, snapping, and tying.

*Toys for Children From Two to Three Years*

Your child's imaginative play skills are beginning to develop at this age, and you may often hear him talking with a toy or with an imaginary companion. Using adult-like tools and appliances to imitate grown-ups will be appealing; the more realistic the toy, the more apt it is to stimulate the creative play skills developing at this stage.

Other favorites will be large-size riding toys with pedals, and toys and equipment that call for throwing, jumping, climbing, and running actions, which strengthen the large muscles. Your child will be able to concentrate on a quiet task and will find the small-muscle activities required in painting, doing puzzles, and using interlocking block sets enjoyable because of his increasingly improved eye-hand coordination.

*Talking toys and dolls* have a great appeal for children from two to three and over. Talking boxes describe a picture to which a pointer is directed, and talking dolls repeat short, clever phrases. The strings on most talking toys must be pulled out all the way if a child is to hear the entire message, but most children don't seem to mind if they don't get it all. When buying a talking toy, it is important to make sure the phrases are distinctly spoken and clearly enunciated.

*Trucks* are especially good for outdoor play in sand. Those that have movable parts, such as dump trucks, fire trucks, and cement mixers, are favorites. Be sure that metal trucks do not have sharp edges and that they are rustproof. They should be easy to operate, so your child won't become frustrated. Check trucks for stability, easy maneuverability, and securely attached wheels.

*Trains* may be of the push or the wind-up variety. Some trains that can be independently operated by a child must first have tracks assembled by an adult. A child should be able to easily place the train's cars on the track. In wind-up models, the winding mechanism must be easy to operate, and the train must move smoothly along the track without getting stuck.

*Kitchen equipment* is favored by both boys and girls. Durability is an important feature, and compactness may be a consideration for storage. Some appliances come separately; some are attached in models that include stove, sink, and refrigerator, all with intriguing details. The most expensive separate appliances are of molded plastic and very realistic, with doors that open and knobs that turn and click. Accessories may be included. At least some assembly by adults is required on most sets and single appliances.

*Realistic tools and toys* help children imitate adults. In selecting tools, which range from play drills and saws to complete tool chests, look for safety, durability, and manageability. Some tools can be made to "run" by pulling a cord and pushing a starter button, and some make realistic vibrating noises. Check stability and maneuverability in toys like baby strollers, shopping baskets, and wheelbarrows. Metal toys should be rustproof, and wheels should roll easily. Among other popular realistic toys are telephones, both talking and nontalking. Talking phones are battery-operated, and some have viewing screens on which characters are seen as they speak. Dashboards, reminiscent of the activity boxes babies love, are also popular. They may include such features as steering wheels with horns, clocks, windshield wipers, ignition keys, rearview mirrors, glove compartments, gear selectors, and speedometers.

*Puzzles* strengthen and enhance a child's eye-hand coordination, matching skills, and shape recognition. Be careful to match the intricacy of a puzzle with a child's development; a puzzle with too many pieces frustrates a child and discourages future attempts. Good first puzzles are sturdy, of plastic or wood, and have only a very few large pieces, sometimes with small plastic knobs attached to each.

*Play scenes* provide children with opportunities to use their imaginations. Available in addition to regular dollhouses are such settings as garages, farms, and nursery schools. Accessories include family figures, cars, furniture, animals, and play equipment. The more familiar a child is with a particular setting, the more appealing it is. Play scenes should be easy to assemble, provide storage for their own individual pieces and have moving features. The structure should be sturdy, and the number of pieces should not overwhelm the child.

*Quiet-play toys* encourage children close to three to concentrate as they develop motor and manipulatory skills. Children of this age can understand and enjoy simple games and can use fairly complicated realistic toys. Some toys for this age group help children understand money, tell time, or count. They should be challenging enough to maintain interest, but not so difficult as to be frustrating. If a toy seems beyond your child's capability, put it away for a while and try it again later. Some quiet-play toys are interlocking blocks, play boards with adherent plastic or felt pieces, cameras, realistic household toys, puzzles, play scenes, and simple games that can be played alone. Now is the time for a variety of art materials, too: washable colored markers, crayons, paper, and finger paints. Artwork will require your supervision at first, but it is an important and necessary part of your child's development. Art fosters imagination and encourages creativity.

## Reading to Your Child

Besides providing hours of enjoyment and a storehouse of knowledge and memories that will last a lifetime, reading will help your child develop four basic thinking skills: the ability to pay attention, a good memory, capability in problem solving, and proficiency in language. The single best way you can encourage your child to love books and reading is to read aloud to her. You can't start too early; you can't continue too long. Reading experts recommend that you start reading to your

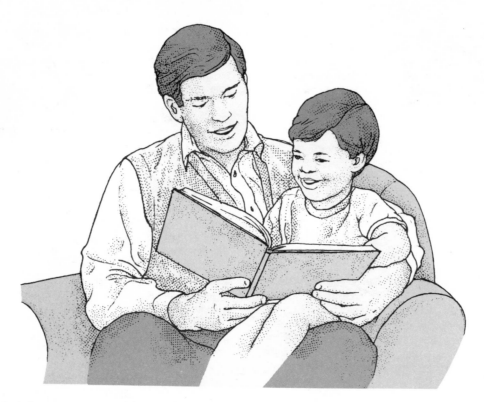

*By reading regularly to your child, you will aid the development of his reading skills, and cultivate his love of books.*

child at birth and continue into the teenage years, perhaps in family sessions. Your infant will not understand the words you read, and indeed, you need not even read children's stories. A parenting book, the daily newspaper, or a new novel will be equally enchanting to your baby, who loves the sound of your voice and the concentration of your attention. If you love poetry, read it to your infant and continue to read it as the child grows. Many children love the rhythm and cadence of adult poetry long before they can understand it.

A half hour a day is a reasonable amount of time to spend reading to your child, probably divided into a few short sessions for a small child. Any time of day is good for reading. Most parents like to make it part of the bedtime ritual; it's a way to help a child relax and get ready for sleep. Morning, at the breakfast table, is another favorite time for many parents and children. The main thing is to take the time for reading and to skip a day for only the most important of reasons.

## Choosing Books

There are thousands of children's books on the market. Many of the best children's books have been around for years. With so many books on the market, it makes sense that only the best ones survive over time. One way to sort through them is to ask your local children's librarian for suggestions and get the name of the local retailer who has the best selection of children's books. If you're fortunate enough to have access to a university library that has a noncirculating children's collection, you'll be able to read the latest and most popular children's books before you buy them. Though your local library will have these, they will often be circulating and unavailable.

Your child's first books should be short, simple picture books, brightly illustrated. They should be small enough for a baby to handle, and toughly constructed of cloth or cardboard, because they will be chewed and pulled apart and thrown. Your child will be two or over before she begins to take care of books; until then they will be treated as toys, so you may want to buy inexpensive editions of most. Be sure the books you buy for even the youngest child are well written, not artificial sounding, and well illustrated. Otherwise, they will bore you, and your child will catch your feeling.

It will be at the age of about two years that your child begins really to appreciate books. Besides beginning to take good care of them, she will have figured out how they "work"—from front to back, from left to right—and will have learned to turn the pages one at a time. Your toddler will have memorized some stories and nursery rhymes, and will be able to recite surprisingly long sections or whole verses and to "read" along with you. You will be required to read the same book over and over and over, and you will be caught if you don't do it justice every time or if you skip a word or change a name. Comfort yourself with the knowledge that you are fulfilling a necessary function in your child's development: experts say that repetition is a stimulator of interest and important to the process whereby brain cells make connections.

Between the ages of two and three, stories that involve some kind of confrontation are popular, such as "The Three Billy Goats Gruff." At this age, children also like stories about holidays and seasons because this helps them understand family traditions.

One way to stimulate your child's interest in reading and to supplement the reading material you have on hand is to tell her your own stories. A story can be as long or as short as the time you have to tell it in, and it can be especially tailored to your child. It can be about a toy or the family pet, a picnic or a walk in the woods, a little boy or girl just like yours with a parent just like you. Whatever the topic, make your story lively; have something happen right in the beginning, and keep things moving. Don't be afraid to use some words your child doesn't understand because hearing new words is the way vocabularies are expanded. It's fine to have your main character struggle against fierce odds, but be sure to give your story a happy ending. Fairness must prevail; the good must win, and the bad must lose.

## Books From the Library

Your child will probably own ten or more books of his own by age two, and it is at about this time that you will need to begin supplementing the supply with books from the library. At first you may find it easiest and best to visit the library alone, since you'll be able to take your time in selecting the books that best suit your child's interests and level of understanding. But sometimes take your child with you; the weekly or biweekly library habit is one you want to start early and encourage forever. You'll want to continue to choose some of the books you'll be reading, but let your child pick

some out, too, even if they don't seem appropriate to you.

Unfortunately, not all libraries allow children under school age to have library cards; if yours does, help your child sign up for his own—having one's own library card is a sure sign of growing up. Check into other privileges and services the children's department of your library offers. At toddler "story periods" of a half hour or so, to which a parent accompanies each child, librarians sometimes read very short stories and lead the children in finger plays and action singing games. Regular story hours and other programs are often available for children of two and a half or three.

## Selecting the "Best" Books for Your Child

You'll want your child to be exposed to a variety of books, but you will notice before long that she is developing definite preferences. One child likes exciting stories with true-to-life characters, another loves anything silly, and still another prefers fantasy. Of course, tastes change, as a child is exposed to different kinds of books and to different experiences in daily life. For example, your three-year-old, who understands perfectly the difference between being naughty and behaving well, will enjoy books about mischievous children for a while. If you're expecting a new baby, your toddler or preschooler will want to see a lot of books about how babies are born and what it's like to have a little brother or sister.

Your librarian and the clerks in bookstores will lead you to the books all children should know. Some will be brand-new, some relatively new, and some so old that your own parents knew them as children. Among the latter, and probably some of your own favorites, will be the classic fairy tales—beautifully illustrated stories about unforgettable characters like the wicked witch who tries to cook the children and the dragons that threatened the castle. Some parents feel fairy tales are too violent for children at any age, but librarians and reading experts recommend them for children six or over who can understand the difference between reality and fantasy.

No periodicals especially for children three and under are available, but the adult magazines and catalogs that come into your home will be interesting. Look through them with your child, pointing out pictures of babies, grandparents, animals, foods, and toys. With those pictures, you can make up scrapbooks that your child will cherish, and when the child is about three, she can help you with the cutting and pasting.

---

### Reading "Don'ts"

- Don't continue to read a book once it is obvious your child doesn't like it.

- Don't use reading as a reward or punishment. It should be something that's done every day, whether your child has been an angel or something less.

- Don't start reading a long book when you know you won't have time to do it justice. Every book deserves to be given a good reading, and children aren't ready for continued stories until they are four or five.

- Don't feel your child must sit quietly beside you or in your lap while you read. An active child may be able to listen better while she colors or strings beads.

---

## The World of Music

Early development specialists believe that the youngest of babies should be exposed to music, and not only lullabies and children's songs. It has been well established that fetuses can hear, and some have said that infants have shown definite signs of recognizing music that their mothers heard before giving birth. A French obstetrician, interested in knowing just what an unborn baby hears, inserted a hydrophone (an instrument for listening to sound transmitted through water) into the uterus of a woman about to give birth and tape-recorded the sounds. Besides the mother's heartbeat and the whooshing sounds of the womb, the voices of the mother and her doctor and the strains of a Beethoven symphony were clearly heard in the background.

As children exposed to books can be counted upon to grow up loving reading, those exposed to music will almost surely appreciate it all their lives. Many of your infant's favorite toys will probably be musical, and he will enjoy whatever music you listen to on the radio or stereo, the music you play yourself on any instrument, and the humming, whistling, and singing with which you accompany your work.

At about one year, your baby will try to accompany the music you provide by clapping his hands and bouncing to the beat. By two, he will enjoy going to outdoor concerts with you. Provide short pieces of music that your child will listen to from start to finish sometimes. Use soothing chamber music at night to induce sleep and patriotic songs and marches to get the morning routine under way. Try folk songs and some of the music of other cultures. Try to give your child the best of whatever kind of music you select by shopping carefully.

Unfortunately, many of the best records are rarely available at local record and department stores. If your favorite stores do not stock a good selection of children's records, you may be able to borrow them from your library. Also, there are a number of mail-order catalog companies that carry children's records, including the following:

- Better Books Company
  P. O. Box 9770
  Fort Worth, TX 76107-0770
  (books, cassette read-alongs, video)

- Listening Library
  P. O. Box L
  Old Greenwich, CT 06870
  (cassettes, LP's, and films, many with manuals)

- Clarus Music, Ltd.
  340 Bellevue Avenue
  Yonkers, NY 10703
  (records, cassettes, preschool materials)

- Children's Book & Music Center
  2500 Santa Monica Boulevard
  Santa Monica, CA 90404
  (educational materials, LP's, cassettes, videos, rhythm instruments)

Toddlers enjoy folk songs, music from other cultures, records that call for activities like exercises and play-acting, and stories read aloud. Some records come with accompanying storybooks.

Children enjoy nothing more than making their own music, especially if it involves making up a band and parading around the house or the yard with another child or two. You can buy toys that make sounds, such as a toy piano or a children's guitar, but simple, real instruments are better. Some very suitable for toddlers are bongo drums and tom-toms, marimbas, cymbals, triangles, bells, and tambourines.

## Creative Play

Your child is being creative when she shakes a tambourine or bangs a drum to the beat of the dishwasher or makes something where nothing was before—a drawing, a finger painting, a clay animal. Creative imagination is also at work when she puts on your old shoes and plays house, insists that you set a place for an imaginary friend at the dinner table, tells you a tall tale about how the milk really got spilled, or begs you to get rid of the monsters that inhabit the bedroom closet.

Nurturing your child's creative abilities involves a bit of a paradox. You need to let go a little, to back off and leave artistic and inventive decisions up to her. However, you can trigger imagination by asking thought-provoking questions concerning the whys, hows, and whats of things. It's very important that you be available to provide reassurance when things don't go right and praise for trying, as well as for completion.

Some concrete help is required. For example, it's your job to offer your child experiences from which to take off in creative ventures. Without having seen and heard and participated in many of the wonders of the world, she does not have a base upon which to build or play. Offering these experiences does not mean a tour of Europe; it means, for example, long and careful looks at everyday things and places and people, picnics in the park, and visits to woods and streams.

Sometimes actual instruction is called for. You will need to teach your child how to use the art materials you supply; your suggestions will be helpful in first efforts at drawing and painting, and your supervision will definitely be required in many situations. Art supplies are fun to buy, and you may be surprised at the number of them that even a baby can handle and enjoy. Before the age of one, your child will love to scribble on a big piece of paper with a fat graphite pencil. He can move up soon to colored pencils, jumbo crayons, chalk, and, by age two, water-based felt-tip pens.

When your child is ready to paint, probably at about two, think first of protection—one of your old shirts to cover the child and newspaper sheets or a special mat to cover the floor. A two-year-old can help you make finger paint a few times, then do it alone. Mix a quarter cup of liquid laundry starch with two drops of food coloring or one teaspoon of tempera paint powder. For easel painting, poster paints are the smoothest flowing and most satisfying for a small child.

Paper for drawing and painting can become expensive in the quantities some eager artists require. Consider using the closely printed want-ad pages of the newspaper, plain newsprint (which you may be able to buy from the newspaper office or art supply store in a roll), shelf paper, and the white insides of cut-open disposable-diaper boxes. Beginning painters sometimes do better with pastry brushes or trim-painting brushes from a paint store; they hold more paint and are easy to handle.

From the age of two, your child will love to pound, roll, and flatten whatever kind of clay you supply, as her sense of touch develops. The most practical first clay is a plasticized variety you can buy or a flour or baking soda and cornstarch clay you make yourself.

---

**Flour Clay**

4 cups flour                 food coloring
1 1/2 cups salt
2 cups water

Add water *slowly.* Knead ten minutes (coat your hands with vegetable oil to protect them from the salt). Separate into batches and add food coloring to each batch. Refrigerate in airtight containers between uses. Oil your children's hands every time they use the clay. When dried for twenty-four hours, flour clay sculptures can be painted.

**Baking Soda and Cornstarch Clay**

2 cups baking soda         food coloring
1 cup cornstarch
1 1/4 cups cold water

Add water slowly. Cook six minutes (medium heat, stirring constantly). Spread on a cookie sheet to cool, covering with a damp cloth to keep clay moist. Knead ten minutes. Divide into small batches and add food coloring. Store in airtight containers.

---

*Coloring books*
Should you let your child use coloring books, or will they discourage creativity? They're fine, say educators, as long as you supply plain, blank pa-

per too and don't insist that your child stay inside the lines. They say coloring books help a child develop dexterity with crayons and offer a chance to explore color and color combinations. With a coloring book, a child can turn out a creditable picture, perhaps on a day when she hasn't the energy to start from scratch.

## Imagination at Work

You'll see your child's first attempts at make-believe before he can walk, when the two of you play peek-a-boo with a handkerchief. At six months, your baby will pretend to groom his head, bald or not, with a hairbrush. Your early walker will imitate your floor sweeping with a push-toy, if there's no little broom handy. Your child will amaze you with his inventiveness about finding props—a receiving blanket will be a swirling cape for dancing or a knapsack for carrying supplies to a hiding place blocked off with a pile of books under the dining room table. You can contribute props, too, including such castoffs as hats and shoes and other dress-up clothes, costume jewelry, and a briefcase or small suitcase. You'll learn not to discard big cardboard boxes, the cores from rolls of toilet tissue or paper towels, the plastic eggs panty hose come in, or almost anything else that is clean and whole.

Sometimes your child will bring his dolls, stuffed animals, and puppets into imaginative play. Long conversations may take place as your child reenacts interesting or worrisome situations. You will see and hear versions of punishments and scoldings that you will recognize as having originated with you.

Other times these dramas may include an imaginary playmate who comes and goes or who is with your child day and night. Only children are more apt than others to have these imaginary friends, but many later siblings have them, too. The friend may cause you some annoyance when your child insists upon a good-night kiss or a seat at the table for him or her, but there are advantages, too. The most important is companionship, whenever and wherever your child wants it.

## The Proper Role of Television

Television, some say, is responsible for a new and different kind of American child: a little "addict" who is pale, listless, apathetic, and lacking in appetite, whose fate is to become a passive adult who has serious gaps in language, reading, and communication skills. These critics believe that TV is all bad, that it destroys family life and discourages reading and conversation. Some go so far as to banish television from their lives altogether, in an effort to pretend that it does not exist. And in homes where the set is on from early morning until late at night, where children are allowed to watch television for hours and hours every day, it *is* bad. At its worst, it is used as a pacifier, a convenient, round-the-clock babysitter that never needs to be paid.

Many parents are convinced, however, that at its best, television is superb in its capabilities as both entertainer and educator. They believe that TV is so much a part of society today that children should start early to learn to use it wisely and get the most out of it. Five hours a week is suggested by some of these parents as a reasonable amount of time for a child of two or three to watch television. Before that age, your child will probably watch only fleetingly, if at all, noticing only movement and color and not following a plot. As well as controlling the hours of viewing, you should select age-appropriate offerings on public, network, and local television, choosing topics to which you want your child exposed.

Rather than using TV as a babysitter, watch at least some programs with your child. Watching together can be a little like reading a story. As you cuddle in a big chair, you can point out things about the action or characters that you want her to notice, as you would if you were reading a story. When a program is over, you can talk about it with your child, answering questions and asking some of your own about her perceptions of the action.

Two of the main criticisms of television for children concern violence and advertising. Statistics tell us that by the time she graduates from high school, the average American child has watched 350,000 commercials and has seen eighteen thousand murders on television. For toddlers and preschoolers, the Saturday morning cartoon programs are probably the worst offenders. One study has shown that some eighteen violent acts occur during a given hour on these programs; another, that only about three percent of the characters injured in outlandish and unrealistic accidents ever require any kind of treatment. Physical and verbal aggressiveness have been found to increase noticeably among three- and four-year-olds who consistently watch the cartoons; it seems that the more they watch, the more accepting they become of aggressive behavior.

In the area of advertising, the plain fact is that the foods advertised most during children's programming are among the least nutritional—heavily sweetened cereals, candy, and chewing gum—and sometimes the most costly. Ads for toys are accused of warping children's values and suggesting that all children *need* and *must have* certain objects. Recent programs have featured stories with characters drawn directly from toys, so that, as some say, children cannot possibly distinguish the ads from the program itself.

Parents of small children can control the least desirable aspects of television to a high degree simply by not allowing viewing of the programs they dislike. "No" can and should be used; parents have the right, and the duty, to pass on their values. They can also join forces with groups that put pressure on advertisers and children's programmers and that lobby for the passage of suitable regulatory laws. For several years, one such group, Action for Children's Television (ACT) has worked to decommercialize and improve the quality of television, with considerable success in some areas. To join, or for more information, write ACT at 20 University Road, Cambridge, MA 02138.

## Exploring the Natural World

Your baby's first really good look at the wonders of nature will probably be taken from the seat of the stroller. There's a lot to be seen, heard, and smelled from that vantage point, but children need to touch, prod, poke, and fondle, too. The best way for that investigating to be carried on is from ground level, during walks, which you can start taking as soon as your baby can walk reasonably well. Your first excursions may be in your own backyard, where there's a great deal to be explored with the help of an attentive parent, but soon you'll want to go farther afield. At the changing of the seasons, if not more often, try to take walks in "real" woods where there is a stream, where things you don't see in your neighborhood grow and live, and where there are few, if any, people around.

When you're going to take the baby for a ride in the stroller, you can decide just where you'll go and how long you'll be gone, but walks are different. You can't set time or distance goals, because your toddler won't necessarily keep to the straight path you choose and will alternate bumbling along at a good clip with stopping completely. Every leaf and twig will need inspection, every insect and every object on the ground, appropriate or not. Everything in the world is new and interesting and needs minute inspection. You'll ruin the whole experience if you try to set a steady pace and "accomplish" anything at all.

Take along a few simple supplies on your nature walks: a small pail for pebbles and other finds, a magnifying glass to examine the ground and everything in or on it in detail, a jar with a lid for a bug or a worm, and perhaps even a pair of garden clippers, if you'll be where a blossom or a branch may be taken. The items your child brings home from a walk will be very important to her, at least for a little while, and some may be the beginning of collections that will have lifetime interest. When you get home from any woodsy place, bathe your child, in case he or she has managed to get into poison ivy or poison oak. It is best to launder clothes, too.

The toddler who lives in a climate where all four seasons can be experienced outdoors is fortunate, for each has its special attractions. Summer can be enjoyed anywhere, and two of its most enjoyable aspects are water and sand. A small plastic swimming pool with about six inches of lukewarm water in it or a backyard sandbox with a supply of sand, plus an assortment of unbreakable cups, bowls, and utensils for pouring and measuring, will keep the most restless toddler occupied for long periods of time. For safety's sake, a child in any amount of water must, of course, be closely supervised. Since a portable pool must be emptied every time it's used, a small one is easier. For a very small child, a plastic bathtub is suitable. And for your own convenience, use fairly coarse sand in the sandbox; the beautiful and more expensive white sand is very difficult to brush off damp skin. Sunburn is a real danger for delicate skin; put a hat on your child, and use a sunscreen containing para-aminobenzoic acid (PABA).

Fluffy new snow is as attractive to a toddler as a pool of water. Show your child how to make angels in the snow and roll up snowballs big enough to make snowmen, then give a little science lesson. Pour a very little water in a flat pan outdoors on a cold day and watch it freeze. Continue to add just a little more and see it freeze, layer by layer. Let your child prove that each snowflake is different from every other by examining flakes with a magnifying glass. Melt some snow to see how little water it makes and how dirty that water is. Your toddler probably won't be out so long that you have to worry about frostbite, but you can prevent chapped lips and cheeks by applying a coat of petroleum jelly. If it's too cold to go out at all, bring

## LEARNING AND COGNITIVE DEVELOPMENT

### *Language Development*

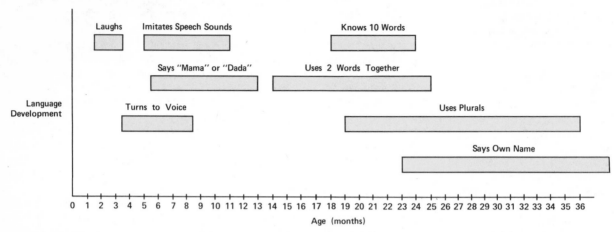

Keep in mind that babies vary greatly in their language development. The indicated age ranges are guidelines, not absolute requirements.

a big pan full of snow inside and let your child stand at the sink on a sturdy chair to play in it.

Most children like to watch things grow if they grow quickly. You can almost see a tablespoon of birdseed sprout on a wet sponge in a dish. Mung beans will begin to sprout in forty-eight hours in a screw-top jar of water, and they'll be edible in a week. If you roll up a dampened paper towel or piece of blotting paper inside a glass jar and put a lima bean between the paper and the jar, your child will be able to see roots reaching down and shoots growing up. When your child has developed a little more patience, let her watch the top of a carrot grow in a dish of water or a grapefruit seed grow in a paper cup filled with potting soil.

Living creatures of all kinds are endlessly attractive to children. When yours can understand that some pets aren't meant to be cuddled and that none can be eaten, you may wish to try some pets other than dogs or cats—fish, gerbils, or birds from a pet shop, for example; an ant farm that you can order through the mail; earthworms, hermit crabs, or even crickets from outdoors. The best thing about those you bring in from the yard or garden is that they can be returned to their natural environments when your child tires of them.

Always supervise your child's investigations of animals; undomesticated creatures could hurt your child—and your child could harm them! Teach your child that she is a part of—not master of—her environment. Show her how to smell, feel, look, and listen to the world around her. Teach her

to *respect* living organisms, plant and animal, and to never destroy them intentionally (don't stomp on the flowers, never pull the wings off insects, don't pull the kitten's tail). Some accidents will happen—but explain that, in general, one should try to be gentle and careful.

## Language Development

*Language* means a great deal more than *talking*. From the day your baby is born, you and he will communicate, carrying on "conversations" through eye contact, smiles, and body language. Your baby will react to your voice and the sound of your heartbeat. His primary tool of communication will be crying. By the age of two months, your baby will probably have developed different cries to indicate hunger, pain, fatigue, and discomfort.

Your baby's earliest noncrying speech sounds will be the throaty noises that come with increased production of saliva—the gurgling, sputtering, cooing, and squealing that begin at about three months. Soon he will begin to string together and repeat consonant and vowel combinations, like "ba-ba-ba." Be aware that it's a rare baby who follows any timetable for developing talking skills; children vary in this as in any other area of development. It may be at any time between six months and a year that your baby will be calling one or two very important people by name (most likely, "Mama" and "Dada"). In fact, an early talker will likely know and use as many as

364

a dozen words at one year old. They'll probably all be nouns, his versions of the words for such familiar objects as cookie, juice, dog, and cup.

You'll know your child really is anxious to talk as adults do when you begin to hear continuous jargon, strings of meaningless gibberish, complete with inflections that make them sound like a stream of talk in a foreign language. This kind of talk may go on for a long time after your child is able to make himself very well understood with real words, usually when he is playing alone. Between the ages of one and two years, your child will probably have a vocabulary of about fifty words (you can plan on one of them being "no") and will enjoy singing along with you to familiar and repetitive songs. Don't be surprised if your child seems to hit a plateau in speech development when he learns to walk; it's difficult to work hard on two skills at once. Children usually begin to string nouns and verbs together to make sentences of two or more words sometime between the ages of two and two and a half years, and an early talker may even add a preposition ("*under* the table") or an adjective ("*big* dog"). By the time your child is three, he may have a vocabulary of as many as three hundred words. You'll perhaps notice that the frequency of temper tantrums and periods of frustration decreases as your child finds the words to express anger and desires.

### Encouraging Your Child to Talk

Encourage your child to talk all the time you're together, as you go about your daily activities. A few ways in which you may wish to consciously aid language development are these:

- Speak directly to your baby often, giving total attention to her. Get down to your child's level physically, and look her in the eye.

- Speak slowly and distinctly, using all the words that apply to what you are doing with and for the baby—parts of the body, pieces of clothing, kinds of food, favorite toys. Use the same words for things every time when your child is under two; call all footgear *shoes* for example, not *sandals* or *sneakers*.

- Keep explanations and directions simple. By about fifteen months, your child will be able to do what you ask if you say something like "Bring me a diaper." You'll cause confusion if you use a long sentence that begins with "Run into the bedroom, will you, and . . . ."

- Use picture books to help your child develop word-object associations, pointing out familiar objects often and asking her to find the dog, the baby, or the house in pictures. Play word games, teach your child finger plays, and sing action songs.

- Give your child your attention when she speaks to you. Wait patiently for her to get out the right words to finish a thought instead of finishing it yourself or giving what's asked for before the words are out.

- Be equally patient in answering your child's questions, however endless they seem to be. Practice expanding a bit on a question by giving additional information. For example, if your child asks "What's that?" about a squirrel, add to your answer the fact that the animal is in the tree because it's looking for acorns to eat.

- Discourage baby talk and incorrect grammar, not by correcting your child, which is discouraging and will make her hesitant about talking at all, but by repeating the words or the sentence correctly.

### Speech Problems and Stuttering

There are many reasons why your child may talk a little later, or even much later, than other children her age. Few of them are serious, and most kids eventually catch up. For one thing, most girls talk earlier than most boys. A child's environment can affect the development of speech, too. If your family is not one in which a great deal of talking takes place, your child will probably be a late talker, and will probably talk less than some other children. If she spends days in a day care center or nursery school where one care-giver is responsible for several children, development of speech may be slowed. Competition for individual attention at home may be responsible for late talking, also. For example, if you have two children very close in age, or twins, you will not be able to devote a great deal of individual time to each. The "private language" that twins sometimes develop is more often the result of lack of one-on-one time with a parent than a desire to talk only to each other.

Other factors that affect speech development are a child's intelligence, hearing, and control of the muscles involved in speaking. Speech may be delayed or impaired if the speech centers in the brain are not normal, or if there is any abnormality of the larynx, throat, nose, tongue, or lips. Speech that does not develop normally may also be due to partial or complete deafness, mental retardation, brain damage, or malfunction of the speech centers in the brain.

Children between two and five years of age often lack fluency in speech and may stutter and stammer sometimes when they can't find words to express themselves. There may be involuntary pauses or blocks in speaking and rapid repetition of syllables or initial sounds of a word. These problems can be temporary, occurring only occasionally when a child is excited, impatient, or embarrassed, or they may be chronic, due to muscle spasms or underlying mental or emotional conflicts that may need to be resolved before speech is likely to improve.

Stuttering in children from two to five can be disregarded unless it is still a problem several months after its onset. The child may not even be aware of it unless it is pointed out to him. To help a child who stutters, do not show anger or impatience by refusing to understand, finishing the child's thought, or trying to force him to speak slowly and more clearly. Ignore the stuttering yourself, and don't allow siblings or other children to tease or laugh at the child. Read, sing, and speak to your child as much as you can.

Consult your doctor if your child speaks only in a monotone or with a marked nasal quality, if his vocabulary and ability to pronounce words seem to be diminishing instead of improving, or if stuttering is severe, constant, or prolonged. In addition to testing the child's hearing, the doctor will perform a physical examination, checking the child's throat, palate, and tongue. If your child is under five, you may be referred to a speech pathologist for evaluation and treatment if the stuttering is considered to be a severe problem, if the child seems to be extremely frustrated in his efforts to speak clearly, or if you yourself need assistance in handling your child's speech development. If your child continues to substitute sounds (*th* for *s*, for example) or stutters after the age of five or six, the doctor may suggest a consultation and possibly treatment by a speech pathologist.

## Ear Infections and Deafness

Deafness, or impaired hearing, is a partial or complete loss of the sense of hearing in one or both ears. A child may be born with a hearing loss, or it may develop at any age. Since children learn to speak by imitation, one who can't hear speech can't produce it.

Normal hearing occurs when sound waves pass down the ear canal and cause the eardrum to vibrate. Vibrations of the eardrum in turn move the three tiny bones in the middle ear. This motion of the bones transmits the vibrations across the middle ear to the inner ear, where they are changed to electrical impulses that are carried to the brain through the eighth cranial nerve. The brain interprets these electrical impulses as sound. Damage, disease, or malfunction of any of these structures can result in deafness. Any of the following problems may lead to hearing difficulties, which are likely to lead to learning difficulties.

*Ear canal problems* that may cause hearing loss include a buildup of earwax, a foreign object in the canal, and an infection known as "swimmer's ear."

*Eardrum and middle ear problems* may be caused by an inflammation of the middle ear or a blockage in the eustachian tube, which connects the throat and the middle ear. Middle ear infection *(otitis media)* occurs most commonly in the first two years of life, especially among children who receive frequent exposure to it in day care centers. The infection often involves a fluid buildup that causes mild to moderate, intermittent hearing loss for as long as nine months, threatening proper development of language skills.

*Inner ear problems* may be caused by injuries or infections.

*Eighth cranial nerve problems* have several possible causes. (This nerve is responsible for carrying all signals from the ears and balance structures to the brain.) A child may be born with a nerve that has not developed properly or that was damaged before birth. For example, if a pregnant woman has rubella (German measles), the virus may infect the eighth cranial nerve in her unborn child. After birth, this nerve can be damaged by an injury or an infection by a virus (mumps or measles) or a bacterium (meningitis). This nerve can also be affected by certain medications.

Signs of a child's hearing loss are often first detected by the parents. You can suspect a hearing loss if any of the following behavior occurs: an infant over three months old ignores sounds or does not turn her head toward sound; a baby over one year old does not speak at least a few words; a child over two does not speak in at least two- or three-word sentences; or a child simply does not seem to hear well. Any of these symptoms may be caused by a hearing loss, but they also may have other causes. If you think your child may have a hearing problem, see your doctor. He or she may refer you to a center that specializes in speech and hearing. A child with impaired hearing should start special education as soon as the condition is discovered, even if she is as young as one year old.

You may be able to prevent hearing problems for your child by taking proper precautions. *Never* put any object, including cotton swabs, into your child's ear canal for any reason; you may force earwax to become packed into the canal, or you may damage the eardrum. See that your child has the recommended immunizations against measles and mumps, the side effects of which can cause deafness. If you are a woman of child-bearing age, consult your doctor about rubella immunization for yourself.

## Answering Your Child's Difficult Questions

Over the years, you will give your child a great deal of information in answer to his questions about things both trivial and serious. Some of your answers will be very brief, just "yes" or "no"; others will be longer. A great many will begin with the word "because." Some will consist of facts, plain and simple, and others will express emotions, values, or philosophy. Your answers will all have something in common, though, whether they concern why the sky is blue, where babies come from, or how a beloved grandparent can pass from life to death. With the first "why" question you answer, you will establish your own unique style of giving information, and your child will know from then on what to expect from you.

To foster your child's trust in you and his confidence that the answers you give are reasonable and valid, consider following these guidelines:

- Be willing to answer questions when your child asks them. If the timing is very inconvenient, promise that you'll talk later, then bring up the subject yourself as soon as you can.

- Take your child's questions seriously; even those that seem frivolous or unimportant to you are worth your attention. Answer them candidly and matter-of-factly, avoiding sentimentality.

- Don't lie or try to whitewash facts, but don't feel that you have to go into every topic completely, especially for a young child. Remember that your answer must fit a short attention span; try to respond only to the question that is asked, giving your child just the information he asks for and can handle.

- Be prepared to repeat your answers many times, especially those on the most important topics. Children need repetition to test facts, to be sure they remain the same from day to day.

- Notice how a repeated question is phrased. It may seem to be the same one that has been asked before, but your child may be returning for slightly expanded information, after having digested one or two facts.

- Be aware that children under four have a very imperfect sense of time and no understanding at all of permanence. "Forever" really means almost nothing to them, and you will have to repeat it often when it is part of an answer you give.

- Remember that children are often unable to give the proper weight to the importance of information. They frequently ask what seem to adults to be trivial or insensitive questions about important things, some apparently almost designed to hurt, when they simply don't have enough information or experience to be tactful or considerate.

### Questions About Death

Parents today often find death harder to talk about with their children than sex—a reversal from Victorian days, when sex was never discussed among "nice" people, but death was accepted as a matter of fact. Children learned about death when they saw their relatives die at home and attended wakes and family funerals in the parlor. Today people die in hospitals or rest homes, and many children grow up having never seen a dead body or attended a funeral. Death has become a taboo subject, a shameful secret that we ignore, hoping with futile foolishness that it won't come close to us.

Ideally, your child will have some comprehension of death before a loved person dies. When you come across dead birds and insects on nature walks or when a family pet dies, you will have an opportunity to explain that everything that lives eventually dies. Facts will need repeating, of course, but in the course of a few brief experiences, you can talk about how things live on different time scales; how dead bodies disintegrate and return to nature; how the old wears out and is replaced by the new; and how dead things do not return. One simple way to help children grasp the reality of death is to discuss it in terms of the absence of certain functions: dead flowers no longer grow and bloom; the dead dog no longer breathes, barks, or eats.

You can also make use of deaths in stories you read to your child. Your library or bookstore will offer many excellent children's books that deal specifically with death. Remind your child, when you watch television together, that cartoons are make-believe; they usually give the impression that death is reversible, temporary, and impersonal; characters rise up whole and go about their business after having been smashed or blown to pieces. Another misconception your child can pick up from television programs and books is that only the wicked die. Your aim in all this will not be to fill your child's head with depressing facts, but simply to prepare her a little for the inevitable death of a loved person.

Most of your child's questions about death will undoubtedly be asked when a friend or family member has died and you yourself are upset and grieving. Talking about the death and formulating the answers that will most help your child will be very difficult for you. Try to remember that you want to be honest with your child, that "protecting" her will ultimately be harmful for you both. The normal steps of grief are denial, anger, guilt, and, finally, acceptance. Your child's questions will probably be related to them, and you will be asked to repeat the answers often.

To counter denial, tell your child as often as necessary that yes, Grandpa is dead, and will not return, but that those who loved him will always remember him. Do not use misleading terms like "sleeping" and "gone away"; the first may well make your child afraid to go to bed, and the second will lead her to expect Grandpa's return. And do not use confusing euphemisms like "called home" and "happy in heaven"; your child will find it hard to understand why people are sad when death sounds so good.

If your child shows anger at the doctor for not curing Grandpa or at God for letting him die, it is probably best to be empathetic. Other family members are angry, too, you can explain, but anger won't change things. You can also encourage play therapy if your child is old enough to act out roles with dolls or stuffed animals.

It is in the area of guilt that a vital but not verbalized question may occur: Is your child responsible for Grandpa's death? Children often feel responsible for a death because they have not been "good" or have told someone to go away. Your reassurance is called for. Continue to talk about Grandpa, stressing always the fun your child had with him and how much he loved the child.

When your child seems to have accepted the reality of the death, allow her to cry with you, to share your sadness, in order to complete the grieving process. Continue to talk about Grandpa; visit the grave together, if you wish; explain and let your child share in any commemorative activities you perform, such as contributing to an organization or planting a tree.

At some point after the death, your child may feel a great deal of fear—fear that she will die; fear that you will die and leave her alone and uncared for; nameless fear that if Grandpa can die, anything terrifying and horrible can happen. In spite of your constant reassurance, your child may regress in areas in which strides forward had recently been made, such as night waking, toilet training, or eating. Bear with her; the stage will pass.

## Questions About Reproduction and Anatomy

Any time after the age of about two and a half, your child will probably surprise you with the question, "Where do babies come from?" The question itself will not be so surprising, especially if you or someone close to your family is pregnant, but your child will probably pick a most inconvenient time to ask. The best answer, wherever and whenever the question comes up, is brief and factual: "They grow inside their mothers." Later, when your child has absorbed this bit of information and comes back with more questions, you should be equally matter-of-fact in explaining, probably in the following order, that the baby grows in the mother's uterus, a special place in the mother's body; comes out through a birth passage called the vagina; and is conceived when a cell from the father's body joins a cell in the mother's body.

This interest in reproduction did not spring up the instant before your child asked the first question. A child's education in sexuality begins at birth, with the mother's touch, and continues as he is held and cuddled while being fed, bathed, changed, and rocked. Shortly after a baby's discovery of hands and feet as the wonderful and ever-present entertainers they are, he or she finds the genitals, and the pleasures of self-stimulation are revealed. Toilet training is another milestone; a child handles his or her genitals frequently and discovers that some of the functions of that part of the body can be "controlled."

Toddlers go through a period of curiosity and concern about gender identity at some point between two and three, and they have a good many questions. They ask about the differences between boys and girls, about the possibility of somehow losing a penis (or getting one), about why boys stand up to urinate and girls sit down. Both facts and reassurance are demanded of you at this point. Your little girl may feel that her comparatively "plain" sex organs are less special and will need to be comforted by learning that, because of the way they are organized, she, but not her brother or any other male person, can someday give birth to a baby. Your little boy will worry that somehow he may lose his penis and will need to be convinced that this will not happen, that he will forever be male, just as his sister will forever be female.

Children's questions are more easily answered if their parents have healthy attitudes about sex and nudity and are reasonably open about appearing naked before them. It's not necessary, or advisable, to run a nudist colony in your home, but showing alarm or disapproval about perfectly normal curiosity will make both you and your child uncomfortable about a natural subject. Curiosity about the opposite sex can also be satisfied if there are siblings of both sexes in the family or if a child has opportunities to see other children going to the bathroom or being bathed.

In sharing the facts with your child, use the correct terminology for the body parts. Your child can handle the words *penis, testes, breasts, vulva, vagina,* and *uterus* as easily as any others, and will not have to learn them later. Keep answers short and simple for toddlers, going into no more detail than is asked for. Sometimes asking a question yourself to check on your child's comprehension will turn up an area that needs clarification. Small children often put isolated bits of information together to come up with some startling misconceptions about pregnancy: for example, mothers become pregnant by eating a lot or by swallow-

ing a seed; a baby is born through the mother's anus or navel; and pregnancy is an illness.

Your hesitancy about explaining sexuality and reproduction to your child is natural and common among most parents. It will disappear as you become more accustomed to answering the questions and giving the information so important for your child to have. Do remember to include the roles of love and intimacy and respect in your talks about reproduction with a child of any age. If you do not, you are telling only half the story.

## Questions About Divorce and Domestic Strife

A mistake that many parents make during a separation or divorce is to think that a child under two years old, too young to ask questions, will not be much affected. Your baby will, of course, not understand much of what is going on, but he will realize that things are different, will be upset, and will need special attention at a time when it is hard for you to give it.

Even very young children should be told that the parents are separating before the departing spouse moves out, if possible. They should be told the truth—that the parent who is leaving will not come back to live. However young they are, they should *not* be told that Daddy is going on a business trip or that Mommy is going to visit Grandma. Divorce is somewhat similar to death in that it is final; euphemisms and lies or half-truths do more harm than good and ultimately have to be corrected.

It's best for both spouses to be present when children old enough to understand (children almost never do really understand divorce—how can the two people they love the most not love each other?) are informed of the coming separation. They should share this responsibility, and each can answer the questions pertaining most directly to him or her. If there are two or more children, it's also best to tell them at the same time, however widely separated they are in age. They supply a base of familiarity for each other, and an older child may be able to help a younger one deal with the confusion. Those old enough to handle additional information can be given it at another time.

Probably the first question a child of any age will ask will be "Why?" Your answer will probably be something like this: "Because we aren't happy living together, and think it would be best for all of us if we lived apart." The second question may be unasked, but it will be in your child's mind: "If you can stop being happy together, can you stop being happy with me?" At this point, it is very important for you to say to your child, "We will both always love you; that will never change." Another question most children will ask is, "What will happen to me?" It's normal for children to be concerned primarily about themselves. Be as specific in your answer as you possibly can.

The next question children will ask may concern the departing parent. Tell them where this parent will live, and how and when they will be able to see him or her. Postpone giving information about changes in financial conditions that may cause a change in your lifestyle or news that one or both parents will be remarrying soon. Do encourage questions about any other aspect of the separation, however, even if they are painful.

You may find that your child will go through a process similar to grieving before he accepts the reality of your separation. You may be surprised, and perhaps even hurt, if your child appears to take your announcement very lightly and not to care. In reality, the child may be denying what will have to be accepted later, operating on the principle that if he ignores the problem, it will go away. Anger is common among children whose parents separate or divorce—they are angry at their parents and at a world in which such an unbelievable disaster can occur. Children are apt to look upon one parent as the victim and the other as the villain. If anger is directed at one parent, it will be up to the other to discourage it.

Guilt is an almost universal problem for children whose parents separate or divorce. They think that if they had behaved better, had done what they were told, one parent would not be leaving. They need constant reassurance that this is not so. Acceptance of the situation, when it comes, should be treated much like acceptance of a death. Grieving is natural when a marriage dies and a family is broken up, and your child should not be prevented from sharing your sadness and disappointment by the mistaken notion that he is being "spared."

## Toilet Training

Toilet training is a developmental skill that your child cannot master until he or she is physically and mentally ready, however anxious you may be

to have a "grown-up" child and be through with diapers. Actually, the process of training is perhaps more properly called toilet *learning,* since your child will teach himself or herself. Your part is to provide the setting and materials, the methods to be used, and the necessary encouragement.

The age at which their children were toilet trained is almost as important as the age at which they slept through the night among parents who keep close track of such events and brag a bit. Some studies show that the average child is usually toilet trained at about thirty months, but comparing your child with another is a waste of time; the differences among children in mastering this skill are vast. Girls are usually trained before boys of the same age, but an "early" boy may be trained at two and a "late" girl not until four. The advantages of having a toilet-trained child are obvious, and many parents consider starting training at about age two, if their children seem to be ready. It's advisable to back off quickly, though, if your timing seems to be wrong; the self-esteem of a child who "fails" this test of control suffers, and the anxiety engendered may lead to extended bed-wetting problems.

### Readiness

You will suspect that your child is ready for toilet training if wearing a wet or soiled diaper has become uncomfortable and distasteful to him or if he sometimes tells you or lets you know in some other way that urination or defecation is about to take place. Before you start, let the child observe you and any sibling in the bathroom; an older brother or sister is usually a great role model and an enthusiastic one. Get several pairs of underpants—the looser, the better—and let your child practice pulling them up and down. Look in your bookstore or library for some of the excellent potty-training books available for children, and read them to your child.

Decide whether your child will use a potty chair or the big toilet, with or without an adapter. The potty chair has the advantages of being child-sized, close to the floor, and easy to get on and off; the adapter takes no extra space, doesn't need emptying, and allows your child to skip the middle step of changing from the chair to the big toilet. Simply teaching your child to use the big toilet is, of course, easiest of all, if the child is large enough and not frightened. If you choose the potty chair, look for one in which the pot is easily removed for emptying; you will want your child to take over this task as soon as possible. If you opt for the seat adapter, consider one that folds up conveniently for travel. If your child is a boy, you will need a shield, either built-in or attachable, to deflect the flow of urine, because boys do not stand up to urinate at first. Do not use a chair or adapter that has a shield for a little girl; instances of injury to the labia have been reported. If you decide on the potty chair, set it up some time before you start training your child so that it will become familiar. Let the child sit on it, fully clothed, if he or she wishes, when you are in the bathroom together.

Another decision you will have to make concerns terminology. Children can handle the words for body parts easily enough, but *urinate* and *defecate* are more difficult, and they or substitutes for them will of course be used far more frequently. Most families settle on more casual words, such as *pee* and *BM*. Remember that there is a fine line between the acceptable and the crude; a word or term that sounds cute coming from a two-year-old may not be so at all from a five-year-old.

Still another decision to make is that about rewards for successful performance during toilet training. Parents disagree; some disapprove heartily of using material rewards for the accomplishment of what they see as a natural and normal step in development, while others see no harm in the practice and think it helps inspire a child to earlier success. Among the latter, there are those who reward their children with treats, such as candies, nuts, or raisins, and those who prefer to use small, inexpensive presents instead of food. One material gift that all children get is a supply of "big girl" or "big boy" pants, often introduced with some fanfare by parents and usually thrilling to a child. Some parents who don't believe in any kind of concrete reward other than training pants like to mark a child's progress with colored stars on a calendar. One thing all do agree upon is that praise is a highly suitable and effective reward. Praise generously, they say, but not so lavishly that your child begins to think of bowel and bladder control as earth-shaking achievements, more important than they really are and, possibly, as tools to manipulate their parents.

### Starting Toilet Training

The most common order for toilet training is bowel control first, then daytime bladder control, and, later, nighttime bladder control, but all children do not follow that pattern. If your child has bowel movements at a regular time most days,

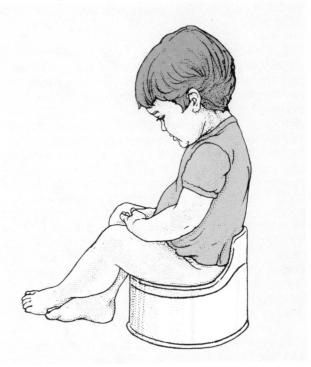

*Toilet training is a developmental milestone in the life of your child.*

you may have him, trained in that department long before you try for bladder control; some parents try with good success when their children are about fifteen months old. A good time for a child who is not regular to try is about a half hour after a meal. Sit with your child for a few minutes, perhaps reading a book as you wait, but only as long as the child is willing. Be prepared for your child to feel proprietary about his feces, and be careful not to imply that they are dirty or bad in any way. Some children are upset when their feces are flushed away, and some are frightened of the flushing noise. If your child is one of these, you may decide to flush only after he has left the bathroom.

One reason some children have trouble managing bowel control is that they are constipated. Constipation is not so much a matter of infrequency of bowel movements (having as few as three or four normal movements a week is perfectly natural for some children) as it is of hard stools that are painful and difficult for a child to pass. Discomfort will make a child hold back and compound the problem. To help a constipated child, decrease his intake of milk and milk products and increase whole grain and dried fruit in the diet. Prune juice is helpful for a child who will take it. If constipation continues, see your doctor for advice.

Summer is the best time to start toilet training, if you have a choice, because the fewer clothes a child must bother with, the easier the process will be. As often as you can, let your child wear underpants only, to cut down the problems of dealing with outer pants or skirts and shirts. You may find it helpful to plan to concentrate heavily on training for about a week, staying close to home with your child and not trying to accomplish much of anything else. The twenty-four-hour method of training, advanced a few years ago by two psychologists, who designed it first to help the retarded (Nathan Azrin and Richard Foxx, *Toilet Training in Less Than a Day*, Pocket Books, 1974), is championed by some parents and disapproved of by others. It involves very concentrated effort from both child and parent, and some feel that it is overly manipulative and somewhat punitive. Reports of the timing of success vary.

Your ultimate objective is to get your child to go into the bathroom alone, when he needs to; pull down his pants; clean himself when finished; pull up his pants; empty the pot, if one is used; and flush the toilet. Obviously, all this self-care will not occur at first, and perhaps you will be helping, reminding, and even leading your child physically to the bathroom for some time. The best times to give reminders or to take a child to the bathroom are the first thing in the morning, before and after naps, a half hour after meals, and before bed. Children usually urinate about eight times a day, and more often when they are excited or tired. Remember that part of toilet training is teaching your child good habits of hygiene—careful and thorough hand-washing and, for girls especially, wiping from front to back instead of the reverse (to prevent possible urinary tract infections).

## Accidents and Regression

Accidents will happen, whatever method you use and however quickly your child learns. When one does, clean up quickly, making very little of it. Console your child if she is upset, and do not punish, scold, or shame her. If accidents are so frequent that you can see training is going to be unsuccessful, stop at once and put your child back in diapers. Try again in a few weeks or a month, when you think the child is ready.

A child who is completely toilet trained will sometimes have accidents when she is ill or coming down with an illness. Sometimes a child will regress, and control of bowels or bladder, or both, will seem to be entirely forgotten. Regression sometimes accompanies or follows an illness. A child who regresses (or one who can't seem to master the control training requires, though apparently ready) may have a lactose intolerance or other food allergy or a urinary infection. The latter is usually accompanied by pain and a burning sensation when urinating and sometimes also by changed color or a foul odor in the urine. If you suspect a physical problem, consult your doctor.

In most cases, regression has an emotional, rather than a physical, cause. It may occur when a new baby comes into the house, when someone close to the family dies, when parents separate or divorce, or at some other stressful time. It's best to go along with it as best you can, not showing anger or scolding, but putting your child back into diapers without comment.

Nighttime bladder control usually comes later than daytime control, though some children go through the night dry even before they are daytime-trained. Good control is needed, for a child who sleeps through the night may have to wait as long as twelve hours. You may want to encourage nighttime control by holding back on liquids before bedtime and getting her up when you go to bed. Bed-wetting (*enuresis*) is considered to be a real problem only after a child is about six.

## Discipline: The Difference Between Right and Wrong

*Discipline* is a stern-sounding word; it smacks of the military, of the submission of one's will to that of another person. To parents of an earlier generation, the word was synonymous with *punishment*. These strict authoritarians, concerned with securing unquestioning obedience, felt they would spoil their children if they paid them too much attention or showed them excessive affection. Today we know that warmth and love are necessary if children are to have full lives, and that a better definition for discipline is "learning how to behave." Our long-range aim is to teach our children to discipline themselves, to have self-control rather than to be blindly obedient to laws laid down by those who are bigger and stronger than they.

Good behavior is relative, of course. Standards are personal, and conduct and manners unacceptable in your family may be seen as satisfac-

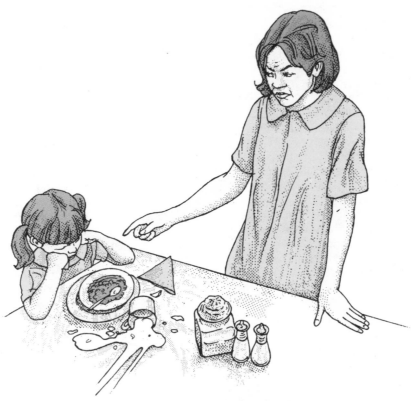

*Appropriate discipline will teach your child the difference between right and wrong.*

tory in other families. And times change. You may not require exactly the same behavior of your child that your parents required of you, but you may insist on certain other attitudes and actions. As your child grows, he will gradually absorb the principles that form the basis of your value system.

Obviously, your child will have to mind you without question as early safety lessons are learned. Self-discipline cannot be expected of a toddler, and your "No!" to running into the street or hitting the baby must be obeyed instantly. Your child will be learning, though, and with every similar experience the lesson will be reinforced, until it is he, instead of you, who takes responsibility for his actions. Another example of beginning understanding of self-control might occur when you stop your three-year-old from throwing a ball in the house. Your aim is not to show the child who's boss or even simply to prevent balls from being thrown in the house. It is to teach the child to respect and protect property, and eventually your child will learn this. With self-control, he will not only refrain from throwing balls in the house, but will also not knock over lamps, bang on the furniture with a hammer, or carry on other destructive activities.

## General Guidelines for Loving Discipline

• *Be sure your expectations are reasonable.* It's easy for parents to expect too much from their children, especially from their first children. No one would expect a nine-month-old baby to show self-control about what goes into her mouth; a child that young obviously needs total and constant protection from the environment. But you may be tempted to treat your bright toddler, who walks well, understands what you say, and speaks in sentences, as a sort of miniature adult. You don't understand why she rebels and defiantly tests every limit you set. The truth is that nature is pushing this child to separate from you, to become independent, and the child is going about fulfilling that drive in the only ways she knows. Her defiance means she is growing up. For the time being, give as few commands as possible, offer two choices whenever you can, and use diplomacy instead of pressure to get the child to behave acceptably.

continued

continued

- *Reward good behavior, not misbehavior.* Give a "good" child more attention than a "bad" one. When your toddler pats the dog gently, reward with praise and a hug. When he throws a tantrum because you save the dog from mistreatment by putting it out, step over the screaming child and pay no attention. For a small child, love and praise are better than material rewards of food, toys, or money. Be careful, though, not to spoil a compliment, even to a toddler, by partially invalidating it—congratulating your toddler on picking up toys, for example, and then pointing out that they have not been arranged neatly on the shelves. Remember that the most thrilling compliment of all is the "overheard" one, especially when it is being related to the child's other parent.

- *Don't overreact to misbehavior.* It's easy to get into the habit of scolding and punishing with the same intensity for a minor offense as for a serious one, in order to get your child's instant attention and obedience. Save your sharpest tone of voice for real emergencies and your most severe punishments for actions dangerous to your child or someone else.

- *Be brief, be clear.* Keep your rules simple and repeat them often. Speak plainly, in words of one syllable. Look into your child's eyes, and hold her hands as you give a command. Be sure not to make rules that can't be enforced because they're based on actions that can't be regimented or on emotions. You can't make a child sleep, for example, or force her to love someone. When your child breaks a rule, tell her briefly and succinctly what has been done wrong and why it was wrong. Holding your child's hands or touching her on the shoulder as you reprimand shows your love and may also get closer attention.

## Punishment to Fit the "Crime"

Small children need guidance more than punishment, but when your child is between two and two and a half, he will begin to understand the difference between right and wrong, and you will find yourself searching for a way to punish misbehavior fairly and effectively. The way you punish your child will depend upon his age, both of your personalities, and, probably, the way you yourself were punished as a child. Your tender-hearted and adoring one-year-old will most likely wilt under even a cross look from you, while your defiant toddler's feelings seemingly can't be hurt by the most severe scolding. One two-year-old will respond positively to your quiet verbal correction; another might deliberately repeat an offense no matter what you say or do. Try to remember, in the most trying of situations, that your purpose in punishing your child is not to get even but to teach, and that it is the *act* you dislike, not the child. Mete out punishment immediately (not leaving it until "Daddy gets home"), and follow it very shortly with evidence that you love your child.

"Time-out" is an effective punishment for children of almost any age, as suitable for an angry, overwrought toddler as for a rebellious preadolescent. The only difference will be that you'll settle your toddler into a little chair in the corner for a very short time—perhaps two or three minutes—and you'll isolate an older child for as long as it takes him to accept your requirements. One of the best things about a time-out is that it provides a cooling-off period for both child and parent.

Allowing logical consequences to follow misbehavior probably provides the fairest and most reasonable punishment. You'll make good use of logical consequences later, when your older child oversleeps and misses the bus—and walks to school. Or when he doesn't get chores done on time—and doesn't watch television. But even a child under three can understand that if he rides a tricycle into the street, after being specifically warned not to, the tricycle will not be ridden at all for one whole day. Or that if he uses a toy as a weapon, the toy will be taken away. The logical consequence of hitting, biting, or kicking is to be separated from the playmate or adult under attack.

Eventually, the question of corporal punishment will arise: should you or shouldn't you spank your child? Some parents feel that a child should never be spanked, that spanking is more a vent for their own bad moods than a teaching tool. The lesson it does teach, they say, is that hitting is the way to solve problems. The one exception they are likely to make is the quick spank they will give a toddler for running into the street or otherwise risking harm to himself or to others.

Do not ever shake a child or hit her about the head—you risk brain damage and even death. A child's neck muscles are still weak; when the head snaps back, the brain hits the skull, and blood vessels stretch or break. A blood vessel in the eye may also be damaged, causing partial or total vision loss.

Finally, it is wise to instruct any and all care-givers that they must never physically discipline your child. This type of punishment, if used at all, is best and most safely administered by you.

## Discipline for the "Difficult Child"

Every parent knows that some children are harder to handle than others. Sometimes problems occur because of personality differences between a parent and a child, but there are children with whom any parent would have trouble. The truly difficult child has probably been so from infancy, given to troubled sleep, feeding problems, and perhaps many minor illnesses. The challenge grows as the child does. She is strong-willed, with powerful needs and unyielding determination, and often intensely curious about every aspect of her surroundings. Parents of a child like this can comfort themselves somewhat in knowing that many difficult children are unusually intelligent. Some can be classified as hyperactive, but that diagnosis is not usually made before the child is of school age. Drug therapy is sometimes recommended for hyperactive children. Some doctors and nutritionists feel that the condition can be controlled by a diet that omits sweets and food colorings. (See Chapter 9 for additional information on diet.)

It is important to accept this strong-willed child as she is and to convey your love often and sincerely. Avoid confrontation when you can by distracting the child or heading off a situation you know will cause trouble. Be firm when you have to, but save your energy for major problems by letting your child win a battle now and then. There will be periods when your child will be especially hard to handle and you will feel stressed. Try to find time for yourself during these periods, if only for an afternoon or evening.

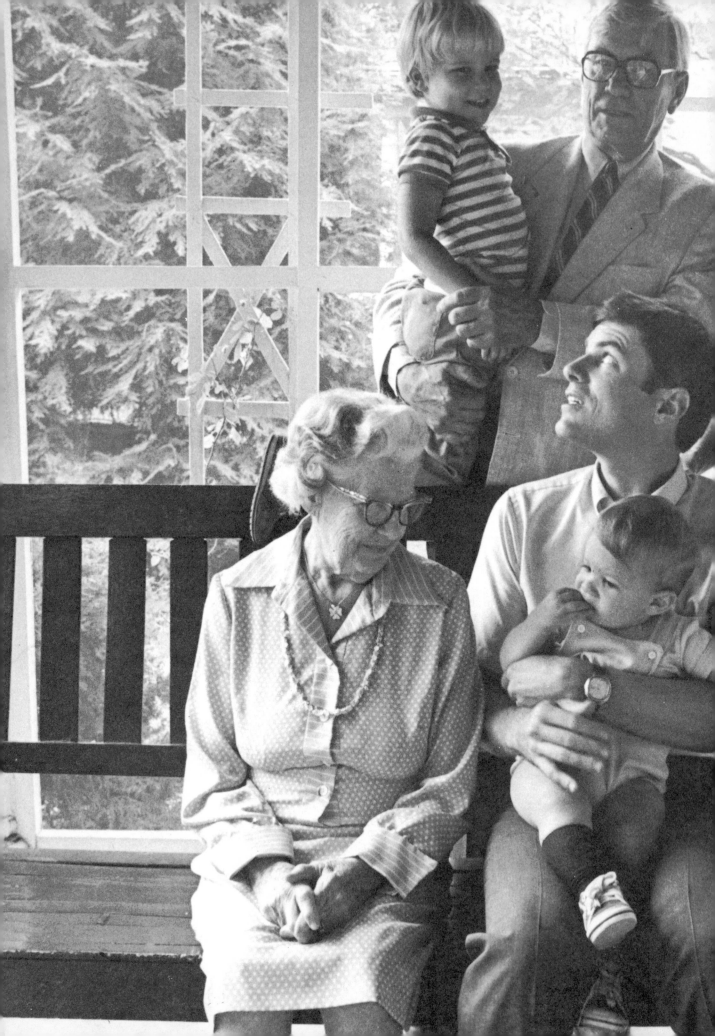

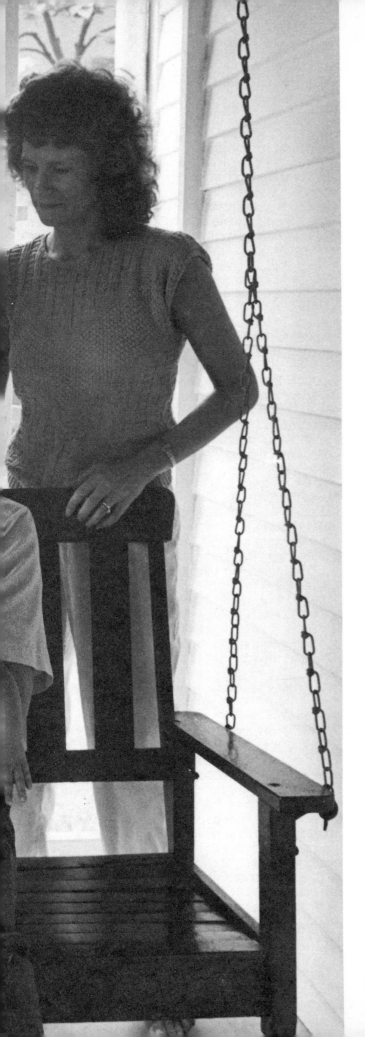

# Chapter 12:
# Family
# Structure

## The Evolving Family Unit

Despite the changing lifestyles and ever-increasing personal mobility that characterize modern society, the family remains the central element of contemporary life. Families offer warmth, security, and a measure of protection against an often uncaring world. But family structure, like society at large, has undergone significant changes in the years since World War II. While the nuclear family—with Dad, Mom, and offspring happily co-existing beneath one roof—remains the ideal, variations in family structure are plentiful—and often successful. Whatever your particular family situation, it will have tremendous influence upon your baby's happiness, development, and future life.

377

# FAMILY STRUCTURE

## The Nuclear Family Unit

### Spacing

A majority of parents want more than one child, and once the first child is here or on the way, it's natural to wonder how long you should wait to have another. It's really a personal decision.

On the one hand, many parents opt to wait a few years, until the first child is no longer in the demanding infant stage. These parents might tell you that the thought of dealing with two infants at once was just too overwhelming for them. On the other hand, parents who had their children in quick succession might tell you that they didn't have time to lose their touch between children, and that having two infants at a time is easier than having an infant and perhaps a toddler or even an older child, whose conflicting needs and demands involve a lot of gear-switching.

One thing to consider when you're exploring the question of how many years to leave between brothers and sisters is what you want their roles with one another to be. If siblings are born several years apart, the older siblings often adopt a care-taking role with the younger siblings. When siblings are born closer together, they're more likely to relate as peers and playmates. All siblings are going to fight from time to time, and whether they're of the same or opposite sex is going to influence their relationships, too.

### Birth Order Factor

If you've read any pop psychology, you've probably already come across the term *birth order factor*. It refers to a child's place in the family. There are certain traits that seem to go hand in hand with birth order. Birth order affects not only how your child sees herself, but also how you will parent your child. For instance, parents often have greater expectations of firstborn children.

Research has shown consistent responses among children when they were asked for their perceptions and feelings about their "rank" in the birth order, so it's important for parents to be aware of how birth order may affect each child, and how it may cause you to overlook some things each child might be needing.

The firstborn child is the "pioneer" in the family and, unless there's a remarriage into a family with other children, always enjoys the position of being the oldest. Firstborn children are often very dependable, responsible, loyal, and protective. They often assume a "little parent" role in the family. Among adults, a high percentage of firstborns can be found in such demanding professions as medicine and politics. Firstborns often say that their parents place too much responsibility on them in the family, and that parental expectations for them are too high.

Since the firstborn child is an only child, at least for a while, she is the one child in the family who will ever know what it's like not to have to share attention with a sibling. For this reason, it's especially difficult for firstborns to deal with the birth of the second child. The second child is always going to be seen as a threat by a firstborn, since if it wasn't for him, the firstborn would still have exclusive claim to parental attention and energy. It's not unusual for a firstborn to plot ways to get rid of the second child. This may involve backbiting or actual physical attacks against the second child, or attention-getting behaviors like whining and crying.

The second child experiences a much different world than the first, who has already paved the way for him. Second children often take the role of rebel, clown, entertainer, artist, troublemaker, loser, peacemaker, or negotiator in families. As adults, they often become lawyers and entertainers, continuing the roles they played as kids.

Second children often feel that they don't get enough attention from their parents and, unlike firstborns, that their parents don't expect much from them. They complain about being compared to their older siblings, and often wish they would just be appreciated for who they are. They resent being bossed around by their older siblings.

Middle children often express relief about being in the middle. Their parents are accustomed to parenting by the time they arrive, so some of the pressure is off. But middle children often feel unappreciated by and uninvolved with the rest of the family. They usually end up with all the hand-me-downs from the older child, which doesn't help them feel very special either (unless they happen to be the first sister or brother born into the family, a situation that would change the family dynamics a great deal). Middle children often see themselves as being dependable, self-reliant, diplomatic, and easygoing. Because they do tend to be very independent, they often end up in very independent sorts of jobs. As children, they often wish their parents would get more excited about their achievements, spend more time alone with them, and for heaven's sake, buy them something *new* once in a while.

The baby, or youngest child in a family, usually has special status. The parents' expectations of the youngest child may be low, and this child doesn't have to do much to get all her needs met. For one thing, by the time the baby of the family is born, the parents have usually attained a healthy earning power, so things may be considerably easier than they were when the first child was born. The baby is showered with material possessions and special attention. She knows she has a special place in the family and learns to charm and manipulate other family members to get what she wants. Nonetheless, babies don't like being called babies; they want to be taken seriously. They often see themselves playing the role of the little one, the cute one, the spoiled one, or the one with the temper. Because they are surrounded by so many authority figures as children, they may end up in passive and submissive fields as adults. Some babies don't ever really grow up, and this is because their parents don't ever really *allow* them to, wanting them to forever remain their cute, precious, final child.

## Only Children

There are lots of reasons for having only one child—sometimes the parents plan it that way; sometimes stillbirths, miscarriages, deaths, or medical problems prevent parents from having other children. These factors will affect how an only child views himself and how his parents view him.

Most only children relish their position, even if they occasionally wish they had the companionship of brothers and sisters. Unfortunately, as parents age, an only child often becomes the sole caretaker, with no siblings to help out.

Only children are often seen as being loners, overly responsible, lucky, perfect, fragile, strange, or very special. Only children themselves may feel lonely for lack of peer interaction. Due to their extensive exposure to adults, they might have difficulty being around other kids even when the opportunities exist. They often feel incredible pressure from their parents, since they're the last and only hope in the family. While parents of larger families may try to fulfill their own dreams through several children, when there's only one child, all of these wishes are focused on that child.

## Late-Born "Only" Children

A child born several years after other siblings experiences some of the same things as an only child, especially if the older children have already grown up and left home. But he is also the baby of the family, and his role reflects this dual situation. Parents aren't as likely to pressure this child as much as they might a true only child. He does not have to share attention with his siblings, but can experience the loneliness and differentness that the only child feels, particularly if his parents are much older. This latter situation will come into play with special clarity when the child reaches school age and meets other children's parents.

Advantages to having so-called "late" children are that there is little sibling rivalry, and the older siblings may be able to help their parents with the baby. Many of the anxieties of first-time parenting are gone, and parents are free to enjoy. For the older children, having a baby in the house may teach nurturing skills and increase their appreciation for what was once done for them. What often ensues is more open affection among everyone in the household.

## Forging the Family Unit

What can family members do to enhance their bonding to each other, in an age when isolation of people in general may inhibit bonding within the family unit?

Let's start at the beginning. Studies have shown that when a father is present for the birth of his child, the child's relationship with him in the first months of life is enhanced. If this is not the first child, it's important for siblings to be involved, too. Many hospitals are beginning to recognize this; many offer sibling programs to help prepare children for new brothers and sisters.

Families can maximize closeness and reap practical benefits by having regular family meetings where plans are made and problems are discussed. Even small children can take part in some family decision-making and problem-solving: where to go on vacation, how to paper-train the puppy, and so forth. When all family members feel that they are valued and that their ideas are listened to, they are more likely to cooperate with each other. When families plan and do things together, they have more shared memories, which enhances their sense of family. Families can establish their own traditions and festive occasions

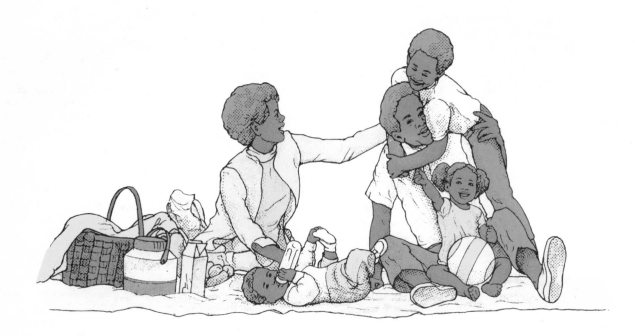

*Planned outings that involve the entire family foster communication and feelings of togetherness.*

when they enjoy particular activities, like visiting Grandma on Sundays or having a picnic on the Fourth of July. When family members plan and interact together, each experiences a sense of belonging, wholeness, and dignity.

## The Extended Family

In days past, extended families played a big part in helping new parents. Grandparents were often present to help with the new baby. Extended-family members often lived under one roof, or just down the road; children saw their relatives often enough to know who was who. Today, this is frequently not the case. Modern extended families are often unlike extended families of years past.

### The New Extended Family

While it's true that today's extended family is often spread out across the country, and Susie or Johnny may be walking—or even driving—before they meet some of the extended-family members, most families still have some extended family nearby. Geographical isolation is far more common among upper-middle-class families, who move for occupational opportunity, than it is among middle- and lower-class families, who tend to move to cities where they already have relatives.

But even when extended-family members are relatively close by, there is no escaping the fact that families do live more privately than they once did. In some cases, extended families still give each other day-to-day assistance with shopping, child care, and household tasks. More often, though, each branch of the family retains its basic independence, but at some time may assist another branch with gifts, low- or no-interest loans, or advice.

What does all this mean for kids? Essentially, children become more emotionally dependent on their parents when there are few significant adults in their lives. Don't expect your child to consider a seldom-seen relative important. Unless you find a way to open up your family's network, your children will probably be isolated from the extended family.

Some families hold regular family get-togethers or large reunions to reestablish a more integrated sense of family. You can help your toddler begin to understand the idea of extended family by creating a special "My Family" photo album with pictures and names. When he or she is a little older, you can begin to illustrate the nature of the relationships with a family tree.

Other families today are experimenting with alternative ways to open up the family. For instance, some form babysitting, food, and other kinds of cooperatives. This simply means that several couples pool specific resources. This lessens the burden of couples having to do everything solo.

A family cluster is a way to create a surrogate extended family. Several families meet regularly and become emotionally close. They share values, attitudes, and tasks. Often, family clusters share possessions, like vacation homes and cars. For children, this provides an enlarged number of significant adults and "cousins."

## Working Parents

### The Workplace

While many people *prefer* to work, it's no surprise that many new parents go back to work for financial reasons. Many return a lot sooner after childbirth than they may want to. A recent survey found that fewer than twenty-five percent of 153 national companies offered a sixteen-week maternity leave with a full salary. Most companies base the length of paid maternity leave on the amount of accumulated sick leave. *Paternity* leave—time off for the new father—is a wonderful concept. Unfortunately, it has yet to gain popularity with personnel benefits administrators.

But there may be other options. You may be able to negotiate returning to work part-time at first, so you'll be a little less pressured until you and your baby have your routine down. Job sharing is another option that is gaining ground; it means that you and someone else, possibly another mother, share a full-time position. Also, take another look at your budget. Is it really going to be worthwhile to return to work when you consider the cost of child care? Or could you come out even by tightening up a little?

As more and more parents work full-time, corporations are becoming increasingly involved in the problems of working parents. Corporations are not altruistic; they provide benefits when it costs them more money not to. Companies are adversely affected by parental problems of finding and paying for adequate day care and sick-child care when they result in troubled and unproductive employees and in absenteeism.

Most child-care benefits are provided in the form of resource and referral services, and as op-tional child care financial assistance in employee benefits packages. (When employees pick and choose a package of benefits out of many options, the program is said to offer cafeteria-style benefits.) Some companies in larger cities are also paying for sick-child care both in and out of the home, and a few firms actually run on-site day care centers or buy slots in nearby consortium centers; a consortium is formed when several organizations buy space in and support a day care center.

Unfortunately, the majority of workers are not employed by these larger companies. At this writing, smaller employers just aren't providing these benefits. However, smaller companies *are* beginning to respond by offering *flex-time* (flexible working hours), flexible benefits (which may include financial help with child care), and work-at-home options.

Assuming that you have decided to return to work and that you have some latitude about the timing, the next question is *when*. If you decide to go back in the first six to twelve weeks, make sure you properly introduce your baby to her caretaker(s), and make sure she gets used to being held and fed by that person while you're still present. Babies can tell the difference between one person and another almost as soon as they're born. In the first six to twelve weeks you will already know some of your baby's idiosyncrasies, and you can relate these to her caretaker(s).

If you return to work when your child is about six months old, keep in mind that your child already has a sense of who you are, and a sense of his separateness. He may really fuss when you turn him over to the day care center, and he may cling to the teacher when you come to get him at the end of the day. It will help to find ways to make these daily transitions easier; perhaps a familiar toy or blanket or just a distraction will do the trick.

Waiting a year to return to work will meet your need for time to get to know your child and share her first glimpses of the world. But at this point, going back to work may actually be more of a problem than it would have been early on. Your one-year-old is extremely possessive of you, and won't yet be able to understand why you're leaving. You may need to phase her into child care gradually. Your spouse may be able to ease the transaction by being there at times when you're not. It will be important to see that the caretaker is going to give your child the same kinds of stimulation that you've been providing; continuity is important to your child's emotional and developmental well-being. See Chapter 7 for information about day care options and selection.

### Quality Time

As a working parent, you have many demands and little time at the end of the day. How can you get all the household chores done, have time to spend with your child, and maybe even have some time left over for yourself?

Creativity is the key. Small children don't necessarily know the difference between work and play, so any way you can find to incorporate the two may help. For instance, one woman puts her baby in a backpack, turns on rock music, and "dances" while she vacuums the house. Taking your baby along while you do errands can be fun; if it's a nice day, why not take the stroller and walk? You might (watchfully) allow a toddler to play with the bubbles in the sink as you do the dishes.

Toddlers can learn to set the table, and they take great pride in it. If your child begins to learn to pitch in with household responsibilities at an early age, there will be more time for everyone. The time you spend teaching her to do these things can be quality time, and your child will feel more valued and grown up.

The thing to remember is that quality time does not have to be a major scheduled event. It might be the time you spend reading to your child right before bedtime, or the time you spend helping her build something with her blocks. Every task you must do with your child can be quality time—putting her to bed, getting her dressed, feeding her. The trip to and from the day care center can be a good time for you to hear about your child's day. You can use these moments for sharing feelings, or for laughing, and even arguing. Yes, you're going to argue, since your goals and your child's are going to conflict at times. When you aren't able to spend much time with your child, this will be painful for both of you, so it's important to sit down and talk about the conflict.

Try to save some of your sick time so you can be available to be home with your child when she is ill. If the illness is nothing major, this time can be special for both of you. Your child will cherish being cuddled, being read to, and being listened to.

Make your vacations family events, but don't schedule them so heavily that they are as stressful

as everyday life! Establish weekend family routines or plans. Let your child contribute to those plans as early as possible.

Trying to be a Supermom or Superdad while your children are very young can be draining. You can alleviate some of the stress by accepting that these years will be over sooner than you think. Focusing now on trying to have a perfectly kept house will rob you of time you could be reserving for yourself and your children. Make the most of this special time of early childhood. You'll miss it when it's gone.

## Single Parents

If you've just experienced a divorce, a separation, or the death of your spouse, you may be totally overwhelmed with your loss and the new responsibilities of being a single parent. There you are, totally in charge of decision-making, finances, breadwinning, and nurturing. It's no wonder newly single parents often feel fatigue and depression.

Most single parents today are women, who face a substantially lower income than their male counterparts. They often must rely on child support and government subsidies. Often, they must move to smaller, less expensive quarters in order to make ends meet. Coupled with the financial problems that they may already have is the fact that many employers are biased against single parents, because they think they're less reliable.

The newly divorced or widowed parent doesn't face these changes alone; children also experience loss and a disruption of routine. Toddlers are affected more by how the parent is coping and by changes in routine than by the fact of the divorce or the death.

When a parent dies or leaves, children need attention, affection, and reassurance; they need to be told how important they are. Without such assurance, your child may fear losing *you*, as well. Do your best to maintain schedules and routines as much as possible, and don't be lax about rules because you think things are already hard on your child—children need limits to feel secure; dispensing with rules is like dispensing with routine—it's unsettling.

After a divorce, try to make sure your child sees his other parent regularly. It's important for you to try to maintain a relationship with your ex-spouse for the sake of coordinating visitation; cooperation and flexibility are essential, no matter what your personal feelings may be. It's also important that you don't say anything negative about your ex-partner to your child. You need to support your child's contact with him (here we're assuming the mother has custody) and with your former in-laws.

If you can, seek support for yourself from relatives, your church, and social groups. If you have no support, the stress of being a single parent will be especially high. Parents Without Partners is a support group for single parents, with chapters in most communities.

If you are what is referred to as the noncustodial parent (you don't have custody), you must also be willing to maintain contact with your ex-partner, despite your personal feelings. You must support your child in his relationship with her. If she is not allowing visitation, you must continue to let your child know you are there for him. This may seem futile, but at some point, when he is old enough to do things for himself, he will know how to contact you—and he will. If you have been granted visitation, you must find ways to continue having a parenting relationship with your child. Don't structure every moment spent with him as fun time; if you do, time spent won't be very real, and you and your child will never really know each other. The two of you need to talk quietly, and be reflective and honest. An unending succession of ball games and amusement parks will make this difficult.

The concept of co-parenting, or *joint custody,* is gaining momentum. It works best when both parents live in the same community and when they are able to maintain a very cooperative relationship, with high levels of communication. Joint custody is emotionally easier on fathers, who traditionally have not been granted custody. It allows them to remain involved in decision-making about their children; as a result, they remain financially responsible, because they feel as though they are part of their children's lives. Noncustodial fathers often back out of visitation and child support payments because they feel uninvolved with and unable to have an impact on their children's lives.

Sometimes the noncustodial parent lives in another state; and though he may still be involved with his child, contact is limited to infrequent visits, telephone calls, and letters. For his contact to have much of an impact, he must master the arts of letter writing and phone calling. Writing crea-

tive, entertaining notes that the child can easily read and providing stamped return envelopes can keep communication going. Phone calls should be made at times convenient for everyone.

When an ex-spouse is completely uninvolved, the single parent often doesn't know what to tell the child. It's important to allow a child to continue trying to contact a parent until she realizes the parent isn't going to respond. Often, the inclination is to prevent this in order to protect the child from being hurt; this backfires because the child will interpret this to mean that Mommy is trying to keep her away from Daddy. Once your child realizes that Daddy is gone and isn't coming back, you can help by allowing her to talk about him, as a way of working through her grief.

## Never-Married Single Mothers

Many of today's single mothers have never been married. An increasing number of women have spent their twenties establishing themselves in their careers, and have not seriously desired to have children until they reached their thirties. By then they may feel that their "biological clock is ticking," and that if they wait until they meet a suitable marriage partner, it may be too late for childbearing. There is also increasing acceptance among younger women of the idea of having a child outside of marriage.

Some women who opt for motherhood without marriage choose to become pregnant through artificial insemination. Many, however, discover that a lot of doctors are unwilling to artificially inseminate an unmarried woman. Some who choose artificial insemination genuinely do not want to become emotionally involved with the father of the child, and feel this would be inevitable if they knew him. Others, predominantly gay women, choose artificial insemination simply because it does not require a personal relationship with a male partner. Still others want to raise the child alone and fear that if they knew the father, he might later make claims on the child.

Some women who want a child without getting married select a partner who is willing to father the child with no strings attached. Others agree that the "acknowledged father" will be involved in the child's life although the parents will not marry. There is also a practical side to knowing the man who will father the child: the prospective mother might fear contracting AIDS through artificial insemination by an unknown donor.

Whatever their choice, however, these mothers are free to raise their children according to their own ideas and values, and they reap many of the rewards of parenting. On the other hand, they undertake heavy responsibilities, and risk the loneliness of parenting without a partner with whom to share both the burdens and the good times. For this reason, support groups for such single mothers have begun to spring up—at least in several major cities.

### Widowed Parents

How well a family adjusts to the death of a parent depends a lot on how the parent died. When a parent dies after a short-term illness, the family may adjust more quickly than it would if the death were sudden or from a long-term illness. Other families may find that dealing with a long-term illness has given them time to work through some of their grief before the family member dies.

Children go through essentially the same stages of grief as adults: shock and numbness, followed by grief and depression; then an emotional distancing from the loss; and finally creative adaptation to the loss. The thing to remember is that children display these feelings differently than do adults. Even children under the age of three feel the loss, though they may not understand the finality of death. Children may deny the death, they may act angry toward the deceased parent, and they may feel guilty, thinking they did something to make the parent go away.

To help children, it's important to explain the death to them in language they can understand. Don't use euphemisms; they add to confusion and lead to questions like, "If we lost Daddy, why aren't we going to look for him?" Explanations that are too gentle can be confusing and even frightening; your child could fear that if he ever gets sick again, he will die, too.

When children become depressed, they often come down with minor illnesses like colds and intestinal upsets, or they play less, or they become more clinging and dependent. You can help by understanding that your child is feeling a loss and needs to feel more secure. Be open and willing to talk to your child about his fears.

You will undoubtedly need to find support for yourself, as well. You may get some from the children, depending on their ages, but you will also need adult support. If you can't rely on family—

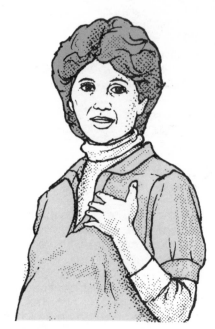

*More older women than before are becoming first-time mothers.*

who may be telling you that you should be over your grief and carrying on with your life after a certain amount of time—we urge you to contact your local Widowed to Widowed group, where you can open up and find support in dealing with the changes you are experiencing in widowhood. It's not uncommon to need two to three years to adjust to the loss of a spouse.

## Older Parents

It used to be that very few women had their first children after the age of thirty-five, though it was not uncommon for women to bear additional children in their middle years. Today, many women are not beginning to have children until they are in their thirties; there are a number of reasons for this. Many women are choosing to become established in their lives and careers before turning their thoughts to childbearing and to their biological clocks. Many see their twenties as a time to experiment and experience freedom. At this age, some women don't feel psychologically ready for the commitment of having children. Still other women, immersed in their careers, have such high expectations for themselves—and others—that they're unable to find mates who meet their qualifications for fatherhood. Though these women might opt to have children sooner, they often don't find a suitable situation for doing so until they're approaching forty. And then there are the couples who, for some reason, appear to be biologically unable to conceive until, just when they have about given up, they finally conceive.

There are a number of positive aspects to having a first child in mid-life. There are also some drawbacks. First, the positives:

- A new parent who is around age forty has fifteen to twenty years of adult life experience, and so has a lot more inner resources to draw on in times of stress than does a younger parent.

- Middle-aged adults are usually at the height of their earning power, so there's more financial stability to support a child.

- Having had time to sow their wild oats, middle-aged adults are ripe for being parents. They have a sense of identity—the child is not going to have to provide them with it.

- Having a first child in mid-life provides a real sense of renewal.

- Adults in mid-life have a deeper sense of the value of life itself, and so tend to place high value on the time they can spend with their children.

While many of the positive things about having a baby in mid-life involve the joys of raising a small child, the drawbacks have mostly to do with the future, and with the parents' concerns about aging:

- Older parents may have lower energy levels. They may wonder if they will have the energy to enjoy doing things with a child, or if they will have to hobble behind.

- They wonder if they will live to see their child become an adult. Will they ever see their grandchildren? Will they very quickly become a burden to a child just as he is trying to get on his feet as a young adult?

- When the age difference is forty or more years, quite a schism is created; parents worry whether their values will be at all relevant to their child.

- Often when a child becomes a teenager—a difficult period for even young parents to deal

with—older parents find themselves becoming impatient to return to the privacy they knew before their child was born, and longing for solitude and freedom from daily child care responsibility. This can create a lot of additional stress.

## Parents Who Have Late Babies

Parents who have late babies—babies born ten or more years after their siblings—have a few advantages over parents who just start their families in their middle years.

Often, the older children in these families can be relied on to take semi-parental roles with their new brothers and sisters. They can become built-in babysitters, making it easier for the parents to maintain their routines with less disruption.

Having a late baby is less stressful than having a firstborn. Parents of late babies have plenty of experience in parenting and lots of confidence. They find they can enjoy their late-born children even more than their firstborns.

A late child is a good lesson in sex education for the other children. Pregnancy will force adolescents to acknowledge their parents' sexuality; this may be uncomfortable for them and may cause them to become distant and even hostile. However, these feelings usually disappear when the baby comes along and Mom returns to a normal state and everyone is pampering the new baby. When all the children in the family are involved in preparing and caring for the baby, a late baby can provide a splendid lesson in parenting. In fact, parents often notice that their teens become more gentle, and the family closer, as a result. The new baby becomes a unifying influence, a point of common pleasure and concern.

The drawbacks of having a firstborn in your middle years, however, still apply here. When that last-born child hits her teens, it's likely that the other kids will have grown up and moved out, and it's even more likely that after so many years of parenting, the parents will be tired and anxious to move to an empty nest. Another, more initial drawback to having a late baby is that a working mother may be kept from her job at a time when her income is especially needed for other children who may be approaching college age. Nonworking mothers, too, may have difficulty adjusting to spending time at home with a baby.

## Adolescent Parents

You have probably read how dismal the picture is for teenagers who choose to raise children in our society. We can't paint a pretty picture, either. If you're going to have a child and you're under twenty, there are some things you can do to enhance the picture, but you'll still be faced with lots of difficulties.

Make sure you seek medical advice as soon as you know you're pregnant. It's unfortunate that most teens don't; often, they're embarrassed, don't know where to go to find advice, or just want to deny the pregnancy. Age, nutrition, and quality of care are all factors in maternal and baby health. Poor diet and lack of prenatal care can lead to complications like anemia, premature birth, and low birth weight.

There is a long-term impact on the child when teens have and raise children. Because of poor prenatal care, there is often a high incidence of illness and mortality. Children often have educational and emotional problems later on. Research has shown that the younger the mother, the more likely it is that her child will have a lower IQ score. Children of teens often become victims of child abuse or neglect, simply because their parents are too immature to understand infant and child behaviors, and may get frustrated very easily. Or the parents simply tire of having a child around and want to go out and have some fun—because they're still kids themselves. They can be resentful at having to grow up in a hurry.

Financially, teens who have children are more likely to end up living below the poverty level. Research shows that teen mothers tend to have additional children more rapidly, which means that they're even less likely to be able to offset childcare costs with income. This is compounded by the fact that teen mothers often terminate their education prematurely, and qualify only for poorly paying jobs; often they are financially better off on welfare. As a result, welfare dependency is widespread among single teen mothers. Unable to achieve financial independence, teens who have children often end up living with one or both of their parents.

Statistics show that when teen fathers remain with their mates and children, their educational attainment is also reduced, and their long-term earning power is less than that of their peers. Most often, teen fathers are *not* involved, and it has been assumed that they don't want to be. Yet a recent study has found this to be a myth. Teen fathers want to help the mother and child, but they themselves need assistance and support. Unfortunately, until recently little or no attention has been paid to the problems of the teen father. Many of these young men have never had father figures themselves, and just don't know how to father. Some pilot programs now provide counseling and job training for teen fathers, and have been very successful in encouraging young fathers to stay involved with their children and provide the necessary financial support. Though there are presently only a few such programs, they are growing in number.

We can tell you about all the perils of having a child as a teen, but if you have already made the choice, you need to seek help for yourself. Find out about teen pregnancy classes in your area by calling a hospital or family planning center. Such classes will prepare you for labor and provide support. Some classes will help you develop life skills and decision-making skills. If there are no teen pregnancy classes available, check your local YMCA or YWCA for other kinds of parenting classes and support groups.

One program is the Minnesota Early Learning Design (MELD) for Young Moms (MYM). This program provides self-help groups led by former teen mothers. The groups meet one evening a week; teens are welcome to bring their babies. The evening includes a free meal, education, and time for sharing. The exact focus is determined by the needs of each group, but the objectives are: 1) to enhance understanding of child development, 2) heighten self-awareness and involvement in the outside world to help establish future goals, 3) develop assertiveness and information-seeking skills, and 4) improve the physical well-being of mother and child. If your community does not have an MYM group, you can find out how to start one by contacting Minnesota Early Learning Design, 123 N. 3rd Street, Eighth Floor, Minneapolis, MN 55401; 612-332-7563.

The best way to eliminate the problems of being a teenage parent, or to prevent having more children, is to learn about and use contraceptives. The capacity to reproduce is at its highest between the ages of fifteen and eighteen, so it's no wonder that many teens who may think it's safe not to use contraception all the time, or to use it just once in a while, end up getting pregnant.

For contraception to work, you must anticipate sexual activity and recognize the risk of preg-

**More Support Organizations for Young Parents**

- Alan Guttmacher Institute, 111 5th Avenue, New York, NY 10003; 212-254-5656.

- Center for Population Options, 1012 14th Street NW, Suite 1200, Washington, DC 20005; 202-347-5700.

- Child Welfare League of America, Inc., 67 Irving Place, New York, NY 10003; 212-254-7410.

- Family Focus, 2300 Green Bay Road, Evanston, IL 60201; 312-869-4700.

- Joseph P. Kennedy, Jr. Foundation, 1350 New York Avenue NW, Suite 500, Washington, DC 20005; 202-393-1250.

- March of Dimes, 1275 Mamaroneck Avenue, White Plains, NY 10605; 914-428-7100.

- National Organization of Adolescent Pregnancy and Parenting, P. O. Box 2365, Reston, VA 22090; 703-435-3948.

- Office of Adolescent Pregnancy Programs, Grants Management Division, Room 736-E Humphrey Building, 200 Independence Avenue SW, Washington, DC 20201; 202-245-7473.

- Teen Fathers Collaboration, c/o Bank Street College of Education, 610 112th Street, New York, NY 10025; 212-663-7200.

nancy. Then you must obtain a contraceptive and talk to your partner about your intention to use it. And you *must* use it, and use it *every* time.

If you need more information about contraceptives, ask your doctor. If that's not comfortable, find your local family planning center. Family planning centers generally have counselors who are patient and understanding and very willing to help; they won't think you're stupid for asking questions. On the contrary, they recognize that your questions are a reflection of your concern and your need to be informed, so that you can make responsible, mature decisions. Many family planning centers will provide you with contraceptives if you don't have the money to buy them, or they will

sell them to you at a reduced rate. Take advantage of the opportunity.

## Step-Families

While we still tend to think of families as consisting of a mother, a father, and their children, the reality is that with all the divorces and remarriages that occur in our society, a large number of families are actually step-families, or blended families. Unfortunately, in our society, the word "step" has gained a lot of negative connotations; we all read *Cinderella*, right?

When parents remarry, they often have hopes that their new family will be a lot like the old one. Unfortunately, there are going to be some real differences between your new family and your old one. That's not to say that it can't be a happy family, but it's important to understand some of the wrinkles you'll be dealing with.

In a remarried family, parenting is no longer solely the domain of the married couple; there's going to be at least one biological parent and possibly other stepparents in different households, not to mention both grandparents and step-grandparents. In this way, the remarried family is a more open system than a nuclear family. Typically, there are children moving in and out of the household for visitation, so the question of who's actually in the family is not always crystal clear.

Not all the members of a remarried family have always been together, so it's likely they have different ways of doing things. In a nuclear family, kids don't question that their parents are indeed the parents. In a remarried family, the parents may not have been together long enough to reach a consensus about parenting issues; the kids may not accept parenting from the stepparents. This can be hard on adults as well as children.

In a nuclear family, relatives and friends usually recognize all family members as a family. When you remarry, they may see you and your children as family, but not "him and those kids of his." That your new family isn't accepted by your extended family is hard. It's also important to know that the law doesn't recognize stepparent relationships. You can grow close to a stepchild over a number of years, but if you divorce the stepchild's biological parent, the law gives you no rights to visitation.

Strong themes of loss recur in remarried families. Both parents and children come from other families that are no longer intact. If these losses have not been worked through, there may be continued fears of loss and abandonment, and emotional scars. If the parents are still at odds with their ex-spouses, the children will suffer from conflicting loyalties, and the new marriage can suffer as well. What often happens is that the children end up in the middle, often being used as spies between one household and the other. It's extremely important for all adults involved—the married couple and their ex-spouses—to cooperate with each other in a fair and frank manner with regard to the children.

When children enter a remarried family where there are other children, their rank in the family is often changed. For instance, the oldest child may become the second child. Suddenly, the role of each child is unclear. It's also important to note that because step-siblings are not blood relatives, the incest taboo is not as clear.

These are just a few of the dynamics that can make a remarried family very different from a nuclear family. We aren't trying to scare you away from entering into a remarried family, but we are trying to help you see that some of the intense feelings and complications that will come up are entirely normal. And there are some things you can do to minimize the difficulties.

Before entering into a remarried family, it's important that all members have recovered from past losses. Your children may need to talk about your ex-spouse, and you may need to let them, regardless of how you feel about him or her.

Before you all move in together, there are some steps you can take to ease the transition:

- All individuals who will make up the new family need to be open about their fears. You all need to listen to each other. Know that it's going to take time for all of you to adjust to new roles and a different household.

- Co-parenting relationships need to be maintained in a cooperative way with ex-spouses. This is important if loyalty conflicts are to be prevented. Kids need to hear that even though Mommy and Daddy don't want to be together anymore, they both love and care about their children.

- Plan space for children in all households where they will be staying; it's very disconcerting for them not to have a space of their own.

- Make sure everyone on all sides of the family (your family, your ex-spouse's family, and your new spouse's family) understands your new situation.

- Make emotional room for all the new relationships and roles.

To complete a healthy transition once you have all moved in together, you will need to accept that this is a different sort of family, one where roles will shift as different family members (for example, ex-spouses, and children who may not live with you all the time) come in and out of your life. Allow and encourage your new family to share memories and histories together. This will help all of you to integrate and become a family. It's important for children to know that the past has not been forgotten or negated by this new family. Don't overreact and become defensive if your stepchild compares you with his biological parent. Take time to establish a friendly relationship with stepchildren; don't jump into a disciplinary role too quickly, especially with older children. It's also important that you and your spouse support each other in parenting roles; if you don't, the children will sense it and play each of you against the other.

## The Development of Love

It's not uncommon to enter into remarriage with the expectation that if you love your spouse, you will of course love his or her children. There are many reasons why "instant love" between parent and stepchild doesn't necessarily happen. The most basic is that those who have never had children may not have experienced being close to a child.

Very often, "instant love" is an unrealistic expectation that causes us to try to be Superparents. It's not uncommon to feel guilty about loving your own children more than your stepchildren. If you find yourself in this situation, it might be helpful to talk to a counselor or other supportive professional who can help you clarify the discrepancies that may exist between your beliefs and expectations and what is realistic. It may also be helpful for your spouse to consider whether his or her expectations may be inhibiting you from establishing a genuine relationship with your spouse's children. A stepparent is not a parent, but ultimately you and your stepchildren will build bonds that will reflect the unique relationship you have with them.

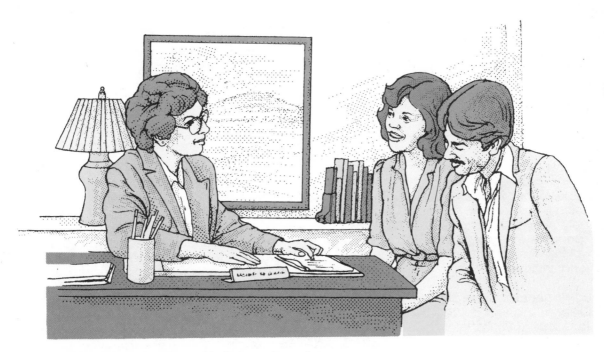

*Adoption agencies are useful, but stringent in their requirements.*

### Yours, Mine, Ours, and Theirs

The decision of a remarried couple to have children of their own often helps harmonize relationships between step-siblings, probably because the blood relationship that all the siblings now have in common with the new child strengthens bonds. However, sometimes the step-siblings feel unimportant or left out. Complicating things further, about the same time you and your new spouse are having children, your ex-spouses may have remarried and may also be having children. So your biological child now has a half-sibling by your remarriage, a half-sibling by your ex-spouse's remarriage, and step-siblings by your spouse's ex-spouse's remarriage. If this is confusing for you to read, imagine what it's like for the children, especially if they're young! It may be helpful to sit down and map out a family tree. This will help the children better understand who's who, and will also help clear up some of your own confusion.

Remarried families are very complex. Each additional member of the family system allows for another relationship or another role with every other member in the system. There can be biological parents and grandparents, stepparents and step-grandparents, siblings, half-siblings, and step-siblings. No wonder this becomes confusing! With this many people in a family and so many differ-ent kinds of relationships between these people, there's a lot of potential for stress. There's also an increased potential for a large support network if everyone communicates and cooperates. The rewards can be enormous.

## Adoption

It used to be that there were hundreds of abandoned infants who needed parents. Due to legalized abortion, more widespread use of birth control, and decreased stigma for unwed mothers, this is no longer the case. If you want to take the traditional route of adopting a child through an agency, there may be several years' wait—*if* you qualify. But there are other avenues—private adoption, foreign adoption, open adoption, and independent adoption—none of them without perils. You'll need to ask yourself how much money you're willing to spend and what you're willing to endure.

Before you begin, contact someone you know who has already adopted. If you don't know any adoptive parents, contact your local library or human services agency for information on a local adoption support group. You will get lots of time-saving information from others who have been through the process. They'll tell you which agencies to avoid, and which agencies can best serve your set of circumstances.

## Adoption Agencies

Don't kid yourself. If you're going to go through an adoption agency, know that each agency has its own profile of what it considers to be the "perfect parents." If you don't fit that profile—and an interviewer can tell with a few pointed questions—you won't even be given an application. The agency's profile will weigh factors pertaining to your age, stability, and parenting ability. If your application is satisfactory, you will be interviewed extensively. A social worker will be sent to your home, perhaps for several visits to do a home study, which involves being asked for a great deal of personal information.

Though agencies generally won't arrange for nontraditional parents (older couples, singles, gays) to adopt, if you're interested in a special-needs child (defined as a child who is older, or handicapped in some way), an agency may be willing to work with you.

Agency fees usually work on a sliding scale and range from a few hundred dollars to about five thousand dollars.

## Private Adoptions

Private adoptions are usually arranged by lawyers who bring together parents who want to adopt and mothers who plan to give up their babies. Before considering this route, know the law. In some states, it is illegal to have an intermediate party search for the child, even though it may be legal for *you* to search for the child.

A private adoption is sometimes the fastest way to locate an infant, and it often gives the biological mother a way to learn something about the adoptive parents. However, some agencies say that private adoption does not allow for a good home study, since the lawyers involved are chiefly concerned with the money that will change hands. In many cases, the lawyer represents both the adoptive parents and the birth mother, which usually means the birth mother doesn't get proper counseling or legal representation.

Private adoption fees range from $3,500 to ten thousand dollars. Additionally, you often have to pay the birth mother's medical expenses.

## Foreign Adoptions

Foreign adoptions can be arranged through traditional as well as specialized agencies. They can also be arranged by dealing directly with foreign agencies or intermediaries. Most recent foreign adoptions were from India, Latin America, the Philippines, and South Korea. Western European babies are even more scarce than babies from the United States.

Because there are more layers of bureaucracy to cut through—lawyers in both countries, both governments, and, most likely, an orphanage—there's a greater potential for problems in foreign adoption. And foreign adoptions can be quite costly—up to fifteen thousand dollars. Worse, there is occasional fraud in the foreign adoption business, and you could stand to lose your money. However, if all goes well, a foreign adoption can be arranged in as little as nine months.

The best route to take for a foreign adoption is to work through well-established organizations. There are several publications that will guide you:

- The Latin America Parents Association (P. O. Box 72, Seaford, NY 11783) will send you a list of dependable adoption agencies and orphanages in Central and South America.

- If you want to deal directly with agencies that specialize in South Korean adoptions, write to: Holt International Children's Services, P. O. Box 2880, Eugene, OR 97402.

- The U.S. Government Printing Office publishes a booklet entitled "The Immigration of Adopted and Prospective Adoptive Children." Write to the Superintendent of Documents, U.S. Government Printing Office, Washington, DC 20402-9325. Current price is $1.75. The office recommends you call (202-783-3238) before writing for the booklet to check availability and price.

If you're a single or otherwise nontraditional parent, foreign adoption will be more open to you in some countries than in others.

## Open Adoptions

Open adoption means something different to every agency. For instance, the birth mother and the adoptive parents can conceivably have an ongoing relationship after the adoption. In most instances, though; open adoption means that the birth mother is allowed to write a letter to her child that the adoptive parents will present to the child at a certain time, or that an agreement is made to exchange pictures without names and addresses.

Open adoption is easier on the birth mother, since her existence is acknowledged. This may help reduce her grief after the adoption has taken place because she knows at least a little bit about her baby's situation. When birth mothers have less apprehension, they're less likely to try to find their children later on.

## Independent Adoptions

Independent adoption means that you pay the medical and legal expenses for a pregnant woman who will be giving up her child. While this can be fast, allowing you to bypass agency red tape and restrictions, it can be emotionally devastating if the biological mother changes her mind at the last minute. Also, the adoption is not final until a judge signs the adoption papers when the baby is between six months and a year old. Keep in mind that each state has different laws about how long birth parents have the right to change their minds. If things work out, though, independent adoption can be a beautiful experience. You may get to take the baby home right from the hospital, whereas with most other adoption methods you may not see the chid before she's a month old. You also have greater intimacy and control, since you will know the birth mother during her pregnancy. Some adopting couples have actually assisted in the delivery!

The first step in an independent adoption is to find a birth mother. This is easier said than done, but you can start by notifying relatives and friends. Other connections might be social workers, members of the clergy, and doctors. The important thing is to let lots of people know you're looking. If you contact the National Adoption Exchange (1218 Chestnut Street, Philadelphia, PA 19107), they'll put you in touch with local independent adoption groups.

*Know your state law.* We can't stress this enough. An oversight with regard to the law can overturn an adoption. How long do birth parents have a right to change their minds in your state? Is it permissible to bring a baby into your state from another? With interstate adoptions, it's likely you'll need to be in compliance with the Interstate Compact on the Placement of Children, which oper-

ates in all parts of the country except New Jersey and Washington, DC. Does the law allow for you to have an intermediary (someone to help you connect with the birth mother) in your state? Whether or not you can have a lawyer as an intermediary, you'll need one to advise you about the law and to do the paperwork.

Costs for independent adoptions can be less than those for private agency adoptions. Usually, you will pay the birth mother's medical and legal expenses. Some state laws allow you to pay her living expenses. Whatever you do pay, make sure you document it, because things like new cars for the biological mother may suggest baby-buying to a judge, and that's illegal.

## Explaining Adoption

While an adopted infant does not inquire about her origins, an adopted toddler—like any toddler—may. Direct answers to the queries of adopted children are always best, but remember that a child under the age of three hasn't the comprehension of an older child. Simple, truthful answers to your toddler's questions will satisfy her. "You grew inside your mother, and now you're our little girl," is one example. As your child grows older, your answers to her questions will become progressively more complex.

Other family members—especially an adopted child's siblings, and particularly those who are your natural children—should be included in your plan of simple truthfulness. Never try to hide facts about adoption from any of your children. To do so invites misunderstanding and painful future revelations.

## Finding a Support Group

At some point, you're probably going to want more information about some aspect of childbirth, parenthood, child development, or family life. For that reason, we've included this list of contacts. Keep in mind that our list provides the names of national organizations. If you can't find the local chapter of an organization in your phone book, the national office will be able to give you addresses and phone numbers. Many of these organizations maintain extensive libraries in their areas of interest, so they can be a very good source of information. More often than not, if they don't have the information you're looking for, they will know where you can get it.

# FAMILY STRUCTURE

| ORGANIZATION | PURPOSE |
|---|---|
| **Action for Children's Television**<br>20 University Road<br>Cambridge, MA 02138<br>617-876-6620 | National organization with local groups supporting and advocating quality children's TV programming. |
| **ALMA (Adoptees' Liberty Movement Association) Society**<br>P. O. Box 154<br>Washington Bridge Station<br>New York, NY 10033<br>212-581-1568 | Helps adoptees and natural parents search for each other. |
| **American Academy of Pediatrics**<br>141 Northwest Point Road<br>Elk Grove, IL 60007<br>312-228-5005 | Doctors engaged in health care and medical treatment of children and youth. |
| **American Red Cross**<br>17th and D Streets NW<br>Washington, DC 20006<br>202-737-8300 | International and community emergency services. |
| **American Speech and Hearing Association**<br>10801 Rockville Pike<br>Rockville, MD 20852<br>301-897-5700 | Specialists in speech and language pathology and audiology. |
| **Association for Childbirth at Home, International**<br>P. O. Box 39498<br>Los Angeles, CA 90039<br>213-667-0839 | Provides referral service to doctors, nurses, and midwives, and classes for home birth. |
| **Association for Retarded Citizens**<br>P. O. Box 6109<br>Arlington, TX 76005<br>817-640-0204 | Promotes treatment, research, understanding, and legislation; advocates family services. |
| **C/SEC, Inc. (Cesarean/Support, Education and Concern)**<br>22 Forest Road<br>Framingham, MA 01701<br>617-877-8266 | Provides emotional and physical support and education, and addresses of local support groups to parents who have had cesarean births. |
| **Child Help USA**<br>Box 630<br>Hollywood, CA 90028<br>800-422-4453 | Offers child-abuse counseling and referrals to legal services. |
| **Child Welfare League of America, Inc.**<br>67 Irving Place<br>New York, NY 10003<br>212-254-7410 | Advocates improved services for deprived, dependent, or neglected children and families. |
| **Committee for Single Adoptive Parents**<br>P. O. Box 15084<br>Chevy Chase, MD 20815 | Publishes source list and handbook for single adoptive parents. |

| ORGANIZATION | PURPOSE |
|---|---|
| **Compassionate Friends**<br>P. O. Box 3696<br>Oak Brook, IL 60522-3696<br>312-990-0010 | Chapters provide informal self-help for parents who have experienced the death of a child; aids parents in positive resolution of grief. |
| **Council for Exceptional Children**<br>1920 Association Drive<br>Reston, VA 22091<br>703-620-3660 | Concerned with education of handicapped and gifted children; provides information and sponsors workshops, conferences, and advocates. Their Division for Early Childhood (same address) is dedicated to education and development issues concerning handicapped children and infants. |
| **Family Services Association of America, Inc.**<br>254 W. 31st Street<br>New York, NY 10001<br>212-967-2740 | Federation of local agencies and groups that provide family counseling, family life education, advocacy, and programs focusing on parenting, mental health, and marital issues. |
| **Fatherhood Project**<br>c/o Bank Street College<br>of Education<br>610 W. 112th Street<br>New York, NY 10025<br>212-663-7200 | Encourages male involvement with childbearing and serves as a national clearinghouse for information on father-participation programs. |
| **International Childbirth Education Association**<br>P. O. Box 20048<br>Minneapolis, MN 55420<br>612-854-8660 | Furthers educational, physical, and emotional preparation for childbirth and breast-feeding. |
| **La Leche League International**<br>9616 Minneapolis Avenue<br>P. O. Box 1209<br>Franklin Park, IL 60131-8209<br>312-455-7730 | Advocate of breast-feeding; local groups emphasize good mothering through breast-feeding. |
| **Maternity Center Association**<br>48 E. 92nd Street<br>New York, NY 10128<br>212-369-7300 | For improvement of maternal care, mother and infant health, and family life. |
| **Mothers at Home**<br>P. O. Box 2208<br>Merrifield, VA 22116<br>703-352-2292 | Supports mothers who choose to stay home to raise families. |
| **Mothers Without Custody**<br>P. O. Box 56762<br>Houston, TX 77027<br>713-840-1622 | Supports mothers living apart from minor children; helps establish local self-help groups. |
| **National Adoption Hotline**<br>2025 M Street NW Suite 512<br>Washington, DC 20036<br>202-463-7563 (hotline)<br>202-463-7559 (office) | Offers agency resource list to prospective adoptive couples, and to mothers who wish to give up their children for adoption. |

continued

# FAMILY STRUCTURE

continued

| ORGANIZATION | PURPOSE |
|---|---|
| **National Association of Parents and Professionals for Safe Alternatives in Childbirth (NAPSAC)**<br>P. O. Box 428<br>Marble Hill, MO 63764<br>314-238-2010 | Dedicated to establishing family-centered, medically safe childbirth programs. Promotes natural childbirth education. |
| **National Committee for Prevention of Child Abuse**<br>332 S. Michigan Avenue<br>Suite 950<br>Chicago, IL 60604<br>312-663-3520 | Provides information dealing with child abuse prevention and parenting. |
| **National Congress of Parents and Teachers (PTA)**<br>700 N. Rush Street<br>Chicago, IL 60611<br>312-787-0977 | Interested in cooperation among home, school, and community on behalf of youth and children. Advocates of legislation to benefit children. |
| **National Easter Seal Society**<br>2023 W. Ogden Avenue<br>Chicago, IL 60612<br>312-243-8400 | State and local societies support people with disabilities. Disseminates information. |
| **National Foundation–The March of Dimes**<br>1275 Mamaroneck Avenue<br>White Plains, NY 10605<br>914-428-7100 | Promotes prevention of birth defects. Offers educational programs and helps local groups establish prenatal care and related services. |
| **National Organization of Adolescent Pregnancy and Parenting**<br>P. O. Box 2365<br>Reston, VA 22090<br>703-435-3948 | Promotes services, prevention, and resolution of teen parenting problems. |
| **National Organization of Mothers of Twins Club**<br>12404 Princess Jeanne NE<br>Albuquerque, NM 87112<br>505-275-0955 | Will help you locate local support groups for mothers who have had multiple births. |
| **National Sudden Infant Death Syndrome Foundation**<br>Two Metro Plaza, Suite 205<br>8240 Professional Place<br>Landover, MD 20785<br>301-459-3388 | Concerned with SIDS; assists bereaved parents and families of high-risk infants; supports research. |

| ORGANIZATION | PURPOSE |
|---|---|
| **North American Council on Adoptive Children**<br>P.O. Box 14808<br>Minneapolis, MN 55414<br>Send self-addressed stamped envelope for reply. | Supports adoptions of special-needs children, including older, handicapped, and disabled youngsters. Refers individuals to local support groups. |
| **Parents of Premature and High-Risk Infants International**<br>University of Utah Health Sciences Center<br>50 N. Medical Drive<br>Room 2A210<br>Salt Lake City, UT 84132<br>801-581-5323 | Supports efforts of parents forming and maintaining local groups; facilitates communication between groups; offers resources and information. |
| **Parents Without Partners**<br>8807 Colesville Road<br>Silver Spring, MD 20910<br>301-588-9354 | Local support groups for single parents; provides information and publishes manuals, bibliographies, resource lists, and brochures, as well as a monthly magazine. |
| **Planned Parenthood Federation of America**<br>810 7th Avenue<br>New York, NY 10019<br>212-541-7800 | Operates 750 centers across the U.S. Centers offer counseling, contraceptives, and practical information. |
| **Self-Help Center**<br>1600 Dodge Avenue<br>Evanston, IL 60201<br>312-328-0470 | Provides information and publishes directory of numerous self-help organizations. |
| **Single Mothers by Choice**<br>P. O. Box 7788 FDR Station<br>New York, NY 10150<br>212-988-0993 | Support and information for single women who have decided to have children outside marriage. Also provides support and information for single men and women considering adoption. |
| **Stepfamily Association of America, Inc.**<br>602 E. Joppa Road<br>Baltimore, MD 21204<br>301-823-7570 | Educational organization providing information and support for step-families. Acts as support network and national advocate for stepparents, remarried parents, and their children. |
| **United Cerebral Palsy Association**<br>66 E. 34th St.<br>New York, NY 10016<br>212-481-6300 | National organization of state and local affiliates helping individuals with cerebral palsy and their families. |
| **U.S. Consumer Product Safety Commission**<br>Washington, DC 20207<br>800-638-CPSC | Call their toll-free number for information on safety standards for cribs, toys, and other children's accessories. Area offices in major cities. |

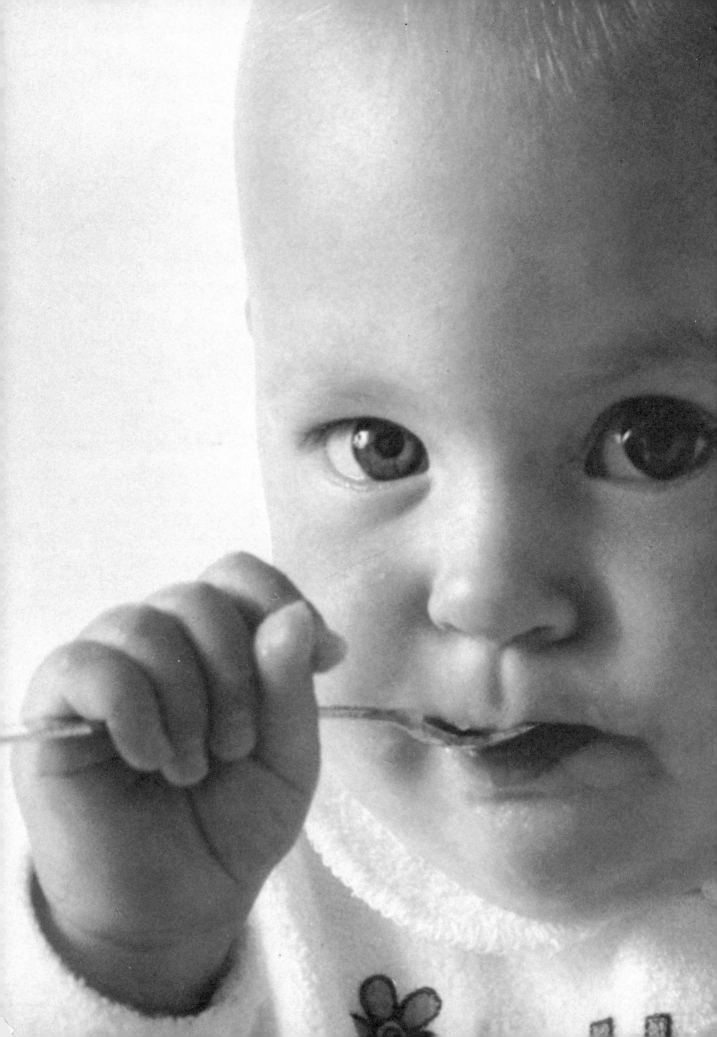

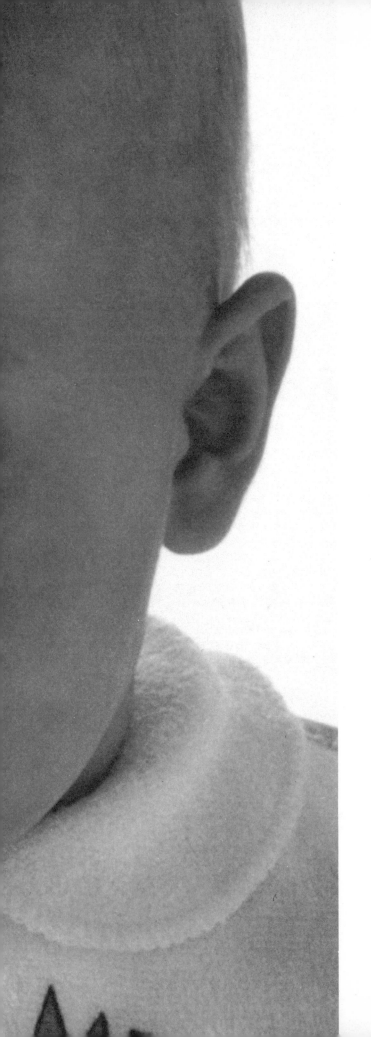

# Chapter 13:
# The Road to
# Independence

## Becoming a Person

For your child, the journey to independence is an exciting, frequently frustrating, and sometimes frightening adventure. By the time your child is three years old, she will have made remarkable developmental strides—some willingly, others less so. These strides are not only intellectual (as discussed in Chapter 11), but social and emotional as well. Though still dependent upon you for many things, your three-year-old will have begun to establish her sense of self. She will have tested the limits and boundaries in her life, and will have left many of them behind. In her first three years, she will establish many of the elements of her adult personality. In short, she will become a person.

As your baby grows and progresses, you will change, in her eyes, as surely as her self-concept will change. As she becomes more perceptive and more aware of herself as a separate entity, she will cast you in a variety of roles. Some of these roles, such as care-giver and disciplinarian, will continue for many years. Other roles you'll play—such as that of the omnipotent creature who "ceases to exist" when your baby cannot see you—are transitory.

Your awareness of the whys and hows of your child's ever-changing concept of herself and of you can make your child's journey to a healthy independence an easier one for all concerned.

## The Parent-Infant Bond

Given the opportunity, parents and babies naturally form a strong relationship with each other. This relationship is often called the parent-infant bond. For the parent, this bond is woven of love and responsibility. For the infant, it is his first—and perhaps most important—relationship.

Psychoanalysts have theorized that the first love relationship a baby experiences with a parent sets the stage for all later interpersonal relationships. They contend that if you don't have this necessary relationship in your formative years, you won't be able to love as an adult. A number of psychologists and psychiatrists have found support for this view. For example, John Bowlby, a British psychoanalyst, studied children growing up without parents in the first years of life; these children often had problems relating with others and forming bonds later in life. From such studies, psychologists have recognized what parents knew all along—how important sensitive, responsive, and consistent parenting is to the healthy development of a child.

However, it is also important to point out that babies may not have to be with their parents all the time, despite the current emphasis in Lamaze classes and parents' magazines on the position that there is a "critical period" for parents to bond to their babies. Supporters of this position state that parents who are separated from their newborns after birth will have difficulty forming that essential parent-infant bond. Citing studies conducted with animals, they point out that mother mice will often refuse to care for their young if they are separated right after birth. Fortunately, humans are not mice, and more recent research suggests that human mothers generally are quite able to go on to be good mothers even if they have to be separated from their babies as a result of prematurity, illness, or other reasons.

Nonetheless, positive changes have occurred because of recent recognition of the process of bonding. Many hospitals have dramatically humanized the way in which parents and babies are treated. Parents are allowed greater contact with babies, particularly in intensive care nurseries. There, parents can now often participate in the feeding, handling, and general care of their babies right away, instead of waiting until their infants are released from the hospital.

## Birth to Two Months

From the moment of birth, there are already characteristics of both you and your baby that allow you to begin developing a special relationship. Newborn babies themselves are very effective at getting their parents and other adults to take care of them.

### Physical Appearance

Have you ever noticed that most animal babies are considered cute and cuddly? Some scientists believe that this is nature's way of ensuring that animals (including human beings) care for their young. This is why your baby's physical appearance alone makes you feel warm and good inside. His large head and rounded features make him look "cuter" and more "babyish." In fact, the more any baby has these kinds of features, the more positively he is seen by adults in general. Studies report that adults look at chubbier babies more and express a greater desire to play with and take care of them. Even parents have been found to be more responsive to their children when they are "cute" than when they are not. Apparently, new babies endear themselves to their parents and grandparents, in part at least, just by the way they look.

### Reflexes

Many of a newborn's reflexes (unlearned behavior patterns) serve to ensure physical proximity to his mother. During your baby's first examination, your pediatrician may demonstrate how your baby's hand forms into a tight grasp around your fingers. In the early months, the grasp reflex is so strong that your baby can almost support his own weight. When a newborn is startled by a loud noise or a sudden change in position, his arms flail out to the side and then are quickly brought together, as if he were trying to grab onto his mother. This reflex is called the Moro, or startle, reflex. This and other reflexes are believed to be remnants from our evolutionary ancestry.

## The Cry

Any parent can tell you that a baby's crying is a very unsettling sound, one that is not easy to tune out. Although annoying, your baby's cry should be thought of as her first means of communicating with you.

Crying is a highly adaptive response from an evolutionary viewpoint, probably designed to get the care-giver to attend to the baby's needs. In fact, four out of five times that a parent interacts with her baby, it is because the baby cried. Crying alerts you to your baby's needs. Most parents quickly respond by trying to find out what is wrong, checking to see if the baby is cold, wet, or hungry, or if she is just bored. In fact, babies may have different cries for different reasons. Parents can often recognize what their babies' cries mean.

Many parents think they can actually identify their newborns by their cries. This may be an accurate perception. Psychologists have studied the acoustical features of individual babies' cries with sophisticated technology—spectrographs that record sound patterns. They have found that babies may be identifiable by unique "cryprints."

Although all babies cry, wide variations occur in how much time a baby spends crying. Some babies may have "three-month colic"; others may cry only when distressed, hungry, angry, or in pain. Fortunately, by three months most babies will dramatically reduce the amount of time they spend crying.

You can help your baby to cry less. It has been found that parents who quickly attend to their babies' crying by picking them up during the first three months seem to have babies who cry less at nine months. Contrary to old wives' tales, you are not "spoiling" your baby by comforting her and relieving her crying.

What works to soothe a crying baby varies depending on your baby's age. Once you have determined that your baby is warm, dry, and fed, age-old soothing techniques can be employed; and these will change with your child's developmental changes. Of course, the best way to quiet a young baby is to pick her up. Next comes hold-ing a very young baby so that she can look over your shoulder, combining closeness and distraction. Newborns also like to be swaddled in receiving blankets. Rocking, giving something to suck, and providing some sort of auditory stimulation, like music, will help reduce newborns' crying about half the time. Sometimes, touching your baby or just being nearby can make her stop crying.

## Looking Patterns

Although a newborn baby can't see things very clearly from a distance, he is quite able to see your face when you hold him in your arms. In fact, that's about all he can see. Newborns tend to look at areas of high contrast (like a black object against a white background) and the outside of images (like a hairline on a face). Thus, a parent's face is an optimal visual stimulus for a baby.

## "Cuddliness"

When you hold your new baby, you may notice that he naturally molds his body to cuddle with you. This molding ensures maximal body contact between the two of you and makes you feel warm and tingly.

Unfortunately, not all babies like to cuddle as much as their parents would like, but may squirm in their parents' arms. This may just be their nature—and not a reflection of parenting skills. Developmental tests of infants, such as the Brazelton Neonatal Behavioral Assessment Scale, measure newborns' reactions. In one of the tests babies are rated from "very resistant to being held" to "extremely cuddly and clinging." One study indicated that mothers had difficulty teaching "resistive" newborn babies to cuddle. The more a mother tried to cuddle an unwilling baby, the less the baby cuddled. If your baby does not want to be cuddled all the time, don't be alarmed or assume you're doing something wrong. Remember that your baby is an individual, and adjust your desire to cuddle him to his responsiveness to being cuddled.

## Two to Three Months

### Your Baby Begins to Look More at You

At two to three months, babies look more at their parents than at strangers. This helps you feel that your baby has formed a preference for you, which, in turn, strengthens your affection and love for your baby.

In actuality, of course, babies begin to look more at their parents because they see them the most—they recognize them. Hence, you become one of the first memories your baby constructs. Babies also like to watch things that change a little bit each time they look at them. Because faces change all the time, your face is an ideal stimulus.

Babies at this age are beginning to "understand" what faces are. Two-month-olds can differentiate pictures with scrambled faces from those with faces with correctly placed features. By three months, babies may be able to discriminate facial expressions well enough to identify the eyes, nose, and mouth. Also, your baby will start to remember you and recognize you in other ways.

### The Social Smile

Not only do babies smile more, they begin to smile socially—that is, they smile at people more than at things. These early smiles probably reflect more the fact that faces are familiar objects than that a truly social process is taking place. Nevertheless, when you smile at your baby, your baby can smile in response. There is nothing like those first smiles to make you fall in love with your baby all over again.

### Your Baby Becomes a More Active Participant

In "talking" to their infants, parents perform what in adult conversations would be socially inappropriate behaviors just to get their babies to look and smile at them. We make all sorts of exaggerated, funny faces when we look at our babies. The routine parents go through with their babies has been described as a "dance." Your baby looks at you, locks his eyes on yours, and then looks away. You then use your routine of funny faces to get your baby to look back at you. It is as if the two of you are taking turns in a finely tuned conversation or dialogue.

By three months, your baby will assume a greater role as the initiator of the sequences of play and interaction. In the first month, your baby followed your lead; at three months your baby can begin the dance as well.

### Your Baby Becomes Adjusted to Your Rhythms

Your two-month-old is beginning to adjust to your biological rhythms. Most babies will now sleep through the night and feed more regularly and less often. Failure to make these adjustments to your sleeping and waking patterns can be a major source of strain on your relationship with your baby and your spouse. Especially fatigued parents have a hard time enjoying their babies. If your baby continues crying excessively and does not seem to be falling into any sort of routine with you, a call to the pediatrician might be in order.

## Four to Five Months

### Special Smiles

Special smiles just for parents begin appearing at four months. A smile will spread across your baby's face when he sees you, but not anyone else. This behavior implies not only recognition of you—a cognitive skill—but also recognition of your specialness—a social skill. This, of course, produces an incredibly strong emotional response from you. It makes it more fun for you to be with your baby and play with him. In fact, it may be hard for you to pull yourself away to do household chores or return to work. This, in turn, brings great benefits to your baby, providing him with two ready playmates to teach him the many things he needs to learn.

### Babbling and Cooing

Isn't it wonderful to hear a baby beginning to make sounds, to coo and babble as you jiggle him up and down? Your baby's babbling and cooing evoke a strong response from you, just as his smiling does. Your play begins to take on a real conversational quality. Now, each of you is more likely to take a turn—you respond to your baby's cooing with words and funny faces, and your baby answers with more cooing and babbling.

### Laughing

Some babies begin to laugh even before four months, some as early as five weeks. Laughing occurs about a month after your baby first smiles. A sudden, intense (perhaps surprising) stimulus can make a baby laugh.

But you may notice that sometimes your baby is not sure whether to laugh or cry. Laughter appears to be an emotion on the cutting edge of fear. Theories regarding laughter suggest that babies laugh at things that are almost, but not entirely, understandable to them. Things that are too confusing, however, will make them cry. Four- to six-month-olds tend to laugh more at things that touch them (like tickling) and talk to them (like you saying silly things).

Your baby's laughing helps form an emotional link between the two of you, making your play a lot of fun. We like to see babies laugh, so we repeat whatever we did to get them to laugh again and again. By doing this, your baby is learning to gain some control over his environment. Through laughing, babies can also learn the kind of effect they have on other people.

## Feeding and Sucking

By four months, in all probability, either your baby has found his fingers or thumb to suck on between feedings or you have offered him a pacifier. Several factors may influence the amount of time your baby spends sucking just for fun. More sucking is likely to occur, particularly with breast-fed babies, when you begin to wean your baby. (Oftentimes, weaning is more difficult for the mother than the baby. That special dependency relationship may be difficult to leave behind.)

When teeth begin to erupt, you may see your baby chew more on hands, fingers, and any available toys. Weaning and teething frequently take place simultaneously because of baby's biting.

Most babies like to suck on something between and during meals. If babies have the good fortune to find their own thumbs—some do this as early as three weeks—they may be able to calm themselves down. Nonnutritive sucking (sucking for pleasure and not for nutrition) is one of your baby's first means of exploration. Babies use their mouths for exploring the world by touching and tasting all sorts of things.

People used to think that the amount of sucking that babies did would have lasting effects on their personalities and behavioral patterns. For example, some thought that babies who didn't suck enough because of bottle-feeding (or because the holes in the nipples were running too fast) would grow up to have "oral" personalities and would be thumb-sucking school-age children and smoking adolescents.

These early theories have not been upheld. How babies were fed or weaned makes little difference in their later personality development. Frequent sucking also doesn't seem to have any effect on emotional development (or on dental development, until the permanent teeth start coming in), so there is no need to continually remove your baby's thumb from his mouth or deny him a pacifier. In fact, it is impossible to keep babies from sucking when they want to; some babies will suck even when they have nothing in their mouths.

The upshot of professional studies is that a child's emotional development and stability are not related to how she was fed. Also, weaning has not been found to have long-term, resounding ill effects, either psychological or physical, on well-fed babies. Rather, such issues as parental warmth, maternal responsiveness, and the level of conflict in the home are related to development of secure relationships.

## Problems in Interaction

By as early as four months, your baby is beginning to develop a specific relationship with you. Your patterns of play with your baby help you to form a lasting bond. But problems can occur in parent-baby play.

Problems in interaction can best be viewed as a breakdown in the play sequence—a misstep in the dance—such that mutuality (a back-and-forth togetherness) and turn-taking are inhibited. Sometimes, the break is obvious to all concerned—as in child neglect and abuse. More often, problems may be very subtle and can be identified only through frame-by-frame analysis of videotapes of parents with their babies. Some babies and parents show a beautiful rhythmicity and "dance" in their play, while others appear "out of step." The misstep appears when what you expect to happen next just doesn't happen. An example of this kind of misstep is seen with a mother who turns away just as her baby starts to smile at her. Problems can arise because the baby isn't learning that he can control his mother's behavior through appropriate social behaviors of his own. Psychologists would say that the partners in such an interaction are "noncontingent"—that is, one partner's response has nothing to do with the other partner's signal. Babies experiencing this type of interaction can "learn helplessness": no matter what their signal is, they are unable to adequately control their environment (in this example, the mother's response). For this reason, it is essential that all parents react sensitively to their babies' signals.

Another problem can occur if one partner in the interaction is overwhelming. Some parents "turn off" their babies by working too hard to sustain their attention. If, for example, a mother continues to intrude on her baby, moving closer and trying to coax a smile, even while the baby signals that she doesn't want to play, the mother is dominating the interaction by not allowing her baby a chance to be an equal partner.

There can also be a problem with the match between the personality style of the parent and the activity level of the baby.

Unfortunately, there are no set rules or easy answers for the "right way" to play with your baby, except to be sensitive to your baby's particular characteristics. Some babies are far more difficult to parent than others. Sometimes, just knowing why babies respond in the way that they do is enough to free parents from any misgivings they may be having and help them get back on the right track. The best advice you may ever receive as first-time parents is to relax, have fun, and enjoy your baby!

### Recognizing Your Child's Uniqueness

Every baby is different. Some of these differences come from you and the kind of environment you provide. But some of these differences seem to come with the baby at birth. One of these inborn differences is in his temperament, or behavioral style—that is, whether a child is "easy" or "difficult" or "slow to warm up." Considering temperament is important because, unfortunately, gross mismatches occur occasionally between the temperaments of parents and their infants. These parents are bound, therefore, to "go against the grain" when trying to set limits for their children.

An "easy" baby shows biological regularity (in feeding, sleeping, and eliminating), predictable behavior, and adaptability. Almost any parent finds this kind of baby easy to get along with because she quickly adjusts to parental routines and expectations.

The "difficult" child, on the other hand, withdraws from new situations, has negative and intense moods, and adapts slowly. Although some parents take great pleasure in this type of baby, describing their baby's difficultness as "vigor" and "lustiness," more frequently, parents and teachers of "difficult" children feel threatened, anxious, and inept. If yours is such a child, it is important to keep in mind that your baby's personality is probably not your fault. A difficult baby's temperament often exists independent of parental attitudes and of management techniques.

Although the "slow-to-warm-up" child is somewhere in the middle, this baby sometimes causes more confusion for parents than either the "easy" or the "difficult" baby. These babies may be frustrating because their behavior is often so unpredictable. At times, they are a joy to be with, but changes in routine seem to throw them, causing great difficulty for their parents.

Your child's temperament influences the behavior and attitudes of peers, siblings, children, parents, and teachers. How your child "fits" with these significant people in his daily life will dictate his patterns of adjustment to new situations. If you think that a poor "fit" may be detracting from your baby's opportunities for growth and development, you might ask your pediatrician about the available parent-infant programs in your community. Parent-infant educators can often suggest some techniques to help make parenting easier.

## Six to Twelve Months

### Face Recognition

By seven months, your baby may have begun to respond differently to different people. This happens as babies sharpen their visual perceptual skills and learn to recognize people by their faces, by seeing either a full face or a profile. Face recognition is a gradual process acquired over the first eight months of life. Some babies can read their parents' facial expressions too, because they are able to see subtle differences in faces. As with many developmental acquisitions, visual discrimination and perception of faces help your baby to maintain contact with you.

### Stranger Anxiety

By six months (sometimes earlier), your baby may have developed a very clear and strong

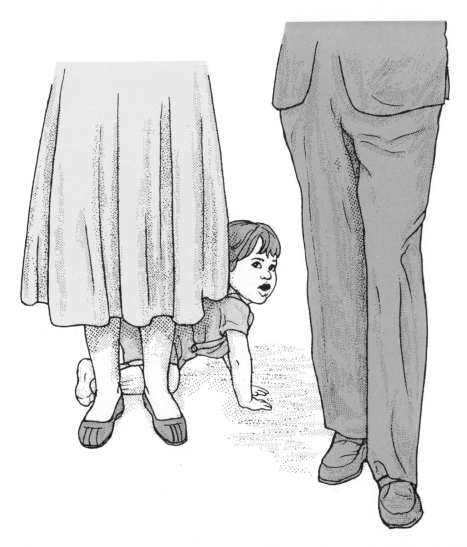

*Stranger anxiety of one sort or another is common among children aged six months to twelve months.*

preference for one parent or the other. This preference is exemplified by your baby's crying and clinging to you as a new adult approaches—"stranger anxiety." Babies in our culture often show at least some form of stranger anxiety.

One baby who had to be hospitalized for a short period of time quickly learned to cry hysterically at all people in blue coats because some of them were doctors and nurses who were sticking him with needles. Just think how much cognitive processing occurred inside the baby's head for him to make those associations.

Another baby who only infrequently saw his grandmother cried as she approached to hold him. It is natural for grandparents to feel rejected

by a grandchild's crying, but if the phenomenon is placed in the context of normal development, they should understand. If you have this problem, suggest that they wait a while to become reacquainted with your baby before picking him up.

There are wide variations in the time when stranger anxiety develops and in the strength of reactions. Some babies always react more strongly than others. They scream hysterically, look terrified, and cling tightly to you. Another baby may give you a dirty look, as if to say, "Are you sure you want to hand me over to this strange person?"

When your baby's fear of strangers is at its peak, it is very tempting to sneak out of the room when you want to leave him with a babysitter. However, if you do this, your baby may become more upset than if you tell him that you are leaving. Forewarning older babies and children, telling them what is going to happen next, is a useful technique to lessen and sometimes prevent distress reactions.

Stranger anxiety may peak, seem to disappear, then reappear again and again over the course of the next year, depending on your baby's experiences, temperament, and way of handling new situations. The process of becoming independent is begun at birth but is certainly not finished within the first three years of life; it continues in different forms throughout your and your child's lifetimes.

Babies' temperamental qualities may affect differences in the strength of reactions to strangers, but other factors—the setting's familiarity, the tiredness of the baby, and past experience with strangers—may also come into play. Parents who bring their babies to work with them may find that their babies exhibit little stranger anxiety, because they are used to seeing so many new faces every day. What is important to understand is that your baby's fear of strangers is a healthy reaction and a part of your child's normal emotional development.

## Parents as "Refueling Centers"

With your baby's ability to crawl and move away from you comes the desire to use you as a secure base from which to explore. A developmental progression can be observed—your baby will first cling tightly to you, then move away, return for an occasional hug (or "refueling"), and then move off but continue visually checking in to make sure you haven't gone anywhere.

While younger babies require a lot of holding, feeding, and playing on your lap, mobile babies no longer need as much of your continued, close-at-hand attention. You may even be able to leave the baby in another room as long as you remain available and maintain some verbal communication. (Of course, you want to make sure that the room is sufficiently "baby-proofed" so your baby's safety is not in danger.) In one study with mothers and babies conducted in a two-room laboratory, the babies would not let their mothers leave them behind in one of the rooms; however, as long as the situation was under the babies' control, and they were the ones who chose to go into the next room, the babies ventured out of their mothers' sight and explored.

Your availability and occasional reassurance should be supportive of your baby's exploratory behavior. Babies of this age who are allowed this controlled freedom to explore, with the reassurance of verbal contact with the parent when out of sight, seem to fare better on later tests of emotional and cognitive abilities. Allowing your baby some freedom of exploration and control over the environment and not interfering unnecessarily with what she wants to do will enhance your relationship with her.

## Executive Dependence

Some psychologists have called this exploratory stage at six to twelve months one of *executive dependence*, when a baby continues to be very dependent on his care-givers, but also has some control over them. Your baby may easily become a tyrant in this stage—for example, he may cry because he wants a cookie and then become frustrated because he no longer remembers what he wanted. Your baby can keep you hopping, trying to second-guess what his needs are.

While your baby's continued dependence on you may be annoying and frustrating at times, meeting his basic needs is essential for healthy emotional and cognitive growth. Your responsiveness and your habit of attending to and appropriately acknowledging your baby's signals, requests, and demands will enable him to become effective in his interactions with the world. That kind of attention teaches your baby to think, "If I do something, I can have an effect. I can make something happen!"

## Twelve to Eighteen Months

### Separation Anxiety

Your baby's protest at your leaving the room—sometimes referred to as separation anxiety—is a healthy reaction. Rest assured, it does not mean your baby will become an overly dependent adult. It is part and parcel of normal development.

Separation anxiety requires both cognitive advances involved in the development of *object permanence* (you continue to exist in your baby's mind even when you are out of sight) and a special need for you that cannot be met by someone else. Separation anxiety represents your baby's fear of losing you. In the earlier months, your baby probably woke up from a nap screaming; a year later, just calling to your baby from another room may be enough to help her wait for you. This change happens when your baby can remember who you are (even when you are not with her) and is confident that you will come back to take care of her. Before your baby develops object permanence, when you leave the room it is as if you no longer exist—it's little wonder that she screams when you are gone.

By twelve to eighteen months, your baby understands that you are a distinct entity. (On one day you may wear a suit and on another day you may wear blue jeans, but you are still the same person.) At the same time, your baby begins to realize that you exist even while you are no longer in the same room. As babies develop greater motor control, they can move away from their parents and can see them from a distance, which helps babies to perceive themselves as separate individuals. This separateness helps babies begin to develop a sense of self.

Peek-a-boo, one of the most delightful games played with babies, is supportive of your baby's beginning differentiation of "self" as separate from you. When you cover up your face, to a young baby, you really have disappeared. To a baby at the beginning of this stage, the absence of your visual presence is cognitively interpreted as your disappearance. When you uncover your face, you magically return. For an infant, the emotions of surprise and the joy of being reunited are very real in these games.

Peek-a-boo continues to hold magical powers for the eighteen-month-old. Toddlers cover up their faces with their hands so that they no longer can see us. What is so amusing is the toddler's belief that if she cannot see you, you cannot see her either. Although the toddler has begun to recognize her existence as separate from you, she is not yet able to take on another person's perspective (that is, put herself in someone else's shoes).

## A Secure Attachment to You

By twelve months of age, your baby has formed a meaningful relationship with you. (Here we are speaking to mothers, because women have traditionally been the primary care-givers for babies. But much of what is discussed here applies to fathers, as well.) Psychologists refer to this as a baby's "specific attachment." Not only does your baby clearly prefer you, but he also strives to avoid your absence and can use your presence to give himself security.

People used to talk about this relationship in terms of its intensity—how much and how loudly did a baby cry when his mother left the room. They believed that babies with more intense reactions loved their mothers more. We now realize that the intensity of a child's response to separation from his mother is less important than the degree of security that he can gain from her presence. In fact, psychologists now classify children in terms of whether their attachment is secure. A secure attachment is shown with babies who seek closeness with their mothers. After a separation, when their mothers return to the room, these securely attached babies approach and look up to their moms.

Having a secure attachment is good for babies' long-term development. Securely attached babies end up having better peer relationships and emotional stability during the first six years. Of course, the seeds of this relationship begin early in life with the mothers' handling of their babies. Studies find that mothers who responded sensitively and appropriately to their babies in the first two to six months of life are more likely to have babies with these secure relationships. Surprisingly, the baby's characteristics early on seem to play little role.

## Recognition of Self

About this time, babies can also recognize themselves in the mirror. One study examined how babies reacted to their mirror reflections. Lipstick was put on their noses, and observers watched to see if the babies would try to wipe the lipstick off. The babies all learned to recognize themselves in the mirror and wipe off the lipstick sometime between nine and twenty-four months.

Because babies are becoming more aware of their separateness, they begin to recognize how vulnerable they really are without you there to take care of them. Try to think about how it feels to have your feet pulled out from under you. That's how your baby feels as she starts to realize that she is not you.

This happens right before your baby takes her first independent steps. Tolerance for frustration

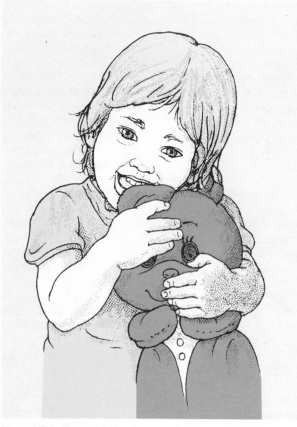

*Your child's "lovey" helps her manage her transition to independence.*

and stressful events diminishes. At times, your baby seems like an "emotional wreck"—quick to cry and not easily pacifiable. You wonder what happened to your nice, calm baby. Some psychiatrists have suggested that the apprehension associated with walking may be fear of loss of support from the parent. All of a sudden, your baby is alone and separate. Independent walking, perhaps, marks the discovery of the solitary "self."

## Conflicting Feelings

Your baby will experience conflicting emotions as he masters walking. At the same time he is hanging onto you, he is pushing you away. With his first steps, striving toward greater independence, he seems to be saying, "Look at all the things I can do! I can walk and go where I want!" In the next breath, showing his extreme dependency, your baby seems to say, "Stay here. I can't be without you for a moment." All of this is healthy and normal.

## Development of Attachment to a Transitional Object

By this time, your baby may have established a specially loved blanket or stuffed animal (a "lovey") that accompanies her to bed and to "scary" places. This lovey is called a transitional object because it helps your baby in the transition between extreme dependency on you and the move toward independence.

Your baby's lovey provides security and comfort, particularly in fearful situations. For your baby, this selected object is said to serve the purpose of keeping a part of you with her even while you are gone. It is important to respect your baby's desire to have this lovey with her.

Some babies maintain this attachment to a special lovey into the preschool years and beyond. There is no predetermined time for abandonment of a lovey; your child will put hers aside when she is ready. In most cases, the attachment is normal, and will be outgrown naturally.

## Eighteen Months to Two Years

### Language Makes Life Easier for Everyone

When your baby can communicate some ideas to you, your parenting job becomes a bit easier. You can ask what's wrong. You no longer are required to be a mind-reader and try to second-guess your toddler to figure out what is bothering him.

Much younger babies use gestures and single words to make their wants and needs known. Your baby may have developed some of his own unique gestures to express different wants. Many eighteen-month-olds have command over a number of words. These single words can mean whole sentences. Some eighteen-month-olds put words together in two- and three-word combinations.

Wise parents make use of their babies' natural ability to acquire language to make their jobs easier. For example, one mother was so quick to get everything for her toddler that he didn't need to talk. All his needs were being met without much effort on his part. When her pediatrician suggested that she wait for her son to ask for things, the little boy started talking in five-word sentences. In this situation, the mother had been *too* good at reading her son's signals.

If you have concerns about your baby's development of language, be sure to discuss them with your pediatrician. Babies prone to frequent ear infections occasionally have fluctuating hearing losses. If you suspect your baby isn't listening to you or doesn't understand what you say, you might want to check this out. Sometimes children have behavior problems because of poor hearing. Kids can be particularly difficult to manage when they don't hear what you say.

For some babies, having the words in one's head but not having the words come out right can be a very frustrating experience. There is so much that they want to say, but they don't know how to say it. Try not to place too much pressure on your baby to say the words correctly. A lot of internal and external demands are being placed on the almost-two-year-old. Not only are these youngsters trying to master an upright world, they are also trying to become competent users of language. This is a time when gentle encouragement, assurance, and firm limits are needed.

## Egocentricity

At eighteen months, your baby has an egocentric view of the world—that is, she sees herself as the center of the world and is unable to see things through other people's eyes. The term "egocentric" is often used to refer to self-centered adults, but it also depicts a baby's view of her position of power in the world: she, too, thinks that the world revolves around her.

At this age, your baby recognizes that parents can do things for her. Adults serve a purpose for babies: they are a means to an end. However, while adults can give babies what they want, they can also make demands and set limits, which can be a source of conflict. For example, a mother can ask her toddler to begin to master independent living skills (such as giving up the nighttime bottle, using a cup and a spoon, and using the potty) before the toddler feels she is ready.

Feeding can be a potential battleground for parents and babies—with the baby often winning. Babies can use the feeding situation as a way to control parents. A laid-back approach—allowing the baby some selection of food and not forcing her to eat detested foods—can prevent later feeding problems. There are also some tricks that you can use, such as disguising the disliked foods with preferred tastes.

Conflicts about self-care skills often center on dependence-independence issues. Some sort of balance must be achieved between your baby's dependence on you, the care-giver, and your desire for your baby's increased independence. Some of these skills—such as toilet training—may be best dealt with at a later date since some readiness skills may be needed. There is no single timetable because children master developmental skills at their own rates.

## No!

One of a baby's first words is *no.* Babies often say no to your requests even when they mean *yes.* Some say it is easier for a baby to shake his head from side to side than up and down, but defiance is certainly also the name of the game. We have all seen many a two-year-old throw a temper tantrum right in the middle of the store because he didn't get what he wanted. These temper tantrums are disruptive and embarrassing but are all part of growing up. Though never easy to deal with, they are inevitable, and are faced by every parent. The difficulty is not yours alone. And yes, the phase will pass!

Although toddlers do have more language available to them, this stage is characterized by a great deal of opposition. It's as if the toddler has to do the opposite just as a statement of his independence. This is a very important developmental step for your child. It is an assertion of your child's sense of himself as an individual. These difficult times are important for your child to separate from you and move toward becoming a distinct person.

Like everything else in development, the timetable varies from child to child. Some very verbal children don't hit the "terrible twos" until they are three. This is a consequence of the child's and parents' ability to talk about what the child is feeling, thinking, or wanting. Parents can explain a lot of different kinds of things to toddlers; sometimes what appear to be quite rational explanations can defuse a potentially explosive situation. Other times, these explanations are totally useless, partly because the baby doesn't have the necessary level of understanding to know what you are talking about. Also, there are times when your child just won't give in. It is very important for parents to sit down and talk with each other so that they can establish priorities as to what's worth a fight and what isn't.

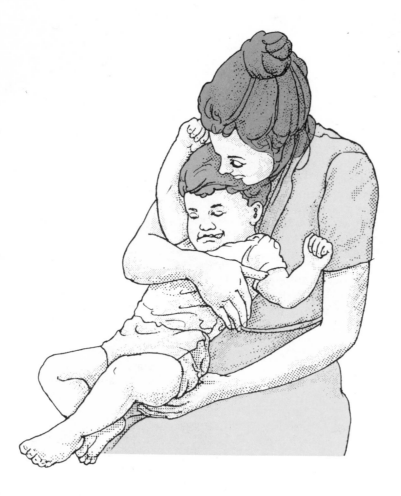

*Your toddler's progression to independence will bring tantrums and even defiance.*

## Intense Separation Reactions

Even though your baby has already experienced some stranger anxiety, it is likely that she will develop more intense reactions to separation at this developmental stage. Leaving her with a babysitter or dropping her off at the day care center may be more difficult. Remembering to take a favorite toy or lovey along may help with these leave-takings. Fear of new situations results partly because of your child's inexperience with them.

Easy sleep patterns that have been established may be disrupted in this stage. So much time during the day is spent in motor activity—walking and running—that by the time evening rolls around, your toddler is likely to be too overtired to go to bed easily. In addition, you shouldn't be surprised if your baby starts to wake up again in the middle of the night. This may be because your baby is afraid of being alone. Night fears begin around eighteen months. They may continue through the third and fourth year, changing in intensity and content. Three-year-olds can often tell you about dreams that wake them up.

At these early ages, your baby doesn't know what's real and what's fantasy, so nighttime, being alone, and dreams can be frightening experiences. You can relieve some of your baby's fearfulness by comforting her and telling her that you are there and will protect her. On occasion, even letting your baby crawl into bed with you can give her a sense of security and you a good night's sleep.

Children's fears can be lessened through imaginative play and books. Play is a terrific means of working out difficulties your child may be experiencing. Some of your baby's fears and worries can be worked out through your playing together. Each of you can take turns pretending to be the "scary monster," which the other one banishes. Some delightful children's books cast triumphant little boys or girls as conquerors of nighttime monsters.

In addition to books, parents can use puppets to engage their toddlers, and older children too, in lively reenactments of daily concerns and fears. Playing with puppets removes some of the tension associated with real-life discussions about upsetting issues. By giving the worries to the puppets in the realm of your play, some forbidding topics are no longer as unthinkable.

Toddlers need a regular bedtime routine. Many parents use the hour before bedtime to read books with their children. Not only is reading to your child known to be beneficial to her later reading readiness, but eighteen-month-olds find the same routine night after night comforting. Thus, a consistent bedtime "ritual" is good for your child's emotional growth and cognitive development and may provide a better night's sleep for both parents and child.

## New Advances

As a parent, your role is to support your baby's move toward independence while at the same time recognizing his need to be dependent on you. Some children have great difficulty struggling to reach the next developmental milestone. Others make smooth transitions from milestone to milestone. Some experts believe that development is mainly dependent on the child's growth or maturation, with maturation moving in an upward, cyclical manner. Occasionally, peaks and valleys do occur.

With this cyclical view of development, parents can see how new advances can be upsetting for children. Thus, with advances to each new stage of development, notably with walking, your baby's behavior may seem disorganized until he is sure of himself and has consolidated his new skills.

## Sharing Toys With Other Children

Neither eighteen-month-olds nor two-year-olds are very good at sharing toys. This, too, is a part of normal development and should be accepted as such. From your baby's perspective, her toys are an extension of herself. For someone to take a toy from her is a direct affront to her integrity. It's as if a part of her has been taken away. Parents are probably unrealistic to request a child of this age to share with other children. You can start to work toward that goal, but it may be too soon to reasonably expect to achieve it.

One helpful hint is to have a special set of toys designated for the play group. This way the toys don't seem to belong to any one person. Aggression and fighting over toys can also be reduced with planned activities. The activities should be ones that are creative, messy, and fun, such as painting, or playing with blocks, sand, and molding material.

## Difficulties With Changes in the Routine

Eighteen-month-olds are very ritualistic. Often routines must be carried out in exactly the same way or the toddler is upset. Recognizing this, you can help your toddler by trying to maintain as consistent a routine as possible. By doing this, your toddler doesn't have to try to figure out what's going to happen next. Transitions are also eased by letting children know what to expect.

Toddlers' typical ritualistic behavior may be due to their limited understanding of language. Sometimes we are fooled into thinking that eighteen-month-olds know more than they do. On occasion, parents should stand back and reevaluate why the child acted the way he did. Perhaps he did not understand what was said or asked. While toddlers understand a great deal, not all ideas hold the same meaning for eighteen-month-olds as they do for adults.

Because of this, your child's reactions to disruptions in his routine are likely to be more intense than they were earlier in his life. The toddler's distress and obstinacy are said to be, in part, related to the beginning development of his sense of self. To the toddler, parent and child are becoming two separate people, which may be a stressful adjustment.

The emotions of fear and worry may seem more apparent with toddlers than with young babies. Some two-year-olds appear quite wary when confronted with new situations. In particular, such things as firecrackers, loud noises, and vacuum cleaners can be pretty frightening. Toddlers don't understand the relationship between cause and effect yet and may attribute magical or lifelike properties to noises and machines. The toddler may even think that these strange occurrences happened because of something he did.

Some children hold onto their parents until they are comfortable and secure in a new setting. Yet at home, if all is going well, your child should be able to leave your side to play by himself in another room. Your child's caution and his checking in on you represent a beginning sense of reality. It is part of the normal developmental process, without which your child would not develop into a healthy, independent person.

Although at times your toddler will be difficult to manage, this is the age when it is even more important to be firm in setting limits, consistent in your demands, and nurturing during the bad as well as the good moments. Your role is to balance the toddler's desire for independence with his continued need for reassurance, love, and affection.

## The Third Year

### Control and Dependency

The first half of the third year may remain difficult for you and your child as far as issues of control and dependency are concerned. Although your child's language and self-care skills are more advanced, in some ways your child continues to feel like a tightrope walker, occasionally teetering with uncertainty over what she can and cannot do. Try to recognize your child's need for independence. By promoting independence along with emotional support, parents can help their children through this stage. An extra cuddle or more lavish praise for the good things that the child is doing helps to counteract some of the normal negativism.

One management technique that works quite well with toddlers is the use of praise. To help your child develop a positive self-image, you should encourage and delight in your child's new accomplishments and achievements. Praise ("That's good! I like that block tower"), hugs, and kisses are important ingredients in promoting a good self-image. At two and three, a child's self-esteem—how she feels about herself—is often a reflection of her perception of her parents' opinions of her. Interest in and enjoyment of your child's play set the tone for a healthy self-concept.

One of the most difficult jobs parents have is setting reasonable limits for their children. Letting your child know what's expected, what's tolerable, and what's unacceptable is a long-term process that continues well into the teenage years. As early as in the first year, for example, you are setting some limits by not letting your child stick her fingers into the electrical outlets.

Some potential conflicts can be defused by rearranging the environment, so that you don't have to worry about your child's hurting herself, breaking your valuable vase, or eating a poisonous plant. Child-proofing the major living quarters in your house allows your child to safely explore many interesting and different objects.

Of course, changing the environment will not take care of those times when a direct confrontation is necessary. It helps to quickly and adeptly address the situation. Tell your child what you don't like about what she is doing. Give her a simple reason why, for example, pulling the tail on the cat hurts the cat. Parents don't need to use more than one or two sentences of explanation. Ask the child to stop. If that doesn't work, put the child on a chair for a few minutes either in the same room with you or in a different room. After the allotted time has elapsed, you can then talk about what happened. Later in the day, but not immediately afterward, be sure to let your child know you still love her by giving her a hug and a kiss. On a particularly bad day, you may even want to engage her in a very special time just for the two of you. The earlier you begin to set aside a special chair or place to be used for thinking about unacceptable behavior, the sooner your child will learn that some things just mustn't be done.

In the early years, parents take on the roles of care-giver, teacher, and playmate. Creating an emotionally supportive environment is essential for your child to become independent yet aware of her parents' love and acceptance. On occasion, behavioral extremes are acceptable for two-year-olds. As a regular pattern, however, the child who is always out of control or overly compliant is telling you something. These are warning signals that suggest that you should take a good, hard look at your disciplining techniques. Ask yourself: Are my methods so loose that the boundaries of acceptable and unacceptable behaviors are unclear? Am I so rigid in setting limits that my child is afraid to upset me by resisting my controls? Am I providing enough time for relaxed activities and play with my child?

By the end of the third year, with increased growth, maturity, and confidence, your child will become willing to relinquish some of her insistence on being independent. She may even give up some of her executive independence ("I want to do it myself!") for your love and affection. Great pleasure is obtained from praise and attention.

Participation in such body management activities as feeding, toilet training, and dressing becomes a matter of routine. Although many three-year-olds continue to have high activity levels, their activity begins to be more directed, with a far less frenetic quality.

The secure three-year-old may be willing to allow you to help her set limits. This new stage has been called the stage of *volitional dependence* because the child's dependency needs can now be brought under her control. Your child will be less impulsive and more manageable; an occasional explanation of rules will be understood—and actually followed, too. For example, when you are working in one room, you may no longer have to worry about leaving your child to play in another, but instead may be able to trust her not to misbehave.

## Feelings and Emotions

Of particular importance, but sometimes overlooked, is talking to your children about how they feel. By the age of three, children have a wide range of emotions available to them: they feel afraid, mad, sad, and glad. While children may not have exactly the same meanings for these feelings that adults do, children can learn to label and identify "good" and "bad" feelings. Don't underestimate their capacity for understanding emotions and feelings.

Parents can help their children develop a language for expressing and dealing with feelings by giving the feelings names. While doing so, parents have a responsibility to manage their own feelings to help children deal with theirs. Sometimes, our own childhood experiences creep into how we handle emotions with our children. For all of us, there are some feelings that give us trouble. For instance, difficulties with such feelings as anger and aggression may spill into our parenting. If we cannot tolerate angry feelings, we might try to prevent our children from displaying anger by saying "That's no reason to be angry!" when in fact a child may have good reason to be angry. Through the use of play, you can provide children with some emotional avenues for anger, fear, and anxiety.

## A Self-concept Emerges

Between their second and third birthdays, most children become fairly competent language users. They readily use the personal pronouns "I," "me," and "mine," particularly to defend ownership of their toys and possessions. They have great difficulty letting anyone else play with something that is theirs.

Around this time, your toddler can refer to himself by his own name. Sometimes, when playing with dolls or superheroes, your toddler may reenact earlier events. Different roles may even be assigned to the dolls. If you sit down and play directly with your toddler, you can get a glimpse of the inner workings of his mind. This glimpse may be both delightful and unnerving, since you may observe firsthand how your child views your parenting style. Many parents have heard their sweet little girl harshly send her favorite doll to her room because she didn't "behave."

By three years of age, your child has a good sense of "me" and "you" and of "self" versus "nonself." With better cognitive capacities and a wider repertoire of experiences, the three-year-old has internalized memories of the significant people in his life—his parents. As their sense of self grows, children's personalities become more representative of what they will be like as they grow older. Preferences and dislikes are readily displayed in how they interact with the world: for example, some children already prefer very physical activities, while others choose quiet, sedentary play.

## Aggression and Fighting

Fighting usually centers on wanting to have a toy that someone else has. Aggression is a normal part of growing up and may be related to our survival instincts. Most children are fairly aggressive when trying to defend their belongings and themselves.

There are no easy answers for how to handle excessive aggression. However, it certainly doesn't make sense to the child or to the parent to handle aggression with aggression. Imagine this scenario: Two sisters are fighting over a toy. One parent comes in, yells at them to stop fighting, and hits one of them because the child won't give the toy back. What does this teach the children? There's quite a mixed message here—it's all right to fight and to hit, but only if you are bigger and more powerful than your adversary.

# THE ROAD TO INDEPENDENCE

Parental handling does influence how aggressive a child will be. Children in families where physical violence, such as hitting or spanking, is used as punishment generally turn out to be more aggressive than other children. The least aggressive children come from families that are nonpunitive, nonpermissive, and nonrejecting. The parents in such families are consistent in their handling of aggression. They don't use physical punishment or unnecessarily harsh language. They set firm and clear limits as to what is expected of their children, and they are accepting of their children.

Consistency is important in whatever intervention technique you use in dealing with your child's aggression. A useful technique is to remove the child from the fight and isolate her for a few minutes. Quick handling of the situation, before the fighting gets out of hand, is helpful. Once your two-year-old can talk, asking her to talk about how she feels or what she wants will help her learn to express herself verbally instead of physically.

Sometimes, providing your child with an outlet for her pent-up energy helps reduce the level of her aggression. Particularly in wintertime, just as with adults, active physical exercise will help release the tension and reduce the level of stress. Imaginative play also helps to work through aggressive tendencies. The age-old fairy tales can be used to work through some anxieties. Parents can capitalize on the child's imagination to help work out conflicts.

## Imagination

Imagination is especially wonderful and exciting to watch develop in your child. Through the windows of your child's play and the talking he does to himself, you can actually follow your child, the "movie director," casting a set of characters into their various roles. Fantasy develops along with your child's more sophisticated knowledge of the world, although he cannot yet totally differentiate fantasy from reality.

Some children have such great imaginations that they tell the most unbelievable stories—and sometimes get in trouble for doing so. One child we know had an imaginary friend; whenever he did something really bad that he didn't want to catch the blame for, his imaginary friend was there to cover for him. Usually, the presence of an imaginary friend is just a sign of a healthy, imaginative child. But imaginary friends can become too powerful: they can interfere with your child's ability to accept responsibility, can be present to the exclusion of other friends, and can do all your child's talking. Luckily, this doesn't happen very often. If you're concerned about your child's imaginary companion, you may want to consult with a professional.

By three, your child has internal pictures of the people in his world, the television shows he watches, and daytime events. The world is no longer viewed as a place filled with magical powers: cause-and-effect relationships are becoming explainable to him. Earlier, his parents were omnipotent; now there are some chinks in their armor. Before your child was able to connect cause-and-effect relationships, he thought things happened because of the things he did. Imagine how powerful and scared a two-year-old might feel if he thought he caused lightning to appear. This kind of thinking takes years to change into the logical form it will acquire in adulthood.

## Television

Presidential commissions have confirmed the profound effects of television violence on children's aggressive behavior. These reports indicate that violent television programming is related to an increase in children's fighting. If you do not want to have a physically aggressive child, you may consider monitoring your child's television viewing habits. One way to do this is to count the number of aggressive acts in your child's Saturday morning cartoons. Then you can decide if you would like her to continue to watch them.

Cartoon-watching also seems to have a negative impact on children's activity levels. While they sit and stare at the television set, they appear zombie-like; afterward, these same children act overexcited, running helter-skelter with little direction or content in their play. In all likelihood, a steady diet of superheroes and monsters is harmful. Also, because two- and three-year-olds are unable to distinguish between fantasy and reality, the evil warriors and monsters may seem real to them, and the characters in some of these daytime "entertainments" can come back to haunt toddlers at nighttime. To make matters worse, it is often difficult to tell where the cartoons end and the commercials begin.

However, television can be used for positive ends as well. Good educational programs, like *Sesame Street* and *Mr. Rogers' Neighborhood*, can teach your toddler many interesting things.

See Chapter 11 for additional discussion of the proper role of television.

## Multiple Attachments: Expanding Horizons

By three years of age, your child is likely to have a number of relationships with people other than his parents. He may have a favorite babysitter or just a good friend. He will prefer to play with children his own age rather than to play with you, though he still enjoys and needs you. Long periods of time can be spent in play without any fighting and with some sharing of toys.

As your child's world expands—for example, when he goes to a day care center or nursery school—the influences on your child's self-esteem will also include new people's attitudes toward him. As parents, it's essential to provide him with the security he needs so he can go out and explore his surroundings.

While your child may be quite ready to go off to nursery school, once in a while he may slip back to his less-sure former self and not want to leave your side. These are considered to be normal separation reactions. His going to nursery school is a big emotional step for both of you.

Here is an example of a three-year-old boy we knew. It was the first week of nursery school. Every day the boy's mother walked him to the classroom, gave him a hug and a kiss, and said goodbye. Each time, the boy cried uncontrollably, refusing to take his jacket off for the whole day. Knowingly, the teachers respected the child's need to hold onto his jacket. For this child, removing his jacket meant that he was going to stay at this place without his mother. In a way, he was unsure that he was ready for all this independence. Both mother and child benefited from the teachers' warm assurance that everything would be all right. Gradually, the teachers enticed the child into the fun the others were having. Some nursery schools are quite aware of children's difficulties with separation and build this into their programs by slowly introducing children into the classroom. For some children, nursery school is the first time for them to be on their own. It is, on the one hand, an obvious milestone, but on the other hand, it is just one of the many steps that take your baby gradually toward independence.

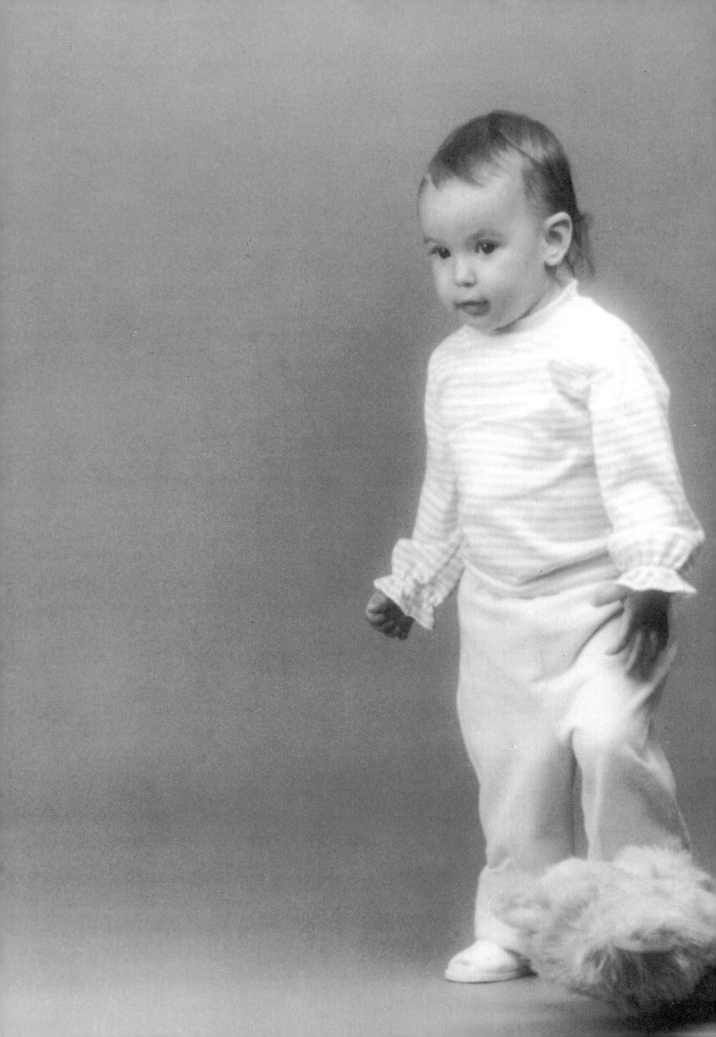

# Chapter 14:
# Planning
# for Baby's
# Future

## Your Financial Responsibilities

Now that you're parents, another human being will be dependent on you for all of his or her needs for at least the next eighteen years.

Hugs and kisses are free, but other things such as food, clothing, housing, medical care, and education cost money—lots of it. To raise one child from birth to age eighteen will cost an average of nearly $100,000. That figure covers just the basic necessities through high school, but many parents today want more for their children.

At age five, when most children begin school, the costs of child-rearing begin to escalate. About forty percent of the total expense of raising a child occurs between the ages of twelve and seventeen, which is good news for early planners who will benefit by beginning a savings program when their children are preschoolers.

# PLANNING FOR BABY'S FUTURE

Now is the time to arm yourself with information about how to prepare for your family's future and to begin the steps to turn your plans into reality.

*Begin by determining your financial condition.* Before you can plan intelligently for your child's future, it's necessary to have a firm grasp of your present financial situation. It's impossible to plan for the future if you don't know what's going on now.

Figuring out your net worth can be a very revealing exercise. Draw a line down the center of a piece of paper. Label *assets* on the left side and list them; include cash in checking and savings accounts, equity in owner-occupied real estate, bonds, stocks, cars, and investment real estate.

Under *liabilities* on the right side, list mortgages outstanding, installment loans for cars, appliances, or furniture, revolving credit card balances for department stores, and professional services such as medical and dental. Include past-due accounts and charity donations.

Then add up each column. If you subtract your liabilities from your assets, you'll have your net worth. Don't worry if your figures aren't precise; just the fact that you're sitting down with pen, paper, and calculator makes it all the more likely that you'll take firm action when planning your child's financial future.

Making a simple monthly budget to determine how you are spending your income can be another eye-opener. By listing your income and your spending, you can highlight the areas where changes can be made. For example, you may be surprised to find out how much you spend on long-distance phone calls or how often you eat out. Seeing those figures in black and white may spur you to reduce your expenditures, and channel the money to your savings account instead.

## Insurance

Next, review your insurance policies. For many people, life insurance is a kind of instant estate; it's guaranteed financial protection for your family.

Term life insurance (temporary; bought for a specified period of time, or *term*) is often purchased by younger people who like the low initial premiums. Remember that premiums for term insurance rise slowly through your thirties and more quickly thereafter. For people in their sixties and beyond, term insurance rates may be out of reach.

Whole-life insurance (permanent; for your "whole life") rates are about five times higher than for term insurance, but the premium remains level from the date of issue. Additionally, the whole-life policy acquires a cash value that increases over time.

You may want to look into newer types of life insurance that combine term and whole-life. Such a policy typically will combine at least $10,000 of whole-life upon the head of the household with at least $50,000 of term insurance, all for a single premium. Another innovative policy is adjustable life insurance, which allows the policyholder to raise or lower the amount of insurance and vary the type of insurance between whole-life and term, as life's circumstances change.

If you or your spouse is staying home or working part-time, that person should also consider buying a term policy that will cover the day-care expenses that would result in case the stay-home parent dies.

What about your health insurance? Many companies now offer membership in a health maintenance organization (HMO) as an option to the usual health insurance. HMOs are corporations that contract with physicians and hospitals to deliver health care under a prepaid plan. With these plans, employers can offer their workers enhanced benefits at prices comparable to traditional insurance. Joining an HMO can make sense, particularly to a family whose members seem to be running to the doctor's office every other week. The costs of office visits, prescriptions, vaccinations, diagnostic tests, and hospitalization are often covered by an HMO plan. Keep in mind that you have to use the HMO's doctors and hospitals, so if you have a doctor you particularly like, an HMO may not be for you.

A new wrinkle in employer- or insurance-plan-sponsored health care is the Preferred Provider Organization (PPO). As with an HMO, a PPO plan provides discount health care to members, offering co-payment arrangements and other incentives. Typically, members contribute through payroll deductions. As a PPO member, you can choose your physician and hospital from those included in the PPO group. Fees for services are covered one hundred percent. If you wish, you can choose an outside (nonmember) physician or hospital, in which case you will be liable for a percentage of any fees. Obviously, what makes PPOs appealing is that a member can select his or her care-givers.

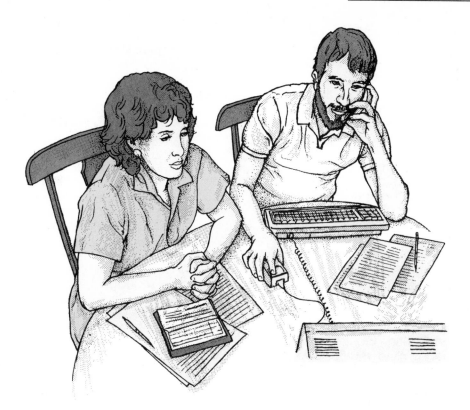

*Your establishment of goals and priorities is vital to successful financial planning for your child's future.*

Check to see if you have adequate protection through work or Social Security in the event you become disabled. If not, find out if you qualify for auto insurance that provides benefits for disability from traffic accidents, or for special private insurance programs that pay monthly loan or mortgage payments during a disability. There are different definitions of what "disabled" means; an insurance agent should explain exactly what "disability" means in the policy. The agent should also explain the policy's "renewability," or the conditions of extending the policy beyond its expiration date.

The whole point of insurance is to cover the "just in case" situations; you want to be sure your policies are appropriate for a family with young children.

## Setting Your Goals

An important component of planning for your child's future is having something definite to reach for. Setting goals gives your planning form and shape. Rank your goals by priority. A college education for your child? Ballet lessons? Braces? A two-week vacation every year?

How are you going to pay for what you need and want? Since saving money under the mattress probably won't help you to achieve your goals, most people look for a way their money will grow—that means *investing*.

Simply put, investing means committing money with the expectation of a profit. All the planning you've done up to now will determine the kinds of investments you choose. Successful investors will analyze their own situations in terms of income, monthly cash requirements, and net worth over the years. They will also determine how much risk they can live with comfortably. If you want liquidity and safety, stick with money market funds, insured certificates of deposit, U.S. Treasury bills and bonds, fixed annuities, and equity in your home.

High-quality stocks, high-grade corporate and municipal bonds, and investment real estate traditionally provide income and/or long-term growth. High-risk investments include options, futures, tax investments, and undeveloped land.

Because there are so many investment choices available, it's important to educate yourself on which ones are best suited for your situation. Resources for self-education include seminars and classes offered through adult education programs at local high schools and junior colleges, YMCAs, and public libraries. Newspapers and magazine articles probably provide the most timely written information on investments. It's imperative to educate yourself, because no one will look after your family's interests as well as you will.

Unless you have a large income (over $100,000) and a complicated tax situation, you probably don't need to hire a financial planner. If you decide you *do* need a financial planner, be wary of know-it-all types. No one person can be an expert in all aspects of investing and estate planning. Use the same caution you employed when choosing your doctor and attorney.

If you do decide to invest, commercial banks, brokerage firms, and savings and loans will be competing for your business. Since deregulation, U.S. banks and thrift institutions (noncommercial banks, savings and loans, and mutual savings banks) have expanded their lending and investment opportunities to become more competitive with brokerage firms, which traditionally have offered a wide variety of financial services.

Since saving for their children's college education is a common goal of many parents, investment programs specifically geared to that end are springing up everywhere. Some institutions will send you a computerized education savings analysis based on information you give them. The analysis is usually free, but of course the bank is hoping you will use its services.

A typical analysis will look at your child's age, number of years before his college education begins, the percentage of college costs that you will pay, your estimated taxable income and its probable rate of growth, and other factors. This information is the basis for the institution's analysis of how much money you will need, and when you will need it.

A certificate of deposit (CD) is one investment vehicle available. A CD is a time deposit that cannot be withdrawn without penalty before a specified maturity date. The minimum deposit for seven- to thirty-one-day accounts is $1,000. The law requires no minimum deposit in accounts with maturities of more than thirty-one days, but individual banks may have their own minimum deposit requirements.

Other financial instruments you may encounter include:

- *Bonds.* A fixed-income security that represents a loan to the bond issuer. The bondholder usually receives semiannual interest payments. *Corporate bonds* are issued by private companies; *municipal bonds* are backed by specific revenues and are exempt from federal income taxes.

- *Money Market Deposit Accounts.* These enable banks and thrift institutions to compete with money market mutual funds. These interest-bearing accounts are insured and offer limited transaction privileges, such as check writing.

- *Mutual Funds.* Pooled investments that are professionally managed. A money market fund is a mutual fund that typically invests in short-term securities, such as Treasury bills. Mutual funds are not insured.

- *Stocks.* Ownership interests in a corporation, entitling the stockholder to voting rights and a part of the corporation's earnings (dividends).

- *Treasury Securities.* The U.S. Treasury issues bills, bonds, and notes. Each is sold at a discounted face amount and cashed in for full face value at maturity. Lengths of maturity vary.

- *Zero-Coupon Bonds.* These corporate or government-issued bonds are sold at deep discounts from face value and pay no interest until maturity (hence their name). Zeros have become popular for college investing because the maturities can be staggered, so that some will mature during each of the years you'll have children in college.

## Safeguard Your Child; Make a Will

By making a last will and testament, you are getting the final word on who gets what part of your estate, and, more importantly, who will care for your child when you are gone.

Though a will is a valuable document, people often procrastinate about putting one together. It's easy to put off making a will because it isn't a pleasant pursuit for most people. But for parents, a will is, at the least, peace of mind insurance.

A common misconception about wills is that they're only for wealthy people. Because jointly-owned real estate, bank accounts, life insurance benefits, and pension proceeds are typically not covered under a will, many people believe that a will is probably not necessary if they don't have extensive personal property. But from a parent's point of view, the most important aspect of a will is the designation of a guardian in the event both parents die at the same time. Maybe you don't really care how your personal property is divvied up, but you *do* care about how your child is reared.

Therefore, discussions about the person or persons best-suited to raise your child are important. Do you want someone who knows your child well, who has similar values and religious beliefs? Take into consideration the age of the potential guardians and their interest in taking on responsibility for a child. This is important; if they feel they wouldn't be good parent substitutes, consider someone else. It is imperative to discuss everything with the guardians you have in mind.

Another question is *guardian of the person* versus *guardian of the property*. The person who will watch over your child does not necessarily have to be the one who will take care of your child's financial needs. Of course, one person can do both, but if you have a relative who you feel would be a wonderful substitute for you and your spouse, but not as equipped to manage the child's property, you can name both a guardian of the person and one for the property.

You will also have to name an *executor* (male) or *executrix* (female) of your will. That person is responsible for gathering together your assets, paying any outstanding bills, paying the death taxes, and then distributing whatever assets remain, according to the specifications of the will. Your executor can be a relative, friend, attorney, or an institution such as a bank or trust company. Some people choose an individual *and* an institution, in order to have the personal approach of a trusted friend and the knowledge of an organization. Either way, trustworthiness, reliability, and organization are attributes your executor should possess.

Although state laws vary, some common principles apply regardless of where you live. Though there's no law that says you must have a lawyer draw up your will, if you want to make sure you have a *valid* will, hire a competent attorney who is familiar with state law and, to some degree, with applicable federal and state estate-tax laws.

The written document prepared by your lawyer must be signed by you in the presence of two (or sometimes three) witnesses, although many states allow you to verbally state to the witnesses that you have previously signed the will. *The witnesses should not be persons who are beneficiaries under the will.*

Two of the most important requirements in making your will valid are that you tell the witnesses the document they are signing is in fact your will (not just some random legal document) and that each witness sign the will at your specific request. This may sound quirky, but the failure to observe these requirements has led to the invalidation of many wills.

The original will should be kept in a safe place, but *not* in a safe-deposit box, since these are often sealed upon notice of death.

Your planning will go a long way toward creating a happy and successful future for your children. But don't fall so in love with your plans that you never review or change them. Remember to be flexible; if your financial outlook has changed, perhaps some of your plans should change as well.

# Appendix

## Tips for Traveling With Infants and Young Children

Traveling with infants and young children need not be a formidable task, though any trip—even across town—requires common sense, planning, and organization. You must always keep three important factors in mind: the child's safety, physical comfort, and contentment.

### Safety Restraints

Even before the baby's birth, parents should buy a quality child safety restraint for use in the family car. Several good models are on the market, but each of them must be installed properly to be effective. See Chapters 4 and 8 for helpful consumer information about car seats and other safety restraints.

Beginning with baby's first trip home, develop the habit of using the safety restraint each time the child rides in the car, regardless of the distance involved. Under no circumstances should any child be allowed to ride "loose;" the lap of an adult passenger is an especially dangerous place for a baby or young child.

### Planning Your Trip

When including your baby in major traveling, begin planning for your trip several weeks before departure. Tell your pediatrician about it and ask for his advice. A few doctors do restrict infant travel.

If you will be traveling by commercial carrier—plane, train, or bus—ask the ticket agent about infant passengers and special services. One domestic airline, for example, requires a doctor's written consent before it will transport an infant under seven days old. Most carriers need advance notice to supply children's meals and to provide bassinets for use en route.

Prepare separate lists—the things you will need for the baby during the trip, the things you will want at your destination, the things you might like to have easily accessible (in the trunk of your car, for example, if you are planning to drive). Then organize your packing according to your lists, using a lightweight carry-along bag for traveling and a separate suitcase for the rest of the baby's things.

Gather the necessary items in a single spot so that they will not be forgotten. As you locate and pack each item, check it off the appropriate list and take the lists with you—they perform admirably for the return trip too.

### What to Pack

What you take with you is mostly a matter of common sense; it depends primarily on the age of your child and your mode of transportation.

Formula can be refrigerated in insulated coolers packed with ice, although commercial carriers frequently have refrigerator space for a bottle or two. If necessary, you can warm bottles under a hot water faucet.

Traveling is infinitely easier since the advent of disposable diapers. Even if you use washable ones at home, consider taking throwaways with you on the trip. You need only take a few since the supply can be replenished readily while traveling and after you arrive at your destination. Disposable diapers eliminate the problem of storing soiled ones. Soiled washable diapers should be rinsed out in a restroom before being stowed in a plastic bag until laundry facilities are available.

Dress your youngster in loose, comfortable clothing suitable to the particular travel environment; if the vehicle is air-conditioned, take along a sweater or lightweight blanket for the child's comfort.

Facial tissues are "musts" when traveling with young children. Commercially packaged, moistened towels are handy, but you can also carry washcloths in a plastic bag.

A plastic trash bag functions well as a laundry bag, and a plastic sheet protects beds from accidents, but be sure to place the plastic *under* the bedsheet to avoid the danger of suffocation. Take a large bedsheet with you—it provides a clean infant play area on a motel floor or bed or even on a grassy area by the side of the road.

## The Contented Traveler

Infants and young children do not tolerate restraint for extended lengths of time, and since a cranky child can distract the driver, it's wise to stop frequently, get out, and stretch. Encourage toddlers to run around in a safe area, to play ball or tag. Place an infant on a flat surface or across your thighs so he can kick for a few minutes. On commercial carriers, walk your toddler in the aisle, holding his hand to protect him in case of sudden lurches.

It is also wise to purchase the best commercial travel accommodations you can afford when young children are involved; the increased space provides greater freedom of movement, and the service is usually better.

Keeping children content while confined in close quarters is often a real challenge. Having an adult ride in the back seat of a car alongside a restrained toddler is often a good idea. The child with adult companionship will be happier and less likely to demand a place on the front seat.

Take along your child's favorite stuffed animal or blanket, a bag of small, soft-plastic toys, or cloth books. Crayons and a coloring book or pad of paper will help keep an older child occupied. Avoid hard or pointed objects that could become dangerous in a moving vehicle.

Playing games helps to pass the time. For example, look for cows and trucks in magazines or by the side of the road. An occasional snack provides distraction and may alleviate motion sickness. Cookies or crackers may be a little messy, but they are preferable to ice pops, lollipops, and hard candies, which could prove dangerous.

If your trip is by car, limit your daily mileage to what your child can tolerate. It is always a good idea to end your driving by late afternoon. This prevents undue fatigue, ensures a night's lodging for a tired and possibly cranky child, and provides the time for him to adjust to new surroundings before bedtime.

Your young child's safety, comfort, and contentment help to make any family trip an enriching experience. By using common sense to organize and plan ahead, what might have been a formidable task could be a pleasant interval in your daily routine.

# HISTORY OF PREGNANCY AND DELIVERY

| Obstetrician | Pediatrician |
|---|---|
| Name _____ | Name _____ |
| Address _____ | Address _____ |
| City/State _____ | City/State _____ |

**Length of pregnancy** (full term, eight months, other) _____

_____

**Medications taken during pregnancy, if any**
(sleeping pills, aspirin, cough medicine, other) _____

_____

**Complications during pregnancy**
(bleeding, swelling, high blood pressure,
infections, illness, exposure to German
measles or other infectious diseases) _____

_____

**Onset of labor** (specify premature,
spontaneous, induced) _____

**Length of labor** _____

**Medical assistance during delivery**
(specify forceps, episiotomy, anesthesia) _____

_____

**Type of delivery** (vaginal, cesarean) _____

**Position of baby during birth**
(head first, breech) _____

**Condition of baby at birth** (specify color,
spontaneous respiration, immediate crying) _____

**Medical treatment necessary** (oxygen,
resuscitation, blood transfusion, other) _____

_____

**Congenital abnormalities** _____

**Hospital nursery used** (specify
newborn, premature, high risk) _____

# BIRTH STATISTICS

Baby's name _____ Sex _____

Birth date _____ Time _____

Weight _____ Length _____

Birthplace (Hospital) _____

(Street address) _____

(City) _____ (County) _____ (State) _____

Blood type _____ Rh factor _____

Mother's maiden name _____

Father's name _____

Home address (Street) _____

(City) _____ (County) _____ (State) _____

# RELIGIOUS CEREMONY

Date of ceremony _____

Place of ceremony (church or synagogue) _____

(Street address) _____

(City) _____ (County) _____ (State) _____

Godmother _____

Godfather _____

Maternal Grandmother (maiden name) _____

Maternal Grandfather _____

Paternal Grandmother (maiden name) _____

Paternal Grandfather _____

# DEVELOPMENT HISTORY

| New Activity | Age | Height | Weight |
|---|---|---|---|
|  |  |  |  |
|  |  |  |  |
|  |  |  |  |
|  |  |  |  |
|  |  |  |  |
|  |  |  |  |
|  |  |  |  |
|  |  |  |  |
|  |  |  |  |
|  |  |  |  |
|  |  |  |  |
|  |  |  |  |
|  |  |  |  |
|  |  |  |  |
|  |  |  |  |
|  |  |  |  |
|  |  |  |  |
|  |  |  |  |
|  |  |  |  |
|  |  |  |  |
|  |  |  |  |
|  |  |  |  |
|  |  |  |  |
|  |  |  |  |
|  |  |  |  |
|  |  |  |  |
|  |  |  |  |
|  |  |  |  |

# IMMUNIZATION RECORD

| Type | Initial | Booster | Remarks |
|---|---|---|---|
| DPT* | | | |
| DT** | | | |
| Oral Polio | | | |
| Measles† | | | |
| Rubella† | | | |
| Mumps† | | | |
| Smallpox†† | | | |
| Other | | | |
| Tuberculin Test††† | | | |

*Diphtheria, Pertussis (Whooping Cough), Tetanus (Lockjaw)—combined inoculation given in three initial doses spaced one to two months apart.
**Diphtheria and Tetanus—combined inoculation given after age six.
†Measles, Mumps, and Rubella—sometimes a combined inoculation (MMR).
††A nonroutine inoculation given at the doctor's option.
†††Not an inoculation but a test for the presence of tuberculosis.

# ILLNESS/INJURY RECORD

| Illness or Injury | Date | Symptoms | Medical Treatment |
|---|---|---|---|
| | | | |
| | | | |
| | | | |
| | | | |
| | | | |

# Glossary

**Abortion**
The termination of a pregnancy through expulsion of the fetus from the uterus, generally before it can survive independently.

**Abortion, spontaneous**
Miscarriage that has not been induced artificially, but rather occurs due to natural causes.

**Abscess**
A collection of pus surrounded by inflamed tissue, caused by local infection and accompanied by pain, heat, and swelling.

**Afterbirth**
The placenta and other special tissues associated with fetal development that are expelled from the uterus after the birth of an infant.

**Amino acid**
A building block of protein, which is used by the body to build muscle and other tissue.

**Amniocentesis**
A prenatal diagnostic technique by which a sample of the amniotic fluid may be removed for laboratory analysis to determine whether chromosomal abnormalities are present in the fetus.

**Amniotic fluid**
The fluid that surrounds the developing fetus before birth.

**Amniotic sac**
The "bag of waters" in which the fetus and the amniotic fluid are contained during pregnancy.

**Anemia**
Any condition in which the number or volume of red blood cells or the amount of hemoglobin in the blood is inadequate.

**Anesthesia**
Loss of sensation, induced medically to permit a painless surgical procedure. General anesthesia involves the entire body and produces loss of consciousness; local or regional anesthesia involves only a particular area.

**Anesthesiologist**
A physician who specializes in the administration of anesthesia.

**Anomaly**
Malformation or abnormality of a body part.

**Anorexia nervosa**
An eating disorder characterized by compulsive self-starvation, which may result in life-threatening weight loss.

**Antibiotic**
A drug, usually derived from living organisms, used to combat bacterial and fungal infections.

**Antibody**
A special kind of protein produced by the body's immune system to counteract or destroy foreign substances or organisms.

**Antigen**
A substance that stimulates the production of antibodies to combat it.

**Antitoxin**
An antibody either produced by or introduced into the body to counteract a poison.

**Anus**
The opening at the end of the rectum, through which feces pass.

**Apgar scoring system**
A method of evaluating a baby's physical condition (on the basis of ratings for heart rate, breathing, skin color, muscle tone, and reflex responses) immediately after birth.

**Apnea**
Temporary involuntary cessation of breathing.

## Areola (plural, **areolae**)
The pink or brown circular area of skin around the nipple of the breast.

## Aspirate
1. To inhale a liquid or solid into the lungs. 2. To remove fluid from the lungs by means of a suction device.

## Aural
Relating to the ear or the sense of hearing.

## Bile
The fluid secreted by the liver to aid in digestion, especially of fatty foods.

## Bilirubin
A reddish-yellow pigment in the blood, urine, and bile that results from the normal breakdown of hemoglobin in the red blood cells. When present in the blood in excessive amounts, as in jaundice, it gives the skin and the whites of the eyes a yellowish tinge.

## Biopsy
The surgical removal of a small sample of tissue, which is then examined microscopically to establish a diagnosis.

## Botulism
A severe form of food poisoning, caused by a bacterium *(Clostridium botulinum)* often found in improperly canned or preserved foods. The early symptoms (vomiting, abdominal pain, and double vision) may progress to muscle weakness, respiratory difficulties, and even death.

## Breech presentation
Position in which the fetus' feet or buttocks, instead of the head, are nearest the cervix when labor begins.

## Bronchi
Plural of **bronchus.**

## Bronchiole
One of the progressively narrower branches of the airway between the bronchi and the tiny air sacs (alveoli) of the lungs.

## Bronchiolitis
Inflammation of the bronchioles, usually due to bacterial or viral infection.

## Bronchitis
Inflammation of the mucous membranes lining the bronchi, usually due to bacterial or viral infection.

## Bronchus
One of the larger passageways that carry air between the trachea and the air sacs of the lungs. The trachea divides first into two main bronchi, which in turn divide into five lobar bronchi, which divide into twenty segmental bronchi, and so on for two or three further subdivisions of progressively smaller diameter.

## Bulimia
An eating disorder characterized by episodes of binge-eating (rapidly consuming large amounts of food) followed by purging (getting rid of the food by causing vomiting, using laxatives or diuretics, or other means).

## Carbohydrate
Any of the organic compounds, including starches, cellulose, and sugars, that are an important dietary source of energy and fiber.

## Caries
Tooth decay; dental cavities.

## Cerebrospinal fluid
Fluid that surrounds and cushions the brain and spinal cord.

## Cervix
The lower portion of the uterus, which extends into the vagina.

## Cesarean section
Delivery of an infant through a cut in the abdominal and uterine walls when vaginal delivery is inadvisable or impossible.

## *Chlamydia*
A family of bacteria that cause a variety of diseases in man and animals, including eye and urogenital infections.

## Chloasma
A patchy, brownish discoloration of the skin, especially on the face, during pregnancy.

## Chorionic villi sampling
A technique for prenatal diagnosis of chromosomal abnormalities, whereby samples of the projections of the membrane surrounding the fetus (the chorionic villi) are collected for laboratory analysis.

## Chromosomes
The cellular structures that contain the genes.

## Circumcision
Surgical removal of the foreskin from the penis.

## Cleft lip
Congenital defect in which the structures that form the upper lip fail to merge.

## Cleft palate
Congenital defect in which the bones that form the sides of the roof of the mouth fail to fuse.

## Colostrum
The milk secreted shortly before and for a few days after childbirth.

## Congenital
Present at the time of birth or before.

## Convulsion
Involuntary, violent, and uncontrolled muscle contractions of the face, trunk, or extremities.

## CT scanning
A diagnostic imaging technique whereby a computer generates cross-sectional images of an organ or part of the body based on x-ray images taken in a series of planes through the body.

## Culture
To cultivate microorganisms from an infected area on a special substance that encourages growth.

## Curette
A scoop-shaped instrument used to scrape the internal surface of an organ or cavity.

## D & C (dilatation and curettage)
A surgical procedure in which the uterine cervix is expanded with an instrument called a dilator and the lining of the uterus is scraped with a curette, usually performed to remove abnormal tissue or to obtain a specimen for diagnostic purposes.

## Defecate
Pass feces from the bowels.

## Dehydration
Excessive loss of water from the body, often due to severe vomiting, diarrhea, exertion, or extreme environmental temperatures.

## Diabetes mellitus
A chronic disease in which the body cannot properly utilize carbohydrates because of insufficient production of insulin by the pancreas.

## Dilatation
The expansion or stretching of any organ or opening beyond its normal dimensions.

## Dilation
The state of being expanded or stretched beyond normal dimensions.

## DNA
Deoxyribonucleic acid. The molecular material, present in nearly all living cells, that makes up the genes and chromosomes. DNA is responsible for the transmission of inherited traits.

## Eclampsia
A serious (potentially fatal) complication of pregnancy, characterized by high blood pressure, edema, presence of protein in the urine, and convulsions.

## Ectopic
Occurring in an abnormal location.

## Ectopic pregnancy
Pregnancy in which the fertilized egg begins to develop outside the uterus, usually in one of the fallopian tubes.

## Edema
Swelling; excessive accumulation of fluid in body tissues.

## Embryo
In humans, the growing organism from the moment of fertilization until eight weeks after conception.

## Emetic
An agent that induces vomiting.

## Endometriosis
A condition in which tissue that normally lines the uterus grows in another area of the body, most commonly in the lower abdomen.

## Endometrium
The lining of the uterus, in which the fertilized egg is implanted and which is shed during menstruation if conception has not taken place.

## Engorgement
Overdistension of the breast with milk.

## Enuresis
Bed-wetting; inability to control urination, especially while sleeping.

## Enzyme
A substance, usually protein, that speeds a chemical reaction in the body without being used up itself.

## Epidural

A form of regional anesthesia used in both vaginal and cesarean deliveries, achieved by injecting an anesthetic into an area of the lower spine.

## Episiotomy

An incision made in the tissues around the vagina in the final stages of childbirth to make delivery easier and to avoid more extensive tearing.

## Erythroblastosis fetalis

A form of anemia that develops in Rh-positive infants of Rh-negative women. Because the blood of the child contains an antigen that is not present in the mother's blood, antibodies are formed in the mother's blood that attack the child's red blood cells. It is seen only rarely in first babies because the mother usually is not exposed to the baby's blood until delivery.

## Esophagus

The tube through which food moves from the mouth to the stomach.

## Fallopian tube

One of the two tubes that extend from each side of the uterus, through which an egg must pass after release from the ovary.

## Fatty acid

Any of the substances obtained by the breakdown of fats in the digestive process, which play an essential role in providing energy and in maintaining cell membranes throughout the body.

## Feces

The waste matter discharged from the large intestine; a bowel movement.

## Fetoscopy

A technique by which the fetus can be directly examined for anatomical defects while still within the uterus. At about fourteen to twenty weeks' gestation, a hollow tube is inserted through an incision in the abdomen of a pregnant woman, and a light source and special lens are inserted to allow visualization of the structures within the uterus. A separate channel in the tube may be used to obtain, under direct guidance, blood or tissue samples for laboratory analysis.

## Fetus

An unborn developing human from the eighth week of gestation until birth.

## Fissure

A gap or groove.

## Fontanel

A soft space, covered by a membrane, on a baby's head where the skull bones have not yet come together.

## Fungi

Plural form of fungus.

## Fungus

A lower form of plant life, some species of which can cause disorders in humans.

## Gene

The unit in the chromosome that is responsible for transmission of hereditary characteristics.

## Genitalia

The sex organs.

## Gestation

Pregnancy.

## Gestational age

Duration of a pregnancy, measured from the first day of the last menstrual period.

## Gonorrhea

A contagious venereal disease caused by the gonococcus bacterium and characterized by inflammation of the genital mucous membranes.

## Gravid

Pregnant.

## Gynecologist

A physician who specializes in disorders of the female reproductive system.

## Hemoglobin

The red pigment contained in red blood cells, responsible for transporting oxygen from the air sacs of the lungs to other body tissues.

## Hemorrhage

Bleeding, especially an abnormally large amount.

## Heredity

The transmission of traits from parents to offspring.

## Heritable

Relating to a trait that can be passed on from parent to offspring.

## Hernia

Abnormal protrusion of part or all of a structure through surrounding tissues.

## Herpes
A recurring inflammation of the skin and mucous membranes caused by the herpes virus. A mild form causes blister-like sores ("cold sores" or "fever blisters"), usually around the mouth. A more severe form causes painful blisters, usually on the external genitalia. In some cases, infection of the eyes and brain is possible. Transmission is by direct contact, sexual contact, or from mother to offspring in the birth canal during labor.

## Hormone
A chemical secreted in one part of the body and transported to another, where it regulates certain vital functions and processes.

## Hydrocephalus
A condition in which the head becomes enlarged because of excessive accumulation of cerebrospinal fluid within the skull.

## Hyperemesis gravidarum
Excessive vomiting during pregnancy.

## Immunity
The body's ability to resist infection. Active immunity is acquired by vaccination against a disease or by recovery from a previous infection. Passive immunity, which is only temporary, is acquired from antibodies obtained either from the mother through the placenta during gestation or by injection of serum from an immune person or animal that has active immunity.

## Immunization
The production of immunity to a disease either by injecting antibodies into the body or by stimulating the body to produce its own antibodies.

## Immunoglobulin
A naturally occurring or artificially introduced protein that plays an important role in the immune response of the body to antigens.

## Inoculation
Artificial induction of immunity by introducing a disease agent into the body.

## Jaundice
A condition characterized by an elevated level of bilirubin in the blood, indicated by a yellowish discoloration of the skin and the whites of the eyes, often caused by some degree of malfunction of the liver.

## Labia
The folds of skin and fatty tissue that enclose the vaginal opening.

## Laceration
A cut or wound caused by tearing of tissue.

## Lactation
The production and secretion of milk by the breasts.

## Lanugo
The fine hair on the body of a fetus, which is sometimes seen on the forehead, shoulders, and back of a newborn infant, especially a preterm infant.

## Laparoscope
An illuminated, tubular instrument that may be inserted through the abdominal wall to visualize the organs in the abdomen.

## Legumes
Seeds of the bean and pea family, including dry beans, peas, and lentils, which are a good source of protein.

## Lochia
The discharge of blood, mucus, and other tissue from the vagina after childbirth.

## Lymph
The transparent, slightly yellowish liquid found in the lymphatic system of vessels and nodes, which contains a type of white blood cell, the lymphocyte.

## Lymph node
Any of the oval-shaped organs located throughout the body that manufacture lymphocytes and filter germs and foreign bodies from the lymph fluid as it passes through.

## Meconium
The contents of the intestines of the fetus, which usually start being passed as bowel movements soon after birth.

## Meninges
The membranes that cover the brain and spinal cord.

## Meningitis
Inflammation of the meninges.

## Metabolism
The sum of all the chemical processes in the body by which food is converted into living tissue and energy.

## Miscarriage
Spontaneous ending of a pregnancy prior to 24 weeks' gestation.

## Motor skills, fine
Ability to perform movements that require precise coordination of the small muscles, such as picking up and manipulating small objects.

## Motor skills, gross
Ability to perform movements that require coordination of the large muscles, such as sitting, crawling, and walking.

## Natural childbirth
Giving birth without the use of drugs.

## Neonatal
Pertaining to the newborn infant (up to one month old).

## Neonate
An infant during the first four weeks after birth.

## Obstetrician
A physician who specializes in the care of women during pregnancy, childbirth, and the postnatal period.

## Ovulation
The release of an egg from the ovary.

## Oxytocin
A hormone secreted by the pituitary gland during labor to stimulate uterine contractions and milk secretion. A synthetic form is sometimes administered to bring on or speed labor.

## Pediatrician
A physician who specializes in the care of children.

## Penis
The external male sex organ, through which urine and semen are passed.

## Perineal
Of or relating to the perineum.

## Perineum
The region between the anus and the genital organs.

## Pertussis
Whooping cough.

## Perinatal
The period from twenty-eight weeks' gestation to the end of the first week of life.

## Petechiae
Small hemorrhages under the skin.

## Phenylketonuria (PKU)
An inherited congenital disorder of protein metabolism, which, if untreated by dietary management, can lead to mental retardation.

## Placenta
The structure through which the fetus receives nourishment and oxygen and eliminates waste products. It also produces hormones that regulate many of the changes in the mother's body that occur during pregnancy and childbirth.

## Placenta previa
A condition in which the placenta partially or completely covers the cervix, hindering or preventing vaginal delivery.

## Placental abruption
Premature separation of the placenta from the uterine wall.

## Plasma
The liquid portion of the blood, in which the blood cells are suspended.

## Postpartum
Relating to the period after childbirth.

## Pre-eclampsia
A disorder of pregnancy, characterized by elevated blood pressure, edema, and kidney malfunction, that may precede the development of eclampsia.

## Pregravid
Of or relating to the period before pregnancy.

## Prepared childbirth
A method of childbirth education in which expectant mothers are informed about the anatomical, physiological, and psychological aspects of pregnancy and childbirth and are trained in physical and mental responses to labor.

## Presentation
The position of the fetus in relation to the cervix when labor begins.

## Prolapse
Downward displacement of an organ or structure from its usual position.

## Prolapse of the cord
Situation preceding or during labor in which the umbilical cord passes through the cervix before the fetus, which can result in compression of the cord and resultant reduction in the amount of oxygen available to the fetus.

## Pudendal
Of or relating to the pudendum.

## Pudendum
The external genital organs, especially those of the female.

## Pyelonephritis
An infection, usually bacterial, of the kidney.

## Quickening
The first fetal movements felt by the mother (usually around the eighteenth week of pregnancy).

## Radiography
The technique of examining the body by projecting x-rays through it to produce images on photographic film.

## Rectum
The portion of the large intestine closest to the anal opening.

## Rh factor
A group of antigens in the blood. Persons who have the Rh factor are designated Rh-positive; those who lack the Rh factor are designated Rh-negative. Erythroblastosis fetalis can occur if an Rh-negative mother bears an Rh-positive baby.

## Rickets
A condition caused by a deficiency of vitamin D in the diet, beginning most often during infancy and early childhood, which is characterized by defective bone growth and sometimes results in skeletal deformities. An adequate diet containing sufficient vitamin D, coupled with exposure to ultraviolet light (such as sunlight), will generally both prevent and cure rickets.

## RNA
Ribonucleic acid. A material that, along with DNA, is present in all living cells and is responsible for the transmission of inherited traits.

## Rubella
German measles. A highly contagious viral infection, characterized by fever, a widespread pink rash, and enlargement of the lymph nodes in the neck. Although generally mild, if contracted by a woman early in pregnancy, it may cause serious birth defects in the fetus.

## Scurvy
A condition due to deficiency of ascorbic acid (vitamin C) in the diet, characterized by anemia, extreme weakness, spongy gums, and hemorrhaging under the skin and in the mucous membranes.

## Semen
The secretion produced by the male sex glands that contains the sperm.

## Shock
A condition that results when the circulatory system slows down or ceases to function in response to injury, infection, or profound emotional disturbance. Symptoms include rapid pulse, low blood pressure, paleness, and cold, clammy skin.

## Stillbirth
Delivery of a dead fetus after the twenty-eighth week of gestation.

## Stool
Feces.

## Strabismus
Condition in which the eyes are not aligned and are unable to focus simultaneously.

## Striae
Streaks ("stretch marks") seen on the abdomen of a pregnant woman, due to stretching of the skin to accommodate the enlarging uterus.

## Syphilis
An infectious venereal disease caused by the microorganism *Treponema pallidum*. Transmission may be either congenital (from mother to offspring in the vagina during childbirth) or by sexual contact. The degenerative course of the disease begins with the appearance of a primary sore and, if left untreated, eventually involves all the organs of the body.

## Toxemia of pregnancy
A serious disorder of pregnancy (encompassing pre-eclampsia and eclampsia) in which poisonous compounds are present in the bloodstream.

## Toxoid
A poison that has been altered so that it is no longer poisonous but still stimulates the formation of antibodies, as in vaccinations.

## Toxoplasmosis
A disease caused by the one-celled parasite *Toxoplasma gondii*, which is transmitted from animals (especially cats) to humans who handle parasite-infected feces (for example, cat litter) or who eat undercooked meat containing the parasite. Infection during pregnancy can cause death

of the fetus or birth defects, especially mental retardation and blindness, in the newborn.

## Trachea
The tube that extends from the larynx to the bronchi; the windpipe.

## Transverse presentation
Position in which the fetus is lying at right angles to the cervix when labor begins.

## Trimester
One of three approximately equal periods of time. (Pregnancy is traditionally divided into three trimesters, each three months in length.)

## Tubal pregnancy
The most common form of ectopic pregnancy, in which the fertilized egg starts to develop in one of the fallopian tubes rather than in the uterus.

## Ultrasound imaging
A technique for displaying and recording the echoes from high-frequency sound waves reflected from the various tissues within the body, used to produce images of organs and other structures.

## Umbilical cord
The structure through which the fetus' blood flows to and from the placenta, to obtain oxygen and nutrients and to dispose of waste products.

## Umbilicus
The navel ("belly button"), where the umbilical cord is attached to the fetus.

## Umbilical hernia
Protrusion of abdominal contents through a defect in the abdominal wall near the navel.

## Urethra
The tube through which the urine passes from the bladder to the outside.

## Urinate
To pass urine from the bladder through the urethra to the outside of the body.

## Urologist
A physician who specializes in disorders of the female urinary tract and the male genitourinary system.

## Uterus
The hollow, muscular organ in which the fertilized egg becomes implanted and grows; the womb.

## Vaccination
Introduction of an antigenic substance (a solution containing dead or weakened microorganisms or specially treated toxins) to stimulate the production of antibodies, creating immunity to a disease.

## Vagina
The muscular canal, lined with mucous membrane, that leads from the vulva to the uterine cervix; the birth canal.

## Varicose
Abnormally swollen or dilated. Often used to describe veins in which the valves are weakened, allowing backflow of blood; most commonly seen in the rectum (hemorrhoids) and in the legs (varicose veins).

## Varicosity
An area of abnormal dilatation of a structure.

## Vernix
Protective, fatty substance that covers the skin of the fetus and is still present at birth.

## Vulva
The external female genitalia, surrounding the openings of the vagina and the urethra.

## Whooping cough
An infectious disease, primarily affecting children, that is due to bacterial infection. Symptoms include inflammation of the mucous membranes of the air passages, excessive secretion of mucus, mild fever, and attacks of explosive coughing followed by gasping breaths (which produce the characteristic whooping sound). Protection against the disease is obtained by receiving the diphtheria-pertussis-tetanus vaccination.

# Index

fitness. *See* exercise
fixed annuities, 417
fluid retention, 152, 153
fluids, during pregnancy, 24–25
fluoride
    and breast-feeding, 290, 296
    and tooth decay prevention, 290–91
flushing, and niacin, 31
focus, and vision in newborn, 310
folate, 28–29
    and citrus fruit, 24
    and vegetables, 22
folic acid, 25–26
fontanels. *See* soft spots
forceps-assisted delivery, 65, 116–17
    anesthesia and, 126, 127
foreign adoption, 390
formal operational stage, in child development, 339
formula, 221, 281–83
fractures, 234–35
fraternal twins, 144
fruits, and pregnancy, 24–25
furniture, baby and child, 75–83, 94–95

**G**

gallstones, 19
gastroenteritis
    and dehydration, 227
    and stomachache, 249
    and vomiting, 254
gates, 90–91, 270
general anesthesia. *See* anesthesia
genetic counseling, 150, 259
genitals, in newborn, 128, 307. *See also* circumcision
German measles. *See* rubella
Gesell, Arnold, 339, 352
gestational diabetes, 152–53
gifted children, 351–52
goat's milk, 296, 297
goiter, and iodine, 31
gonorrhea
    and ectopic pregnancy, 141
    and newborn eye care, 120–21
grains, and pregnancy, 22–23
grandparents, 181–82, 343
grasping reflex, 308. *See also* reflexes
gross motor development, 313–15
growth patterns, 311–13
guardian, 419

gums
    and dental care, 290–92, 312–13
    and leukemia, 240
    during pregnancy, 18

**H**

habitual aborters, 143. *See also* miscarriage
hair, in newborn, 308
handicapped children, 264–67, 347–51
    impact on parents, 150–51, 265–66
hand-to-mouth reflex, 308. *See also* reflexes
harelip. *See* cleft lip
HCG. *See* human chorionic gonadotropin
head
    and labor, 111
    birth defects of, 148
    fetal, 15
    in newborn, 148, 307, 313
headache
    and encephalitis, 233
    and meningitis, 241
    and mumps, 241
    and pneumonia, 241
    and postpartum depression, 159
    and strep throat, 250
    and toxemia, 152
head lice, 235
health aids for baby, 91
health maintenance organization (HMO), 74–75, 416
hearing
    fetal, 360
    in newborn, 310
    problems with, 235–36, 264–65, 366–67
    *See also* deafness
heart
    and alcohol, 34
    and miscarriage, 143
    and rubella, 154
    and stillbirth, 142
    and ultrasound study, 149–50
    birth defects of, 148
    murmurs, 17, 236
    treatment of abnormalities in, 150
heart attack
    and Rh incompatibility, 151
    and stillbirth, 142
heartbeat
    and ectopic pregnancy, 142

and placental abruption, 146
    newborn, 130
heartburn, during pregnancy, 18, 19, 32, 107
heat rash, 236–37
heart rate
    abnormal fetal, 155
    and exercise, 37
Heimlich maneuver, and choking, 218–19
hemangiomas, 212
hematocrit, 211
hemoglobin
    and folate, 28
    and iron, 23, 30
    levels, 281
hemophilia, 258, 264
hemophilus influenza type B (HiB) vaccine, 204
hemorrhage
    and ectopic pregnancy, 142
    and out-of-hospital birth, 65
    and placental abruption, 146, 155
    and placenta previa, 146, 155
    and shock, 247
hemorrhoids, 19, 125, 133
hepatitis
    and stomachache, 248
    viral, 153
herbal teas, and pregnancy, 33
hereditary illnesses, 254–59
heredity, and birth defects, 149
hernia, 237
    during pregnancy, 18
herpes virus, 154
hiatal hernia, 18
HiB vaccine. *See* hemophilus influenza type B vaccine
high chairs, 79–81
hips, during pregnancy, 18, 107
hives, 237
HMO. *See* health maintenance organization
hoarseness
    and croup, 226
    and laryngitis, 239
Holt International Children's Services, 390
home birth. *See* out-of-hospital birth
honey, 296, 297, 301
hormonal changes, 15, 16, 18, 108
    and nausea and vomiting, 32
hormone imbalance, and fertility, 53, 54

mouth-to-mouth resuscitation, 229–31
mucus plug, cervical, 17
multiple births, 33, 144–45, 183–85
  and cesarean section, 119, 147
  and fertility drugs, 54
  and labor, 109
  and nutrition, 33
  and out-of-hospital birth, 65
municipal bonds. *See* bonds
muscles
  abdominal, 17, 18, 193–95
  and exercise, 34–48, 188–200, 316–33
  pelvic, 45, 192–93
  spasms, 225
  tone, in newborn, 129
muscular dystrophy, 264
music for children, 360
mutual funds, 418

## N

naming the baby, 73–74
  with multiple births, 183–84
nasal congestion, and common cold, 222
nasal discharge, and common cold, 222
National Adoption Hotline, 393
National Association of Parents and Professionals for Safe Alternatives in Childbirth (NAPSAC), 394
National Center for Education in Maternal and Child Health, 266
National Committee for Prevention of Child Abuse, 394
National Congress of Parents and Teachers (PTA), 394
National Easter Seal Society, 394
National Foundation—The March of Dimes. *See* March of Dimes
National Information Center for Handicapped Children and Youth, 266
National Organization of Adolescent Pregnancy and Parenting, 387, 394
National Organization of Mothers of Twins Clubs, 185, 394
National Sudden Infant Death Syndrome Foundation, 264, 394

natural childbirth, 58, 66–67, 126–128
nature exploration for children, 363–64
nausea
  and anesthesia, 126–27
  and anxiety, 48
  and appetite, 19, 27
  and exercise, 36
  and gastroenteritis, 249
  and iron supplements, 24
  and poisoning, 244
  and pregnancy, 12, 19, 27, 32
  and stomachache, 248–49
  and toxemia, 152
  *See also* morning sickness; vomiting
neck pain
  and encephalitis, 233
  and measles, 240
  and meningitis, 241
neonatal jaundice. *See* jaundice
nephritis, 250
nervous system
  and pregnancy, 153
  and stillbirth, 142
  and zinc, 31
nesting urge, 110
newborn
  Apgar score, 129–30
  care plan, 70–71
  decisions concerning, 61–62
  examination, 130–31
  immediate care, 128–32
  physical appearance, 306–8
  reflexes and responses, 308–9
  senses, 309–11
niacin, 30–31
nipples, 92–93
  and breast-feeding, 285
  during pregnancy, 12, 17, 18
  *See also* baby bottles
nipple shields, 93
nitrous oxide, 128
noncustodial parent, 383
North American Council on Adoptive Children, 395
nose
  congested, 222
  fetal, 15
  in newborn, 306
nosebleeds, 241–42
  and leukemia, 240
Novocain (procaine), 127
nuclear family, 378–80
nurse practitioner, as care-giver, 14, 202
nursers, 92

nursery, hospital, 61–62, 64, 122, 123
  intensive-care, 13
nursery school, 353
nursing bras, 93
Nutrients for Pregnancy chart, 26–31
nutrition
  during pregnancy, 14, 19–33, 106
  postpartum, 279–81

## O

obesity
  in mother, 27
  preventing, in children, 302–3
object permanence, 404–5
obstetrician-gynecologist, selecting an, 13–14, 59–60, 61
Office of Adolescent Pregnancy Programs, 387
older mothers, 138–39, 384–85
  and infertility, 53, 138
  and placental abruption, 146
  and toxemia, 151
only children, 379
open adoption, 390–91
oral health, children's, 289–92
orchitis, and mumps, 241
osteopathic physician, 60
out-of-hospital birth, 58, 60, 61, 64–65
ovaries, during pregnancy, 17
overeating, 302–3
overexcitement
  and poisoning, 244
  and Reye's syndrome, 245
ovulation, and fertility, 52, 53, 54, 138. *See also* fertility drugs
oxytocin, 116, 117
  and fetal monitoring, 115
  and intravenous fluids, 113
  and labor, 155
  and out-of-hospital birth, 65
  and postterm delivery, 141
  and stillbirth, 143
  and uterus, 107–8
  decisions concerning, 117

## P

pacifiers, 93, 164–65
pain medications, 58
  and out-of-hospital birth, 64–65
  *See also* analgesics; anesthesia
paleness
  and anemia, 211

and leukemia, 240
and shock, 247
palms, reddening of, 18–19
parallel play, 344
parental responsibilities,
163–66, 415–16
parent-child interaction,
problems with, 401–2
Parent Effectiveness Training
(PET), 162
parent-infant bond, 61–62, 67,
132, 398
and breast-feeding, 284
Parents of Multiple Births
Association of Canada, 185
Parents of Premature and
High-Risk Infants
International, 395
parent support groups, 162,
264, 266, 387,
391–95
Parents Without Partners, 383,
395
pediatric cardiologist, 236
pediatrician, selecting a, 62
pediatric nurse practitioner, 62
peeling skin, in newborn, 307
peers, and social
development, 343–45
pellagra, 31
pelvic exam, 14, 142
pelvic floor, 192–93
pelvic floor squeeze (Kegel
exercise), 45, 47
pelvic inflammatory disease
(PID)
and ectopic pregnancy, 141
and infertility, 53
pelvic pain, during pregnancy,
19
pelvic tumors
and ectopic pregnancy, 142
and fallopian tube
obstruction, 53
pelvis, and pregnancy, 18, 107,
111
in teenage mothers, 139
Penthrane (methoxyflurane),
128
perinatologist, 60, 62
perineum
and episiotomy, 118–19
and local anesthesia, 128
care of, 133
damage to, during delivery,
125
peritonsillar abscess, 252–53
pernicious anemia, 29
pertussis, 254
and DTP vaccine, 204

PET. See Parent Effectiveness
Training
petechia, 214
and meningitis, 241
See also bruises
pets, 182–83
pharyngitis. See sore throat
phenylketonuria, 256, 264, 346
and bottle-feeding, 121
See also PKU test
phlegm, and measles, 240
phosphorus
and dairy products, 22–23
and pregnancy, 22–23, 28,
30–31
and vitamin D, 28
phototherapy, 131
physical changes in mother
after pregnancy, 133–34
during pregnancy, 14–15,
16–19, 107–8
physical development, 304–34
exercises to encourage,
318–333
fine motor, 315–16
gross motor, 313–15
growth patterns, 311–21
reflexes and senses, 308–10
physician, 59–60
physician extenders, 202
physician's assistant, 202
Piaget, Jean, 329
PID. See pelvic inflammatory
disease
pillows, baby, 77
pinworms, 242
Pitocin. See oxytocin
pituitary gland, fetal, 15
PKU test, 130, 256, 346
placenta, 15
and weight gain, 19, 21
during pregnancy, 26, 106–7,
109
expulsion of, 125
functions of, 106–7
placental abruption, 139,
146–47
and cocaine, 34
and preterm delivery, 140
and stillbirth, 142
placenta previa, 35,
145–46
and cesarean section, 119
and preterm delivery, 140
and stillbirth, 142
Planned Parenthood
Federation of America, 395
plastic pants,97
play groups, 345
playmates, 343–45

playpens, 81–83
play yards. See playpens
pneumonia, 243, 261
and measles, 240
and postterm pregnancy, 141
and stomachache, 248
and sudden infant death
syndrome (SIDS), 263–64
walking, 243
poisoning, 243–45, 254
emergency care for, 244
preventing, 270–72
poisons, common household,
271
polio vaccine, 204
portable cribs. See cribs
port-wine stains, 212–13
position, baby's, and labor, 111
positions for labor and
childbirth, 122, 125
post-delivery blues. See
postpartum, depression
postpartum
care of mother, 132–34
depression, 157–60, 280
diet, 279–80
exercises, 41–46, 187–200
postterm pregnancy, 141
potties. See toilet training,
equipment
PPO. See Preferred Provider
Organization
precipitate labor, and
marijuana, 34
pre-eclampsia, 21. See also
toxemia
Preferred Provider Organization
(PPO), 416
pregnancy
and birth plan, 68–71
attitudes toward, 57–58
complications of, 137–55
dreams during, 48–49
exercises during, 34–48
exercises following, 41–46,
187–200
father's role in, 51–52, 134–35
informed consent and, 58–59
physical changes of mother
and fetus during, 14–19
signs and symptoms of,
11–13
See also childbirth; labor
pregnancy-induced diabetes.
See diabetes
pregnancy tests, 11, 12
home, 12
prelabor. See false labor
preliminary signs of labor, 109,
110

444

sunburn, 250
support groups, 162, 264, 266, 387, 391–95
suppositories, 19
surfactant, 16
swallowed objects, 250–51. *See also* choking
swallowing, and tonsillitis, 252
sweat
    and fever, 207
    and shock, 247
swelling
    and bone fractures, 234
    and insect bites and stings, 238
    and toxemia, 151
swimmer's ear, 232
swimming lessons, 276
swings, baby, 89–90
swing sets, 101
swollen glands. *See* lymph nodes
symphysis pubis. *See* pelvis, and pregnancy
syphilis, during pregnancy, 154
syrup of ipecac, 243, 244–45
Systematic Training for Effective Parenting (STEP), 162

**T**
tables, toddler, 94–95
talking. *See* speech development
target heart rate zone, 37–38
Task Force on Mental Retardation, 20
taste, sense of, in newborn, 309–10, 336
Tay-Sachs disease, 256, 264
TB test. *See* tuberculosis test
tear ducts, blocked, 213–14
teenage pregnancy, 32–33, 139–40, 386–87
    and nutrition, 21
    and toxemia, 151
Teen Fathers Collaboration, 387
teeth
    and calcium, 30–31
    and phosphorus, 30
    and vitamin A, 26
    and vitamin D, 28
    caring for, 290–92
    development of, 15, 312–13
teething, 290–91
telangiectasias, 19
television, 362–63, 412–13
temperature, taking a child's, 208–9. *See also* fever
term life insurance, 416

testicles
    and mumps, 241
    examination of, 205
    undescended, 252
testosterone, and fertility, 53, 54
test-tube fertilization. *See in vitro* fertilization
tetanus, 213
    and bites, 213
    and burns, 216
    and cuts, 226–27
    vaccine, 204
tetracycline, 129
thallassemia, 264
thiamin. *See* vitamins, B₁
thinning of cervix, 108, 110. *See also* cervix
threatened miscarriage, 143
throat, and tonsillitis, 252. *See also* sore throat
thumb-sucking, 93, 164–65, 291, 401
thyroid gland
    and iodine, 30, 31
    and miscarriage, 143
    and preterm delivery, 140
    fetal, 15
    *See also* hypothyroidism
thyroid medication, and pregnancy test, 12
ticks, 238–39
tissue growth
    and magnesium, 30, 31
    and vitamins C and E, 28
toiletries, for baby, 91
toilet training, 369, 371–72, 411
    and constipation, 224
    equipment, 94
tonic neck reflex, 308. *See also* reflexes
tonsillitis, 248, 252–53
toothbrushing, 291
tooth decay, 290–91
TOPV. *See* trivalent oral polio vaccine
touch, sense of, in newborn, 309
toxemia, 139, 151–52
    and calcium, 31
    and diabetes, 152
    and multiple births, 144
    and stillbirth, 142
    and weight gain, 21
    in older mothers, 139
    in teenage mothers, 139
toxoplasmosis, 154
toy chest, 95
toys, 354–57
    and safety, 100–3

training cups, 93
training pants, 94
tranquilizers
    and pregnancy tests, 12
    during labor, 126
transitional object, 406
transition phase of labor, 123
traveling with children, 420–21
Treasury bills, 417, 418
Treasury securities, 417
trichloroethylene, 128
Trilene (trichloroethylene), 128
trimester, 15
trivalent oral polio vaccine (TOPV), 204
trust period in child development, 340
tubal pregnancy. *See* ectopic pregnancy
tuberculosis test, 204
twins
    caring for, 183–85
    naming, 183–84
    Siamese, 144
    special concerns of, 183–85
    support groups for parents of, 185
    *See also* multiple births

**U**
ultrasonography, diagnostic
    and birth defects, 149–50
    and ectopic pregnancy, 142
    and gestational age, 13
    and placental abruption, 146
    and placenta previa, 146
    and spina bifida, 258
    and stillbirth, 143
ultrasound study. *See* ultrasonography, diagnostic
umbilical cord, 129, 155
    and stillbirth, 142
    care of, 132, 307–8
    prolapsed, 119, 155
unconsciousness
    and convulsions, 225
    and poisoning, 244
    and Reye's syndrome, 245
    and shock, 247
underactive thyroid gland. *See* hypothyroidism
United Cerebral Palsy Association, 395
urinary tract
    during pregnancy, 17–18
    infections, 249, 253
urination
    and dehydration, 227
    and urinary tract infections, 249, 253